DAVIS ESSENTIAL NURSING CONTENT
+ PRACTICE QUESTIONS

Psychiatric Mental Health

Cathy Melfi Curtis, MSN, RN-BC
Psychiatric Mental Health Nurse
Charleston, South Carolina

Carol Norton Tuzo, MSN, RN-BC
Psychiatric Mental Health Nurse
Charleston, South Carolina

F.A. Davis Company · Philadelphia

F. A. Davis Company
1915 Arch Street
Philadelphia, PA 19103
www.fadavis.com

Copyright © 2017 by F. A. Davis Company

Printed in the United States of America

Last digit indicates print number: 10 9 8 7 6 5 4 3 2 1

Publisher, Nursing: Terri Wood Allen
Content Project Manager II: Amy M. Romano
Illustration and Design Manager: Carolyn O'Brien

Library of Congress Cataloging-in-Publication Data

Names: Curtis, Cathy Melfi, author. | Tuzo, Carol Norton, author.
Title: Davis essential nursing content + practice questions psychiatric
  mental health / Cathy Melfi Curtis, Carol Norton Tuzo.
Other titles: Davis essential nursing content plus practice questions
  psychiatric mental health
Description: Philadelphia : F.A. Davis Company, [2017] | Includes
  bibliographical references and index.
Identifiers: LCCN 2016010592 | ISBN 9780803633162 (paperback : alk. paper)
Subjects: | MESH: Psychiatric Nursing | Mental Disorders—nursing |
  Examination Questions
Classification: LCC RC440 | NLM WY 18.2 | DDC 616.89/0231—dc23 LC record available at
http://lccn.loc.gov/2016010592

The authors dedicate this book to Mary Townsend. She has provided, through her published works, the essential concepts of psychiatric mental health to nursing students and has been a role model for the authors of this text. Guided by her expertise, the authors of this book were able to produce a product to further assist nursing students in their quest for success in both classroom testing and the NCLEX®.

Why This Book Is Necessary

Most beginning nursing students have information overload. They must possess knowledge about a variety of subjects, including anatomy and physiology, psychology, sociology, medical terminology, diagnostic and laboratory tests, and growth and development, to mention a few. In addition, with the expanding roles and responsibilities of the nursing profession, the nursing information that beginning nursing students must learn is growing exponentially in depth and breadth. Psychiatric nursing concepts are either taught in abbreviated sessions as a specialty course or integrated into the entire nursing curriculum. Therefore, additional educational support is critical to promote the understanding of psychiatric mental health nursing concepts. These concepts can be applied in all fields of nursing. *Davis Essential Nursing Content + Practice Questions Psychiatric Mental Health* provides that additional educational support.

Who Should Use This Book

Davis Essential Nursing Content + Practice Questions Psychiatric Mental Health provides beginning nursing students with need-to-know information as well as questions to practice their ability to apply the information in a simulated clinical situation. This textbook is designed to:

- Be required by a nursing program as the sole textbook for a psychiatric mental health nursing course to be used in conjunction with reliable primary Internet sources for nursing information.
- Be required or recommended by a nursing program to be used in conjunction with a traditional psychiatric mental health nursing textbook.
- Be used by beginning nursing students who want to focus on essential information contained in a psychiatric mental health nursing course.
- Be used by nursing students to learn how to be more successful when answering National Council Licensure Examination (NCLEX)–type multiple-choice and alternate-item format nursing questions early in their nursing education.
- Be used by nursing students preparing for the NCLEX-RN® or NCLEX-PN® examination to review basic nursing theory and practice.

What Information Is Presented in This Textbook

This textbook begins with an introduction, which includes information to help students maximize their ability to study effectively and achieve success when studying pediatric contact and when taking nursing examinations. General study strategies, specific study strategies, test-taking tips for answering multiple-choice questions and alternate-format questions, and the test plan categories for the NCLEX® examinations are discussed. The content is divided into 20 chapters.

- The first 19 chapters outline the critical need-to-know information related to psychiatric mental health nursing in outline format, eliminating nice-to-know, extraneous information. Only essential information is included, limiting the challenge of wading through excessive material. This approach assists students to focus on what is most important.
- Each chapter includes definitions of key words to assist the student in understanding the context of the information presented.
- All chapters include at least 20 high-level questions related to the content covered in the chapter. Each question contains rationales for correct and incorrect answers. Studying rationales for the right and wrong answers to practice questions, helps students learn new or solidify previously learned information.
- Multiple-choice questions as well as alternate-type questions included on NCLEX examinations are incorporated.
- Each question is coded according to the NCLEX-RN test plan categories: Integrated Processes, including the Nursing Process, Client Need, and Cognitive Domain.
- For added flexibility, every question in the book appears online at www.DavisPlus.com. Students can create targeted quizzes by sorting the questions by Content Area, Concept, and/or Question Type.
- To provide even more opportunities to practice NCLEX-type questions, the book includes two 75-question comprehensive tests posted online at www.DavisPlus.com. Like the practice questions in the book, each question includes rationales for correct and incorrect answers and coding for the NCLEX test plan categories.

- Chapters focusing on DSM-5 content end with a Putting It All Together case study, encouraging students to put the content into practice. Students are quizzed on the relevant objective and subjective information presented in the scenario and asked to identify a nursing diagnosis, interventions, and client evaluation.
- Chapter 20 is a Comprehensive Final Examination containing a 100-item psychiatric mental health nursing examination that integrates questions spanning content throughout the textbook.

Students should use every resource available to facilitate the learning process. The authors believe that this textbook will assist nursing students to master psychiatric mental health concepts and use this understanding to succeed on the National Council Licensure Examination (NCLEX).

JULIE BERTRAM, RN, MSN, PMHCNS-BC
Assistant Professor
St. Louis University School of Nursing
St. Louis, Missouri

CONNIE BUTTRICK, MSN, RN-BC
Instructor of Nursing
Bellin College
Green Bay, Wisconsin

LORRAINE CHIAPPETTA, RN, MSN, CNE
Professional Faculty, Course Coordinator
Washtenaw Community College
Ann Arbor, Michigan

DR. DIANE CRAYTON, DNP, FNP, RN-BC
Assistant Professor, School of Nursing
California State University
Turlock, California

ELAINE L. DAVI, MSN, RN
Professor
Hudson Valley Community College
Troy, New York

ABIMBOLA FARINDE, PharmD, MS, CGP
Clinical Pharmacist Specialist
Columbia Southern University
Orange Beach, Alabama

BARBARA FICKLEY, RN, MSN, PMHNCS-BC
Professor of Nursing
Valencia College
Orlando, Florida

SHELIA FOSTER, RN, MSN
Assistant Professor of Nursing
Saint Mary's Center for Education, School of Nursing
Huntington, West Virginia

MAVONNE GANSEN, DM, MA, RN
Faculty/Comprehensive Nursing Care of the Mental Health Client
Northeast Iowa Community College
Peosta, Iowa

MELISSA GARNO, EdD, RN
Associate Professor, BSN Program Director
Georgia Southern University
Statesboro, Georgia

MARSHA GERDEMAN, RN, BSN, MS
Associate Professor
Rhodes State College
Lima, Ohio
Adjunct Instructor
Central Ohio Technical College
Newark, Ohio

DIANE GRIFFIN, MSN, RN
Assistant Professor of Nursing
University of Maine at Fort Kent
Fort Kent, Maine

ELIZABETH D. GULLEDGE, PhD, RN, CNE
Associate Dean of Nursing; Assistant Professor
Jacksonville State University
Jacksonville, Alabama

SARAH KATULA, APN, PhD
Associate Professor
Elmhurst College
Elmhurst, Illinois

ELIZABETH KAWECKI, EdD, ARNP, CNE
Associate Professor
South University, College of Nursing and Public Health
Royal Palm Beach, Florida

PAMELA LASKOWSKI, MSN, RN, CNE
Nursing Instructor
Millikin University
Decatur, Illinois

REBECCA LUEBBERT, PhD, RN, PMHCNS-BC
Assistant Professor
Southern Illinois University, Edwardsville
Edwardsville, Illinois

KAREN MARTIN, MSN, RN
Associate Professor
Pennsylvania College of Technology
Williamsport, Pennsylvania

DR. MARYELLEN McBRIDE, PhD, CNS-BC
Assistant Professor
Washburn University
Topeka, Kansas

ELAINE L. McKENNA, MSN, PMHCNS-BC, CNE
Nursing Instructor
Pennsylvania State University
University Park, Pennsylvania

TANYA HARDY MENARD, MS, RN, NPP
Assistant Professor
Hampton University
Hampton, Virginia

CHERYL A. PASSEL, RN, PhD, AHN-BC
Assistant Professor
Marian University
Fond du Lac, Wisconsin

JEAN RODGERS, RN, MASTER IN NURSING
Nursing Faculty
Hesston College, Department of Nursing
Hesston, Kansas

DONNA RYE, MSN, RN
Assistant Professor
Cox College
Springfield, Missouri

MARGARET SHEPARD, PhD, RN
Associate Professor
Rutgers University
Camden, New Jersey

EILEEN M. SMIT, RN, MSN, FNP-BC
Professor
Northern Michigan University
Marquette, Michigan

CLAUDIA STOFFEL, MSN, RN, CNE
Professor, Nursing
West Kentucky Community and Technical College
Paducah, Kentucky

DR. JANET TEACHOUT-WITHERSTY, MS, CNS, DNP, RN
Associate Professor of Nursing
West Virginia Wesleyan College
Buckhannon, West Virginia

DOROTHY A. VARCHOL, MSN, MA, RN-BC
Professor
Cincinnati State Technical and Community College
Cincinnati, Ohio

EDITH WATSON, BA, RN, BSN, MSN, CLNC
RN Crisis Interventionist
Christiana Care Healthcare System (CCHS)
Newark, Deleware

ZANA B. WEBB, RN, BS, MSN
Associate Degree Nursing Instructor
Meridian Community College
Meridian, Mississippi

KHATAZA JESSIE WHEATLEY, MSN, RN
Assistant Professor
Southwest Baptist University, Mercy College of Nursing & Health Sciences
Springfield, Missouri

BONNIE WHITE, MSN, RN, CCM
Assistant Professor
MCPHS University
Worcester, Massachusetts

RODNEY A. WHITE, RN, MSN
Associate Professor
Lewis and Clark Community College
Godfrey, Illinois

WANDA WILLIAMSON, RN, MSN, DNP
Clinical Assistant Professor
North Carolina A&T University
Greensboro, North Carolina

MAUREEN (MIMI) WRIGHT, DNP, RN
Adjunct Professor
University of Connecticut
Stamford, Connecticut

We thank Jacalyn Sharp at F. A. Davis for her assistance with the publication of this book.

CATHY MELFI CURTIS
CAROL NORTON TUZO

I dedicate this book to the memory of my mother, Sarah Harvey Melfi, RN, and my aunt, Francis Xavier Harvey, RN. Being raised with two nurses always made for good dinnertime conversations. I thank my children, Scott, Emily, and Katie, who were supportive during the project development, and my grandchildren, Tessa, Bobby, Eve, Jessie, Willie, Addy, Jamie, Gavin, Megan, and Macie, who seem to be impressed that their names are in the front of a textbook.

—CATHY MELFI CURTIS

I dedicate this book to the memory of my husband, George Lawrence Tuzo, whose support and encouragement saw me through nursing school, and also to the memory of my parents, Astrid and Eric Norton, who always encouraged me to pursue my dreams and have fun along the way. Thanks also to my children, Steve, David, and Monique, and the grandchildren, Elise, Zac, and Alli Rae Tuzo, who inspire me on a daily basis. And lastly to my retired women friends who tolerated my chronic reply, "I can't go. I can't do it. I'm working on the book." (You know who you are.)

—CAROL NORTON TUZO

Contents

Although the functioning of the human brain is still largely a mystery, neuroscientists are coming to a deeper understanding of how it gives rise to consciousness, thought, and emotions. With the advent of this research and the development of new and more effective medications for serious brain disorders, the delivery of psychiatric clinical care moved from the large institutions of the first half of the 20th century to present-day outpatient clinics. The teaching of psychiatric mental health nursing content has, in many cases, also changed from a full-semester course to being a component of courses such as medical/surgical and community health nursing. Some schools of nursing integrate psychiatric concepts throughout the entire curriculum. One thing is certain: nurses need to understand mental health concepts and content as they encounter, in all fields of nursing, clients and families with psychological problems. Both psychological and physical needs should be addressed by the nurse to administer effective holistic care.

Psychiatric content is also tested in curricular courses, whether stand-alone or integrated, as well as on the NCLEX®. Passing grades on course examinations and the NCLEX must be achieved to progress in any nursing program and to earn a nursing license. Many factors influence an individual's ability to learn all this information, such as genetic endowment, maturation level, past experience, self-image, mental attitude, motivation, and readiness to learn. Some of these variables cannot be changed; however, implementing study and test-taking strategies can enhance personal internal control, purposeful learning, and success on nursing examinations.

This text presents various teaching strategies that can help maximize learning. The content of each chapter is concisely presented in outline form, including all the "need-to-know" information, while eliminating extraneous "nice-to-know" content. The questions presented are meant to generate critical thinking as you review both the questions and answer options. It is important to review the rationales for all the answer choices to fully understand the often complex psychiatric content. Don't ignore the rationales for the incorrect answers. Learning has truly occurred when you can explain *why* an answer is incorrect.

In addition, this book presents test-taking tips that will help you understand what a test question is asking, identify key words that affect the meaning of both the question and answer, practice how to examine options in a multiple-choice question, and determine how to eliminate incorrect options (distractors). At the beginning of each chapter, key terms are presented that help you focus on understanding concepts and terminology needed to choose correct answers.

For additional information on the studying and test-taking strategies presented in this introduction, refer to *Test Success: Test-Taking Techniques for Beginning Nursing Students* published by the F. A. Davis Company.

Use General Study Strategies to Maximize Learning
1. Set short- and long-term learning goals because doing so promotes planned learning with a purpose.
2. Control internal and external distractors.
   a. Select a study environment that allows you to focus on your learning and is free from external interruptions.
   b. Limit internally generated distractions by challenging negative thoughts. For example, rather than saying to yourself, "This is going to be a hard test," say, "I can pass this test if I study hard."
   c. Establish a positive internal locus of control. For example, say, "I can get an A on my next test if I study hard and I am prepared," rather than blaming the instructor for designing "hard" tests.
   d. Use controlled-breathing techniques, progressive muscle relaxation, and guided imagery to control anxious feelings.
3. Review content before each class because doing so supports mental organization and purposeful learning.
4. Take class notes.
   a. Review class notes within 48 hours after class because doing so ensures that the information is still fresh in your mind.
   b. Use one side of your notebook for class notes, and use the opposite page to jot down additional, clarifying information from the textbook or other sources.
   c. After reviewing your notes, identify questions that you still have and ask the instructor for clarification.
5. Balance personal sacrifice and time for relaxation. A rigorous course of study requires sacrifices in terms of postponing vacations, having less time to spend with family members and friends, and having less time to engage in personal leisure activities. However, you should find a balance that supports your need to meet course requirements and yet allows you time to rest and reenergize.

6. Treat yourself to a reward when you meet a goal because doing so supports motivation. Your long-term reward is to graduate and become a nurse. However, that reward is in the distance, so to stimulate motivation now, build in rewards when short-term goals are achieved.
    a. An external reward might be watching a television program that you enjoy, having a 10-minute break with a snack, or calling a friend on the phone.
    b. An internal reward might be saying to yourself, "I feel great because I now understand the principles presented in this chapter."
7. Manage time effectively.
    a. Examine your daily and weekly routines to identify and eliminate barriers to your productivity, such as attempting to do too much, lacking organization, or being obsessive-compulsive.
    b. Learn to delegate household tasks.
    c. Learn to say "no" to avoid overcommitting yourself to activities that take you away from what you need to do to meet your learning needs.
    d. Get organized. Identify realistic daily, weekly, and monthly "to do" calendars. Work to achieve deadlines with self-determination and self-discipline.
    e. Maintain a consistent study routine because doing so eliminates procrastination and establishes an internal readiness to learn.
8. Recognize that you do not have to be perfect. If every waking moment is focused on achieving an "A," your relationship with family members and friends will suffer. The key is to find a balance and accept the fact that you do not have to have an "A" in every course to become a nurse.
9. Capitalize on small moments of time to study by carrying flashcards, a vocabulary list, or a small study guide, such as one of the products in the *Notes* series by F. A. Davis Publishing Company.
10. Study in small groups. Sharing and listening increases understanding and allows for correction of misinformation.

Use Specific Study Strategies to Maximize Learning

1. Use acronyms, alphabet cues, acrostics, and mnemonics to help learn information that must be memorized for future recall.
2. When studying, continually ask yourself "how" and "why" because the nurse must comprehend how a process occurs and why a particular intervention is or is not appropriate. Many questions on nursing

examinations require the nurse to comprehend the how and why to decide what the nurse should do first or next or what the nurse should not do.
3. Relate new information to something you already know to enhance learning. When trying to remember the meaning of the "positive" and "negative" symptoms of schizophrenia, relate "positive" to "added" (beyond the normal) and relate "negative" to "missing" (less than the normal).
4. Identify and study principles that are common among different nursing interventions because doing so maximizes the application of information in client situations. For example, trust is the common denominator in all interpersonal relationships. No progress in client care can occur without a mutual feeling of trust.
5. Identify and study differences. For example, three patients may have an increase in blood pressure for three different reasons, such as anxiety, acute pain stimulating the sympathetic nervous system, and side effects of medications.

Use Test-Taking Tips to Maximize Success on Nursing Examinations

1. There is no substitute for being prepared for a test. However, when you are uncertain of a correct answer, test-taking tips are strategies you can use to be test wise.
2. By being test wise, you may be better able to identify what a question is asking and to eliminate one or more distractors. Your chances of selecting the correct answer increase when you are able to eliminate distractors from consideration. For example, when answering a traditional multiple-choice question that has four answer options, if you can eliminate one distractor from further consideration, you increase your chances of selecting the correct answer to 33%. If you are able to eliminate two distractors from further consideration, you increase your chances of selecting the correct answer to 50%.

Test-Taking Tips for Multiple-Choice (One-Answer) Item

1. A traditional multiple-choice item typically presents a statement (stem) that asks a question. Usually, four statements that are potential answers follow the stem (options), one of which is the correct answer and three of which are incorrect answers (distractors). The test-taker must select the option that is the correct answer to receive credit for answering a traditional multiple-choice item correctly.

2. Test-taking tips describe strategies that can be used to analyze a traditional multiple-choice item and improve a test-taker's chances of selecting the correct answer.

Test-Taking Tip 1:
Identify Positive Polarity of a Stem

1. A stem with positive polarity is asking, "What should the nurse do when . . . ?"
2. The correct answer may be based on understanding what is accurate or comprehending the principle underlying the correct answer.
3. For example, a stem with positive polarity might say, "Which nursing action should a nurse implement when a client becomes aggressive toward staff?"
4. **Study tip:** Change the stem so that it reflects a negative focus and then answer the question based on a stem with negative polarity. For example, "Which action should a nurse *not implement* when a client becomes aggressive toward staff?"

Test-Taking Tip 2:
Identify Key Words in the Stem That Indicate Negative Polarity

1. A stem with negative polarity asks such questions as, "What should the nurse not do? What is contraindicated, unacceptable, or false? What is the exception?"
2. Words in a stem that indicate negative polarity include *not, except, never, contraindicated, unacceptable, avoid, unrelated, violate,* and *least.*
3. For example, a negatively worded stem might say, "Which action violates the client's rights when considering the use of seclusion?"
4. **Study tip:** Change the word that indicates negative polarity to a positive word and then answer the question based on a stem with positive polarity. For example, if a stem says, "Which action implemented by the nurse *violates* the client's rights?" change the word *violates* to *reflects.* You have just changed a stem with negative polarity to a stem with positive polarity.

Test-Taking Tip 3:
Identify Words in the Stem That Set a Priority

1. The correct answer is something that the nurse should do first.
2. Words in the stem that set a priority include *first, best, main, greatest, most, initial, primary,* and *priority.*
3. For example, a stem that sets a priority might say, "What should a nurse do first when administering antipsychotic medications to a paranoid client?"

4. **Study tip:** After identifying the first step in a procedure, place the remaining steps in order of importance.

Test-Taking Tip 4:
Identify Options That Are Opposites

1. Options that are opposites generally reflect extremes on a continuum.
2. More often than not, an option that is an opposite is the correct answer.
3. If you are unable to identify the correct answer, select one of the opposite options.
4. Some opposites are easy to identify, such as positive and negative symptoms of schizophrenia, whereas others are more obscure, such as psychosis and neurosis.
5. **Study tip:** Make flashcards that reflect the clinical indicator on one side and identify all situations than can cause that sign or symptom on the other side.

Test-Taking Tip 5:
Identify Client-Centered Options

1. Client-centered options focus on feelings, opportunities for clients to make choices, and actions that empower clients or support client preferences.
2. More often than not, a client-centered option is the correct answer.
3. For example, a client-centered option might say, "What family issues would you like to discuss with your psychiatrist?" This example option gives a client an opportunity to make a choice, which supports independence. A nursing action that supports a client's independence is an example of a client-centered option.
4. **Study tip:** Compose your own client-centered options that would be a correct answer for the scenario presented in your test question.

Test-Taking Tip 6:
Identify Options That Deny Clients' Feelings, Needs, or Concerns

1. Options that avoid clients' feelings, change the subject, offer false reassurance, or encourage optimism cut off communication.
2. Options that deny clients' feelings, needs, or concerns are always distractors unless the stem has negative polarity.
3. For example, an option that says, "You will feel better tomorrow," fails to recognize the client's concerns about the pain that the client is feeling today.
4. If a stem with negative polarity says, "What should the nurse *avoid* saying when clients express concerns about the pain they are experiencing?" the option that says, "You will feel better tomorrow" is the correct

answer. *It is important to ensure that you identify the polarity of the stem.*

5. **Study tip:** Construct additional options that deny clients' feelings, needs, or concerns that relate to the scenario in the stem, such as, "Cheer up because things could be worse," "Don't worry; I promise that the voices will be less and less every passing day," or "The antipsychotic medication you are receiving should stop the voices soon."

Test-Taking Tip 7:
Identify Equally Plausible Options

1. Equally plausible options are options that are so similar that one option is no better than the other.
2. Equally plausible options can both be deleted from further consideration.
3. For example, one option says "Suicidal" and another option says "Risk for self-harm." These two options are saying the same thing; therefore, you can eliminate both from further consideration.
4. Another example is if one option states, "Encourage expression of feelings" and another option states, "Encourage the client to talk about the emotions experienced." Both of these options present interventions that increase verbal expressions. One option is no better than the other; therefore, you can eliminate both options from further consideration. By doing so, you increase your chances of selecting the correct answer to 50%.
5. **Study tip:** Construct equally plausible options for the correct answer and identify equally plausible options for the options that are distractors

Test-Taking Tip 8:
Identify Options With Specific Determiners (Absolutes)

1. A specific determiner is a word or phrase that indicates no exceptions.
2. Words that are specific determiners place a limit on a statement that generally is considered correct.
3. Words in options that are specific determiners include *all, none, only, always,* and *never.*
4. For example, options with a specific determiner might say, "Always use anxiolytics to decrease levels of anxiety"
5. Most of the time, options with specific determiners are distractors. However, there are some exceptions that focus on universal truths in nursing. For example, "Restraints are never to be used as punishment or for the convenience of staff," or "Always check the circulation of a client in restraints every 15 minutes."
6. **Study tip:** Construct examples of options with specific determiners so that you are able to recognize when an option has a specific determiner. Next,

identify whether the option should be deleted or whether the option is an exception to the rule.

Test-Taking Tip 9:
Identify the Unique Option

1. When one option is different from the other three options that are similar, examine the unique option carefully.
2. More often than not, an option that is unique is the correct answer.
3. For example, if a question is asking you to identify an expected client response to a problem and three of the options identify an increase in something and one option identifies a decrease in something, examine the option that identifies the decrease in something because it is unique.
4. **Study tip:** Construct options that are similar to the distractors and construct options that are similar to the unique option. Doing so can help you to distinguish among commonalities and differences.

Test-Taking Tip 10:
Identify the Global Option

1. Global options are more broad and wide-ranging than specific options.
2. One or more of the other options might be included under the umbrella of a global option.
3. Examine global options carefully because they are often the correct answer.
4. For example, a global option might say, "Maintain client confidentiality" versus a specific option, which might say, "Do not release client information over the telephone."
5. **Study tip:** Construct as many specific options as possible that could be included under the umbrella of a global option. Construct as many global options as possible in relation to the content presented in the stem. Doing so will increase your ability to identify a global option.

Test-Taking Tip 11:
Use Client Safety and Maslow's Hierarchy of Needs to Identify the Option That Is the Priority

1. This technique is best used when answering a question that asks what the nurse should do first or which action is most important.
2. Examine each option and identify which level need it meets according to Maslow's hierarchy. Identify whether any of the options are associated with maintaining a client's safety.
3. For example, in a question associated with suicidal ideations, an option that addresses client safety and prevents harm is the priority.

4. **Study tip:** Start by identifying the action that is least important and work backward toward the option with the action that is most important. Then identify the reasoning behind the assigned order. This technique focuses on the how and why and helps you to clarify the reasoning underlying your critical thinking. This technique is often done best when working in a small study group.

Test-Taking Tip 12:
Identify Duplicate Facts in Options

1. Some options contain two or more facts. The more facts that are contained in an option, the greater your chances of selecting the correct answer.
2. If you identify an incorrect term, definition, or dosage, eliminate all options that contain the incorrect item.
3. After you eliminate options that you know are incorrect, move on and identify any fact(s) of which you are sure.
4. Focus on the options that contain at least one fact of which you are sure.
5. By eliminating options, you increase your chances of selecting the correct answer.
6. By the process of elimination, you may arrive at the correct answer even when unsure of all the facts in the correct answer.
7. **Study tip:** Identify all the facts that you can that are associated with what the question is asking.

Test-Taking Tip 13:
Practice Test-Taking Tips

Practicing test taking is an effective way to achieve five outcomes.
1. You can desensitize yourself to the discomfort or fear that you might feel in a testing situation.
2. You can increase your stamina if you gradually increase the time that you spend practicing test taking to 2 to 3 hours. This practice will enable you to concentrate more effectively for a longer period of time.
3. You will learn how to better manage your time during a test so that you have adequate time to answer all the questions.
4. You will increase your learning when studying the rationales for the right and wrong answers. Also, by practicing the application of test-taking techniques and employing the study tips presented, you will learn how to maximize your learning associated with each test-taking tip.
5. You will become more astute in determining what a question is asking and better able to identify when a test-taking tip might help you eliminate a distractor and focus on an option that might be the correct answer.

Test-Taking Tip 14:
Use Multiple Test-Taking Techniques When Examining Test Questions and Options

1. If using one test-taking technique to analyze a question is beneficial, think how much more beneficial it would be to use two or more test-taking techniques to analyze a question.
2. Examine the stem first. For example, ask yourself, "Does the stem have negative polarity?" or "Is the stem setting a priority?" Read closely to see if the language of the stem suggests a test-taking tip to use.
3. Next, examine the answer options. For example, ask yourself, "Do any of the options contain a specific determiner?" or "Is there a global option?" or "Is there a client-centered option?"
4. By using more than one test-taking tip, you can usually increase your success in selecting the correct answer.

Test-Taking Tips for Alternate-Format Items

Alternate-format items are purported by the National Council of State Boards of Nursing to evaluate some nursing knowledge more readily and authentically than is possible with traditional multiple-choice items. To accomplish this, an alternate-format item does not construct a question with the same organization as a multiple-choice item. Each type of alternate-format item presents information along with a question using a distinctive format and requires you to answer the item in a unique manner. Some alternate-format items use multimedia approaches, such as charts, tables, graphics, sound, and video. Understanding the composition of alternate-format items and having strategies to analyze these items can increase your chances of selecting the correct answer.

Multiple-Response Item

1. A multiple-response item presents a stem that asks a question.
2. It presents five or six options as potential answers.
3. You must identify all (two or more) correct answers to the question posed in the stem.
4. On a computer, each answer option is preceded by a circle. You must place the cursor in the circle and click the mouse to select the desired answers.
5. **Test-taking tip:** Before looking at the options, quickly review information you know about the topic. Then compare what you know against the options presented. Another approach is to eliminate

one or two options that you know are wrong; identify one option you know is correct; then eliminate another one or two options that you know are wrong. Finally, you should identify all the options you believe are correct. To do this, you can use some of the test-taking tips that apply to traditional multiple-choice questions, such as identifying options that are opposites; identifying client-centered options; identifying options that deny clients' feelings, needs, or concerns; and identifying options with specific determiners (absolutes) to either eliminate options or to focus on potential correct answers.

Drag-and-Drop (Ordered Response) Item

1. A drag-and-drop item makes a statement or presents a situation and then asks you to prioritize five or six options.
2. The item may ask you to indicate the order in which nursing interventions should be performed, the order of importance of concerns, or actual steps in a procedure.
3. To produce a correct answer, you must place all of the options in the correct order.
4. When answering a drag-and-drop item on a computer, you may highlight and click on the option or actually drag the option from the left side of the screen to a box on the right side of the screen. When practicing a drag-and-drop item in a textbook, you can only indicate the priority order by listing the options in order by number.
5. **Test-taking tip:** Use client safety, Maslow's hierarchy of needs, and the nursing process to help focus your ordering of options. Identify the option that you consider to be the priority option, and identify the option that you consider to be the least important option. Then, from the remaining options, select the next priority option and the next least priority option. Keep progressing along this same line of thinking until all the options have received a placement on the priority list.

Fill-in-the-Blank Calculation Item

1. A fill-in-the-blank calculation item presents information and then asks you a question that requires the manipulation or interpretation of numbers.
2. Computing a medication dosage, intake and output, or the amount of intravenous fluid to be administered are examples of fill-in-the-blank calculation items.
3. You must answer the item with either a whole number or within a specified number of decimal points as requested by the item.
4. **Test-taking tip:** Before answering the question, recall the memorized equivalents or formula that

is required to answer the item; then perform a calculation to answer the item.

Hot-Spot Item

1. A hot-spot item presents an illustration or photograph and asks a question about it.
2. You must identify a location on the visual image presented to answer the question.
3. The answer must mirror the correct answer exactly to be considered a correct answer.
4. When answering a hot-spot item on a computer, you place the cursor on the desired location and left click the mouse. These actions place an X on the desired location to answer the question. When answering a hot-spot item in a textbook, you are asked to either place an X on the desired location or to identify an option indicated by an a, b, c, or d label presented in the illustration or photograph.
5. **Test-taking tip:** Read and reread the item to ensure that you understand what the item is asking. When attempting to answer a question that involves anatomy and physiology, close your eyes and picture in your mind the significant structures and recall their functions before answering the item.

Exhibit Item

1. An exhibit item presents a scenario, usually a client situation.
2. You are then presented with a question.
3. You must access information from a variety of sources. The information must be analyzed to determine its significance in relation to the question being asked to arrive at an answer.
4. These items require the highest level of critical thinking (analysis and synthesis).
5. On a computer, each option is preceded by a circle. You must place the cursor in the circle and click the mouse to select the desired answers.
6. **Test-taking tip:** Identify exactly what the item is asking. Access the collected data and dissect, analyze, and compare and contrast the data collected in relation to what you know and understand in relation to what the item is asking.

Graphic Item

1. A graphic item presents a question with several answer options that are illustrations, pictures, photographs, charts, or graphs rather than text.
2. You must select the option with the illustration that answers the question.
3. On a computer, each option is preceded by a circle. You must place the cursor in the circle and click the mouse to select the desired answer. When answering a graphic item in a textbook, you are presented with an illustration and must select one answer from

among several options, or you are asked a question and must select one answer from among several options, each having an illustration.

4. **Test-taking tip:** When reading your textbook or other resource material, visual images are presented to support written content. Examine these images in relation to the content presented to reinforce your learning. Often times, similar illustrations may be used in either hot-spot or graphic alternate test items.

Audio Item

1. An audio item presents an audio clip that must be accessed through a head set. After listening to the audio clip, you must select the answer from among the options presented.
2. On a computer, each option is preceded by a circle. You must place the cursor in the circle and click the mouse to select the desired answer.
3. **Test-taking tip:** Listen to educational resources that provide audio clips of sounds that you must be able to identify such as breath, heart, and bowel sounds. Engage in learning experiences using simulation mannequins available in the on-campus nursing laboratory. When in the clinical area, use every opportunity to assess these sounds when completing a physical assessment of assigned clients.

NCLEX-RN Test Plan and Classification of Questions

The National Council Licensure Examinations for Registered Nurses (NCLEX-RN) and for Licensed Practical/Vocational Nurses (NCLEX-PN) Test Plans were primarily designed to facilitate the classification of examination items and guide candidates preparing for the examinations. These test plans were developed to ensure the formation of tests that measure the competencies required to perform safe, effective nursing care as newly licensed, entry-level registered nurses or licensed practical/vocational nurses. These test plans are revised every 3 years after an analysis of the activities of practicing nurses, input from experts on the NCLEX Examination Committees, and National Council of State Board of Nursing's content staff and member boards of nursing to ensure that the test plans are relevant and consistent with state nurse practice acts. The detailed test plans for the NCLEX-RN and NCLEX-PN differ because of differences in the scope of practice for these professions. Each of these test plans can be found on the National Council of State Board of Nursing's website at www.ncsbn.org/nclex.htm.

Davis Essential Nursing Content + Practice Questions Psychiatric Mental Health uses the NCLEX-RN 2016 Test Plan categories to analyze every question. This book contains more than 650 questions. The majority of the questions appear in the chapters that reflect the content in the question. In addition, there is a 100-item final examination and two 75-item comprehensive examinations on davisplus.fadavis.com. Each high-level question includes rationales for the correct and incorrect answers; offers a test-taking tip, if applicable; and is classified according to the following categories.

Integrated Processes Categories

Integrated processes are the basic factors essential to the practice of nursing, which are the nursing process, caring, communication and documentation, and teaching and learning. Because the nursing process provides a format for critical thinking, it is included for each question.

Nursing Process

Assessment: Nursing care that collects objective and subjective data from primary and secondary sources.

Nursing Diagnosis (Analysis): Nursing care that groups significant data, interprets data, and comes to conclusions.

Planning: Nursing care that sets goals, objectives, and outcomes; prioritizes interventions; and performs calculations.

Implementation: Nursing care that follows a regimen of care prescribed by a primary health-care provider, such as administration of medications, and procedures, as well as performs nursing care within the legal scope of the nursing profession.

Evaluation: Nursing care that identifies a client's responses to medical and nursing interventions.

Client Need Categories

Client needs reflect activities most commonly performed by entry-level nurses.

Safe and Effective Care Environment

Management of Care: Nursing care that provides or directs the delivery of nursing activities to clients, significant others, and other health-care personnel. Management of care items account for 17% to 23% of the items on the NCLEX-RN examination.

Safety and Infection Control: Nursing care that protects clients, significant others, and health-care personnel from health and environmental hazards. Safety and infection control items account for 9% to 15% of the items on the NCLEX-RN examination.

Health Promotion and Maintenance: Nursing care that assists clients and significant others to prevent or detect health problems and achieve optimal health, particularly in relation to their developmental level. Health promotion and maintenance items account for 6% to 12% of the items on the NCLEX-RN examination.

Psychosocial Integrity: Nursing care that supports and promotes the emotional, mental, and social well-being of clients and significant others as well as those with acute or chronic mental health problems. Psychosocial integrity items account for 6% to 12% of the items on the NCLEX-RN examination.

Physiological Integrity

Basic Care and Comfort: Nursing care that provides support during the performance of the activities of daily living, such as hygiene, rest, sleep, mobility, elimination, hydration, and nutrition. Basic care and comfort items account for 6% to 12% of the items on the NCLEX-RN examination.

Pharmacological and Parenteral Therapies: Nursing care that relates to the administration of medication, intravenous fluids, and blood and blood products. Pharmacological and parenteral therapies items account for 12% to 18% of the items on the NCLEX-RN examination.

Reduction of Risk Potential: Nursing care that limits the development of complications associated with health problems, treatments, or procedures. Reduction of risk potential items account for 9 to 15% of the items on the NCLEX-RN examination.

Physiological Adaptation: Nursing care that meets the needs of clients with acute, chronic, or life-threatening physical health problems. Physiological adaptation items account for 11% to 17% of the items on the NCLEX-RN examination.

Cognitive Level Categories

This category reflects the thinking processes necessary to answer a question.

Knowledge: Information must be recalled from memory, such as facts, terminology, principles, and generalizations.

Comprehension: Information, as well as the implications and potential consequences of information identified, must be understood, interpreted, and paraphrased or summarized. **Application:** Information must be identified, manipulated, or used in a situation, including mathematical calculations.

Analysis: A variety of information must be interpreted, requiring the identification of commonalities, differences, and interrelationship among the data.

Mental Health and Mental Illness

Mental health is a level of psychological well-being or an absence of a mental disorder. It is the psychological state of someone who is functioning at a satisfactory level of emotional and behavioral adjustment. According to the World Health Organization (WHO), mental health includes "subjective well-being, perceived self-efficacy, autonomy, competence, intergenerational dependence, and self-actualization of one's intellectual and emotional potential." **Mental illness** is a mental or behavioral pattern or anomaly that causes either suffering or an impaired ability to function in ordinary life and which is not developmentally or socially normative. Mental disorders are generally defined by a combination of how a person feels, acts, thinks, or perceives. These disorders may be associated with particular regions or functions of the brain. The concepts of mental health and mental illness are culturally defined. Some cultures are quite liberal in the range of behaviors that are considered acceptable, whereas others have little tolerance for behaviors that deviate from cultural norms.

I. Mental Health and Mental Illness

A. Maslow defined mental health and illness in the context of individual functioning and developed a "hierarchy of needs," the lower needs requiring fulfillment before those at higher levels can be achieved, with self-actualization being fulfillment of one's highest potential (Fig. 1.1)

B. Black and Andreasen (2011) define mental health as "a state of being that is relative rather than absolute. The successful performance of mental functions shown by productive activities, fulfilling relationships with other people, and the ability to adapt to change and to cope with adversity" (p. 608)

C. Townsend (2012) defines mental health as "the successful adaptation to stressors from the internal or external environment, evidenced by thoughts, feelings, and behaviors that are age-appropriate and congruent with local and cultural norms" (p. 16)

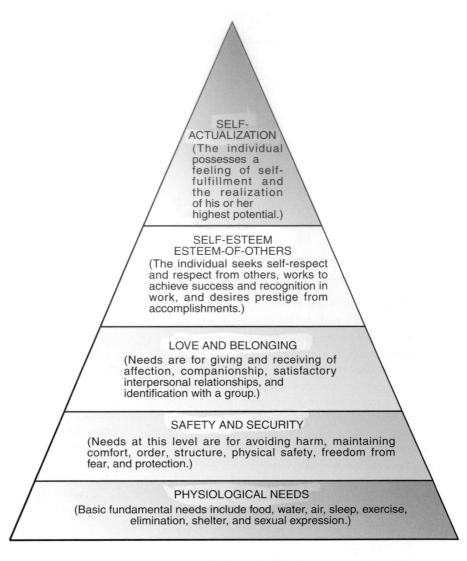

Fig 1.1 Maslow's hierarchy of needs.

The American Psychiatric Association (APA; 2013), in its ***Diagnostic and Statistical Manual of Mental Disorders, Fifth Edition*** (DSM-5), defines a mental disorder as "a health condition characterized by significant dysfunction in an individual's cognitions, emotions, or behaviors that reflect a disturbance in the psychological, biological or developmental processes underlying mental functioning."

II. Physical Responses to Stress

A. Fight-or-flight syndrome
 1. General adaptation syndrome as described by Selye:
    a. Alarm reaction stage: during this stage, the physiological responses of the fight-or-flight syndrome are initiated.
    b. Stage of resistance: the individual uses the physiological responses of the first stage as a defense in the attempt to adapt to the stressor. If adaptation occurs, the third stage is prevented or delayed. Physiological symptoms may disappear.
    c. Stage of exhaustion: this stage occurs when there is a prolonged exposure to the stressor to which the body has become adjusted. The adaptive energy is depleted, and the individual can no longer draw from the resources for adaptation described in the first two stages. Diseases of adaptation (e.g., headaches, mental disorders, coronary artery disease, ulcers, colitis) may occur (Selye, 1956, 1974).
 2. Biological responses to fight or flight.
    a. Senses sharpen. Pupils dilate.
    b. The heart rate increases, and arteries constrict raising blood pressure.
    c. The respiratory rate increases.
    d. The liver increases the metabolism of fat cells and glucose.
    e. Renal and digestive system functions are suppressed.
    f. Dry mouth, diaphoresis, and pallor occur.

g. Endorphins are released to decrease pain.

h. Cognitive responses become primitive.

🛑 When an individual remains under stress for a sustained period of time without intervention for reversal, exhaustion and even death may ensue.

III. Psychological Responses to Stress

A. Anxiety
 1. *Stress* is defined as a state of mental or emotional strain or tension resulting from adverse or very demanding circumstances.
 2. *Fear* is defined as the intellectual appraisal of a threatening stimulus. Fear is caused by the belief that someone or something is dangerous, likely to cause pain, or is a threat.
 3. *Anxiety* is defined as a diffuse apprehension that is vague in nature and is associated with feelings of uncertainty and helplessness.
 4. Levels of anxiety.
    a. Mild anxiety:
       i. Seldom a problem for the individual
       ii. Prepares people for action
       iii. Sharpens the senses
       iv. Increases motivation
       v. Increases the perceptual field
       vi. Enhances learning
    b. Moderate anxiety:
       i. Diminishes the perceptual field
       ii. Decreases alertness
       iii. Decreases attention span and concentration
       iv. Requires problem-solving assistance
       v. Increases muscular tension and restlessness
    c. Severe anxiety:
       i. Greatly diminishes perceptual field and concentration
       ii. Extremely limits attention span
       iii. Causes physical symptoms
          1) Headaches
          2) Palpitations
          3) Insomnia
       iv. Causes emotional symptoms
          1) Confusion
          2) Dread
          3) Horror
       v. Overt behavior is aimed at relieving the anxiety
    d. Panic anxiety can cause:
       i. Inability to focus on any detail
       ii. Possible loss of contact with reality
       iii. Possible hallucinations or delusions
       iv. Desperate actions or extreme withdrawal
       v. Ineffective communication
       vi. Feelings of terror or "going crazy"

🛑 Prolonged panic anxiety can lead to physical and emotional exhaustion and can be life threatening.

 5. Stress adaptation.
    a. Coping behaviors exhibited during mild anxiety:
       i. Sleeping
       ii. Eating
       iii. Physical exercise
       iv. Smoking
       v. Crying
       vi. Drinking
       vii. Laughing
       viii. Cursing
       ix. Pacing
       x. Foot swinging
       xi. Fidgeting
       xii. Nail biting
       xiii. Finger tapping
       xiv. Confiding in others
    b. **Ego defense mechanisms** are used, either consciously or unconsciously, as protective devices for the ego in an effort to relieve anxiety (Table 1.1).

DID YOU KNOW?
Healthy persons normally use different defenses throughout life. An ego defense mechanism becomes pathological only when its persistent use leads to maladaptive behavior such that the physical or mental health of the individual is adversely affected. The purpose of ego defense mechanisms is to protect the mind/self/ego from anxiety or social sanctions and/or to provide a refuge from a situation with which one cannot currently cope.

MAKING THE CONNECTION

Anxiety at the moderate to severe level that remains unresolved over an extended period can contribute to a number of physiological disorders. The *DSM-5* (APA, 2013) describes these disorders under the category of "Psychological Factors Affecting Medical Conditions." The psychological factors may exacerbate symptoms of, delay recovery from, or interfere with treatment of the medical condition. The condition may be initiated or exacerbated by an environmental situation that the individual perceives as stressful. Measurable pathophysiology can be demonstrated. It is thought that psychological and behavioral factors may affect the course of almost every major category of disease, including, but not limited to, cardiovascular, gastrointestinal, neoplastic, neurological, and pulmonary conditions.

Table 1.1 Ego Defense Mechanisms

Defense Mechanism	Description
Compensation	Covering up a real or perceived weakness by emphasizing a trait one considers more desirable Example: A physically handicapped boy is unable to participate in football, so he compensates by becoming a great scholar.
Denial	Refusing to acknowledge the existence of a real situation or the feelings associated with it Example: A woman drinks alcohol every day and cannot stop, failing to acknowledge that she has a problem.
Displacement	The transfer of feelings from one target to another that is considered less threatening or that is neutral Example: A client is angry at his doctor and does not express it but becomes verbally abusive with the nurse.
Identification	An attempt to increase self-worth by acquiring certain attributes and characteristics of an individual one admires Example: A teenaged boy who required lengthy rehabilitation after an accident decides to become a physical therapist as a result of his experiences.
Intellectualization	An attempt to avoid expressing actual emotions associated with a stressful situation by using the intellectual processes of logic, reasoning, and analysis Example: Susan's husband is being transferred with his job to a city far away from her parents. She hides anxiety by explaining to her parents the advantages associated with the move.
Introjection	Integrating the beliefs and values of another individual into one's own ego structure Example: Children integrate their parents' value system into the process of conscience formation. A child says to a friend, "Don't cheat. It's wrong."
Isolation	Separating a thought or memory from the feeling, tone or emotion associated with it Example: Without showing any emotion, a young woman describes being attacked and raped.
Projection	Attributing feelings or impulses unacceptable to oneself to another person. Example: Sue feels a strong sexual attraction to her track coach and tells her friend, "He's coming on to me!"
Rationalization	Attempting to make excuses or formulate logical reasons to justify unacceptable feelings or behaviors Example: John tells the rehab nurse, "I drink because it's the only way I can deal with my bad marriage and my worse job."
Reaction Formation	Preventing unacceptable or undesirable thoughts or behaviors from being expressed by exaggerating opposite thoughts or types of behaviors Example: Jane hates nursing. She attended nursing school to please her parents. During career day, she speaks to prospective students about the excellence of nursing as a career.
Regression	Responding to stress by retreating to an earlier level of development and the comfort measures associated with that level of functioning Example: When 2-year-old Jay is hospitalized for tonsillitis, he will drink only from a bottle, although his mother states he has been drinking from a cup for 6 months.
Repression	Involuntarily blocking unpleasant feelings and experiences from one's awareness Example: An accident victim can remember nothing about the accident.
Sublimation	Rechanneling of drives or impulses that are personally or socially unacceptable into activities that are constructive Example: A mother whose son was killed by a drunk driver channels her anger and energy into being the president of the local chapter of Mothers Against Drunk Drivers.
Suppression	The voluntary blocking of unpleasant feelings and experiences from one's awareness Example: Scarlett O'Hara says, "I don't want to think about that now. I'll think about that tomorrow."
Undoing	Symbolically negating or canceling out an experience that one finds intolerable Example: Joe is nervous about his new job and yells at his wife. On his way home, he stops and buys her some flowers.

6. Consequences of prolonged severe anxiety.
   a. Psychoneurotic responses to severe anxiety as they appear in the DSM-5.
      i. Anxiety disorders: disorders in which the characteristic features are symptoms of anxiety and avoidance behavior (e.g., phobias, panic disorder, generalized anxiety disorder, and separation anxiety disorder).
      ii. Somatic symptom disorders: disorders in which the characteristic features are physical symptoms for which there is no demonstrable organic pathology; psychological factors are judged to play a significant role in the onset, severity, exacerbation, or maintenance of the symptoms (e.g., somatic symptom disorder, illness anxiety disorder, conversion disorder, and factitious disorder).
      iii. Dissociative disorders: disorders in which the characteristic feature is a disruption in the usually integrated functions of consciousness, memory, identity, or perception of the environment (e.g., dissociative amnesia, dissociative identity disorder, and depersonalization-derealization disorder).
B. Grief
   1. *Grief* is defined as a subjective state of emotional, physical, and social responses to the loss of a valued entity.
   2. Stages of grief according to Kübler-Ross (1969):
      a. Stage 1—Denial: This is a stage of shock and disbelief. The reality of the loss is not acknowledged. Denial is a protective mechanism that allows the individual to cope within an immediate time frame while organizing more effective defense strategies.
      b. Stage 2—Anger: Anger may be directed at the self or displaced on loved ones, caregivers, and even God. There may be a preoccupation with an idealized image of the lost entity.
      c. Stage 3—Bargaining: During this stage, which is usually not visible or evident to others, a "bargain" is made with God in an attempt to reverse or postpone the loss. Sometimes the promise is associated with feelings of guilt for not having performed satisfactorily, appropriately, or sufficiently.
      d. Stage 4—Depression: The sense of loss is intense, and feelings of sadness and depression prevail. This stage differs from pathological depression in that it represents advancement toward resolution rather than the fixation in an earlier stage of the grief process.
      e. Stage 5—Acceptance: The final stage brings a feeling of peace regarding the loss that has occurred. It is a time of quiet expectation and resignation.

DID YOU KNOW?
Not all individuals experience each of these stages in response to a loss, nor do they necessarily experience them in this order. Some individuals' grieving behaviors may fluctuate, and even overlap, among the stages.

   3. Resolution of grief.
      a. The grief response can last from weeks to years.
      b. Individuals must progress at their own pace.
      c. Relationship ambivalence and guilt can lengthen the process.
      d. If the loss is sudden and unexpected, mourning may take longer.
      e. Bereavement overload is directly correlated with the number of recent losses and time frame in which they occur.

DID YOU KNOW?
Everyone experiences grief and a sense of loss following the death of a loved one, but the way these feelings are experienced and expressed differs across cultures. Each culture has its own rituals and practices that influence the expression of grief. Carrying out these familiar rituals and customs offers a sense of stability and security and helps people who are dying and their loved ones cope with loss.

   4. Types of grief.
      a. Anticipatory grief: occurs when a loss is anticipated, individuals often begin the work of grieving before the actual loss occurs.
         i. Preparation for the loss can facilitate the process of mourning
         ii. Emotional disengagement may occur resulting in feelings of rejection from the dying person
      b. Maladaptive grief response.
         i. Individuals are not able to progress satisfactorily through the stages of grieving and become fixed in denial or anger
         ii. Prolonged response is characterized by an intense preoccupation with memories of the lost entity for many years after the loss has occurred
         iii. Delayed or inhibited response is characterized by the individual becoming fixed in the denial stage of the grieving process. The emotional pain associated with the loss is not experienced, but anxiety disorders (e.g., phobias, illness anxiety disorder) or sleeping and eating disorders (e.g., insomnia, anorexia) may be evident

IV. Diagnostic and Statistical Manual of Mental Disorders (DSM)

The *Diagnostic and Statistical Manual of Mental Disorders* (DSM) is published by the American Psychiatric Association and provides a common language and standard criteria for the classification of mental disorders.

DID YOU KNOW?
The fifth edition of the *Diagnostic and Statistical Manual of Mental Disorders* (DSM-5) was approved by the Board of Trustees of the American Psychiatric Association on December 1, 2012, and published on May 18, 2013. The DSM-5 is the first major edition of the manual in 20 years.

A. *Diagnostic and Statistical Manual of Mental Disorders, Fifth Edition*
   1. DSM-5 lists all psychiatric and general medical diagnoses.
   2. Dimensional assessment tools are included in Section 3 of the DSM-5 to better incorporate client perspective, as well as cultural differences, into clinical assessment and care.
      a. Goal is to provide additional information that assists the clinician in assessment, treatment planning, and treatment monitoring.
      b. May be specific to a given disorder or relevant to any client's treatment.
      c. Used at an initial evaluation to establish a baseline and on follow-up visits to track changes.
      d. Relies, when possible, on self-report ratings.
   3. Section 3 of DSM-5 includes a number of conditions requiring further research before consideration as official diagnoses.

DID YOU KNOW?
The fifth edition of the *Diagnostic and Statistical Manual of Mental Disorders* (DSM-5) contains, in addition to categorical diagnoses, a dimensional approach allowing clinicians to rate disorders along a continuum of severity. The dimensional diagnostic system also correlates well with treatment planning. Conditions that do not meet DSM-5 criteria are termed "not elsewhere defined" (NED).

REVIEW QUESTIONS

1. A nurse is assessing a client who, over the past 3 years, has experienced feelings of sadness related to the death of a beloved aunt. The client sleeps and eats little and isolates themself. How should the nurse interpret the client's behaviors?
   1. The client's functional impairment indicates a need for psychiatric commitment.
   2. The client's behaviors are part of the normal grief process.
   3. The client's behaviors are not congruent with cultural norms.
   4. The client's functional impairment indicates potential mental illness.

2. A client from India states, "My uncle sinned when he slaughtered his cow for profit." Which data should the nurse consider when assessing this client's mental health?
   1. Delusions are false personal beliefs.
   2. The concepts of mental health and mental illness are defined and influenced by culture and religious beliefs.
   3. Hallucinations are false sensory perceptions not associated with any real external stimuli and may involve any of the five senses.
   4. This client is employing the defense mechanism of projection.

3. According to Maslow's hierarchy of needs, which situation demonstrates the highest level of attainment?
   1. An individual demonstrates an ability to discuss objectively all points of view and possesses a strong sense of ethics.
   2. An individual avoids harm while maintaining comfort, order, and physical safety.
   3. An individual establishes meaningful interpersonal relationships and can identify himself or herself within a group.
   4. An individual desires prestige from personal accomplishments.

4. Order the level of need attainment as described by Maslow from an individual's basic need foundation to the individual's highest fulfillment potential.
   1. _____ Love and Belonging
   2. _____ Self-Actualization
   3. _____ Physiological Needs
   4. _____ Self-esteem, Esteem of Others
   5. _____ Safety and Security

5. Which of the following best exemplifies a client's use of the defense mechanism of displacement? **Select all that apply.**
   1. A student nurse fails a dosage calculation test then arbitrarily picks a fight with a roommate.
   2. An adolescent who feels angry and hostile toward others decides to become a therapist.
   3. A woman is unhappy about being a mother, although others know her as an attentive parent.
   4. A client is drinking 6 to 8 beers a day while still attending Alcoholics Anonymous as a group leader.
   5. After a heated argument with his wife, a husband berates a restaurant waiter for slow service.

6. A nursing instructor is teaching about ego defense mechanisms. Which student statement indicates a need for further instruction?
   1. "Defense mechanisms are used during periods of increased anxiety and when the strength of the ego is tested."
   2. "All individuals who use defense mechanisms to adapt to stress exhibit healthy egos."
   3. "At times of mild to moderate anxiety, defense mechanisms can be used adaptively to deal with stress."
   4. "Some ego defenses are more adaptive than others, but all are used either consciously or unconsciously for ego protection."

7. Clearly depressed about a transfer to Hawaii because of the high cost of living, an Air Force major does research and convinces his family of the great surfing Hawaii offers. A nurse would recognize that the major is using which defense mechanism?
   1. Intellectualization
   2. Denial
   3. Rationalization
   4. Suppression

8. Which of the following situations exemplify the use of the ego defense mechanism of compensation? **Select all that apply.**
   1. With a flat affect and displaying no emotion, a daughter describes her mother's recent suicide.
   2. Failing the college entrance examination due to an inability to comprehend math, the student embarks on a master gardener certification.
   3. A woman recently disbarred from the legal profession takes to her bed and finds comfort in sucking her thumb.
   4. A teacher's aide is reprimanded during school then later criticizes the librarian for a lack of reading materials.
   5. A woman who is unable to bear children applies as a foster parent through the department of social services.

9. Which situation exemplifies the use of the ego defense mechanism of identification?
   1. A veterinarian who dislikes cats begins a specialty in feline medicine.
   2. A self-admitted homosexual tells his parents he has noted homosexual tendencies in his younger brother.
   3. A 10-year-old is rescued from a house fire and later in life decides to become a firefighter.
   4. A singer tells her agent that her heavy smoking will not harm her voice.

10. A war veteran describes having his legs blown off during an attack. His affect is flat, and he shows no emotion during this disclosure. This veteran is using which defense mechanism?
    1. Isolation
    2. Identification
    3. Introjection
    4. Displacement

11. A mother abuses her children and tells the caseworker that it's her husband who abuses the children, even though it has been proven that he's a dutiful father. Which defense mechanism is the mother using?
    1. Compensation
    2. Projection
    3. Displacement
    4. Denial

12. A husband yells at his wife because of her self-indulgent extravagances. Later in the day, he buys her a $1,000 spa gift certificate. The husband is using which defense mechanism?
    1. Denial
    2. Undoing
    3. Compensation
    4. Repression

13. Which of the following is an immediate physical response associated with the "fight-or-flight" syndrome? **Select all that apply.**
    1. Senses sharpen, pupils constrict.
    2. Respiratory rate increases.
    3. Secretions from the sweat glands decrease.
    4. Renal and digestive system functions are suppressed.
    5. Endorphins are released to decrease pain.

14. *Anxiety* may be distinguished from *fear* in that anxiety is an emotional process, whereas fear is a(n) _____ process.

15. Which exhibited symptom would cause a nurse to determine that a client is experiencing a panic level of anxiety?
    1. The client has difficulty concentrating.
    2. The client, without evidence, is convinced his son is planning his murder.
    3. The client requires assistance in decision making.
    4. The client is restless and complains of muscle tension.

16. An anxious client has recently experienced a myocardial infarction. Which of the following are possible problems that may arise from unresolved anxiety? **Select all that apply.**
    1. Anxiety may exacerbate symptoms.
    2. Anxiety may produce genetic anomalies.
    3. Anxiety may delay recovery.
    4. Anxiety may interfere with treatment.
    5. Anxiety may predispose a client to a personality disorder diagnosis.

17. What is the rationale for a nurse to perform a psychosocial assessment on a client with a family history of cardiovascular disease?
    1. Unresolved anxiety can contribute to physiological disorders.
    2. Cardiovascular disease has been associated with mental illness.
    3. It is important to rule out the diagnosis of personality disorder.
    4. Psychosocial assessments can always predict pathophysiology.

18. A widow tells the nurse that her husband died 2 years ago. She continues to feel lonely and vulnerable. Which statement by the widow would indicate that she is considering adaptive coping skill changes?
    1. "I'm going to deal with my situation by moving to California."
    2. "I will find a support group."
    3. "I'm mentally healthy. I can solve my own problems."
    4. "I'll be okay. I'm just not a people person."

19. A nursing instructor is teaching about grief resolution. Which student statement indicates a need for further instruction?
    1. "The grief response can last from weeks to years."
    2. "Individuals must progress through the grieving process at their own pace."
    3. "If loss is sudden and unexpected, mourning may take a shorter period of time."
    4. "Relationship ambivalence and guilt can lengthen the grieving process."

20. A nursing instructor is teaching about the dimensional assessment tools included in Section 3 of the *Diagnostic and Statistical Manual of Mental Disorders, Fifth Edition* (DSM-5). Which student statement indicates a need for further instruction?
    1. "The dimensional assessment tool may be specific to a given disorder."
    2. "The dimensional assessment tool can be used initially to establish a baseline."
    3. "The dimensional assessment tool provides additional data needed for treatment."
    4. "The dimensional assessment tool relies heavily on physician assessment data."

REVIEW ANSWERS

1. ANSWER: 4
Rationale:
1. There is no evidence presented in the question that indicates that the client is a danger to self or others. Therefore, there is no need for psychiatric commitment.
2. The client's behaviors have lasted for 3 years and have affected daily functioning. This indicates abnormal grieving.
3. There is no evidence presented in the question indicating that the client's behavior is not congruent with cultural norms.
4. The client who experiences feelings of sadness for more than 3 years with significant functioning impairment may, after evaluation, be diagnosed with a mental illness.
TEST-TAKING TIP: Clients experiencing prolonged grieving that results in altered functioning need to be evaluated for potential mental illness.
Content Area: Psychosocial Integrity;
Integrated Process: Nursing Process: Assessment;
Client Need: Psychosocial Integrity;
Cognitive Level: Analysis;
Concept: Grief and Loss

2. ANSWER: 2
Rationale: Hinduism, the dominant religion of India, is based on the concept of omnipresence of the Divine, and the presence of a soul in all creatures, including bovines. Thus, by that definition, killing any animal would be a sin.
1. Delusions are false personal beliefs. The client's statement, "My uncle sinned when he slaughtered his cow for profit," should not be immediately assessed as a delusion before a consideration of cultural and religious beliefs.
2. The concepts of mental health and mental illness are defined and influenced by culture and religious beliefs. To properly assess this client's mental health, the nurse must recognize that the client's statement reflects an accepted Hindu religious belief.
3. Hallucinations are false sensory perceptions not associated with any real external stimuli and may involve any of the five senses. The client's statement, "My uncle sinned when he slaughtered his cow for profit," should not be immediately assessed as a hallucination before a consideration of cultural and religious beliefs.
4. Projection is attributing to another person feelings or impulses unacceptable to oneself. There is nothing presented in the question that indicates the use of the defense mechanism of projection.
TEST-TAKING TIP: Culture and religion have a direct bearing on many aspects of mental health and illness.
Content Area: Safe and Effective Care Environment;
Integrated Process: Nursing Process: Assessment;
Client Need: Safe and Effective Care Environment: Management of Care;
Cognitive Level: Analysis;
Concept: Diversity

3. ANSWER: 1
Rationale:
1. Demonstrating an ability to discuss objectively all points of view and possessing a strong sense of ethics

relates to Maslow's description of self-actualization. This is the fifth and highest level of attainment in Maslow's hierarchy of needs. It occurs after the client has met physiological, safety and security, love and belonging, and self-esteem/esteem-of-others needs.
2. Avoiding harm while maintaining comfort, order, and physical safety relates to Maslow's description of safety and security needs, which are the second level of attainment after the client has met physiological needs.
3. Establishing meaningful interpersonal relationships and identifying oneself within a group relates to Maslow's description of love and belonging needs, the third level of attainment, which occurs after the client has met physiological and safety and security needs.
4. Desiring prestige from personal accomplishments relates to Maslow's description of self-esteem/esteem-of-others needs. These occur after the client has met physiological, safety and security, and love and belonging needs.
TEST-TAKING TIP: Recall the hierarchy of needs as described by Maslow and be able to recognize indications of successful completion of the various levels. A review of Figure 1.1 will assist with acquiring this knowledge.
Content Area: Psychosocial Integrity;
Integrated Process: Nursing Process: Assessment;
Client Need: Psychosocial Integrity;
Cognitive Level: Application;
Concept: Critical Thinking

4. ANSWER: 2, 4, 1, 5, 3
Rationale:
1. Physiological needs must be fulfilled before any other higher levels of need can be achieved. These needs include food, water, air, sleep, exercise, elimination, shelter, and sexual expression.
2. Safety and security can be achieved after meeting basic physiological needs. These needs include avoiding harm, maintaining comfort, order, structure, physical safety, freedom from fear, and protection.
3. Love and belonging needs can be achieved after meeting basic physiological needs and safety and security needs. These needs include giving and receiving affection, companionship, satisfactory interpersonal relationships, and identification with a group.
4. Self-esteem and esteem of others' needs can be achieved after meeting basic physiological needs, safety and security needs, and love and belonging needs. These needs include seeking self-respect and respect from others, working to achieve success and recognition, and desiring prestige from accomplishments.
5. Self-actualization is when the individual possesses a feeling of self-fulfillment and the realization of his or her highest potential. Self-actualization needs can be achieved after meeting basic physiological needs, safety and security needs, love and belonging needs, and self-esteem and esteem of others needs.
TEST-TAKING TIP: Recall Maslow's hierarchy of needs theory. A review of Figure 1.1 in this chapter will assist with acquiring this knowledge.
Content Area: Psychological; Integrity
Integrated Process: Nursing Process: Assessment;

Client Need: Psychological Integrity;
Cognitive Level: Application;
Concept: Evidenced based Practice

5. **ANSWER: 1, 5**
Rationale:
1. A student nurse who fails a dosage calculation test and then arbitrarily picks a fight with a roommate is using the defense mechanism of displacement. Displacement is a method of transferring feelings from one threatening target to another target that is considered less threatening or neutral.
2. When an adolescent who feels angry and hostile toward others decides to become a therapist, the adolescent is using the defense mechanism of sublimation. Sublimation is a method of rechanneling drives or impulses that are personally or socially unacceptable into activities that are constructive.
3. When a woman who is unhappy about being a mother is perceived as an attentive parent, the woman is using the defense mechanism of reaction formation. Reaction formation assists in preventing unacceptable or undesirable thoughts or behaviors from being expressed by exaggerating opposite thoughts or types of behaviors.
4. When a client is drinking 6 to 8 beers a day while still attending Alcoholics Anonymous as a group leader, the client is using the defense mechanism of denial. Denial is refusing to acknowledge the existence of a real situation or the feelings associated with it.
5. When a husband berates a restaurant waiter for slow service after a heated argument with his wife, the husband is using the defense mechanism of displacement. Displacement is a method of transferring feelings from one threatening target to another target that is considered less threatening or neutral.
TEST-TAKING TIP: Pair the situation presented in the question with the appropriate defense mechanism. A review of Table 1.1 will give the test taker examples of various defense mechanisms.
Content Area: Psychosocial Integrity;
Integrated Process: Nursing Process: Assessment;
Client Need: Psychosocial Integrity;
Cognitive Level: Analysis;
Concept: Stress

6. **ANSWER: 2**
Rationale:
1. Defense mechanisms are used during periods of increased anxiety and when the strength of the ego is tested. This student statement indicates that learning has occurred.
2. Defense mechanisms can be used adaptively to deal with stress and ego protection. Unhealthy ego development may result from the overuse or maladaptive use of defense mechanisms. Not all individuals who use defense mechanisms as a means of stress adaptation exhibit healthy egos. This student statement indicates that further teaching is needed.
3. At times of mild to moderate anxiety, defense mechanisms can be used adaptively to deal with stress. This student statement indicates that learning has occurred.

4. Some ego defenses are more adaptive than others, but all are used either consciously or unconsciously for ego protection. This student statement indicates that learning has occurred.
TEST-TAKING TIP: Note important words in the answers, such as *all* in Option 2. The use of the word *never, only, all,* or *always* should alert you to reconsider the answer choice and to review all the options again.
Content Area: Psychosocial Integrity;
Integrated Process: Nursing Process: Evaluation;
Client Need: Psychosocial Integrity;
Cognitive Level: Analysis;
Concept: Stress

7. **ANSWER: 1**
Rationale:
1. Intellectualization is when an individual attempts to avoid expressing actual emotions associated with a stressful situation by using the intellectual processes of logic, reasoning, and analysis. The major in this situation is using reasoning to avoid dealing with negative feelings about the high cost of living in Hawaii.
2. Denial is when an individual refuses to acknowledge the existence of a real situation or the feelings associated with it. The major in the question is not exhibiting denial.
3. Rationalization is when an individual attempts to make excuses or formulate logical reasons to justify unacceptable feelings or behaviors. The major in the question is not exhibiting rationalization.
4. Suppression is when an individual voluntarily blocks unpleasant feelings and experiences from awareness. The major in the question is not exhibiting suppression.
TEST-TAKING TIP: Pair the situation presented in the question with the appropriate defense mechanism. Review Table 1.1 for examples of various defense mechanisms.
Content Area: Psychosocial Integrity;
Integrated Process: Nursing Process: Evaluation;
Client Need: Psychosocial Integrity;
Cognitive Level: Analysis;
Concept: Stress

8. **ANSWER: 2, 5**
Rationale:
1. When a daughter describes her mother's recent suicide with a flat affect and no emotion, she is using the defense mechanism of isolation. Isolation is the separation of thought or memory from the feeling tone or emotion associated with the memory or event.
2. Compensation is when a person covers up a real or perceived weakness by emphasizing a trait considered more desirable. The student in the question is compensating for an inability to pursue a college degree by attaining a master gardener certification.
3. When a woman recently disbarred from the legal profession takes to her bed and finds comfort in sucking her thumb, she is exhibiting the defense mechanism of regression. Regression is when a person responding to stress retreats to an earlier level of development and the comfort measures associated with that level of functioning.

4. When a teacher's aide is reprimanded during school then later criticizes the librarian for a lack of reading materials, the aide is exhibiting the defense mechanism of displacement. Displacement is the transferring of feelings from one target to another target that is considered less threatening or neutral.

5. Compensation is when a person covers up a real or perceived weakness by emphasizing a trait considered more desirable. The woman in the question is compensating for an inability to bear children by applying to the department of social services to become a foster parent.

TEST-TAKING TIP: Differentiate between the different defense mechanisms and recognize behaviors that reflect the use of these defenses. Review Table 1.1 for examples of various defense mechanisms.

Content Area: Psychosocial Integrity;
Integrated Process: Nursing Process: Assessment;
Client Need: Psychosocial Integrity;
Cognitive Level: Analysis;
Concept: Stress

9. ANSWER: 3

Rationale:
1. When a veterinarian who dislikes cats begins a specialty in feline medicine, the vet is exhibiting the defense mechanism of reaction formation. Reaction formation prevents unacceptable thoughts or feelings from being expressed by exaggerating the opposite thoughts or feelings.
2. When a self-admitted homosexual tells his parents he has noted homosexual tendencies in his younger brother, he is using the defense mechanism of projection. Projection is attributing feelings or impulses unacceptable to oneself to another person.

3. Identification is an attempt to increase self-esteem by acquiring certain attributes of an admired individual. The 10-year-old in the question has identified with the firefighters by choosing a career as a firefighter in later life.
4. When a singer tells her agent that her heavy smoking will not harm her voice, the singer is exhibiting the defense mechanism of denial. Denial is when an individual refuses to acknowledge the existence of a real situation or the feelings associated with it.

TEST-TAKING TIP: Differentiate between the different defense mechanisms and recognize behaviors that reflect the use of these defenses. Review Table 1.1 for examples of various defense mechanisms.

Content Area: Psychosocial Integrity;
Integrated Process: Nursing Process: Assessment;
Client Need: Psychosocial Integrity;
Cognitive Level: Analysis;
Concept: Stress

10. ANSWER: 1

Rationale:
1. Isolation is the separation of thought or memory from the feeling tone or emotions associated with the memory or event. The veteran in the question showing no emotion related to the loss of both legs is using the ego defense mechanism of isolation.
2. Identification is an attempt to increase self-esteem by acquiring certain attributes of an admired individual. The

situation in the question is not reflective of the defense mechanism of identification.
3. Introjection is integrating the beliefs and values of another individual into one's own ego structure. The situation in the question is not reflective of the defense mechanism of introjection.
4. Displacement is the transferring of feelings from one target to another target that is considered less threatening or neutral. The situation presented in the question does not reflect the defense mechanism of displacement.

TEST-TAKING TIP: The defense mechanism of isolation does not refer to physical seclusion, but rather it refers to an emotional isolation of feelings.

Content Area: Psychosocial Integrity;
Integrated Process: Nursing Process: Assessment;
Client Need: Psychosocial Integrity;
Cognitive Level: Analysis;
Concept: Stress

11. ANSWER: 2

Rationale:
1. Compensation is when a person covers up a real or perceived weakness by emphasizing a trait considered more desirable. The situation presented in the question does not reflect the defense mechanism of compensation.

2. Projection is attributing feelings or impulses unacceptable to oneself to another person. The mother in the question is projecting her unacceptable behavior on to her husband.
3. Displacement is the transferring of feelings from one target to another target that is considered less threatening or neutral. The situation presented in the question does not reflect the defense mechanism of displacement.
4. Denial is when an individual refuses to acknowledge the existence of a real situation or the feelings associated with it. The situation presented in the question does not reflect the defense mechanism of denial.

TEST-TAKING TIP: Projection is a defense mechanism in which the individual "passes the blame" or attributes undesirable feelings or impulses to another, thereby providing relief from associated anxiety.

Content Area: Psychosocial Integrity;
Integrated Process: Nursing Process: Assessment;
Client Need: Psychosocial Integrity;
Cognitive Level: Analysis;
Concept: Stress

12. ANSWER: 2

Rationale:
1. Denial is when an individual refuses to acknowledge the existence of a real situation or the feelings associated with it. The situation presented in the question does not reflect the defense mechanism of denial.

2. Undoing is an act of atonement for one's unacceptable acts or thoughts. The husband in the question is unconsciously attempting to undo his earlier unacceptable actions by giving his wife what she values.
3. Compensation is when a person covers up a real or perceived weakness by emphasizing a trait considered more desirable. The situation presented in the question does not reflect the defense mechanism of compensation.

4. Repression is the unconscious blocking of material that is threatening or painful. The situation in the question is not reflective of the defense mechanism of repression.
TEST-TAKING TIP: Compensation covers up a perceived weakness by emphasizing a more desirable trait, whereas undoing is an act of atonement for unacceptable behaviors.
Content Area: Psychosocial Integrity;
Integrated Process: Nursing Process: Assessment;
Client Need: Psychosocial Integrity;
Cognitive Level: Analysis;
Concept: Stress

13. **ANSWER: 2, 4, 5**
Rationale: During "fight or flight," the hypothalamus stimulates the sympathetic nervous system.
1. During an immediate "flight-or-fight" physical response, senses sharpen, but pupils dilate rather than constrict. This allows for more acute vision.
2. During an immediate "flight-or-fight" physical response, respiratory rate increases to allow for maximum oxygenation.
3. Secretions from the sweat glands increase rather than decrease. This cools the body and regulates the core body temperature.
4. Renal and digestive system functions are suppressed because during the "flight-or-fight" response, these functions are not essential.
5. Endorphins are released to decrease pain. Endorphins act as an opiate and produce analgesia, thus increasing the threshold for pain.
TEST-TAKING TIP: Recall the various physical effects on the body of the "fight-or-flight" syndrome. Note the key words in this question, *immediate physical response,* which determine the correct answers.
Content Area: Physiological Integrity;
Integrated Process: Nursing Process: Assessment;
Client Need: Physiological Integrity: Physiological Adaptation;
Cognitive Level: Application;
Concept: Stress

14. **ANSWER: cognitive**
Rationale: *Anxiety* may be distinguished from *fear* in that anxiety is an emotional process, whereas fear is a cognitive process. Fear involves the intellectual appraisal of a threatening stimulus; anxiety involves the emotional response to that appraisal.
TEST-TAKING TIP: Recall the differences between fear and anxiety.
Content Area: Psychosocial Integrity;
Integrated Process: Nursing Process: Assessment;
Client Need: Psychosocial Integrity;
Cognitive Level: Knowledge;
Concept: Stress

15. **ANSWER: 2**
Rationale:
1. A client who has difficulty concentrating is experiencing moderate, not panic, anxiety.
2. A client who has the delusional belief that his son is planning his murder is experiencing a panic level of anxiety.

3. A client who requires assistance in decision making is experiencing moderate, not panic, anxiety.
4. A client who is restless and complains of muscle tension is experiencing moderate, not panic, anxiety.
TEST-TAKING TIP: Recall the responses to all four levels of anxiety and understand that hallucinations and delusions occur only at the panic level.
Content Area: Psychosocial Integrity;
Integrated Process: Nursing Process: Assessment;
Client Need: Psychosocial Integrity;
Cognitive Level: Application;
Concept: Stress

16. **ANSWER: 1, 3, 4**
Rationale:
1. Exacerbation of symptoms can occur as a result of unresolved anxiety.
2. Genetic predisposition is not affected by unresolved anxiety.
3. A delayed recovery may occur as a result of unresolved anxiety.
4. Unresolved anxiety may interfere with the client's treatment.
5. A personality disorder diagnosis is not the result of unresolved anxiety.
TEST-TAKING TIP: Psychological factors, such as anxiety, may alter recovery of almost every category of physiological disease, including, but not limited to, cardiovascular, gastrointestinal, neoplastic, neurological, and pulmonary conditions.
Content Area: Safe and Effective Care Environment;
Integrated Process: Nursing Process: Assessment;
Client Need: Safe and Effective Care Environment: Management of Care;
Cognitive Level: Application;
Concept: Stress

17. **ANSWER: 1**
Rationale: Anxiety at the moderate to severe level that remains unresolved over an extended period can contribute to a number of physiological disorders. The DSM-5 (APA, 2013) describes these disorders under the category of "Psychological Factors Affecting Medical Conditions."
1. Unresolved moderate to severe anxiety over an extended period can contribute to cardiovascular disease.
2. There is no evidence that cardiovascular disease has been associated with mental illness.
3. Ruling out the diagnosis of personality disorder is not significant to this client's family history.
4. There is no evidence that psychosocial assessments can *always* predict pathophysiology.
TEST-TAKING TIP: The word *always* in Option 4 should cause test takers to question the validity of this statement.
Content Area: Safe and Effective Care Environment;
Integrated Process: Nursing Process: Assessment;
Client Need: Safe and Effective Care Environment: Management of Care;
Cognitive Level: Application;
Concept: Stress

18. ANSWER: 2
Rationale:
1. A move for this client is not an adaptive coping mechanism. Changing the client's external environment does not address the client's ability to deal with her feelings of loneliness and vulnerability. A move at this time may increase the client's stressors.
2. This client understands the importance of a support group, and she is willing to accept help to deal with loneliness and vulnerability. This would indicate adaptive coping.
3. This statement indicates that the client is resisting, not considering, adaptive coping skill changes.
4. This statement reflects denial of the client's true feelings of loneliness and vulnerability. This denial will prevent the client from embracing adaptive coping skill changes.
TEST-TAKING TIP: Recall the differences between a healthy, normal grieving process and a dysfunctional grieving process. Think of examples of each.
Content Area: Psychosocial Integrity;
Integrated Process: Nursing Process: Assessment;
Client Need: Psychosocial Integrity;
Cognitive Level: Analysis;
Concept: Grief and Loss

19. ANSWER: 3
Rationale:
1. The grief response can last from weeks to years. This student statement indicates that learning has occurred.
2. Individuals must progress through the grieving process at their own pace. This student statement indicates that learning has occurred.
3. If loss is sudden and unexpected, mourning may take a longer, not shorter, period of time. This student statement indicates that further instruction is needed.
4. Relationship ambivalence and guilt can lengthen the grieving process. This student statement indicates that learning has occurred.

TEST-TAKING TIP: Recall the concepts related to grief resolution and the importance of time as it relates to the grieving process.
Content Area: Psychosocial Integrity;
Integrated Process: Nursing Process: Evaluation;
Client Need: Psychosocial Integrity;
Cognitive Level: Application;
Concept: Grief and Loss

20. ANSWER: 4
Rationale:
1. The dimensional assessment tool may be specific to a given disorder or relevant to any client's treatment. This student statement indicates that learning has occurred.
2. The dimensional assessment tool can be used at an initial evaluation to establish a baseline and on follow-up visits to track changes. This student statement indicates that learning has occurred.
3. The dimensional assessment tool provides additional information that assists the clinician in assessment, treatment planning, and treatment monitoring. This student statement indicates that learning has occurred.
4. The dimensional assessment tool relies heavily on self-report ratings, not physician assessment data. This student statement indicates that further instruction is needed.
TEST-TAKING TIP: Review the components of the dimensional assessment tool.
Content Area: Psychosocial Integrity;
Integrated Process: Nursing Process: Evaluation;
Client Need: Psychosocial Integrity;
Cognitive Level: Application;
Concept: Promoting Health

Chapter 2

Theoretical Concepts

Aversion therapy—A form of psychological treatment in which the client is exposed to a stimulus while simultaneously being subjected to some form of discomfort; this conditioning is intended to cause the client to associate the stimulus with unpleasant sensations to stop the specific behavior

Behavioral therapy—Therapy that focuses on either behaviors alone or behaviors in combination with thoughts and feelings that might be causing those behaviors; those who practice behavior therapy tend to look more at specific, learned behaviors and environmental effect on these behaviors

Cognitive development—The theory that human intelligence progresses through a series of stages that are related to age, demonstrating at each successive stage a higher level of logical organization than at the previous stage

Developmental task—Activities and challenges that one must accomplish at specific stages in life to achieve appropriate personality development and mental health

Ego—According to Freud, the ego is the part of personality that experiences the reality of the external world, adapts to it, and responds to it; ego functions as a mediator to maintain harmony among the external world, the id, and the superego

Id—According to Freud, the id is the locus of instinctual drives; the id part of personality seeks to satisfy needs and achieve immediate gratification

Libido—According to Freud, the libido is part of the id and is the driving force of all behavior; the term is used to describe the energy created by survival and sexual instincts

Moral development—This theory of development focuses on the emergence, change, and understanding of morality from infancy through adulthood; in the field of moral development, *morality* is defined as principles for how individuals ought to treat one another, with respect to justice, another's well-being, and rights

Nurse-client relationship—Based on knowledge of theories of personality development and human behavior, therapeutic nurse-client relationships are client centered, goal oriented, and directed at learning and growth promotion

Nursing theorists—Nursing professionals who develop theories about the concepts of illness and the unique function of the nurse in providing assistance to clients experiencing alterations in health

Personality—A pattern of relatively permanent traits and unique characteristics that give both consistency and individuality to a person's behavior

Superego—According to Freud, the superego is the part of personality that is made up of all the internalized ideals that come from our parents, society, and culture; the superego works to suppress the urges of the id and tries to make the ego behave morally rather than realistically

Temperament—The unique natural style of interacting with or reacting to people, places, and things; temperament is innate rather than learned

Developmental theories identify behaviors associated with various *stages* through which individuals pass, thereby specifying what is appropriate or inappropriate at each developmental level. Developmental stages are identified by age. Behaviors can then be evaluated for age-appropriateness. Nurses must have a basic knowledge of human personality development to understand maladaptive behavioral responses commonly seen in psychiatric clients. The profession of nursing is based on measurable theoretical concepts. The major goal of nursing theory is the development of nursing knowledge on which to base nursing practice and improve quality of care.

I. Personality

A. Black and Andreasen (2011) define *personality* as "the characteristic way in which a person thinks, feels, and behaves; the ingrained pattern of behavior that each person evolves, both consciously and unconsciously, as his or her style of life or way of being" (p. 612)

B. *Personality* can also be defined as the unique organization of traits, characteristics, and modes of behavior of an individual, setting that individual apart from others, and at the same time determining how others react to the individual

C. *Temperament* is a set of inborn personality characteristics that influences an individual's manner of reacting to the environment and ultimately influences his or her personality development progression

II. Theories of Personality Development

A. Freud's theory of psychosexual personality development (psychoanalytic or intrapersonal theory)
  1. Structure of the personality.
     a. **Id** (pleasure principle).
     b. **Ego** (reality principle).
     c. **Superego** (perfection principle).
     d. **Libido,** a component of the Id, is the psychic energy used to fulfill basic physiological needs or instinctual drives such as hunger, thirst, and sexuality.

MAKING THE CONNECTION

Specialists in child development believe that infancy and early childhood are the major life periods for developmental change. Specialists in life-cycle development believe that people continue to develop and change throughout life, thereby suggesting the possibility for renewal and growth in adults.

---

  2. Categories of the mind.
     a. Conscious (memories within awareness).
     b. Preconscious (memories not in present awareness but easily retrieved).
     c. Unconscious (repressed memories that can only be retrieved through therapy).
  3. Stages of personality development.
     a. Oral stage: birth to 18 months (behavior directed by id, and goal is immediate gratification of needs).
     b. Anal stage: 18 months to 3 years (particular focus on excretory functions).
     c. Phallic stage 3 to 6 years (focus of energy on genital area).
        i. Oedipus complex (males)
        ii. Electra complex (females)
     d. Latency stage: 6 to 12 years (focus on socialization with same-sex peers).
     e. Genital stage: 13 to 20 years (focus on socialization with opposite sex).

DID YOU KNOW?

Developmental theories can be categorized as interpersonal (theories based primarily on relationships or interactions with others), intrapersonal (theories based primarily on genetic predispositions or internal feelings), behavioral (theories based primarily on actions and responses), or cognitive (theories based primarily on thought processes).

MAKING THE CONNECTION

Freud proposed that the development of the *Oedipus complex* or *Electra complex* occurred during the phallic stage of development (Table 2.1). He described this as the child's unconscious desire to eliminate the parent of the same gender and to possess the parent of the opposite gender for himself or herself. Guilt feelings result with the emergence of the superego during these years. Resolution of this internal conflict occurs when the child develops a strong identification with the parent of the same gender and internalizes that parent's attitudes, beliefs, and value system.

Box 2.1 Structure of the Personality

Behavioral Examples

Id	Ego	Superego
"I found this wallet; I will keep the money."	"I already have money. This money doesn't belong to me. Maybe the person who owns this wallet doesn't have any money."	"It is never right to take something that doesn't belong to you."
"Mom and Dad are gone. Let's party!"	"Mom and Dad said no friends over while they are away. Too risky."	"Never disobey your parents."
"I'll have sex with whomever I please, whenever I please."	"Promiscuity can be very dangerous."	"Sex outside of marriage is always wrong."

Table 2.1	Freud's Stages of Psychosexual Development	

Age	Stage	Major Developmental Tasks
Birth–18 months	Oral	Relief from anxiety through oral gratification of needs
18 months–3 years	Anal	Learning independence and control, with focus on the excretory function
3–6 years	Phallic	Identification with parent of same gender; development of sexual identity; focus on genital organs
6–12 years	Latency	Sexuality repressed; focus on relationships with same-gender peers
13–20 years	Genital	Libido reawakened as genital organs mature; focus on relationships with members of the opposite sex

B. Sullivan's interpersonal theory of personality development

1. Major concepts.
   a. Anxiety: the chief disruptive force in interpersonal relations and the main factor in the development of serious difficulties in living.
   b. Satisfaction of needs: fulfillment of all needs. Anything that, when absent, produces discomfort.
   c. Interpersonal security: a sense of total well-being when all needs have been met.
   d. Self-system: experiences or security measures adopted to protect against anxiety.
      i. The "good me" part of the personality that develops in response to positive feedback
      ii. The "bad me" part of the personality that develops in response to negative feedback
      iii. The "not me" part of the personality that develops in response to severe anxiety; emotional withdrawal results, which may lead to mental disorders in adult life
2. Stages of personality development (Table 2.2).
   a. Infancy: birth to 18 months (focus on gratification of needs).
   b. Childhood: 18 months to 6 years (focus on accepting delayed gratification).
   c. Juvenile: 6 to 9 years (focus on peer group relationship development).

   d. Preadolescence: 9 to 12 years (focus on same gender relationship development).
   e. Early adolescence: 12 to 14 years (focus on sense of separate identity from parents).
   f. Late adolescence: 14 to 21 years (focus on interdependence within society and formation of intimate relationships).

C. Erikson's psychosocial theory of personality development

1. Described eight stages of the life cycle during which individuals struggle with developmental "crises." **Developmental tasks** must be successfully completed to achieve positive outcomes and assure healthy personality development.
2. Stages of personality development (Table 2.3).
   a. Trust versus mistrust: birth to 18 months (developmental task: build trust).
      i. Achievement: self-confidence, optimism, drive, and hope
      ii. Nonachievement: emotional self-dissatisfaction, suspiciousness, interpersonal relationship difficulties
   b. Autonomy versus shame and doubt: 18 months to 3 years (developmental task: gain some self-control and independence within environment).
      i. Achievement: self-control, self-confidence, autonomy

Table 2.2	Stages of Development in Sullivan's Interpersonal Theory	

Age	Stage	Major Developmental Tasks
Birth–18 months	Infancy	Relief from anxiety through oral gratification of needs
18 months–6 years	Childhood	Learning to experience a delay in personal gratification without undue anxiety
6–9 years	Juvenile	Learning to form satisfactory peer relationships
9–12 years	Preadolescence	Learning to form satisfactory relationships with persons of same gender; initiating feelings of affection for another person
12–14 years	Early adolescence	Learning to form satisfactory relationships with persons of the opposite gender; developing a sense of identity
14–21 years	Late adolescence	Establishing self-identity; experiencing satisfying relationships; working to develop a lasting, intimate opposite-gender relationship

ii. Nonachievement: lack of pride in abilities, rage against self, sense of being controlled by others

c. Initiative versus guilt: 3 to 6 years (developmental task: develop a sense of purpose and ability to initiate and direct one's own activities).

   i. Achievement: assertiveness and dependability increase, conscience develops and controls impulsive behaviors

   ii. Nonachievement: excessive guilt, inadequacy, and impulsivity

d. Industry versus inferiority: 6 to 12 years (developmental task: achieve sense of self-confidence by learning, competing, and performing successfully).

   i. Achievement: sense of satisfaction, pride in achievement, conscientiousness

   ii. Nonachievement: personal inadequacy, lack of ability to cooperate or compromise, may become passive and meek or overly aggressive

e. Identity versus role confusion: 12 to 20 years (developmental task: integrate mastered tasks into secure sense of self).

   i. Achievement: confidence, emotional stability, self-view as unique, committed value system

   ii. Nonachievement: self-consciousness, doubt, confusion about role in life, absence of values and goals

f. Intimacy versus isolation: 20 to 30 years (developmental task: form intense lasting relationships or a commitment to another person, a cause, an institution, or a creative effort).

   i. Achievement: capacity for mutual love, respect, and total commitment to another

   ii. Nonachievement: withdrawal, social isolation, aloneness

g. Generativity versus stagnation: 30 to 65 years (developmental task: achieve life goals while considering the welfare of future generations).

   i. Achievement: gratification from achievements and meaningful contributions to others and demonstrated responsibility for leaving the world a better place in which to live

   ii. Nonachievement: lack of concern for the welfare of others and total preoccupation with the self

h. Ego integrity versus despair: 65 to death (developmental task: review life and derive meaning from both positive and negative events, while achieving a positive sense of self)

   i. Achievement: self-worth and self-acceptance, sense of dignity without fear of death

   ii. Nonachievement: self-contempt and disgust with how life progressed, worthlessness, helplessness, anger, loneliness, and depression

🛈 Developmental stages are identified by age. An individual's behaviors can then be evaluated for age-appropriateness.

D. Mahler's object relations theory of personality development (Table 2.4)

1. Mahler describes the separation-individuation process of the infant from the maternal figure (primary caregiver).

Table 2.3 Stages of Development in Erikson's Psychosocial Theory

Age	Stage	Major Developmental Tasks
Infancy (Birth–18 months)	Trust vs. mistrust	To develop a basic trust in the mothering figure and learn to generalize it to others
Early childhood (18 months–3 years)	Autonomy vs. shame and doubt	To gain some self-control and independence within the environment
Late childhood (3–6 years)	Initiative vs. guilt	To develop a sense of purpose and the ability to initiate and direct own activities
School age (6–12 years)	Industry vs. inferiority	To achieve a sense of self-confidence by learning, competing, performing successfully, and receiving recognition from significant others, peers, and acquaintances
Adolescence (12–20 years)	Identity vs. role confusion	To integrate the tasks mastered in the previous stages into a secure sense of self
Young adulthood (20–30 years)	Intimacy vs. isolation	To form an intense, lasting relationship or a commitment to another person, cause, institution, or creative effort
Adulthood (30–65 years)	Generativity vs. stagnation	To achieve the life goals established for oneself, while also considering the welfare of future generations
Old age (65 years–death)	Ego integrity vs. despair	To review one's life and derive meaning from both positive and negative events, while achieving a positive sense of self-worth

2. Phases of personality development.
   a. Phase I—normal autistic phase: birth to 1 month (focus: fulfillment of basic needs for survival and comfort).
   b. Phase II—symbiotic phase: 1 to 5 months (psychic fusion of mother and child, with mother fulfilling all needs).

🛑 Mahler suggests that absence of or rejection by the maternal figure at the symbiotic phase can lead to symbiotic psychosis. This can occur between the ages of 2 to 5 years. During symbiotic psychosis, the child is completely emotionally attached to mother and reacts stressfully if the possibility of separation occurs.

   c. Phase III—separation-individuation: 5 to 36 months (four subphases through which the child evolves in his or her progression from a symbiotic extension of the mothering figure to a distinct and separate being).
      i. Subphase 1—differentiation: 5 to 10 months (infant moves away from mother figure and recognizes separateness)
      ii. Subphase 2—practicing: 10 to 16 months (child experiences exhilaration and omnipotence from increased independence)
      iii. Subphase 3—rapprochement: 16 to 24 months (child demonstrates independence with mother figure's encouragement and develops a sense of security and belonging; if mother figure withholds nurturing and fosters dependency, feelings of rage and fear of abandonment develop; a child with unresolved fear of abandonment is thought to be fixed in the rapprochement phase, often leading to a diagnosis of **borderline personality disorder** in later life)
      iv. Subphase 4—consolidation: 24 to 36 months (child relates to objects in an effective constant manner; child establishes a sense

of separateness and can internalize a sustained image of a loved person when out of sight)

E. Piaget's stages of **cognitive development** (Table 2.5)
   1. The development of children's thinking progresses through a sequence of stages that do not vary and are somewhat related to chronological age.
   2. Stages of cognitive development.
      a. Sensorimotor (0–2 years): development proceeds from reflex activity to representation and sensorimotor solutions to problems.
      b. Preoperational (2–7 years): development proceeds from sensorimotor representation to prelogical thought and solutions to problems.
      c. Concrete operational (7–11 years): development proceeds from prelogical thought to logical solutions to concrete problems.
      d. Formal operational (11 years to adulthood): development proceeds from logical solutions to concrete problems to logical solutions to all classes of problems. In this stage the individual is able to think and reason in abstract terms.

F. Behavioral theorists
   1. The principles of **behavioral therapy** are based on the early studies of classical conditioning by Pavlov and operant conditioning by Skinner.
      a. *Classical conditioning* is a learning process that occurs when two stimuli are repeatedly paired; a response that is at first elicited by the second stimulus is eventually elicited by the first stimulus alone (Pavlov's dogs).
      b. *Operant conditioning* is a method of learning that occurs through rewards and punishments for behavior. Through these rewards and punishments, an association is made between a behavior and a consequence for that behavior.
   2. Basic assumptions: based on learning theory; behavioral responses are learned and can be modified in a particular environment.

Table 2.4 Stages of Development in Mahler's Theory of Object Relations

Age	Phase/Subphase	Major Developmental Tasks
Birth–1 month	I. Normal autism	Fulfillment of basic needs for survival and comfort
1–5 months	II. Symbiosis	Development of awareness of external source of need fulfillment
	III. Separation-Individuation	
5–10 months	a. Differentiation	Commencement of a primary recognition of separateness from the mothering figure
10–16 months	b. Practicing	Increased independence through locomotor functioning; increased sense of separateness of self
16–24 months	c. Rapprochement	Acute awareness of separateness of self; learning to seek "emotional refueling" from mothering figure to maintain feeling of security
24–36 months	d. Consolidation	Sense of separateness established; on the way to object constancy (i.e., able to internalize a sustained image of loved object/person when it is out of sight); resolution of separation anxiety

Table 2.5 Piaget's Stages of Cognitive Development

Age	Stage	Major Developmental Tasks
Birth–2 years	Sensorimotor	With increased mobility and awareness, development of a sense of self as separate from the external environment; the concept of object permanence emerges as the ability to form mental images evolves
2–6 years	Preoperational	Learning to express self with language; development of understanding of symbolic gestures; achievement of object permanence
6–12 years	Concrete operations	Learning to apply logic to thinking; development of understanding of reversibility and spatiality; learning to differentiate and classify; increased socialization and application of rules
12–15+ years	Formal operations	Learning to think and reason in abstract terms; making and testing hypotheses; capability of logical thinking and reasoning expand and are refined; cognitive maturity achieved

3. Techniques for modifying client behavior.
   a. *Shaping:* shaping the behavior of another by giving reinforcements for increasingly closer approximations to the desired behavior.
   b. *Modeling:* imitating the behaviors of others to learn new behaviors.
   c. *Premack principle:* using behavior that happens reliably as a reinforcer for a behavior that occurs less reliably.
   d. *Extinction:* withholding positive reinforcement to gain a gradual decrease in frequency or disappearance of an undesired response.
   e. *Contingency contracting:* developing a contract among all parties involved that delineates positive reinforcements and consequences of behavior.
   f. *Token economy:* presenting significant reinforcers for desired behaviors in the form of tokens, which may be exchanged for designated privileges.
   g. *Time-out:* isolating the client so that reinforcement from the attention of others is absent.
   h. *Reciprocal inhibition:* introducing a more adaptive behavior that is incompatible with the unacceptable behavior.
   i. *Overt sensitization:* producing unpleasant consequences for undesirable behavior—a type of **aversion therapy**.
   j. *Covert sensitization:* using mental imagery and imagination to produce unpleasant symptoms to modify maladaptive behavior.
   k. *Systematic desensitization:* presenting a hierarchy of anxiety producing events through which the individual progresses during therapy. Used in the treatment of phobias.
   l. *Flooding or implosion therapy:* flooding with a continuous presentation of the phobic stimulus until it no longer elicits anxiety.

DID YOU KNOW?
Behavior therapy is a form of psychotherapy, the goal of which is to modify maladaptive behavior patterns by reinforcing more adaptive behaviors. Behavioral change procedures are often combined with cognitive procedures, and many behavior therapies are referred to as *cognitive-behavioral* therapies.

G. Kohlberg's theory of **moral development** (Table 2.6)
   1. Moral behavior reflects the way a person interprets basic respect for other persons, such as the respect for human life, freedom, justice, or confidentiality.
   2. Stages of moral development.
      a. Preconventional/Level I (prominent from ages 4–10 years).
         i. Stage 1: punishment and obedience orientation (fear of punishment is likely to be incentive for conformity)
         ii. Stage 2: instrumental relativist orientation (behavior is motivated by concern for self and personal gain)
      b. Conventional/Level II (prominent from ages 10–13 years and into adulthood).
         i. Stage 3: interpersonal concordance orientation (behavior is guided by expectations of others and need for approval)
         ii. Stage 4: law and order orientation (behavior is motivated by respect for laws and authority)
      c. Postconventional/Level III (can occur from adolescence onward).
         i. Stage 5: social contact legalistic orientation (behavior is based on a system of internal values and principles)
         ii. Stage 6: universal ethical principle orientation (behavior is guided by the conscience regardless of negative consequences)

Table 2.6 Kohlberg's Stages of Moral Development

Level/Age*	Stage	Developmental Focus
I. Preconventional (common from ages 4–10 years)	1. Punishment and obedience orientation	Behavior motivated by fear of punishment
	2. Instrumental relativist orientation	Behavior motivated by egocentrism and concern for self
II. Conventional (common from ages 10–13 years, and into adulthood)	3. Interpersonal concordance orientation	Behavior motivated by expectations of others; strong desire for approval and acceptance
	4. Law and order orientation	Behavior motivated by respect for authority
III. Postconventional (can occur from adolescence on)	5. Social contract legalistic orientation	Behavior motivated by respect for universal laws and moral principles; guided by internal set of values
	6. Universal ethical principle orientation	Behavior motivated by internalized principles of honor, justice, and respect for human dignity; guided by the conscience

*Ages in Kohlberg's theory are not well defined. The stage of development is determined by the motivation behind the individual's behavior.

H. Peplau's nursing theory of personality development (Table 2.7)

1. Major concepts:
   a. Nursing is a human relationship in which the nurse recognizes and responds to a client's need for help.
   b. Nurse must understand "self" to respond appropriately to client's problems and needs.
2. Peplau's phases of the **nurse-client relationship:**
   a. Orientation: client, nurse, and family work together to recognize, clarify, and define the existing problem.
   b. Identification: client responds selectively to persons who seem to offer needed help.
      i. Responds by participation or interdependent relations with the nurse
      ii. Responds with independence or isolation from the nurse
      iii. Responds with helplessness or dependence on the nurse
   c. Exploitation: client takes full advantage of offered services and actively participates in own health care, exploring all possibilities for change.

   d. Resolution: client assumes independence. Resolution is the direct result of successful completion of the other three phases.
3. Psychological tasks of personality development.
   a. Learning to count on others: infancy. Newborn learns to communicate feelings, seeking to fulfill dependency needs. Regression occurs if needs are not met. Nurse's role can be that of surrogate mother.
   b. Learning to delay satisfaction: toddlerhood. Toddler learns to delay gratification and please mother figure in the context of toilet training. With rigid training and conditional approval, toddler may exhibit rebellious behaviors to counteract powerlessness. Nurse's role is to convey unconditional acceptance and encourage full expression of feelings.

DID YOU KNOW?

According to Peplau, the potential behaviors of individuals who have failed to complete the tasks of toddlerhood include exploitation and manipulation of others, suspiciousness and envy of others, hoarding, inordinate neatness and punctuality, inability to relate to others, and molding personality characteristics to meet expectations of others.

Table 2.7 Stages of Development in Peplau's Interpersonal Theory

Age	Stage	Major Developmental Tasks
Infancy	Learning to count on others	Learning to communicate in various ways with the primary caregiver to have comfort needs fulfilled
Toddlerhood	Learning to delay satisfaction	Learning the satisfaction of pleasing others by delaying self-gratification in small ways
Early childhood	Identifying oneself	Learning appropriate roles and behaviors by acquiring the ability to perceive the expectations of others
Late childhood	Developing skills in participation	Learning the skills of compromise, competition, and cooperation with others; establishing a more realistic view of the world and a feeling of one's place in it

c. Identifying oneself: early childhood. Child re-acts to low parental expectations by perceiving himself or herself as helpless and dependent. High expectations deprive child of emotional and growth need fulfillment. Age-appropriate, unconditional expectations generate ability for the child to effectively develop at his or her own pace. Nurse's role is to recognize client behaviors indicating unfulfilled needs and to provide experiences that promote growth.

d. Developing skills in participation: late child-hood. Child develops capacity to compromise, compete, and cooperate with others. If these skills are not developed appropriately, progres-sion results in difficulty dealing with the reoc-curring problems of life. Nurse's role is to help clients improve problem-solving skills.

III. Other Nursing Theorists

All of the following nursing theories can be applied to the care of psychiatric clients either through direct nursing interventions or the establishment of an effective nurse-client relationship.

1. Betty Neuman's systems model focuses on concepts related to stress and reaction to stress. Nursing inter-ventions are classified as primary prevention (occurs before stressors invade the normal line of defense and problems occur), secondary prevention (occurs after the system has reacted to the invasion of a stressor and problems are present), and tertiary prevention (occurs after secondary prevention and focuses on rehabilitation).

2. Dorothea Orem developed a general self-care deficit theory of nursing composed of three interrelated concepts: self-care, self-care deficit, and nursing sys-tems. Nursing interventions described in this theory consist of activities needed to meet self-care demands and solve self-care deficits.

3. Martha Rogers believed the science of nursing is the "science of unitary human beings." Rogers believed humans are in constant interaction with the environment and described interactions *with* versus *for* the client to achieve maximum potential.

4. Callista Roy developed the "Roy adaptation model," which consists of four essential elements: humans as adaptive systems, environment, health, and the goal of nursing. Roy describes nursing actions as interven-tions that seek to alter or manage stimuli so that adaptive responses can occur.

5. Madeleine Leininger developed the theory of cul-tural care diversity and universality based on the belief that across cultures there are health-care practices and beliefs that are diverse and similar. The nurse must understand the client's culture to provide care.

6. Jean Watson developed her theory based on the be-lief that curing disease is the domain of medicine, whereas caring is the domain of nursing. She devel-oped seven assumptions about the science of car-ing, which allows the nurse to deliver integrated holistic care.

7. Rizzo Parse developed her theory of "human becom-ing" from existential theory. Parse believes that peo-ple create reality for themselves through the choices they make at many levels, and nurses intervene by assisting the client to examine and understand the meaning of life experiences.

MAKING THE CONNECTION

Personality development is unique to each individual. When psychological tasks are successfully learned and developmental milestones met in each era of personality development, interpersonal skills are acquired that are necessary to establish relationships with others. This leads to a positive, productive lifestyle. When these milestones are not successfully met, unfulfilled needs carry over into adulthood, hindering the establishment of interpersonal relationships, which may result in dis-satisfaction with life and possible mental illness.

REVIEW QUESTIONS

1. A mother brings her 2-year-old child to a well-baby clinic. The child does not attempt to do things independently and continually looks to the mother for meeting all needs. According to Erikson, which of the following describes this child's developmental task assessment?
   1. Mistrust
   2. Guilt
   3. Inferiority
   4. Shame and doubt

2. A suicidal woman is admitted to the hospital. Her father reveals that his perfectionistic ex-wife scolded and punished his daughter during toilet training. How would Freud describe this client's psychosexual development?
   1. The client is fixated in the *oral* stage of development.
   2. The client is fixated in the *anal* stage of development.
   3. The client is fixated in the *phallic* stage of development.
   4. The client is fixated in the *latency* stage of development.

3. According to Erikson's developmental theory, when planning care for a 70-year-old client, which developmental task should a nurse identify as appropriate for this client?
   1. To develop a basic trust in others.
   2. To achieve a sense of self-confidence and recognition from others.
   3. To reflect back on life events to derive pleasure and meaning.
   4. To achieve established life goals and consider the welfare of future generations.

4. Which of the following are examples of an intrapersonal intervention for a client on an inpatient psychiatric unit? **Select all that apply.**
   1. Assist the client in noting which common defense mechanisms he or she frequently uses.
   2. Discuss "acting-out" behaviors and assist the client in understanding why they occur.
   3. Ask the client to use a journal to record thoughts he or she is having before acting-out behaviors occur.
   4. Ask the client to acknowledge one positive person in his or her life to assist the client after discharge.
   5. Encourage the client to openly discuss his or her feelings about an impending divorce.

5. Which of the following is an example of appropriate psychosexual development? **Select all that apply.**
   1. A 24-month-old relieves anxiety through the use of a pacifier.
   2. A 4-year-old boy focuses on relationships with other boys.
   3. A 5-year-old girl identifies with her mother.
   4. A 12-month-old begins learning about independence and control.
   5. A 10-year-old boy excludes all girls from his newly formed neighborhood club.

6. An angry 70-year-old man states, "My life was a joke. Nothing turned out the way I wanted." In evaluating this man's developmental stage according to Erikson, which would be a correct nursing assessment?
   1. Initiative versus guilt with a negative outcome of guilt.
   2. Generativity versus stagnation with a negative outcome of stagnation.
   3. Identity versus role confusion with a negative outcome of role confusion.
   4. Ego integrity versus despair with a negative outcome of despair.

7. Freud described the _____ as the psychic energy used to fulfill basic needs such as hunger, thirst, and sexuality.

8. According to Mahler, the separation-individuation phase occurs when a child 5 to 36 months of age progresses from a symbiotic extension of the mothering figure to a distinct and separate being. Correctly order the subphases of this phase.
   _____ 1. Rapprochement
   _____ 2. Differentiation
   _____ 3. Consolidation
   _____ 4. Practicing

9. Which of the following is an example of a behavioral intervention for a client on an inpatient psychiatric unit? **Select all that apply.**
   1. "Every time you consider purging, snap the rubber band on your wrist."
   2. "When you start to put yourself down, consider all of your strengths."
   3. "Write down your feelings to develop insight."
   4. "The next time you crave a beer, try talking with your sponsor."
   5. "You will receive a gold star each time you obey the unit rules."

10. A nursing instructor is teaching about cognitive theory. Which statement by the student indicates that learning has occurred?
    1. "Interventions related to this theory use a system of reinforcements to achieve adaptive behavior."
    2. "Cognitive theory is based on adaptive interactions and mutual relationships."
    3. "Cognitive theory involves knowledge and thought processes within the individual's intellectual ability."
    4. "This theory states genetic predispositions may affect future mental health."

11. Which of the following are major concepts in Sullivan's interpersonal theory of personality development? **Select all that apply.**
    1. Anxiety
    2. Self-system
    3. Self-confidence
    4. Satisfaction of needs
    5. Interpersonal security

12. A 5-year-old child decides not to draw on the bedroom wall for fear of an extended "time-out." According to Lawrence Kohlberg's theory of moral development, which stage of developmental orientation would the nurse assign this child?
    1. Punishment and obedience orientation
    2. Interpersonal concordance orientation
    3. Law and order orientation
    4. Social contract legalistic orientation

13. A 17-year-old explains that the saying "Don't cry over spilt milk" refers to accepting situations that cannot be reversed. According to Jean Piaget's theory of cognitive development, which stage would the nurse assign this adolescent?
    1. Preoperational
    2. Formal operations
    3. Sensorimotor
    4. Concrete operations

14. A client is diagnosed with borderline personality disorder. According to Margaret Mahler's developmental theory of object relations, fixation in which subphase of the separation-individuation phase would contribute to this diagnosis?
    1. Differentiation
    2. Rapprochement
    3. Consolidation
    4. Practicing

15. Order the stages of moral development, according to Lawrence Kohlberg.
    _____ 1. Social contract legalistic orientation
    _____ 2. Punishment and obedience orientation
    _____ 3. Law and order orientation
    _____ 4. Universal ethical principle orientation
    _____ 5. Interpersonal concordance orientation
    _____ 6. Instrumental relativist orientation

16. After a thorough assessment, a nurse has determined that a client has failed to complete the developmental tasks of Peplau's second stage. Which of the following behaviors may have led to this evaluation? **Select all that apply.**
    1. Suspiciousness and envy of others.
    2. Inability to relate to others.
    3. Inordinate disorganization and tardiness.
    4. Hoarding and miserliness.
    5. Flamboyance and eccentricity.

17. A nurse uses active listening to facilitate a client's problem solving related to financial issues. According to Peplau's framework for psychodynamic nursing, what therapeutic role is this nurse assuming?
    1. The role of a counselor.
    2. The role of a resource person.
    3. The role of a teacher.
    4. The role of a leader.

18. After studying the concepts of nursing theory, the nursing student understands that Watson is to the seven assumptions about the science of caring as Peplau is to:
    1. The phases of the nurse-client relationship.
    2. Cultural care diversity and universality.
    3. Modeling and role modeling.
    4. Human energy fields.

19. Which nursing theorist classifies nursing interventions as "primary prevention," "secondary prevention," and "tertiary prevention?"
    1. Jean Watson
    2. Callista Roy
    3. Betty Neuman
    4. Dorothea Orem

20. Which principles are associated with Madeleine Leininger's nursing theory?
    1. Nurses intervene by assisting the client to examine and understand the meaning of life experiences.
    2. Nursing interventions seek to alter or manage stimuli so that adaptive responses can occur.
    3. Nursing interventions meet self-care demands and solve self-care deficits.
    4. The nurse must understand the client's culture to provide care.

21. Nursing theorist _____ developed a general self-care deficit theory of nursing.

22. What is the nurse's role in the "developing skills in participation" stage of Peplau's psychological tasks of personality development?
    1. To recognize unfulfilled needs and provide experiences that promote growth.
    2. To convey unconditional acceptance and encourage full expression of feelings.
    3. To function as a surrogate mother.
    4. To help clients improve problem-solving skills.

23. Nursing theorist _____ developed an adaptation model that describes nursing actions that seek to alter or manage stimuli so that adaptive responses can occur.

REVIEW ANSWERS

1. ANSWER: 4

Rationale:

1. Mistrust is the negative outcome of Erikson's "infancy" stage of development, trust versus mistrust. This stage ranges from birth to 18 months of age. The major developmental task for infancy is to develop a basic trust in the parenting figure and to be able to generalize it to others. The child described does not fall within the age range of the infancy stage.

2. Guilt is the negative outcome of Erikson's "late-childhood" stage of development, initiative versus guilt. This stage ranges from 3 to 6 years of age. The major developmental task for late childhood is to develop a sense of purpose and the ability to initiate and direct one's own activities. The child described does not fall within the age range of the late childhood stage.

3. Inferiority is the negative outcome of Erikson's "school-age" stage of development, industry versus inferiority. This stage ranges from 6 to 12 years of age. The major developmental task for school age is to achieve a sense of self-confidence by learning, competing, performing successfully, and receiving recognition from significant others, peers, and acquaintances. The child described does not fall within the age range of the school age stage.

4. Shame and doubt is the negative outcome of Erikson's "early-childhood" stage of development, autonomy versus shame and doubt. This stage ranges from 18 months through 3 years of age. The major developmental task for early childhood is to gain some self-control and independence within the environment. The 2-year-old child described falls within the age range of early childhood and is exhibiting behaviors reflective of a negative outcome of shame and doubt.

TEST-TAKING TIP: When assessing for signs of shame and doubt, look for lack of self-confidence, lack of pride, a sense of being controlled by others, and potential rage against self. The age of the client presented in the question is a clue to the developmental task conflict experienced. Review Table 2.3 if necessary.

Content Area: Psychosocial Integrity;
Integrated Process: Nursing Process: Assessment;
Client Need: Psychosocial Integrity;
Cognitive Level: Application;
Concept: Evidenced-based Practice

2. ANSWER: 2

Rationale:

1. Freud described the oral stage of development as a time during infancy when a sense of security and trust develop in the environment and self. The situation presented in the question does not describe inconsistent parenting during infancy that would fixate the client in the oral stage of development.

2. Freud believed that the manner in which children were toilet trained had far-reaching effects on the child's personality development. He described this as the anal phase of personality development. Freud would postulate that this woman's suicidal ideations indicate a negative evaluation of self due to fixation in the anal phase of personality development due to punitive toilet training.

3. Freud believed that during the phallic stage, children developed sexual identity and identified with the same-sex parent. The situation presented in the question does not describe a problem with sexual identity that would indicate fixation in the phallic stage of personality development.

4. Freud believed that the latency period was the time of development of relationships with same-sex peers. The situation presented in the question does not describe a relationship concern between the client and same-sex peers that would indicate fixation in the latency stage of personality development.

TEST-TAKING TIP: Freud's theory of the formation of the personality includes five stages of psychosexual development. Fixation in the anal stage almost certainly results in psychopathology. Review Table 2.1 if necessary.

Content Area: Psychosocial Integrity;
Integrated Process: Nursing Process: Assessment;
Client Need: Psychosocial Integrity;
Cognitive Level: Application;
Concept: Evidenced-based Practice

3. ANSWER: 3

Rationale:

1. Erikson's "infancy" stage of development is *trust versus mistrust*. This stage ranges from birth to 18 months of age. The major developmental task for this stage is to develop a basic trust in the parenting figure and to be able to generalize it to others. The age of the client presented in the question rules out the *trust versus mistrust stage*.

2. Erikson's "school age" stage of development is *industry versus inferiority*. This stage ranges from 6 to 12 years of age. The major developmental task for this stage is to achieve a sense of self-confidence. The age of the client presented in the question rules out the *industry versus inferiority* stage.

3. Erikson's "old age" stage of development is *ego integrity versus despair*. This stage ranges from 65 years to death. The major developmental task for this stage is to review one's life and to derive meaning from both positive and negative events while achieving a positive sense of self-worth. The age of the client presented in the question meets the criteria for the *ego integrity versus despair* stage.

4. Erikson's "adulthood" stage of development is *generativity versus stagnation*. This stage ranges from 30 to 65 years of age. The major developmental task for this stage is to achieve the life goals established for one's self, while also considering the welfare of future generations. The age of the client presented in the question rules out the *generativity versus stagnation* stage.

TEST-TAKING TIP: To correctly answer this question, the test taker must be familiar with Erikson's eight stages of the life cycle during which individuals struggle with developmental "crises." A review of Table 2.3 will assist with acquiring this information.

Content Area: Psychosocial Integrity;
Integrated Process: Nursing Process: Evaluation;
Client Need: Psychosocial Integrity;
Cognitive Level: Analysis;
Concept: Evidenced-based Practice

4. **ANSWER: 1, 5**
Rationale:
1. Intrapersonal theory deals with conflicts within the individual and internal emotional responses. Assisting clients to note defense mechanisms most frequently used is an example of interventions that reflect the use of intrapersonal theory.
2. Discussing acting-out behaviors and why they occur is an intervention reflective of behavioral, not intrapersonal, theory. A major concept of this theory is that all behavior has meaning.
3. Journaling to become aware of how thoughts affect acing-out behaviors is an intervention reflective of cognitive, not intrapersonal theory. Cognitive theory is based on the principle that thoughts affect feelings and behaviors.
4. Interpersonal theory states that individual behavior and personality development are the direct result of interpersonal relationships. The identification of a positive relationship would be an intervention that reflects interpersonal, not intrapersonal, theory.
5. Intrapersonal theory deals with conflicts within the individual and internal emotional responses. Encouraging the client to openly discuss his or her feelings about an impending divorce is an example of an intervention that reflects the use of intrapersonal theory.
TEST-TAKING TIP: Remember intrapersonal theory by thinking "intra" and "personal," meaning "within oneself." "Interpersonal" is between people.
Content Area: Safe and Effective Care Environment: Management of Care;
Integrated Process: Nursing Process: Implementation;
Client Need: Safe and Effective Care Environment: Management of Care;
Cognitive Level: Application;
Concept: Nursing

5. **ANSWER: 3, 5**
Rationale:
1. From birth to 18 months of age, a child is in the oral stage of Freud's psychosexual development. During this stage, an infant would attempt to decrease anxiety by finding relief using oral gratification. A 24-month-old is outside the age range for the oral stage of development.
2. Focusing on relationships with same-sex peers happens during the latency stage, which occurs from 6 to 12 years of age. A 4-year-old is outside the age range for the latency stage of development.
3. From the age of 3 to 6 years, a child is in the phallic stage of Freud's psychosexual development. During this stage, a child is looking to identify with the parent of the same sex and developing his or her own sexual identity by focusing on genital organs. This is an example of appropriate psychosexual development.
4. Learning about independence and control happens in Freud's anal phase of psychosexual development, which occurs from 18 months to 3 years of age. A 12-month-old is outside the age range for the anal stage of development.
5. From the age of 6 to 12 years, a child is in the latency stage of Freud's psychosexual development. During this stage, a child is sexually repressed and focuses on

relationships with same-gender peers. This is an example of appropriate psychosexual development.
TEST-TAKING TIP: Freud placed much emphasis on the first 5 years of life and believed that characteristics developed during these early years bore heavily on one's adaptation patterns and personality traits in adulthood. Review Table 2.1 as needed.
Content Area: Psychosocial Integrity;
Integrated Process: Nursing Process: Assessment;
Client Need: Psychosocial Integrity;
Cognitive Level: Application;
Concept: Evidenced-based Practice

6. **ANSWER: 4**
Rationale:
1. In Erikson's theory of psychosocial development, *initiative versus guilt* occurs between the ages of 3 and 6 years. The scenario in the question is not reflective of this stage.
2. In Erikson's theory of psychosocial development, *generativity versus stagnation* occurs between the ages of 30 and 65 years. The scenario in the question is not reflective of this stage.
3. In Erikson's theory of psychosocial development, *identity versus role confusion* occurs between the ages of 12 and 20 years. The scenario in the question is not reflective of this stage.
4. According to Erikson, the *ego integrity versus despair* stage occurs in old age (65 years to death). The major developmental task of this stage is to review one's life and derive meaning from both positive and negative events, while achieving a positive sense of self-worth. A nurse would assess this angry 70-year-old man as realizing the negative outcome of despair.
TEST-TAKING TIP: Erikson described the eight stages of the life cycle, during which individuals struggle with developmental challenges. Being able to recognize the developmental conflicts of each stage will allow you to recognize despair as a negative outcome. Remember that Erikson based his psychosocial theory on chronological age, which is significant information needed to answer this question correctly. Review Table 2.3 as necessary.
Content Area: Psychosocial Integrity;
Integrated Process: Nursing Process: Evaluation;
Client Need: Psychosocial Integrity;
Cognitive Level: Analysis;
Concept: Evidenced-based Practice

7. **ANSWER: libido**
Rationale: *Libido*, a component of the id, is the psychic energy used to fulfill basic physiological needs or instinctual drives such as hunger, thirst, and sexuality
TEST-TAKING TIP: Recall the structure of the personality according to Freud and recognize libido as a component of the id. Review Box 2.1 as needed.
Content Area: Psychosocial Integrity;
Integrated Process: Nursing Process: Assessment;
Client Need: Psychosocial Integrity;
Cognitive Level: Knowledge;
Concept: Evidenced-based Practice

8. **ANSWER: The correct order is: 3, 1, 4, 2**
   Rationale: Mahler described *separation-individuation*, through which a child 5 to 36 months in age evolves, as a progression from a symbiotic extension of the mothering figure to a distinct and separate being in the following four subphases.
   1. Differentiation (5–10 months)
   2. Practicing (10–16 months)
   3. Rapprochement (16–24 months)
   4. Consolidation (24–36 months)
   TEST-TAKING TIP: Recall the stages of development in Mahler's theory of object relations. Review Table 2.4 as needed.
   Content Area: Psychosocial Integrity;
   Integrated Process: Nursing Process: Assessment;
   Client Need: Psychosocial Integrity;
   Cognitive Level: Analysis;
   Concept: Evidenced-based Practice

9. **ANSWER: 1, 5**
   Rationale:
   1. Behavioral interventions modify maladaptive behavior patterns by reinforcing more adaptive behaviors. Encouraging a client to snap a rubber band instead of purging is an example of a behavioral intervention.
   2. Encouraging a client to think about strengths is a cognitive, not behavioral, intervention. Cognitive theory is based on the principle that thoughts affect feelings and behaviors.
   3. Intrapersonal theory deals with conflicts within the individual. Encouraging a client to write down feelings to develop insight is an example of an intrapersonal, not behavioral, intervention.
   4. Interpersonal theory states that individual behavior and personality development are the direct result of interpersonal relationships. Advising a client to talk with his or her sponsor about alcohol cravings is an interpersonal, not behavioral, intervention.
   5. Behavioral interventions modify maladaptive behavior patterns by reinforcing more adaptive behaviors. Receiving a gold star each time the unit rules are obeyed is an example of a behavioral intervention called token economy.
   TEST-TAKING TIP: Note the key phrase *behavioral intervention* in the question stem. Recall the basic concepts of behavioral theory and compare it to the other theories of personality development in this chapter.
   Content Area: Safe and Effective Care Environment: Management of Care;
   Integrated Process: Nursing Process: Implementation;
   Client Need: Safe and Effective Care Environment: Management of Care;
   Cognitive Level: Application;
   Concept: Evidenced-based Practice

10. **ANSWER: 3**
    Rationale:
    1. Using a system of reinforcements to achieve adaptive behavior is an intervention based on behavioral, not cognitive, theory. Behavioral interventions modify maladaptive behavior patterns by reinforcing more adaptive behaviors. This student statement indicates that further instruction is needed.
    2. Interpersonal, not cognitive, theory is based on adaptive interactions and mutual relationships. This student statement indicates that further instruction is needed.
    3. Cognitive theory involves knowledge and thought processes within the individual's intellectual ability. Cognitive theory is based on the principle that thoughts affect feelings and behaviors. This student statement indicates that learning has occurred.
    4. Intrapersonal, not cognitive, theory deals with conflicts within the individual and any genetic predispositions that may affect mental health. This student statement indicates that further instruction is needed.
    TEST-TAKING TIP: Note the key word *cognitive* in the question stem. Recall the basic concepts of cognitive theory and how it compares and contrasts with the other theories covered in this chapter.
    Content Area: Safe and Effective Care Environment: Management of Care;
    Integrated Process: Nursing Process: Evaluation;
    Client Need: Safe and Effective Care Environment: Management of Care;
    Cognitive Level: Application;
    Concept: Nursing Roles

11. **ANSWER: 1, 2, 4, 5**
    Rationale:
    1. Anxiety, a major concept in Sullivan's interpersonal theory, is the chief disruptive force in interpersonal relations and the main factor in the development of serious difficulties in living.
    2. Self-system, a major concept in Sullivan's interpersonal theory, is a measure adopted by the individual to protect against anxiety.
    3. Self-confidence is the achievement of the developmental task in the trust versus mistrust stage of Erikson's psychosocial theory of personality development, not a major concept in Sullivan's interpersonal theory.
    4. Satisfaction of needs, a major concept in Sullivan's interpersonal theory, is described as anything that, when absent, produces discomfort.
    5. Interpersonal security, a major concept in Sullivan's interpersonal theory, is a sense of total well-being when all needs have been met.
    TEST-TAKING TIP: Recall the major concepts of Sullivan's interpersonal theory of personality development. Review Table 2.2 as needed.
    Content Area: Psychosocial Integrity;
    Integrated Process: Nursing Process: Evaluation;
    Client Need: Psychosocial Integrity;
    Cognitive Level: Analysis;
    Concept: Evidenced-based Practice

12. **ANSWER: 1**
    Rationale: Lawrence Kohlberg believed that each stage of moral development is necessary and basic to the next stage and that all individuals must progress through each stage sequentially. He defined three major levels of moral

development, each of which is further subdivided into two orientation stages, each totaling six.

1. In the *punishment and obedience orientation* stage, fear of punishment is likely to be the incentive for conformity. The child in the question fears a "time-out" and therefore experiences incentive for conformity.

2. In the *interpersonal concordance orientation* stage, behavior is guided by expectations of others and need for approval. The situation presented in the question is not reflective of this stage.

3. In the *law and order orientation* stage, behavior is motivated by respect for laws and authority. The situation presented in the question is not reflective of this stage.

4. In the *social contract legalistic orientation* stage, behavior is based on a system of internal values and principles. The situation presented in the question is not reflective of this stage.

TEST-TAKING TIP: Identify Kohlberg's stages of moral development and match the situation presented in the question with the appropriate stage. Review Table 2.6 as needed.

Content Area: *Psychosocial Integrity;*
Integrated Process: *Nursing Process: Assessment;*
Client Need: *Psychosocial Integrity;*
Cognitive Level: *Application;*
Concept: *Evidenced-based Practice*

13. ANSWER: 2
Rationale: Jean Piaget believed that human intelligence progresses through a series of stages that are related to age, demonstrating at each successive stage a higher level of logical organization than at the previous stages.

1. In the *preoperational* stage (2–7 years), development proceeds from sensorimotor representation to prelogical thought and solutions to problems. The situation presented in the question is not reflective of this stage.

2. In the *formal operational* stage (11 years–adulthood), development proceeds from logical solutions to concrete problems to logical solutions to all classes of problems. In this stage, the individual is able to think and reason in abstract terms. The 17-year-old in the question is demonstrating abstract thinking by the interpretation of the saying "Don't cry over spilt milk."

3. In the *sensorimotor* stage (0–2 years), development proceeds from reflex activity to representation and sensorimotor solutions to problems. The situation presented in the question is not reflective of this stage.

4. In the *concrete operational* stage (7–11 years), development proceeds from prelogical thought to logical solutions to concrete problems. The situation presented in the question is not reflective of this stage.

TEST-TAKING TIP: Identify Piaget's stages of cognitive development and recognize the age ranges designated for each stage. Review Table 2.5 as needed.

Content Area: *Psychosocial Integrity;*
Integrated Process: *Nursing Process: Assessment;*
Client Need: *Psychosocial Integrity;*
Cognitive Level: *Application;*
Concept: *Evidenced-based Practice*

14. ANSWER: 2
Rationale: Mahler described the *separation-individuation* phase through which a child, 5 to 36 months, evolves in his or her progression from a symbiotic extension of the mothering figure to a distinct and separate being in four subphases.

1. In the *differentiation* subphase (5–10 months), an infant moves away from the mother figure and recognizes separateness. An unresolved task in this subphase is not necessarily tied to a future diagnosis of borderline personality disorder.

2. In the *rapprochement* subphase (16–24 months), if the mother figure withholds nurturing and fosters dependency, feelings of rage and fear of abandonment develop. A child with unresolved fear of abandonment is thought to be fixed in the rapprochement phase, often leading to a diagnosis of borderline personality disorder in later life.

3. In the *consolidation* subphase (24–36 months), a child relates to objects in an effective, constant manner. The child establishes a sense of separateness and can internalize a sustained image of a loved person when out of sight. An unresolved task in this subphase is not necessarily tied to a future diagnosis of borderline personality disorder.

4. In the *practicing* subphase (10–16 months), a child experiences exhilaration and omnipotence from increased independence. An unresolved task in this subphase is not necessarily tied to a future diagnosis of borderline personality disorder.

TEST-TAKING TIP: Identify the stages of development in Mahler's theory of object relations. Recognize the connection between unresolved tasks within the rapprochement phase and the diagnosis of borderline personality disorder. Review Table 2.4 as needed.

Content Area: *Psychosocial Integrity;*
Integrated Process: *Nursing Process: Assessment;*
Client Need: *Psychosocial Integrity;*
Cognitive Level: *Analysis;*
Concept: *Evidenced-based Practice*

15. ANSWER: The correct order is: 5, 1, 4, 6, 3, 2
Rationale: Lawrence Kohlberg believed that each stage of moral development is necessary and basic to the next stage and that all individuals must progress through each stage sequentially. He defined three major levels of moral development, each of which is further subdivided into two orientation stages, each totaling six.

1. Punishment and obedience orientation (Level I ages 4–10)
2. Instrumental relativist orientation (Level I ages 4–10)
3. Interpersonal concordance orientation (Level II ages 10–13 and into adulthood)
4. Law and order orientation (Level II ages 10–13 and into adulthood)
5. Social contract legalistic orientation (Level III from adolescence onward)
6. Universal ethical principle orientation (Level III from adolescence onward)

TEST-TAKING TIP: Identify Kohlberg's stages of moral development and how he perceived and described moral progression. Review Table 2.6 as needed.

Content Area: Psychosocial Integrity;
Integrated Process: Nursing Process: Assessment;
Client Need: Psychosocial Integrity;
Cognitive Level: Analysis;
Concept: Evidenced-based Practice

16. **ANSWER: 1, 2, 4**
Rationale:
1. Suspiciousness and envy of others is a potential behavior of individuals who have failed to complete the developmental tasks of Peplau's second stage, *Learning to delay satisfaction*.
2. Inability to relate to others is a potential behavior of individuals who have failed to complete the developmental tasks of Peplau's second stage, *Learning to delay satisfaction*.
3. Inordinate disorganization and tardiness is not a potential behavior of individuals who have failed to complete the developmental tasks of Peplau's second stage, *Learning to delay satisfaction*. A nurse would expect these individual to be inordinately neat and punctual.
4. Hoarding and miserliness are potential behaviors of individuals who have failed to complete the developmental tasks of Peplau's second stage, *Learning to delay satisfaction*.
5. Being flamboyant and eccentric is not characteristic of individuals who have failed to complete the developmental tasks of Peplau's second stage, *Learning to delay satisfaction*.
TEST-TAKING TIP: Recall the *Learning to delay satisfaction* stage of Peplau's interpersonal theory of personality development and recognize the consequences of failure to satisfactorily complete this stage. Review Table 2.7 as needed.
Content Area: Psychosocial Integrity;
Integrated Process: Nursing Process: Evaluation;
Client Need: Psychosocial Integrity;
Cognitive Level: Analysis;
Concept: Evidenced-based Practice

17. **ANSWER: 1**
Rationale:
1. The nurse in the question is assuming the role of a counselor. A counselor is one who listens as the client reviews feelings related to difficulties he or she is experiencing in any aspect of life.
2. A resource person is one who provides specific, needed information that helps the client understand his or her problem and the new situation. The nurse in the question is not acting in the role of a resource person.
3. A teacher is one who identifies learning needs and provides information to the client or family that may aid in improvement of the life situation. The nurse in the question is not acting in the role of a teacher.
4. A leader is one who directs the nurse-client interaction and insures that appropriate actions are undertaken to facilitate achievement of the designated goals. The nurse in the question is not acting in the role of a leader.
TEST-TAKING TIP: Recall the nursing roles that Peplau identified in her framework for psychodynamic nursing.

Content Area: Safe and Effective Care Environment: Management of Care;
Integrated Process: Nursing Process: Implementation;
Client Need: Safe and Effective Care Environment: Management of Care;
Cognitive Level: Application;
Concept: Nursing Roles

18. **ANSWER: 1**
Rationale: Watson believed that curing disease is the domain of medicine, whereas caring is the domain of nursing. She developed seven assumptions about the science of caring that allow the nurse to deliver integrated holistic care.
1. Peplau developed the phases of the nurse-client relationship. This nursing theory promotes the nurse-client relationship by applying interpersonal theory to nursing practice. Key concepts include the nurse as a resource person, a counselor, a teacher, a leader, a technical expert, and a surrogate.
2. Leininger, not Peplau, based her theory of cultural care diversity and universality on the belief that across cultures there are health-care practices and beliefs that are diverse and similar. The nurse must understand the client's culture to provide care.
3. Erickson, Tomlin, and Swain, not Peplau, developed theories that included modeling and role modeling by the use of interpersonal and interactive skills.
4. A variety of nursing theorists based their theories on the concept of a human energy field. These theories share a common view of the individual as an irreducible whole, comprising a physical body surrounded by an aura.
TEST-TAKING TIP: Recall the basic concepts of the theoretical models presented. Assumptions of caring underlie Watson's theoretical model, whereas the concept of the nurse-client relationship is the basis of Peplau's nursing theory model. Review Table 2.7 as needed.
Content Area: Psychosocial Integrity;
Integrated Process: Nursing Process: Evaluation;
Client Need: Psychosocial Integrity;
Cognitive Level: Analysis;
Concept: Evidenced-based Practice

19. **ANSWER: 3**
Rationale:
1. Jean Watson developed her theory based on the belief that curing disease is the domain of medicine, whereas caring is the domain of nursing. Her theory did not include classifying nursing interventions as primary, secondary, or tertiary prevention.
2. Callista Roy developed the "Roy adaptation model," which describes nursing actions as interventions that seek to alter or manage stimuli so that adaptive responses can occur. Her theory did not include classifying nursing interventions as primary, secondary, or tertiary prevention.
3. Betty Neuman's systems model focuses on concepts related to stress and reaction to stress. Nursing interventions are classified as primary prevention (occurs before stressors invade the normal line of defense and problems occur), secondary prevention (occurs after the system has reacted to the invasion of a stressor and problems

are present), and tertiary prevention (occurs after secondary prevention and focuses on rehabilitation).

4. Dorothea Orem developed a general self-care deficit theory of nursing. Nursing interventions described in this theory consist of activities needed to meet self-care demands and solve self-care deficits. Her theory did not include classifying nursing interventions as primary, secondary, or tertiary prevention.

TEST-TAKING TIP: Recall Neuman's systems model and how nursing interventions are described within this theory.
Content Area: Safe and Effective Care Environment: Management of Care;
Integrated Process: Nursing Process: Implementation;
Client Need: Safe and Effective Care Environment: Management of Care;
Cognitive Level: Application;
Concept: Evidenced-based Practice

20. **ANSWER: 4**
Rationale:
1. Rizzo Parse, not Leininger, developed her theory of "human becoming" from existential theory. Parse believes that people create reality for themselves through the choices they make at many levels, and nurses intervene by assisting the client to examine and understand the meaning of life experiences.
2. Callista Roy, not Leininger, developed the "Roy adaptation model," which consists of four essential elements: humans as adaptive systems, environment, health, and the goal of nursing. Roy describes nursing actions as interventions that seek to alter or manage stimuli so that adaptive responses can occur.
3. Dorothea Orem, not Leininger, developed a general self-care deficit theory of nursing composed of three interrelated concepts: self-care, self-care deficit, and nursing systems. Nursing interventions described in this theory consist of activities needed to meet self-care demands and solve self-care deficits.
4. Madeleine Leininger developed the theory of cultural care diversity and universality based on the belief that across cultures there are health-care practices and beliefs that are diverse and similar. The nurse must understand the client's culture to provide care.
TEST-TAKING TIP: Recall Madeleine Leininger's nursing theory of cultural care diversity and universality.
Content Area: Safe and Effective Care Environment: Management of Care;
Integrated Process: Nursing Process: Implementation;
Client Need: Safe and Effective Care Environment: Management of Care;
Cognitive Level: Application;
Concept: Evidenced-based Practice

21. **ANSWER: Orem**
Rationale: Dorothea Orem developed a general self-care deficit theory of nursing composed of three interrelated concepts: self-care, self-care deficit, and nursing systems. Nursing interventions described in this theory consist of activities needed to meet self-care demands and solve self-care deficits.

TEST-TAKING TIP: Recall the principles of Dorothea Orem's nursing theory.
Content Area: Safe and Effective Care Environment: Management of Care;
Integrated Process: Nursing Process: Implementation;
Client Need: Safe and Effective Care Environment: Management of Care;
Cognitive Level: Knowledge;
Concept: Evidenced-based Practice

22. **ANSWER: 4**
Rationale:
1. To recognize unfulfilled needs and provide experiences that promote growth is the nurse's role in the *Identifying Oneself* stage, not the *Developing Skills in Participation* stage, of Peplau's psychological tasks of personality development.
2. To convey unconditional acceptance and to encourage full expression of feelings is the nurse's role in the *learning to delay satisfaction* stage, not the *developing skills in participation* stage, of Peplau's psychological tasks of personality development.
3. To function as a surrogate mother is the nurse's role in the *learning to count on others* stage, not the *developing skills in participation* stage, of Peplau's psychological tasks of personality development.
4. Developing skills in participation is the stage of Peplau's psychological tasks of personality development that occurs in late childhood. The child develops the capacity to compromise, compete, and cooperate with others. If these skills are not developed appropriately, progression results in difficulty dealing with the reoccurring problems of life. The nurse's role is to help clients improve problem-solving skills.
TEST-TAKING TIP: Recall the major concepts and nursing roles found in Peplau's nursing theory of personality development.
Content Area: Psychosocial Integrity;
Integrated Process: Nursing Process: Assessment;
Client Need: Psychosocial Integrity;
Cognitive Level: Application;
Concept: Nursing Roles

23. **ANSWER: Roy**
Rationale: The "Roy adaptation model" consists of four essential elements: humans as adaptive systems, environment, health, and the goal of nursing. Roy describes nursing actions as interventions that seek to alter or manage stimuli so that adaptive responses can occur.
TEST-TAKING TIP: Recall the principles of Callista Roy's nursing theory.
Content Area: Safe and Effective Care Environment: Management of Care;
Integrated Process: Nursing Process: Implementation;
Client Need: Safe and Effective Care Environment: Management of Care;
Cognitive Level: Knowledge;
Concept: Evidenced-based Practice

Chapter 3

Role of the Nurse in the Delivery of Psychiatric Nursing Care

KEY TERMS

Case management—An individualized approach to coordinating client care services, especially when clients with complex needs and chronic problems require multifaceted or interdisciplinary care

Community—A group, population, or cluster of people with at least one common characteristic, such as geographic location, occupation, ethnicity, or health concern

Counter-transference—The overidentification with a client's feelings by a health-care worker because these feelings remind the health-care worker of past or present problems

Deinstitutionalization—The process of replacing long-stay psychiatric hospitals with less isolated community mental health services for those diagnosed with a mental disorder or developmental disability

Group therapy—A form of psychosocial treatment in which a number of clients meet together with a therapist for purposes of sharing, gaining personal insight, and improving interpersonal coping strategies

Institutionalization—Residence in or confinement to a hospital, asylum, or other long-term care setting for an extended period of time

Interdisciplinary treatment team—A group of health-care professionals from diverse fields who work in a coordinated fashion toward a common goal for the client

Medication nonadherence—Doses of prescribed medication not taken or taken incorrectly that jeopardize the client's therapeutic outcome

Primary prevention—Services aimed at reducing the incidence of mental disorders within the population

Recovery—To regain health after illness; to regain a former state of health

Secondary prevention—Interventions aimed at minimizing early symptoms of psychiatric illness and directed toward reducing the prevalence and duration of the illness

Tertiary prevention—Services aimed at reducing the residual defects that are associated with severe and persistent mental illness

Therapeutic milieu—A structured group setting in which the existence of the group is a key force in the outcome of treatment; using the combined elements of positive peer pressure, trust, safety, and repetition, the therapeutic milieu provides an ideal setting for group members to work through their psychological issues

Transference—The unconscious displacement (or transfer) by the client to the nurse of feelings formed toward a person from the client's past

The role of the psychiatric nurse is characterized by interventions that promote and foster health, assess dysfunction, assist clients to regain or improve their coping abilities, and prevent further disability. These interventions include health promotion; preventive management of the therapeutic environment; assisting clients with self-care activities; administering and monitoring psychobiological treatment regimens; health teaching, including psychoeducation; crisis intervention and counseling; and case management.

I. A Brief History of Psychiatric Care

A. **Institutionalization**: In the 19th century, institutionalization of the mentally ill was established to protect society and the affected individuals
   1. Mental illness was stigmatized because of fear and superstitions.
   2. Mental illness was believed to be caused by dysfunctional parenting.
   3. Typical treatments included cold dressings, enemas, electroconvulsive therapy (ECT), purging, lobotomies.
   4. Nursing focused on maintaining order and preventing elopement.
   5. The mentally ill experienced long hospitalizations, resulting in loss of social skills and increased dependency.
   6. Dorothea Dix advocated for humane treatment of persons with mental illness.
   7. After World War II, mental disorders were recognized as illnesses, thereby increasing the need for trained nurses.

DID YOU KNOW?
One in four adults—approximately 61.5 million Americans—experiences mental illness in a given year. One in 17—about 13.6 million—lives with a serious mental illness. Serious mental illness costs Americans $193.2 billion in lost earnings each year.

B. **Deinstitutionalization**
   1. Resulted from inadequate funding, overcrowding, and understaffing in asylums and state hospitals.
   2. Community Mental Health Centers Act of 1963 was to provide funding for community-based mental health centers.
   3. State and federal funding was inadequate to cover costs.
   4. Lack of community resources led to decreased quality of care and homelessness.
      a. Families with children are among the fastest growing segments of the homeless population in the United States.
      b. Research done in 2012 reveals that approximately 30% of the homeless population suffers from some form of mental illness.

5. Treatments included psychotropic medications and interpersonal therapy.
6. Nursing focused on **case management** and **community**-based care with the advent of credentialing and advanced practice nurses.
7. National Alliance on Mental Illness (NAMI) was established to advocate for mentally ill clients and their families.

DID YOU KNOW?
NAMI is the nation's largest grassroots mental health organization dedicated to building better lives for the millions of Americans affected by mental illness. NAMI advocates for access to services and treatment, supports research, and is steadfast in its commitment to raise awareness and build a community of hope for all those in need. NAMI is the foundation for hundreds of NAMI state organizations, NAMI affiliates, and volunteer leaders working in local communities across the country to raise awareness and provide essential and free education, advocacy, and support group programs.

II. Delivery of Care

A. Inpatient hospitalization
   1. Psychiatric services in general hospitals are severely restricted.
   2. Only acute symptoms lead to hospitalization (e.g., acute psychosis, suicidal ideations or attempts, manic exacerbations).
   3. **Interdisciplinary treatment team** (see Table 3.1).
      a. Provides multifaceted assessment to establish the priority of care.
      b. Develops comprehensive treatment plan and goals of therapy.
      c. Assigns intervention responsibilities.
      d. Meets regularly to update plan as needed.
B. Outpatient care/public health model: The trend in psychiatric care is shifting from inpatient hospitalization to outpatient care within the community
   1. Care for client in community is cost-effective.
   2. Case management:
      a. Client is assigned a case manager who negotiates with multiple providers.
      b. Decreases fragmentation of care.
      c. Decreases cost of services.
   3. Levels of prevention in the public health model:
      a. **Primary prevention**: assists individuals to cope effectively with stress, targets and diminishes harmful stressors within the environment to reduce the incidence of mental disorders. Nursing focus is client education.
      b. **Secondary prevention**: early identification of client problems and prompt initiation of

Table 3.1 **The Interdisciplinary Treatment Team in Psychiatry**

Team Member	Responsibilities	Credentials
Psychiatrist	Serves as the leader of the team. Responsible for diagnosis and treatment of mental disorders. Performs psychotherapy; prescribes medication and other somatic therapies.	Medical degree with residency in psychiatry and license to practice medicine.
Clinical psychologist	Conducts individual, group, and family therapy. Administers, interprets, and evaluates psychological tests that assist in the diagnostic process.	Doctorate in clinical psychology with 2- to 3-year internship supervised by a licensed clinical psychologist. State license is required to practice.
Psychiatric clinical nurse specialist	Conducts individual, group, and family therapy. Presents educational programs for nursing staff. Provides consultation services to nurses who require assistance in the planning and implementation of care for individual clients.	Registered nurse with minimum of a master's degree in psychiatric nursing. Some institutions require certification by national credentialing association.
Psychiatric nurse	Provides ongoing assessment of client condition, both mentally and physically. Manages the therapeutic milieu on a 24-hour basis. Administers medications. Assists clients with all therapeutic activities as required. Focus is on one-to-one relationship development.	Registered nurse with hospital diploma, associate degree, or baccalaureate degree. Some psychiatric nurses have national certification.
Mental health technician (also called psychiatric aide or assistant or psychiatric technician)	Functions under the supervision of the psychiatric nurse. Provides assistance to clients in the fulfillment of their activities of daily living. Assists activity therapists as required in conducting their groups. May also participate in one-to-one relationship development.	Varies from state to state. Requirements include high school education, with additional vocational education or on-the-job training. Some hospitals hire individuals with baccalaureate degree in psychology in this capacity. Some states require a licensure examination to practice.
Psychiatric social worker	Conducts individual, group, and family therapy. Is concerned with client's social needs, such as placement, financial support, and community requirements. Conducts in-depth psychosocial history on which the needs assessment is based. Works with client and family to ensure that requirements for discharge are fulfilled and needs can be met by appropriate community resources.	Minimum of a master's degree in social work. Some states require additional supervision and subsequent licensure by examination.
Occupational therapist	Works with clients to help develop (or redevelop) independence in performance of activities of daily living. Focus is on rehabilitation and vocational training in which clients learn to be productive, thereby enhancing self-esteem. Creative activities and therapeutic relationship skills are used.	Baccalaureate or master's degree in occupational therapy.
Recreational therapist	Uses recreational activities to promote clients to redirect their thinking or to rechannel destructive energy in an appropriate manner. Clients learn skills that can be used during leisure time and during times of stress after discharge from treatment. Examples include bowling, volleyball, exercises, and jogging. Some programs include activities such as picnics, swimming, and even group attendance at the state fair when it is in session.	Baccalaureate or master's degree in recreational therapy.
Music therapist	Encourages clients in self-expression through music. Clients listen to music, play instruments, sing, dance, and compose songs that help them get in touch with feelings and emotions that they may not be able to experience in any other way.	Graduate degree with specialty in music therapy.
Art therapist	Uses the client's creative abilities to encourage expression of emotions and feelings through artwork. Helps clients to analyze their own work in an effort to recognize and resolve underlying conflict.	Graduate degree with specialty in art therapy.
Psychodramatist	Directs clients in the creation of a "drama" that portrays real-life situations. Individuals select problems they wish to enact, and other clients play the roles of significant others in the situations. Some clients are able to "act out" problems that they are unable to work through in a more traditional manner. All members benefit through intensive discussion that follows.	Graduate degree in psychology, social work, nursing, or medicine with additional training in group therapy and specialty preparation to become a psychodramatist.
Dietitian	Plans nutritious meals for all clients. Works on consulting basis for clients with specific eating disorders, such as anorexia nervosa, bulimia nervosa, obesity, and pica.	Baccalaureate or master's degree with specialty in dietetics.
Chaplain	Assesses, identifies, and attends to the spiritual needs of clients and their family members. Provides spiritual support and comfort as requested by client or family. May provide counseling if educational background includes this type of preparation.	College degree with advanced education in theology, seminary, or rabbinical studies.

effective treatment to include emergency treatment, hospitalization, and crisis intervention. Nursing focus, in the context of the nursing process, is recognition of symptoms and provision of, or referral for, treatment.

    c. **Tertiary prevention**: prevention of complications, reduction of residual impairment, and promotion of rehabilitation directed toward achievement of maximum functioning. Nursing focus is helping clients learn socially appropriate behaviors leading to community assimilation. Appropriate client referrals are made to aftercare services.

C. Treatment alternatives

  1. Community mental health centers: goal is to improve client coping ability and prevent exacerbation of acute symptoms.

  2. Program of Assertiveness Community Treatment (PACT): a service delivery model that provides comprehensive, locally based treatment to clients with serious and persistent mental illness.

    a. Services provided on a 24 hour a day, 7 days a week, 365 days a year basis.

    b. Services are provided in client homes, local restaurants, parks, stores, or any other place where the client may require living skill assistance.

  3. Day/evening treatment/partial hospitalization programs: designed to prevent institutionalization or to ease the transition from inpatient hospitalization to community living. Programs offer a comprehensive treatment plan formulated by an interdisciplinary team.

  4. Community residential facility (group home, half-way houses, foster homes, boarding homes, sheltered care facilities, transitional housing, independent living programs and others): transitional housing for clients with serious mental

---

MAKING THE CONNECTION

Mental health treatment centers, introduced in the 1960s under federal legislation, were designed to replace large state hospitals located in rural areas. These centers were built in neighborhoods, close to the homes of clients. Features included offering a series of comprehensive services by various mental health professionals. There were provisions for continuity of care, participation of consumers in the centers, and a combination of preventive and direct services. The community mental health center provided program-centered as well as case-centered consultation, program evaluation, and various linkages to a variety of resources.

---

illness has proved to be a successful means of therapeutic support and intervention.

  5. Psychiatric home health care: care provided to clients who are unable to leave the home without considerable difficulty or the assistance of others. Psychiatric home health nurses provide services within the home with an emphasis on medication adherence.

D. Mental health resources

  1. Homeless shelters: provide lodging, food, and clothing to individuals in need of these services.

  2. Storefront clinics: provide medication administration, vital sign assessment, immunizations, communicable disease screenings, dressing changes, first aid, and more.

  3. Mobile outreach units: provide services at various locations to the homeless who refuse to seek treatment elsewhere.

III. The Recovery Model

The substance abuse and mental health services administration (SAMHSA) states: "Recovery from mental health disorders and substance use disorder is a process of change through which individuals improve their health and wellness, live a self-directed life, and strive to reach their full potential" (SAMHSA 2011)

DID YOU KNOW?

The basic concept of a recovery model is empowerment of the consumer. The recovery model is designed to allow consumers primary control over decisions about their own care. "Consumer" terminology reflects this shift from passive client to active consumer of care.

A. Goals of recovery model interventions (Table 3.2)

  1. Changing attitudes of the consumer.

  2. Developing a new meaning and purpose in life.

  3. Empowerment of the consumer.

B. Guiding principles that the consumer needs to understand:

  1. Hope is the catalyst of the recovery process.

  2. Self-determination/self-direction leads to regaining control.

  3. The recovery process is highly personal: builds on strengths, coping abilities, and resources.

  4. **Recovery** is holistic involving mind, body, spirit, and community.

  5. Support includes peers, allies, and professionals.

  6. There is possible need to engage in new roles (e.g., partner, friend, employee).

  7. Must address trauma that might be the precursor to the disorder.

Table 3.2 **Nurse-Client Collaboration in the Mental Health Recovery Process**

	The Tidal Model	The WRAP Model	Psychological Recovery Model
Assessment	• Client tells his/her personal story • Nurse actively listens and expresses interest in the story • Nurse helps client record story in his/her own words • Client identifies specific problems he/she wishes to address • Nurse and client identify client's strengths and weakness	• Client develops a Wellness Toolbox by creating a list of tools, strategies, and skills that have been helpful in the past • Client identifies strengths and weaknesses • Nurse provides assistance and feedback	• Client is feeling hopeless and powerless • Client seeks meaning of the illness • Nurse helps by offering hope • Client begins to develop an awareness of the need to take control of and responsibility for his/her life
Interventions	• Nurse and client determine what has worked in the past • Client suggests new tools he/she would like to try • Client decides what changes he/she would like to make and sets realistic goals • Nurse and client decide what must be done as the first step • Nurse gives positive feedback for client's efforts to make life changes and for successes achieved • Nurse encourages client to be as independent as possible but offers assistance when required • Nurse gives the "gift of time"	• Client creates a Daily Maintenance List -How he/she feels at best -What needs to be done daily to maintain wellness -Reminder list of other things that need to be accomplished • Client identifies "triggers" that cause distress or discomfort and identifies what to do if triggers interfere with wellness • Client identifies signs of worsening of symptoms and develops a plan to prevent escalation • Client identifies when symptoms have worsened and help is needed • Client identifies when he/she can no longer care for self and makes decisions (in writing) about treatment issues (what type, who will provide, who will represent his/her interests) • Nurse offers support, and provides feedback and assistance when needed	• Client resolves to begin work of recovery • Client and nurse identify strengths and weaknesses • Nurse assists client to learn about effects of the illness and how to recognize, monitor, and manage symptoms • Client identifies changes that he/she wishes to occur and sets realistic goals to rebuild a meaningful life • Client examines his/her spirituality and philosophy of life in search of a meaning and purpose—one that gives him/her a "reason to start each day"
Outcomes	• Client acknowledges that change has occurred and is ongoing • Client feels empowered to manage own self-care • Nurse is available for support	• Client develops skills in self-management • Client develops self-confidence and hope for a brighter future	• Client develops a positive self-identity separate from the illness • Client maintains commitment to recovery in the face of setbacks • Client feels a sense of optimism and hope of a rewarding future

8. Must be responsible for self-care, social needs, wants, and desires.
9. Available services promote hope, healing, empowerment, and connection.

C. Models of recovery
1. The tidal model: a person-centered approach that focuses on the consumer's (also known as the apprentice's) personal story. Developed by Barker and Buchanan-Barker, the key concepts of this model include:
   a. A practitioner with genuine interest listens and helps consumer express self.
   b. A practitioner may identify specific problems for consumer to address.

c. A practitioner working with the consumer decides what change is needed as first step to recovery.
d. A practitioner helps consumer identify personal strengths and weaknesses.
e. A practitioner helps consumer develop self-confidence and ability to help self.
f. A practitioner helps consumer understand what is being done and why.
2. The Wellness Recovery Action Plan (WRAP), developed by Copeland et al., is a stepwise process through which the consumer is able to monitor and manage distressing symptoms that occur in daily life. Health care provider, friend, or family

may assist consumer in this process. The steps of WRAP include:
  a. Step 1. Consumer creates a list of tools, strategies, and skills that have been used in the past that assist in relieving disturbing symptoms.
  b. Step 2. Consumer writes a description of how he or she feels (or would like to feel) when experiencing wellness (Part 1). Consumer makes a realistic list of things to do every day to maintain wellness (Part 2). Consumer keeps a list of things that need to be done as a reminder (Part 3).
  c. Step 3. Consumer lists triggers that might cause distress or discomfort (Part 1). Using what has worked before, consumer develops a plan for "what to do" if triggers interfere with wellness (Part 2).
  d. Step 4. Consumer learns signs that indicate a possible worsening of the situation (Part 1). Consumer develops a plan for responding to the early warning signs (Part 2).
  e. Step 5. Consumer lists symptoms that are occurring, indicating a worsening situation. Consumer makes a specific and direct plan to call healthcare provider, friend, or family for assistance.
  f. Step 6. In crisis, support system steps in to keep consumer safe. Support system, using resources, ensures treatments and chooses treatment centers on behalf of consumer.
3. The psychological recovery model: this model, developed by Andresen et al., focuses on the consumer's self-determination in the course of the recovery process. The model identifies *hope, responsibility, self and identity,* and *meaning and purpose* as constants in the recovery process. The stages of the psychological recovery model include:
  a. Stage 1. Moratorium: consumer feels a dark despair, and confusion prevails (hope). Consumer feels powerless and out of control (responsibility), doesn't recognize who he or she is (self and identity), and loses purpose in life (meaning and purpose).
  b. Stage 2. Awareness: consumer realizes recovery is possible and sees a dawn of hope (hope). Consumer sees a need to take control, which leads to personal empowerment (responsibility), sees self as independent of the illness (self and identity), and comprehends illness and gains cognitive control of life (meaning and purpose).
  c. Stage 3. Preparation: consumer resolves to work for recovery (hope). Consumer seeks support groups and finds pathways to goals, manages and monitors symptoms (responsibility), rediscovers a positive sense of self (self and

identity), and leads a valuable and enriching life (meaning and purpose).
  d. Stage 4. Rebuilding: consumer takes on the hard work in rebuilding a meaningful life. Consumer sets realistic goals, and with each success, hope is renewed (hope). Consumer actively takes control of life, enlists social support, and takes control of treatment decisions and illness management (responsibility). Consumer, with a new sense of self-confidence, develops a positive sense of self and a commitment to recovery (self and identity). Consumer, with a newfound sense of identity, begins to examine spirituality or philosophy of life (meaning and purpose).
  e. Stage 5. Growth: consumer accepts this final stage and understands that personal growth is a continuing life process. Consumer feels a sense of optimism and strives for higher levels of well-being (hope). Consumer has confidence in managing illness and feels empowered if a setback should occur (responsibility). Consumer has developed a strong, positive sense of self with a new philosophy of life, resulting in being happier and more carefree (self and identity). Consumer develops a more profound and deeper sense of meaning and may find reward in educating others about the experience of mental illness and recovery (meaning and purpose).

IV. Roles and Responsibilities of the Nurse in Psychiatry

Focuses on helping the client successfully adapt to stressors within the environment
A. Inpatient-setting nursing responsibilities
  1. Safety of the **therapeutic milieu.**
  2. Ongoing assessment of client, family, and situation.

MAKING THE CONNECTION

The New Freedom Commission on Mental Health (2003) has proposed transforming the mental health system by shifting the paradigm of the care of persons with serious mental illness from traditional medical psychiatric treatment toward the concept of recovery. Promotion of wellness has always been a primary goal within the context of a nurse-client relationship. Within the health care system, nurses are in key roles to help individuals with mental illness remain as independent as possible, to manage their illness within the community setting, and to strive to minimize hospitalizations.

3. Problem identification.
4. Planning care and daily activities.
5. Collaboration with client to set realistic outcomes.
B. Nursing roles
   1. Role-modeling agent.
      a. Models positive, realistic attitude.
      b. Models appropriate physical appearance and dress.
      c. Models healthy response to frustration and appropriate conflict resolution.
   2. Discharge planner: nurse provides needed information and access to available resources to meet client needs in outpatient settings.
   3. Reality presenter: distinguishes real (objective reality) from what is not real (hallucinations/delusions).
      a. Validates normal feelings and experiences.
      b. Sets limits based on reality.
   4. Technical expert: nurse performs appropriate client interventions using evidenced-based clinical skills.
      a. Medical treatments.
      b. ECT.
      c. Restraints.
   5. Socializing agent: helps clients learn to socialize
      a. Encourages appropriate dress and hygiene.
      b. Encourages appropriate social behaviors and interpersonal interactions.
      c. Encourages participation in group and recreational activities.
   6. Therapeutic milieu manager
      a. Milieu: scientific manipulation of the environment to produce positive changes in client behavior.
      b. The primary function of the nurse is to provide a therapeutic environment that maintains client safety and is conducive to personal growth and healing.
      c. Purpose of milieu:
         i. Opposes regression
         ii. Fosters personal worth
         iii. Increases ability to interact with others
         iv. Increases social competence
         v. Provides opportunities to adopt positive coping skills
         vi. Provides refuge
         vii. Provides structure and minimizes stressors
         viii. Protects clients from own impulses
      d. Structure of milieu.
         i. Cooperative participation of clients and staff
         ii. Democratic self-government fosters responsibility
         iii. Therapies
            1) Individual counseling
            2) **Group therapy**

            3) Education
            4) Art and recreation
         iv. Physical design
            1) Inviting versus custodial feeling/tone
            2) Open space for socialization
            3) Private rooms for individual and group counseling
            4) Rooms for observation and isolation
      e. Basic assumptions of a therapeutic community.
         i. *Health in each individual is to be realized and encouraged to grow.* The nurse focuses on the client's strengths versus the client's weaknesses
         ii. *Every interaction is an opportunity for therapeutic intervention.* The nurse uses everyday situations as a foundation for providing constructive feedback
         iii. *The client owns his or her own environment.* The nurse encourages client participation in environmental decision making
         iv. *Each client owns his or her own behavior.* The nurse encourages clients to take personal responsibility for personal behaviors
         v. *Peer pressure is a useful and powerful tool.* The nurse uses appropriate group approval to promote adaptive behavior
         vi. *Inappropriate behaviors are dealt with as they occur.* The nurse takes immediate action when maladaptive behavior is demonstrated
         vii. *Restrictions and punishments are to be avoided.* The nurse uses least restrictive measures to intervene when clients exhibit dysfunctional behaviors
      f. Components of a therapeutic community.
         i. *Basic physiological needs are fulfilled.* On the basis of Maslow's hierarchy of needs, the nurse understands that a client's physiological requirements are prioritized over psychological needs
         ii. *The physical facilities are conducive to achievement of the goals of therapy.* The nurse appropriately uses space to assure client privacy and room for therapeutic interactions
         iii. *A democratic form of self-government exists.* The nurse encourages clients to participate in decision-making and problem-solving that affect the management of the treatment setting
         iv. *Responsibilities are assigned according to client capabilities.* The nurse matches client abilities with assigned unit responsibilities,

   providing an opportunity for success experiences, which may enhance self-esteem

   v. *A structured program of social and work-related activities is scheduled as part of the treatment program.* The nurse encourages clients to participate in individualized programs to specifically meet personal needs

   vi. *Community and family are included in the program of therapy in an effort to facilitate discharge from treatment.* The nurse incorporates family and community in discharge planning to facilitate effective transition

7. Medication manager.
   a. Assess client for appropriateness of medication.
   b. Assess client for side effects, toxicity, and allergies.
   c. Assess client for **medication nonadherence.**
      i. "Cheeking"
      ii. Lack of response to medications
      iii. Worsening of client symptoms

🛑 When a client hides an oral medication between his or her cheek and gum, this behavior is referred to as "cheeking." This may be done to avoid ingesting the medication or to accumulate medication to attempt suicide. The nurse should be vigilant about assessing symptoms of nonadherence such as lack of response and checking for "cheeking" by closely examining the client's oral cavity. If this problem has been assessed, the nurse should advocate for an alternative way to administer the medication.

   d. Assess for drug-seeking behaviors.
   e. Nursing implications.
      i. Administer as recommended (e.g., with food)
      ii. Be aware of dietary restrictions
      iii. Recognize drug-drug and drug-herb interactions
      iv. Be aware of drug's effect on the client's sleep/wake cycle
   d. Understand information about psychiatric medications.
      i. Psychiatric medications control but do not cure the disease
      ii. Psychiatric medications can help stop an acute episode
      iii. Psychiatric medications can prevent future episodes
      iv. Psychiatric medication adherence does not always prevent illness exacerbation

🛑 Clients need to remain on their medications even if symptoms begin to abate. Some psychotropic medications may take 4 to 6 weeks to attain full effect. It is extremely important for clients to stay on their medications and not discontinue them without physician approval.

   e. Understand reasons for nonadherence.
      i. Major reasons are adverse side effects and cost
      ii. It may be difficult for client and families to accept chronic illness, especially mental illness
      iii. As symptoms decrease, clients may feel no need for continued medication
      iv. Clients may experience positive rewards from certain aspects of their illness (mania)
      v. Clients may forget or misunderstand medication instructions

8. Teacher: Nurse identifies learning needs and provides information to improve a client's life situation.
   a. Teach client and family to recognize early signs of relapse.
   b. Teach client and family to formulate a plan of action during relapse.
   c. Explain to client and family expected effects of psychiatric medications and treatment.
   d. Teach client and family potential adverse reactions/side effects of medications (avoidance of alcohol, dietary restrictions, sedation, photosensitivity).
   e. Use role-playing to teach interpersonal skills (job interview).
   f. Teach client and family when and where to call for help.

9. Client advocate: speaks in support of clients who may be unable to independently advocate for themselves.

10. Surrogate: serves as a substitute figure for another for the client to process feelings within a safe and nonthreatening environment.

11. Counselor: in the context of the nurse-client relationship, the nurse listens and uses therapeutic communication techniques to facilitate client problem solving and decision making.
   a. The nurse is an attentive listener.
   b. The nurse watches for congruency between verbal and nonverbal messages.
   c. The nurse validates client thoughts and feelings.

12. Therapist: an advanced practice nurse can take the role of therapist, using various therapeutic techniques such as cognitive and behavioral therapies.
   a. *Cognitive therapy* is a type of therapy in which the individual is taught to control thought distortions that are considered to be a factor in the development and maintenance of emotional disorders.
   b. *Behavioral therapy* is a form of psychotherapy the goal of which is to modify maladaptive

---

MAKING THE CONNECTION

To function effectively in leading therapeutic groups, nurses need to be able to recognize various processes that occur in groups (e.g., the phases of group development, the various roles that people play within group situations, and the motivation behind client behavior). The nurse also needs to select the most appropriate leadership style for the type of group being led.

---

behavior patterns by reinforcing more adaptive behaviors.
  13. Group therapy facilitator.
      a. Functions of group.
          i. Socialization (teaching social norms)
         ii. Support (promoting security)
        iii. Task completion (working together to achieve a goal)
         iv. Camaraderie (interacting together to achieve joy and pleasure)
          v. Informational (learning occurs from shared experiences)
         vi. Normative (enforcing established norms)
        vii. Empowerment (providing context for using power to bring about change)
       viii. Governance (developing rules by committees that affect the larger organization)
      b. Types of groups.
          i. Task groups (focus on solving problems)
         ii. Teaching groups (convey knowledge and information)
        iii. Supportive/therapeutic groups (focus on effective ways of dealing with emotional stress)
         iv. Self-help groups (allow clients to discuss fears while receiving comfort and advice from others)

DID YOU KNOW?

The seating in therapeutic groups should have no barriers. An example is a circle of chairs. An ideal group size can range from 2 to 15 members. Larger groups provide less time to devote to individual members. Groups can be open- or closed-ended. *Open-ended groups* are those in which members leave and others join at any time while the group is active. *Closed-ended groups* have a predetermined, fixed time frame. All members join at the time the group is organized and terminate at the end of the designated time period. During group therapy, confidentiality must be maintained by all members at all times, even after therapy has terminated.

c. Curative factors of group therapy.
    i. The instillation of hope (members observe the progress of others, which instills hope)
   ii. Universality (members realize that they are not alone in problems, thoughts, feelings)
  iii. Imparting of information (members gain knowledge from instruction and/or shared experiences)
   iv. Altruism (members mutually share concern for each other)
    v. The corrective recapitulation of the primary family group (members reexperience past family conflict with the goal of resolution)
   vi. The development of socializing techniques (members correct maladaptive behaviors and develop new social skills)
  vii. Imitative behavior (members imitate selected group behaviors that they wish to develop in themselves)
 viii. Interpersonal learning (members learn how they perceive and are perceived by others)
   ix. Group cohesiveness (members develop a sense of belonging and come to value each other and the group)
    x. Catharsis (members openly express both negative and positive feelings)
   xi. Existential factors (members are encouraged to take responsibility for the quality of their own existence)
d. Phases of group development.
    i. Initial or orientation phase (members are introduced to each other; goals are established; leader has dominant role; trust is not yet established; members can be overly polite)
   ii. Middle or working phase (cohesiveness and trust have been established; productive work occurs; role of leader diminishes and becomes that of facilitator; conflict is handled by the group)
  iii. Final or termination phase (should be mentioned from the onset; members may experience a sense of loss and progress through stages of grief; leader encourages review of accomplishments and discussion of feelings of loss)
e. Leadership styles (Table 3.3).
    i. Autocratic ("Do as I say.")
   ii. Democratic ("Let's all decide what to do.")
  iii. Laissez-faire ("Do as you will.")

Table 3.3 Leadership Styles—Similarities and Differences

Characteristics	Autocratic	Democratic	Laissez-Faire
1. Focus	Leader	Members	Undetermined
2. Task strategy	Members are persuaded to adopt leader ideas	Members engage in group problem solving	No defined strategy exists
3. Member participation	Limited	Unlimited	Inconsistent
4. Individual creativity	Stifled	Encouraged	Not addressed
5. Member enthusiasm and morale	Low	High	Low
6. Group cohesiveness	Low	High	Low
7. Productivity	High	High (may not be as high as autocratic)	Low
8. Individual motivation and commitment	Low (tend to work only when leader is present to urge them to do so)	High (satisfaction derived from personal input and participation)	Low (feelings of frustration from lack of direction or guidance)

    f. Member roles within groups.
      i. Categories of roles
        1) Task roles
        2) Maintenance roles
        3) Personal roles
      ii. Purpose of roles (Table 3.4)
        1) Complete the group task
        2) Maintain or enhance group processes
        3) Fulfill personal or individual needs

III. Role Development Challenges/Cautions for the Nurse

A. Novice nurse in a psychiatric setting
  1. Anxiety due to knowledge deficit of psychiatric specialty.
  2. Fear of causing harm through nursing interactions.
  3. Preconceptions of the mentally ill as violent.
  4. Personal experiences that may be projected onto the client.
  5. Potential inappropriate use of sympathy versus empathy.

B. Resistant/testing behaviors of clients
  1. Ambivalence.
  2. Withdrawal.
  3. Tardiness and/or missed appointments.
  4. Threats to terminate therapy.

C. Nurse's use of humor/touch
  1. Use cautiously.
  2. May be misinterpreted.
  3. Can increase or decrease anxiety.

D. Social/sexual overtures by client
  1. May be due to role confusion.
  2. May be used to distance self from nurse.
  3. Nurse must set and maintain boundaries.

E. Transference and counter-transference
  1. **Transference:** Client's unconscious projection of past emotions and experiences into current relationship with the nurse.
  2. Could have positive or negative effect on relationship establishment.
  3. **Counter-Transference:** Nurse's projection of feelings and past experiences into current relationship with the client.
  4. Impedes nurse's ability to be objective and accurately assess and meet client's needs.

Table 3.4 Member Roles Within Groups

Role Behaviors

Task Roles

Coordinator	Clarifies ideas and suggestions that have been made within the group; brings relationships together to pursue common goals
Evaluator	Examines group plans and performance, measuring against group standards and goals
Elaborator	Explains and expands on group plans and ideas
Energizer	Encourages and motivates group to perform at its maximum potential
Initiator	Outlines the task at hand for the group and proposes methods for solution
Orienter	Maintains direction within the group

Maintenance Roles

Compromiser	Relieves conflict within the group by assisting members to reach a compromise agreeable to all
Encourager	Offers recognition and acceptance of others' ideas and contributions
Follower	Listens attentively to group interaction; is a passive participant
Gatekeeper	Encourages acceptance of and participation by all members of the group
Harmonizer	Minimizes tension within the group by intervening when disagreements produce conflict

Individual (Personal) Roles

Aggressor	Expresses negativism and hostility toward other members; may use sarcasm in effort to degrade the status of others
Blocker	Resists group efforts; demonstrates rigid and sometimes irrational behaviors that impede group progress
Dominator	Manipulates others to gain control; behaves in authoritarian manner
Help seeker	Uses the group to gain sympathy from others; seeks to increase self-confidence from group feedback; lacks concern for others or for the group as a whole
Monopolizer	Maintains control of the group by dominating the conversation
Mute or silent member	Does not participate verbally; remains silent for a variety of reasons—may feel uncomfortable with self-disclosure or may be seeking attention through silence
Recognition seeker	Talks about personal accomplishments in an effort to gain attention for self
Seducer	Shares intimate details about self with group; is the least reluctant of the group to do so; may frighten others in the group and inhibit group progress with excessive premature self-disclosure

Adapted from Benne, K. B., & Sheets, P. (1948, Spring). Functional roles of group members. *Journal of Social Issues*, 4(2), 42–49

REVIEW QUESTIONS

1. Which of the following factors contributed to the development of large mental institutions in the 19th century? **Select all that apply.**
   1. The fear of mental illness by the general public.
   2. Superstitions regarding mental illness.
   3. A need to increase the social skills of the mentally ill.
   4. A need to protect society from the affected individuals.
   5. A need to increase independence in the mentally ill.

2. Which of the following led to the deinstitutionalization movement?
   1. Dorothea Dix advocated for deinstitutionalization.
   2. Clients with mental illness were feared by the general population.
   3. The Community Mental Health Centers Act was passed.
   4. The National Institute of Mental Health was established.

3. The _____ therapist, as a member of the interdisciplinary treatment team, focuses on rehabilitation and vocational training in which clients learn to be productive, thereby enhancing self-esteem.

4. A nursing instructor is teaching about the reasons clients are admitted to an inpatient psychiatric unit. Which student statement indicates that more instruction is needed?
   1. "This client should be admitted because he is threatening to kill his mother."
   2. "This client should be admitted because he is convinced that all clergy go first to purgatory and then hell."
   3. "This client should be admitted because of an attempted jump from a bridge."
   4. "The client should be admitted because voices tell him to eliminate all people who look like terrorists."

5. Order the following interventions as they progress through the primary, secondary, and tertiary prevention levels of the public health model.
   1. _____ Identifying client problems early and promptly initiating effective treatment, to include hospitalization, and crisis intervention.
   2. _____ Assisting individuals to cope effectively with stress and targeting and diminishing stressors within the environment.
   3. _____ Preventing complications, reducing residual impairment, and promoting rehabilitation directed toward achievement of maximum functioning.

6. According to the public health model, a service aimed at reducing the incidence of mental disorders within the population is referred to as _____ prevention.

7. A client is interacting with a nurse on an inpatient unit. Which represents a nursing intervention at the tertiary level of prevention?
   1. As part of discharge planning, the nurse teaches strategies for medication adherence.
   2. The nurse assists the client in reducing anxiety with deep-breathing exercises.
   3. The nurse and the client role-play techniques for controlling client anger.
   4. The nurse encourages the client to attend occupational therapy.

8. A nursing instructor is explaining various treatment alternatives to inpatient psychiatric hospitalization. Which student statement indicates a need for further instruction?
   1. "The goal of a community mental health center is to improve client coping ability and prevent exacerbation of acute symptoms."
   2. "A Program of Assertiveness Community Treatment (PACT) provides transitional housing for clients with serious mental illness."
   3. "Day/evening treatment/partial hospitalization programs are designed to prevent institutionalization and/or to ease the transition from inpatient hospitalization to community living."
   4. "Psychiatric home health care nurses provide services to clients who are unable to leave the home without considerable difficulty. The care is provided within the home with an emphasis on medication adherence."

9. The family of a client diagnosed with schizophrenia spectrum disorder asks if a cure is possible. From a recovery model perspective, which is the nurse's most appropriate response?
   1. "Recovery consists of prescribing the correct medications to cure the disorder."
   2. "Recovery aims to provide medications to permanently eliminate hallucinations."
   3. "Recovery focuses on maximum functioning in all areas of living."
   4. "Recovery is a process that involves collaboration between the client and family."

10. A health-care professional who takes a subsidiary role when providing care in the context of the tidal model of recovery would be termed a/an

_____

11. Order the five stages of the psychological recovery model as described by Andresen and associates.
    1. _____ Rebuilding
    2. _____ Preparation
    3. _____ Awareness
    4. _____ Growth
    5. _____ Moratorium

12. Which of the following are included in the goals of "recovery model" interventions? **Select all that apply.**
    1. Changing attitudes of the consumer.
    2. Developing a new meaning and purpose in life.
    3. Empowerment of the consumer.
    4. Creation of a list of tools that have worked in the past.
    5. Listing triggers that might cause distress or discomfort.

13. On an inpatient psychiatric unit, a client diagnosed with major depressive disorder states, "I'm so glad the Zoloft that my doctor just prescribed will quickly help me with my mood." Which nursing response reflects the role of teacher?
    1. "I'll set up a time with your doctor to clarify information about this medication."
    2. "How do you feel about taking this new medication?"
    3. "It's great that you have learned this information about your new medication."
    4. "This medication may take up to 2 to 4 weeks to be effective."

14. _____ occurs when the client unconsciously displaces feelings formed toward a person from his or her past to the nurse therapist.

15. Which is a realistic expectation of clients participating in milieu therapy?
    1. To control or set limits on threats and aggressive acts.
    2. To learn adaptive coping, interaction, and relationship skills.
    3. That all maladaptive behaviors are eliminated and adaptive behaviors substituted.
    4. That trust and rapport are quickly established in the context of the nurse-client relationship.

16. A pediatric RN has recently assumed the role of staff nurse on an inpatient psychiatric unit. Which of the following feelings might the nurse expect to experience? **Select all that apply.**
    1. The informal nature of the setting allows increased creativity for the development of nursing interventions.
    2. The newness of the experience can generate anxious behaviors exhibited by the nurse.
    3. Preconceived thoughts and feelings about psychiatric clients can cause fear of client violence.
    4. A nurse's emotionally painful past experiences can contribute to the nurse's inability to empathize with clients.
    5. The nature of the locked psychiatric unit generates a feeling of security in the novice nurse.

17. A nurse on an inpatient psychiatric unit encourages a client to take a shower and dress appropriately. Which role is the nurse assuming?
    1. Milieu manager
    2. Technical expert
    3. Socializing agent
    4. Role-modeling agent

18. On an inpatient psychiatric unit, which nursing responsibility should be prioritized?
    1. Ongoing assessment of client, family, and situation.
    2. Client problem identification.
    3. Collaboration with client to set realistic outcomes.
    4. Maintaining client safety and security in the therapeutic milieu.

19. The basic assumptions of a therapeutic community guide a nurse's actions when functioning in the role of milieu manager. Which nursing action is correctly matched with the appropriate assumption?
    1. The nurse encourages clients to take personal responsibility for personal behaviors. (Assumption: *Peer pressure is a useful and powerful tool.*)
    2. The nurse takes immediate action when maladaptive behavior is demonstrated. (Assumption: *Restrictions and punishments are to be avoided.*)
    3. The nurse encourages client participation in environmental decision making. (Assumption: *The client owns his or her own environment.*)
    4. The nurse uses least restrictive measures to subdue client anger. (Assumption: *Every interaction is an opportunity for therapeutic intervention.*)

20. A suicidal client has not been responding to pre-scribed antianxiety medications. Which of the following should the nurse functioning in the role of medication manager consider when assessing this client? **Select all that apply.**
    1. The client may be "cheeking" medication.
    2. The client may be trying to accumulate medications for a suicide attempt.
    3. The nurse may need to check the client's mouth after drug administration.
    4. The nurse may need to advocate for an alternative way to administer the drug.
    5. The client may be allergic to the medication.

21. During a therapeutic group, two clients disagree about the appropriate time for "lights out." The nurse leader interrupts the exchange and asks the opinion of other group members. The nurse has demonstrated which leadership style?
    1. Autocratic
    2. Democratic
    3. Laissez-faire
    4. Bureaucratic

22. A nurse believes that the members of a parenting group are in the termination phase of group development. Which group behaviors would support this assumption?
    1. The group members manage conflict within the group.
    2. The group uses denial as part of a grief response.
    3. The group members compliment the leader and compete for various position roles.
    4. The group members trust one another and the leader.

23. A nurse should use which group function to help an extremely ambivalent client join Alcoholics Anonymous?
    1. Socialization
    2. Camaraderie
    3. Empowerment
    4. Governance

24. Which of the following client behaviors would lead a nurse to evaluate a member as assuming a *task* group role? **Select all that apply.**
    1. A client decreases conflict within the group by encouraging compromise.
    2. A client offers recognition and acceptance of others.
    3. A client explains and expands on the group plans and ideas.
    4. A client encourages acceptance of and participation by all group members.
    5. A client maintains direction within the group.

REVIEW ANSWERS

1. ANSWER: 1, 2, 4

Rationale:

1. Mental illness was stigmatized by the general public because of fear. This fear was generated by inappropriate behaviors exhibited by the mentally ill and a knowledge deficit about the etiology of the disease. Placed in large institutions or asylums, the mentally ill were removed from society.

2. Mental illness was stigmatized by the general public because of superstitions. Many individuals believed that the mentally ill were possessed by demons. Placed in large institutions or asylums, the mentally ill were removed from society.

3. In the 19th century, the mentally ill experienced long hospitalizations in large institutions or asylums that resulted in the loss of rather than an increase in social skills.

4. In the 19th century, there were no antipsychotic drugs to control the behaviors of affected individuals. Large institutions or asylums were created to house the mentally ill and protect the public.

5. In the 19th century, the mentally ill experienced long hospitalizations in large institutions or asylums that resulted in the loss of rather than an increase in independence.

TEST-TAKING TIP: Multiple factors contributed to the development of large psychiatric institutions or asylums. Mental illness was not understood and therefore feared, causing a need to isolate these individuals from society.

Content Area: Safe and Effective Care Environment: Management of Care;
Integrated Process: Nursing Process: Assessment;
Client Need: Safe and Effective Care Environment: Management of Care;
Cognitive Level: Application;
Concept: Health Care System

2. ANSWER: 3

Rationale:

1. Dorothea Dix advocated for humane care for the mentally ill in the 1840s when institutions, not deinstitutionalization, were the norm.

2. Fear of the mentally ill generated the establishment of large hospitals or asylums devoted to their care rather than deinstitutionalization, which places clients in the community.

3. The Community Mental Health Centers Act called for the construction of comprehensive community health centers, which began the deinstitutionalization movement.

4. The National Institute of Mental Health was charged with the responsibility for mental health care in the United States, but it did not contribute directly to deinstitutionalization.

TEST-TAKING TIP: The high cost of large asylums and institutions led to the passing of the Community Mental Health Centers Act. This law began the movement of the mentally ill from these large institutions into the community.

Content Area: Safe and Effective Care Environment: Management of Care;

Integrated Process: Nursing Process: Assessment;
Client Need: Safe and Effective Care Environment: Management of Care;
Cognitive Level: Comprehension;
Concept: Health Care System

3. ANSWER: occupational

Rationale: The occupational therapist, as a member of the interdisciplinary treatment team, focuses on rehabilitation and vocational training in which clients learn to be productive, thereby enhancing self-esteem. Besides focusing on rehabilitation and vocational training, the occupational therapist uses creative activities and therapeutic relationship skills to increase client functioning.

TEST-TAKING TIP: Note the key phrase *vocational training* in the question stem. *Vocation* and *occupation* have similar meanings. Recall that an occupational therapist is one of the various members of an interdisciplinary treatment team. Review Table 3.1 as needed.

Content Area: Psychosocial Integrity;
Integrated Process: Nursing Process: Implementation;
Client Need: Psychosocial Integrity;
Cognitive Level: Knowledge;
Concept: Collaboration

4. ANSWER: 2

Rationale:

1. Homicidal thoughts or actions such as "threatening to kill his mother" indicate that the client is a danger to others and would meet admission criteria to an inpatient psychiatric unit. This student statement indicates that learning has occurred.

2. Delusional thinking, such as "being convinced that all clergy go first to purgatory and then hell" would not necessarily meet admission criteria to an in-patient psychiatric unit. If the delusion is threatening to self or others, hospitalization may be necessary. Because this delusion is not threatening, this student statement indicates that more instruction is needed.

3. A suicide attempt like "jumping from a bridge" indicates that the client is a danger to self and would meet admission criteria to an inpatient psychiatric unit. This student statement indicates that learning has occurred.

4. Command hallucinations that direct a client to "eliminate all people who look like terrorists" indicate that the client is a danger to others and would meet admission criteria to an inpatient psychiatric unit. This student statement indicates that learning has occurred.

TEST-TAKING TIP: Recall that acute symptoms that meet certain criteria can lead to admission to a psychiatric facility.

Content Area: Safe and Effective Care Environment: Management of Care;
Integrated Process: Nursing Process: Evaluation;
Client Need: Safe and Effective Care Environment: Management of Care;
Cognitive Level: Application;
Concept: Nursing Roles

5. **ANSWER: The correct order is 2, 1, 3**

   Rationale: The premise of the model of public health is based on the concepts set forth by Gerald Caplan during the initial community health movement in 1964. They include primary prevention, secondary prevention, and tertiary prevention

   2. Primary prevention targets both individuals and the environment. It assists individuals to increase their ability to cope effectively with stress and also targets and diminishes harmful forces (stressors) within the environment in an attempt to prevent illness.

   1. Secondary prevention is accomplished through early identification of problems and initiation of effective treatment.

   3. Tertiary prevention is accomplished by preventing complications of the illness and promoting rehabilitation that is directed toward achievement of each individual's maximum level of functioning.

   TEST-TAKING TIP: Recall the concepts of the public health model and the interventions that occur within each level.

   Content Area: *Safe and Effective Care Environment: Management of Care;*

   Integrated Process: *Nursing Process: Implementation;*
   Client Need: *Safe and Effective Care Environment: Management of Care;*
   Cognitive Level: *Analysis;*
   Concept: *Health Care System*

6. **ANSWER: primary**

   Rationale: Primary prevention is health care that is directed at reduction of the incidence of mental disorders within the population by helping individuals to cope more effectively with stress and target and diminish harmful forces (stressors) within the environment.

   TEST-TAKING TIP: Primary prevention deals with decreasing stress within the environment while increasing the coping skills of the individual in an attempt to prevent illness.

   Content Area: *Safe and Effective Care Environment: Management of Care;*
   Integrated Process: *Nursing Process: Implementation;*
   Client Need: *Safe and Effective Care Environment: Management of Care;*
   Cognitive Level: *Knowledge;*
   Concept: *Health Care System*

7. **ANSWER: 1**

   Rationale:

   1. **Teaching strategies for medication adherence will help to prevent future exacerbations of the client's illness and will promote the client's maximum level of functioning. Tertiary prevention is health care that is directed toward reduction of the residual effects associated with severe or chronic physical or mental illness and achievement of a client's maximum level of functioning.**

   2. When the nurse assists the client in reducing anxiety with deep-breathing exercises, the nurse is employing a secondary prevention intervention. Secondary prevention is accomplished through early identification of problems and prompt initiation of effective treatment. This client's problem has been identified, and the nurse is employing an effective treatment.

3. When the nurse and the client role-play techniques for controlling client anger, the nurse is employing a secondary prevention intervention. Secondary prevention is accomplished through early identification of problems and prompt initiation of effective treatment. This client's problem has been identified, and the nurse is employing an effective treatment.

4. When the nurse encourages the client to attend the occupational therapy group, the nurse is employing a secondary prevention intervention. Secondary prevention is accomplished through early identification of problems and prompt initiation of effective treatment. This client's problem has been identified, and the nurse is employing an effective treatment.

TEST-TAKING TIP: The tertiary level of prevention deals with promoting rehabilitation that is directed toward achievement of each individual's maximum level of functioning.

Content Area: *Safe and Effective Care Environment: Management of Care;*
Integrated Process: *Nursing Process: Implementation;*
Client Need: *Safe and Effective Care Environment: Management of Care;*
Cognitive Level: *Application;*
Concept: *Nursing Roles*

8. **ANSWER: 2**

   Rationale:

   1. "The goal of a community mental health center is to improve client coping ability and prevent exacerbation of acute symptoms." This student statement indicates that learning has occurred.

   2. **A Program of Assertiveness Community Treatment (PACT) is a service delivery model that provides comprehensive, locally based treatment to clients with serious and persistent mental illness. Services are provided on a 24-hour a day, 7 days a week, 365 days a year basis. PACT does not provide transitional housing for clients with serious mental illness. This student statement indicates a need for further instruction.**

   3. "Day/evening treatment/partial hospitalization programs are designed to prevent institutionalization and/or to ease the transition from in-patient hospitalization to community living." This student statement indicates that learning has occurred.

   4. "Psychiatric home health care nurses provide services to clients who are unable to leave the home without considerable difficulty. The care is provided within the home with an emphasis on medication adherence." This student statement indicates that learning has occurred.

   TEST-TAKING TIP: Recall the treatment alternatives to inpatient hospitalization and the services they provide clients diagnosed with mental illness.

   Content Area: *Safe and Effective Care Environment: Management of Care;*
   Integrated Process: *Nursing Process: Evaluation;*
   Client Need: *Safe and Effective Care Environment: Management of Care;*
   Cognitive Level: *Application;*
   Concept: *Collaboration*

9. ANSWER: 3

Rationale:

1. This nursing response is inaccurate because the symptoms of schizophrenia spectrum disorder can be controlled, but the disorder itself cannot be cured.

2. This nursing response is inaccurate because while medications can control the hallucinations that accompany schizophrenia spectrum disorder, there are no medications that permanently eliminate hallucinations.

3. This nursing response is accurate because functional recovery focuses on the individual's level of functioning in such areas as relationships, work, independent living, and other kinds of life functioning.

4. This nursing response is inaccurate because the clinician, not family, and client work together to develop a treatment plan that is in alignment with the goals set forth by the client.

TEST-TAKING TIP: Recall that schizophrenia spectrum disorder is a chronic disorder that can be treated with medications that may control symptoms but will not cure the disorder.

Content Area: Safe and Effective Care Environment: Management of Care;
Integrated Process: Nursing Process: Implementation;
Client Need: Safe and Effective Care Environment: Management of Care;
Cognitive Level: Application;
Concept: Nursing Roles

10. ANSWER: apprentice

Rationale: *Become the Apprentice* is one of the 10 Tidal Commitments in the Tidal Model of Recovery. The consumer is the expert on his or her life story, and he or she must be the leader in deciding what needs to be done. Professionals must be apprentice-minded to learn something of the power of the consumer's story.

TEST-TAKING TIP: Recall the concepts of the Tidal Model of Recovery. Review Table 3.2 as needed.

Content Area: Safe and Effective Care Environment: Management of Care;
Integrated Process: Nursing Process: Implementation;
Client Need: Safe and Effective Care Environment: Management of Care;
Cognitive Level: Knowledge;
Concept: Nursing Roles

11. ANSWER: The correct order is: 4, 3, 2, 5, 1

Rationale: Andresen and associates have conceptualized a five-stage model of recovery called the Psychological Recovery Model. The stages include:

1. Moratorium
2. Awareness
3. Preparation
4. Rebuilding
5. Growth

TEST-TAKING TIP: Recall the five stages of the Psychological Recovery Model as described by Andresen and the order in which the stages occur. Review Table 3.2 as needed.

Content Area: Safe and Effective Care Environment: Management of Care;

Integrated Process: Nursing Process: Implementation;
Client Need: Safe and Effective Care Environment: Management of Care;
Cognitive Level: Analysis;
Concept: Promoting Health

12. ANSWER: 1, 2, 3

Rationale: The basic concept of a recovery model is empowerment of the consumer. The recovery model is designed to allow consumers primary control over decisions about their own care.

1. Changing attitudes of the consumer is a goal of recovery model interventions.

2. Developing a new meaning and purpose in life is a goal of recovery model interventions.

3. Empowerment of the consumer is a goal of recovery model interventions.

4. Creation of a list of tools that have worked in the past is Step 1 in the Wellness Recovery Action Plan, not a goal of recovery model interventions.

5. Listing triggers that might cause distress or discomfort is Step 3 in the Wellness Recovery Action Plan, not a goal of recovery model interventions.

TEST-TAKING TIP: Recall the recovery model and look for answer choices written as goal statements. Review Table 3.2 as needed.

Content Area: Safe and Effective Care Environment: Management of Care;
Integrated Process: Nursing Process: Planning;
Client Need: Safe and Effective Care Environment: Management of Care;
Cognitive Level: Analysis;
Concept: Promoting Health

13. ANSWER: 4

Rationale:

1. The nurse has a responsibility to teach, clarify, and reinforce information related to medications that the client is taking. Transferring this responsibility to the physician negates the nurse's role as a teacher.

2. When the nurse asks the client how he or she feels about taking a new medication, the nurse is assuming the role of counselor and facilitator of the communication process. Here the nurse is not functioning in the role of a teacher.

3. Here the nurse is not functioning in the role of a teacher. By validating erroneous information stated by the client, the nurse's statement is inappropriate.

4. Antidepressive drugs may take up to 2 to 4 weeks to be effective in helping with symptoms of major depressive disorder. When the nurse educates the client about the action and time frame of the medication and what to expect, the nurse is functioning in the role of a teacher.

TEST-TAKING TIP: Note that the client's statement that Zoloft will be quickly effective indicates a knowledge deficit related to this medication. In the role of teacher, the nurse should give accurate information to correct this misperception.

Content Area: Safe and Effective Care Environment: Management of Care;

Integrated Process: Nursing Process: Implementation;
Client Need: Safe and Effective Care Environment:
Management of Care;
Cognitive Level: Application;
Concept: Nursing Roles

14. **ANSWER: Transference**

    Rationale: Transference occurs when the client uncon-
    sciously displaces (or "transfers") feelings formed toward a
    person from his or her past to the nurse therapist. Trans-
    ference is a common phenomenon that often arises during
    the course of therapy.

    TEST-TAKING TIP: Differentiate between when a client
    "transfers" feelings (transference) and when the nurse
    projects feelings (counter-transference).
    Content Area: Psychosocial Integrity;
    Integrated Process: Nursing Process: Assessment;
    Client Need: Psychosocial Integrity;
    Cognitive Level: Knowledge;
    Concept: Assessment

15. **ANSWER: 2**

    Rationale:
    1. It is the nurse's responsibility, not a client expectation,
    to set limits to ensure a safe and therapeutic milieu.
    **2. Milieu therapy is the manipulation of the environ-
    ment so that clients can learn adaptive coping, interac-
    tion, and relationship skills.**
    3. It is the goal of milieu therapy for clients to improve
    maladaptive behaviors, but eliminating all maladaptive
    behaviors is an unrealistic expectation.
    4.It is important that trust and rapport in the context of
    the nurse-client relationship are established, but it is an
    unrealistic expectation that this would occur quickly.

    TEST-TAKING TIP: Recall and differentiate client expecta-
    tions and nursing responsibilities related to milieu therapy.
    Content Area: Safe and Effective Care Environment:
    Management of Care;
    Integrated Process: Nursing Process: Planning;
    Client Need: Safe and Effective Care Environment:
    Management of Care;
    Cognitive Level: Analysis;
    Concept: Promoting Health

16. **ANSWER: 2, 3, 4**

    Rationale:
    1. The informal nature of the psychiatric setting may
    threaten the role identity of a pediatric nurse who may be
    task- and schedule-oriented. The anxiety that this threat
    produces would decrease, rather than increase, the ability
    to be creative.
    **2. The newness of the experience may generate feelings
    of inadequate knowledge of the subject matter and fears
    of harming clients psychologically. This may lead to the
    nurse exhibiting anxious behaviors.**
    **3. Preconceived thoughts and feelings about psychiatric
    clients generated by media portrayal can cause the nurse
    to assume that violence is a major issue, when in fact
    it is not.**
    **4. Emotionally painful past experiences may cause the
    nurse to question his or her own mental health, project**
    personal concerns on the clients, or sympathize versus
    empathize with the clients' situations.
    5. A locked psychiatric unit is more apt to generate feel-
    ings of fear than of security.

    TEST-TAKING TIP: Review the challenges and cautions of
    the novice nurse in a psychiatric setting.
    *Content Area: Safe and Effective Care Environment: Man-
    agement of Care;*
    Integrated Process: Nursing Process: Assessment;
    *Client Need: Safe and Effective Care Environment: Man-
    agement of Care;*
    Cognitive Level: Application;
    Concept: Nursing Roles

17. **ANSWER: 3**

    Rationale:
    1. The primary function of the nurse as a milieu manager
    is to maintain a safe therapeutic environment and provide
    a positive atmosphere for the process of personal growth
    and healing. The situation presented in the question does
    not reflect the role of milieu manager.
    2. Functioning as a technical expert, the nurse performs
    appropriate client interventions using evidenced-based
    clinical skills. The situation presented in the question does
    not reflect the role of technical expert.
    **3. The nurse in the question is functioning as a socializ-
    ing agent by helping the client learn to socialize by en-
    couraging appropriate dress and hygiene. In this role,
    the nurse encourages appropriate social behaviors and
    interpersonal interactions as well as participation in
    group and recreational activities.**
    4. Functioning as a role-modeling agent, the nurse ex-
    hibits a positive and realistic attitude, presents an appro-
    priate physical appearance and dress, and responds in a
    healthy way to frustration and conflict. The situation pre-
    sented in the question does not reflect the role of role-
    modeling agent.

    TEST-TAKING TIP: Recall the various roles a nurse assumes
    in a psychiatric setting and understand the tasks involved
    in the performance of these roles.
    *Content Area: Safe and Effective Care Environment: Man-
    agement of Care;*
    Integrated Process: Nursing Process: Implementation;
    Client Need: Safe and Effective Care Environment:
    Management of Care;
    Cognitive Level: Application;
    Concept: Nursing Roles

18. **ANSWER: 4**

    Rationale:
    1. Ongoing assessment of client, family, and situation is an
    important responsibility of a nurse on an inpatient setting,
    but compared with safety of the milieu, this nursing re-
    sponsibility should not take priority.
    2. Client problem identification is an important responsi-
    bility of a nurse in an inpatient setting, but compared with
    safety of the milieu, this nursing responsibility should not
    take priority.
    3. Collaboration with client to set realistic outcomes is an
    important responsibility of a nurse in an inpatient setting,

but compared with safety of the milieu, this nursing responsibility should not take priority.

4. Safety and security of the client in the therapeutic milieu is the priority responsibility of a nurse in an inpatient setting. Maintaining an environment that provides client safety and security should always be a nurse's priority.

TEST-TAKING TIP: Recall the various roles a nurse assumes in a psychiatric setting and understand that maintaining client safety and security is always a priority.
Content Area: Safe and Effective Care Environment: Management of Care;
Integrated Process: Nursing Process: Implementation;
Client Need: Safe and Effective Care Environment: Management of Care;
Cognitive Level: Application;
Concept: Nursing Roles

19. **ANSWER: 3**
Rationale:
1. When the nurse encourages clients to take personal responsibility for personal behaviors, the nurse is guided by the following basic assumption of the therapeutic community: *Each client owns his or her own behavior.*
2. When the nurse takes immediate action when maladaptive behavior is demonstrated, the nurse is guided by the following basic assumption of the therapeutic community: *Inappropriate behaviors are dealt with as they occur.*
3. When the nurse encourages client participation in environmental decision making, the nurse is guided by the following basic assumption of the therapeutic community: *The client owns his or her own environment.*
4. When the nurse uses least restrictive measures to subdue client anger, the nurse is guided by the following basic assumption of the therapeutic community: *Restrictions and punishments are to be avoided.*
TEST-TAKING TIP: Recall the basic assumptions of a therapeutic community and the nursing interventions that support these assumptions.
Content Area: Safe and Effective Care Environment: Management of Care;
Integrated Process: Nursing Process: Implementation;
Client Need: Safe and Effective Care Environment: Management of Care;
Cognitive Level: Application;
Concept: Promoting Health

20. **ANSWER: 1, 2, 3, 4**
Rationale: "Cheeking" is when a client hides an oral medication between his or her cheek and gum. This may be done to avoid ingesting the medication or to accumulate medication in order to attempt suicide.
1. The nurse should consider that the client may be "cheeking" medication.
2. Not responding to prescribed antianxiety medications is an indication that the client may not be ingesting prescribed drugs. The client may be "cheeking" the medication to accumulate drugs to attempt suicide.
3. If "cheeking" is suspected, the nurse should closely examine the client's mouth after drug administration to ensure that medication has been ingested.

4. If "cheeking" is suspected, the nurse should advocate for an alternate way to administer the drug.
5. There are no client symptoms presented in the question to indicate that the client may be allergic to the medication.
TEST-TAKING TIP: Recall the term "cheeking" and what nursing actions are appropriate if "cheeking" is suspected. Note that the client in the question is suicidal and lacks response to the prescribed medication. These facts should alert you to the possibility that the client is not ingesting the medication.
Content Area: Safe and Effective Care Environment: Management of Care;
Integrated Process: Nursing Process: Implementation;
Client Need: Safe and Effective Care Environment: Management of Care;
Cognitive Level: Application;
Concept: Assessment

21. **ANSWER: 2**
1. The focus of autocratic leadership is on the leader. The message that is conveyed to the group is: "We will do it my way." The nurse's actions presented in the question are not indicative of an autocratic leadership style.
2. The democratic leadership style focuses on the members of the group and group-selected goals. The nurse's actions presented in the question demonstrate a democratic leadership style.
3. The Laissez-faire leadership style allows members of the group to do as they please. There is no direction from the leader. The nurse's actions presented in the question are not indicative of a laissez-faire leadership style.
4. A bureaucrat may use an autocratic leadership style, but bureaucratic is not identified as one of the three common group leadership styles.
TEST-TAKING TIP: Recall the three major group leadership styles and match the nurse's actions presented in the question with the appropriate style of leadership. Review Table 3.3 as needed.
Content Area: Safe and Effective Care Environment: Management of Care;
Integrated Process: Nursing Process: Implementation;
Client Need: Safe and Effective Care Environment: Management of Care;
Cognitive Level: Application;
Concept: Nursing Roles

22. **ANSWER: 2**
Rationale:
1. When group members manage conflict within the group with minimal help from the leader, the group is in the middle or working, not termination phase of group development. During the working phase, cohesiveness has been established within the group. This is when the productive work toward completion of the task is undertaken.
2. When the group uses denial as part of a grief response, the group is most likely in the final or termination phase of group development. Termination should be discussed in depth for several meetings before the final group session. A sense of loss that precipitates the grief process may be in evidence, particularly in groups that have been successful in their stated purpose.

3. The nurse should anticipate that members in the initial, or orientation phase—not the termination phase—of group development will compliment the leader and compete for various position roles. Members in this phase have not yet established trust and have a fear of not being accepted. Power struggles may occur as members compete for their position in the group.

4. When group members initially trust one another and the leader, the group is in the middle or working phase, not the termination phase, of group development. During the working phase, cohesiveness has been established within the group. This is when the productive work toward completion of the task is undertaken.

TEST-TAKING TIP: Recall the three phases of group development and what occurs in each phase.

Content Area: Safe and Effective Care Environment: Management of Care;
Integrated Process: Nursing Process: Assessment;
Client Need: Safe and Effective Care Environment: Management of Care;
Cognitive Level: Application;
Concept: Assessment

23. **ANSWER: 3**
Rationale:
1. The socialization function of group teaches social norms. The situation presented in the question does not reflect the group function of socialization.
2. The camaraderie function of group provides joy and pleasure that individuals seek from interactions with significant others. The situation presented in the question does not reflect the group function of camaraderie.
3. **The nurse should identify that the group function of empowerment would help an extremely ambivalent client to make the decision to join Alcoholics Anonymous. Groups help to bring about improvement in existing conditions by encouraging members to take control of ways to bring about change. Groups have power that individual members alone do not.**
4. The governance function of a group is when rules are made by committees within a larger organization.

The situation presented in the question does not reflect the group function of governance.
TEST-TAKING TIP: Recall the eight functions of group: socialization, support, task completion, camaraderie, informational, normative, empowerment, and governance.
Content Area: Safe and Effective Care Environment: Management of Care;
Integrated Process: Nursing Process: Implementation;
Client Need: Safe and Effective Care Environment: Management of Care;
Cognitive Level: Application;
Concept: Nursing

24. **ANSWERS: 3, 5**
Rationale: *Task* group member roles include coordinator, evaluator, elaborator, energizer, initiator, and orienter.
1. The nurse should identify clients who decrease conflict within the group as assuming the *maintenance* role of compromiser, which is not one of the *task* group roles.
2. The nurse should identify clients who offer recognition and acceptance of others as assuming the *maintenance* role of encourager, which is not one of the *task* group roles.
3. **The nurse should identify a client who explains and expands on the group plans and ideas as assuming the *task* role of elaborator.**
4. The nurse should identify clients who encourage acceptance of and participation by all group members as assuming the *maintenance* role of gatekeeper, which is not one of the *task* group roles.
5. **The nurse should identify a client who maintains direction within the group as assuming the *task* role of orienter.**
TEST-TAKING TIP: Recall the three major types of roles that individuals play within the membership of a group. Review Table 3.4 as needed.
Content Area: Psychosocial Integrity;
Integrated Process: Nursing Process: Evaluation;
Client Need: Psychosocial Integrity;
Cognitive Level: Analysis;
Concept: Assessment

Relationship Development and the Nursing Process

Assessment—The first step of the nursing process in which the nurse collects and analyzes data; assessment may include the following dimensions: physical, psychological, sociocultural, spiritual, cognitive, functional, developmental, economic, and lifestyle

Evaluation—The fifth and last step of the nursing process; this is the process of determining the progress toward attainment of expected outcomes, including the effectiveness of care

Implementation—The fourth step of the nursing process when nursing actions are employed according to the plan of care so that continuity of care can be ensured for the client during hospitalization and in preparation for discharge

Nursing Diagnosis (Analysis)—The second step of the nursing process. Clinical judgments are made about individual, family, or community experiences/responses to actual or potential health problems/life processes. Provides the basis for selection of nursing interventions to achieve outcomes for which the nurse has accountability

Nursing Process (Assessment, Analysis [Diagnosis], Planning, Implementation, Evaluation)—An orderly approach to administering nursing care so that the client's needs are comprehensively and effectively met

Nurse-client relationship—A therapeutic interaction between a nurse and a client in which input from both participants contributes to a climate of healing, growth promotion, and/or illness prevention

Outcomes—End results that are measurable, desirable, and observable and that translate into observable behaviors

Planning—The third step of the nursing process; in this step, based on the assessment and diagnosis, the nurse sets measurable and achievable short- and long-term goals

Professional boundaries—Boundaries that separate therapeutic behavior from any other behavior, which, be it well intentioned or not, could lessen the benefit of care to clients

Religious beliefs—A set of beliefs, values, rites, and rituals adopted by a group of people; the practices are usually grounded in the teachings of a spiritual leader

At the core of nursing is the therapeutic nurse-client relationship. The nurse establishes and maintains this key relationship by using nursing knowledge and skills, as well as applying caring attitudes and behaviors. Therapeutic nursing services contribute to the client's health and well-being. The relationship is based on trust, respect, and empathy and requires appropriate use of the power inherent in the care provider's role. The nursing process consists of five steps (assessment, diagnosis, outcome identification/planning, implementation, and evaluation) and uses a problem-solving approach. This approach has come to be accepted as

nursing's scientific methodology. It is goal directed, with the objective being delivery of quality client care.

I. Nurse-Client Relationship

A. Essential characteristics for establishment of a nurse-client relationship
   1. Rapport: bonding between the nurse and client. Based on acceptance, warmth, friendliness, common interest, trust, nonjudgmental attitude.

2. Trust: a feeling of confidence in another person's presence, reliability, integrity, veracity, and sincere desire to help.

3. Empathy: a process wherein the nurse is able to see beyond a client's outward behavior and sense accurately his or her inner experience.
   a. Feelings are on an objective level.
   b. Unlike sympathy in which the nurse actually shares what the client is feeling and experiences a need to alleviate distress. Sympathy results in loss of objectivity and perspective.

4. Genuineness: the nurse's ability to be open, honest, and "real" in interactions. There is congruence in what is said and what is felt.

5. Respect: valuing the dignity and worth of an individual, regardless of his or her unacceptable behavior.

B. Dynamics of a therapeutic nurse-client relationship
1. Therapeutic use of self.
   a. Ability of the nurse to consciously use his or her personality in an attempt to relate to others.
   b. Ability to effectively help others. This ability is strongly influenced by an internal value system, which is composed of intellect and emotions.

2. Gaining self-awareness.
   a. A nurse needs to recognize and accept what he or she values.
   b. A nurse needs to recognize and accept uniqueness and differences in others.
   c. The nurse can use values clarification to gain self-awareness.

C. Phases of the nurse-client relationship (Table 4.1)
1. Preinteraction phase.
   a. Begins before client contact.
   b. Nurse explores personal feelings, fantasy, fears.
   c. Nurse gathers client data.
   d. Nurse plans for the establishment of a relationship before first meeting.

2. Orientation or introductory phase. Client behavior may be manipulative, and/or regressive during this phase.
   a. Nurse and client meet and get acquainted.
   b. Goal: develop trust and rapport; establish nurse as a significant other.
   c. Determine why client is seeking help.
   d. Explore client's thoughts and feelings.
   e. Establish nurse-client contract: nurse must adhere strictly to agreed upon contract schedule in order to ensure trust.
      i. Mutually set parameters for relationship (what roles are assumed and what responsibilities are established)
      ii. Determine how each will be addressed (e.g., first names, Mr./Ms. Smith)

Table 4.1 Phases of Relationship Development and Major Nursing Goals

Phase	Goals
1. Preinteraction	Explore self-perceptions
2. Orientation (introductory)	Establish trust and formulate contract for intervention
3. Working	Promote client change
4. Termination	Evaluate goal attainment and ensure therapeutic closure

      iii. Set time, place, and duration of interpersonal contact
      iv. Discuss role expectations (what the nurse can and cannot do for client)
      v. Mutually establish goals and discuss termination

3. Working phase
   a. Goal: resolution of client's problem.
   b. Mutually explore relevant stressors.
   c. Therapeutic interventions are individualized.
   d. Assist client to develop insight.
   e. Mutually explore workable solutions.
   f. Assist client to use constructive coping mechanisms.
   g. Set limits if necessary.

4. Termination phase.
   a. Goal: assist client to review what has been learned in the relationship and transfer this learning to interactions with others.
   b. The termination process begins in the orientation phase.
   c. Mutually review progress of therapy and attainment of goals.
   d. Explore client feelings about termination.
      i. Anger
      ii. Loneliness
      iii. Loss
      iv. Rejection (client may reject the nurse as a defense against perceived rejection during termination)
      v. Hostility
      vi. Increased dependency
      vii. Client feelings may be expressed both covertly or overtly (late or missed meetings)
      viii. Client's communication may be shallow and/or superficial

D. Professional boundaries in the nurse-client relationship
1. Boundaries limit and outline expectations for appropriate professional relationships with clients.
2. Boundary crossing can threaten the integrity of the nurse-client relationship.

3. Self-disclosure on the part of the nurse.
   a. May be appropriate when it is judged that the information can therapeutically benefit the client.
   b. Should never be undertaken for the purpose of meeting the nurse's needs.
4. Addressing clients appropriately.
   a. Address clients respectfully.
   b. Begin with a formal approach ("Mrs. Jones").
   c. Respect client wishes ("You can call me Sally").
   d. Never use belittling terms ("Sweetie," "Honey").
5. Gifts.
   a. Accepting financial gifts is never appropriate.
   b. The decision to accept other small gifts may be influenced by a client's cultural beliefs.
   c. Refusing a gift may be interpreted, in some cultures, as an insult.
6. Caring touch (touch when there is no physical need).
   a. Can provide comfort and encouragement.
   b. Clients may be uncomfortable with and/or misinterpret caring touch.
   c. A nurse must be sensitive to vulnerable clients and understand cultural nuances related to touch.

🛑 Romantic, sexual, or similar personal relationships are **never** appropriate between nurse and client.

II. Nursing Process in Psychiatric Nursing (Fig. 4.1)

A. Assessment
1. Begins on admission (intake interview).
   a. Gather *objective data* (data that the nurse collects by the use of all senses. This data can be analyzed, measured, or counted).
   b. Gather *subjective data* (data presented by the client that show his or her perception, understanding, and interpretation of what is happening).
   c. May have to rely on family or significant others for information.
   d. Mental status examination (see Table 4.2).
2. Make observations and note incongruences.
3. Validate specific behaviors.
4. Assess the context or situation that precipitated behavior (precipitating event).
5. Assess the client's thought and feelings.
6. Determine whether the behavior was adaptive or dysfunctional.
7. Determine whether assessment data reflect the typical picture of the client (note changes from the norm).

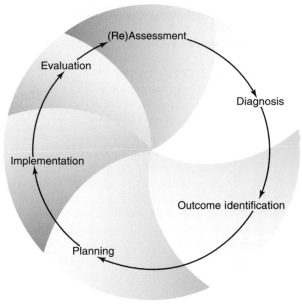

Fig 4.1 The ongoing nursing process.

B. Nursing diagnosis (analysis)
1. Identification of client problems.
2. Based on analysis of:
   a. Verbalizations.
   b. Behaviors.
   c. Assessed data.
3. Problem statement needs to be specific.
4. NANDA-I format used for nursing diagnostic statements.
   a. NANDA-I stem (example: low self-esteem).
   b. Related to (R/T) statement (example: child abuse).
   c. As evidenced by (AEB) statement (example: minimal eye contact, expressions of low self-worth).
5. Actual nursing diagnosis.
   a. Client problem is currently occurring.
   b. Contains all three components of format (NANDA-I stem, R/T, and AEB).
6. Potential "Risk for" nursing diagnosis.
   a. Situation exists to place client at potential risk for a problem to occur.
   b. Contains only first two components of format (NANDA-I stem and R/T statements).
   c. Risk for suicide always prioritized.

C. Planning: the goal is to substitute adaptive for dysfunctional behaviors
1. Client and nurse mutually set **outcomes** that are:
   a. Client centered.
   b. Realistic (achievable).
   c. Measurable (with a time frame).
   d. Culturally relevant.

Table 4.2 Brief Mental Status Evaluation

Area of Mental Function Evaluated	Evaluation Activity
Orientation to time	"What year is it? What month is it? What day is it?" (3 points)
Orientation to place	"Where are you now?" (1 point)
Attention and immediate recall	"Repeat these words now: bell, book, and candle." (3 points) "Remember these words and I will ask you to repeat them in a few minutes."
Abstract thinking	"What does this mean: no use crying over spilled milk"? (3 points)
Recent memory	"Say the three words I asked you to remember earlier." (3 points)
Naming objects	Point to eyeglasses and ask, "What is this?" Repeat with 1 other item (e.g., calendar, watch, pencil). (2 points possible)
Ability to follow simple verbal command	"Tear this piece of paper in half and put it in the trash container." (2 points)
Ability to follow simple written command	Write a command on a piece of paper (e.g., TOUCH YOUR NOSE), give the paper to the patient, and say, "Do what it says on this paper." (1 point for correct action)
Ability to use language correctly	Ask the patient to write a sentence. (3 points if sentence has a subject, a verb, and has valid meaning).
Ability to concentrate	"Say the months of the year in reverse, starting with December." (1 point each for correct answers from November through August. 4 points possible.)
Understanding spatial relationships	Ask the patient to: draw a clock; put in all the numbers; and set the hands on 3 o'clock. (Clock circle = 1 pt; numbers in correct sequence = 1 pt; numbers placed on clock correctly = 1 pt; two hands on the clock = 1 pt; hands set at correct time = 1 pt. (5 points possible)

Scoring: 30–21 = normal; 20–11 = mild cognitive impairment; 10–0 = severe cognitive impairment (scores are not absolute and must be considered within the comprehensive diagnostic assessment).
Sources: *The Merck Manual of Health & Aging* (2005); Folstein, Folstein, & McHugh (1975); Kaufman & Zun (1995); Kokman et al (1991); and Pfeiffer (1975).

2. Types of goals.
   a. Short term.
      i. Achieved during hospitalization
      ii. Client recognition of problems
      iii. Client recognition of strengths, abilities
   b. Long term.
      i. Achieved during outpatient care
      ii. Issues that require follow-up counseling after discharge
      iii. Implementation of actions to deal with assessed problems

D. Implementation: nurse primarily functions as facilitator and as an educator
  1. Routine nursing interventions include limited hands-on actions.
   a. Giving medications.
   b. Monitoring vital signs.
   c. Meeting physical needs.
  2. Main focus is on verbal strategies.

E. Evaluation
  1. Client progress is dependent on realistic goals.
  2. Nurse gathers data and input from the client to evaluate whether goals/outcomes are met/unmet.
  3. If goal(s) is (are) unmet, the nurse should:
   a. Evaluate appropriateness of goal(s).
   b. Evaluate time frame for completion.
   c. Evaluate effectiveness of nursing interventions.
  4. Nurse and client collaborate to modify goals based on evaluation.

III. Cultural and Spiritual Considerations Relevant to Psychiatric Nursing

DID YOU KNOW?

Culture describes a particular society's entire way of living, encompassing shared patterns of belief, feelings, and knowledge that guide an individual's conduct and are passed down from generation to generation. Cultures differ, and it is important for nurses to be aware of the cultural influences that affect an individual's behaviors and beliefs in order to provide culturally sensitive, appropriate, and effective nursing care.

A. Biological variations: The differences that exist among people in various racial groups
  1. Body structure.
   a. Size.
   b. Shape.
   c. Skin color.
  2. Physiological responses.
   a. To medications.
   b. Electrocardiographic pattern differences.
   c. Susceptibility to disease (see "Health Concerns" in Table 5.4 in Chapter 5).

 Caution must be taken not to assume that all individuals who share a cultural or ethnic group are identical or exhibit behaviors perceived as characteristic of the group. This constitutes stereotyping and must be avoided.

B. Dietary restrictions, preferences, and deficiencies common in various cultural groups
   1. Northern European Americans: among English, Irish, Welsh, Finnish, Swedish, Norwegian, Germans, Polish, and the people of Baltic States, the diet may be high in fats and cholesterol and low in fiber.
   2. African Americans: differs little from that of the mainstream culture. Similar to Northern European Americans, but some follow their heritage and enjoy what has come to be called "soul food." This could include collard greens, fried chicken, grits, okra, and cornbread.
   3. Native Americans: nutritional deficiencies are not uncommon among tribal Native Americans. Generally meat and corn products are preferred to fruits and green vegetables.
   4. Asian/Pacific Islander Americans: rice, vegetables, and fish are the main staple foods consumed. Milk is seldom consumed because a large majority of this cultural group experience lactose intolerance.
   5. Latino Americans: diet typically includes maize-based dishes such as tortillas and tamales, and many Latino Americans are lactose intolerant.
   6. Western European Americans: among Italians, Greeks, and French, cuisine is used in a social manner as well as for nutritional purposes.
   7. Muslim Americans: If adhering to a religiously based halal diet, they are prohibited from eating pork and pork products.
   8. Jewish Americans: If adhering to a religiously based kosher diet, they are prohibited from eating pork, pork products, and shellfish. According to kosher guidelines, dairy products and meat may not be mixed together in cooking, serving, or eating.

(!) Assessment of mental illness must be based on what behaviors and beliefs are accepted in a client's culture. It would not be considered delusional in traditional Buddhist culture to believe that an enemy could be reincarnated as a viper.

C. Religious beliefs, attitudes, and practices
   1. Assess any religious requirements or restrictions that limit client care.
   2. Assess dietary limitations related to cultural and/or religious beliefs.
   3. Use caution addressing spiritual needs with a client experiencing religious delusions.
   4. Research has shown that attitudes and emotions have a definite effect on the body.
      a. Hope and optimism produce positive physical changes.

      b. Hope and optimism can influence the immune system and the functioning of specific body organs.
      c. Feelings of despair and pessimism may negatively affect a client's physical condition.
   5. Preexisting conditions that influence communication.
      a. Values, attitudes, and beliefs.
         i. Prejudice
         ii. Negative stereotyping
         iii. Symbolic behaviors (style of clothes)
      b. Culture or religion.
         i. Cultural mores
         ii. Norms
         iii. Ideas
         iv. Customs
         v. Displaying religious symbols
      c. Social status: nonverbal indicators of high-status persons.
         i. Less eye contact
         ii. More relaxed posture
         iii. Louder voice pitch
         iv. Place hands on hips more frequently
         v. Are "power dressers"
         vi. Maintain more distance when communicating with individuals considered to be of a lower-status
      d. Gender.
         i. Influences manner of communication
         ii. Difference in posture
         iii. Male/female roles
         iv. Gender signals and roles are blurring
      e. Age.
         i. Vocabulary and slang vary with age
         ii. Adolescents generate a unique pattern of communication influenced by technology

REVIEW QUESTIONS

1. The nurse's ability to have unconditional positive regard for the client and also to maintain a nonjudgmental attitude is described as which characteristic that enhances the nurse-client relationship?
   1. Genuineness
   2. Empathy
   3. Objectivity
   4. Respect

2. In which stage of the nurse-client relationship is a contract for interaction formulated?
   1. The stage when the nurse explores prejudices related to mental health issues.
   2. The stage when the nurse determines why the client sought help.
   3. The stage when the nurse explores stressors and promotes insight.
   4. The stage when the nurse evaluates the client's progress and goal attainment.

3. When developing a therapeutic relationship with a client, which characteristic is most essential?
   1. Catharsis
   2. Confrontation
   3. Genuineness
   4. Giving advice

4. An interaction between two people (usually a caregiver and a care receiver) in which input from both participants contributes to a climate of healing, growth promotion, and/or illness prevention is defined as a (an) _____ relationship.

5. What should be the nurse's primary goal during the termination phase of the nurse-client relationship?
   1. To evaluate goal attainment and ensure therapeutic closure.
   2. To establish trust and formulate a contract for intervention.
   3. To explore self-perceptions.
   4. To promote client change.

6. A pacing, agitated client diagnosed with bipolar mania is unable to concentrate during an interaction with the nurse. The nurse uses closed-ended questions, offers finger foods, and reassures the client. What is the nurse promoting by these actions?
   1. Sympathy
   2. Trust
   3. Veracity
   4. Congruency

7. A client has recently experienced a second trimester miscarriage and is feeling very depressed. Which therapeutic statement by the nurse conveys empathy?
   1. "You are feeling very depressed. I know how you feel. I felt the same way when I lost my first baby."
   2. "I can understand you are feeling depressed. It is difficult to lose a baby. I'll sit with you."
   3. "You seem depressed. I think it would be helpful if I explained to you the five stages of grief."
   4. "I know this is a difficult time for you. Would you like a prn medication to help you feel better?"

8. In which phase of the nurse-client relationship would a nurse role-play with a client to practice appropriate ways to deal with anger?
   1. Preinteraction
   2. Orientation
   3. Working
   4. Termination

9. Which situation exemplifies rapport, a condition essential to the development of a therapeutic relationship?
   1. The nurse communicates regard for the client as a person of worth who is valued and accepted without qualification.
   2. The nurse communicates an understanding of the client's world from the client's internal frame of reference, with sensitivity to the client's feelings.
   3. The nurse communicates openness, self-congruency, authenticity, and transparency when dealing with the client.
   4. The nurse communicates acceptance, warmth, friendliness, common interests, a sense of trust, and a nonjudgmental attitude when dealing with the client.

10. When being confronted for engaging in dysfunctional behavior during group therapy, a client uses the defense mechanism of projection. Which short-term outcome is appropriate for this client?
    1. The client will not injure himself or herself or someone else.
    2. The client will covertly express feelings of anger in group therapy.
    3. The client will take responsibility for the dysfunctional behavior by the end of shift.
    4. The client will participate in outpatient therapy within 2 weeks of discharge.

11. A client is transported to the emergency department (ED) for head and abdominal trauma sustained in a physical altercation with a family member. In this situation, which nursing diagnosis would take priority?
    1. Risk for other-directed violence R/T anger toward a family member.
    2. Risk for disturbed body image R/T head and abdominal injuries.
    3. Risk for injury R/T possible complications secondary to trauma.
    4. Risk for anxiety R/T injuries AEB tremors and crying.

12. Which expected client outcome should a nurse identify as being correctly formulated?
    1. Client will lose a significant amount of weight by discharge.
    2. Client will write a list of strengths and weaknesses.
    3. Client will resolve marital problems by end of session.
    4. Client will shower, shampoo, and shave by 8:00 a.m. tomorrow.

13. Which nonverbal behavior should a nurse avoid when gathering assessment data on a newly admitted client? **Select all that apply.**
    1. Maintaining indirect eye contact with the client.
    2. Providing space by leaning back away from the client.
    3. Sitting squarely, facing the client.
    4. Sitting with arms and legs in an open posture.
    5. Standing while the client sits.

14. Order the following nursing interventions as they would proceed through the steps of the nursing process.
    1. _____ Analyze attitude after assertiveness training session.
    2. _____ Score a client's alcohol withdrawal symptoms using a Clinical Institute Withdrawal Assessment (CIWA) scale.
    3. _____ Facilitate an assertiveness training session.
    4. _____ Collaborate with client to set a realistic weight loss goal.
    5. _____ Document the client's problem in NANDA-I terms.

15. A client diagnosed with an anxiety disorder tells the nurse, "I'm not sleeping much. My mood is a 4 on that 10-point scale. I hurt all over and feel sad and irritable." Which of the following is subjective assessment data? **Select all that apply.**
    1. "I'm not sleeping much."
    2. "My mood is a 4 on that 10-point scale."
    3. "I hurt all over."
    4. "I'm feeling sad."
    5. "I'm feeling irritable."

16. Which data gathering technique can be employed during the evaluation step of the nursing process? **Select all that apply.**
    1. Asking the client to rate anxiety after administering an anxiolytic.
    2. Asking the client to verbalize understanding of explained unit rules.
    3. Asking the client to describe any thoughts of self-harm.
    4. Asking the client if the group on assertiveness skills was helpful.
    5. Asking the client if a prn medication would be helpful.

17. A nursing instructor is teaching new students about various diseases that occur within cultural groups. For which cultural group is sickle cell disease a health concern?
    1. Asian/Pacific Islander Americans
    2. Jewish Americans
    3. Latino Americans
    4. Arab Americans

18. A nursing educator is teaching newly hired psychiatric nurses about how various cultural groups view mental illness. Which cultural group views mental illness as a social stigma?
    1. Jewish Americans
    2. Arab Americans
    3. Asian/Pacific Islander Americans
    4. Latino Americans

19. A religious Muslim client on a psychiatric unit pushes the tray away without eating any of the ham, rice, and vegetable entrée. To what would the nurse attribute this behavior?
    1. The client is allergic to the rice.
    2. The client is a vegetarian.
    3. The client is following kosher dietary laws.
    4. The client is following halal dietary laws.

20. A nurse, understanding the correlation between cultural groups and genetic disease, should recognize which of the following conditions as more common in the Jewish American population? **Select all that apply.**
    1. Gaucher's disease
    2. Familial dysautonomia
    3. Turner's syndrome
    4. Spondyloschisis
    5. Tay-Sachs disease

21. Based on general knowledge about the culture, which characteristics would the nurse expect to assess from a client who has recently emigrated from Italy?
    1. The client is probably future oriented.
    2. The client's family is probably small.
    3. The client's personality will probably be warm and affectionate.
    4. The client may view touching during communication as unacceptable.

1. ANSWER: 4
Rationale:
1. Genuineness is the ability of the nurse to be open and real in interactions with clients. The nurse's feelings, and the expression of these feelings, must be congruent to establish genuineness. Genuineness is not described as maintaining a nonjudgmental attitude and unconditional positive regard for the client.
2. Empathy is a criterion for the establishment of the nurse-client relationship. Empathy is defined as the ability to sense and appreciate the client's feelings. Empathy is not described as maintaining a nonjudgmental attitude and unconditional positive regard for the client.
3. Objectivity is important to maintain in the nurse-client relationship to assess a client's thoughts and feelings accurately. Objectivity is not described as maintaining a nonjudgmental attitude and unconditional positive regard for the client.
4. Respect is the nurse's ability to have unconditional positive regard for the client along with an attitude that is nonjudgmental. Respect is a criterion for the establishment of the nurse-client relationship.
TEST-TAKING TIP: Review the characteristics that enhance the establishment of the nurse-client relationship: rapport, trust, respect, genuineness, and empathy. What behaviors reflect these characteristics?
Content Area: Psychosocial Integrity;
Integrated Process: Nursing Process: Assessment;
Client Need: Psychosocial Integrity;
Cognitive Level: Application;
Concept: Nursing

2. ANSWER: 2
Rationale:
1. During the preinteraction stage of the nurse-client relationship, the goal is to explore misconceptions and prejudices.
2. During the orientation stage of the nurse-client relationship, the nurse determines why the client sought help. A contract for interaction is formulated during the orientation stage of the nurse-client relationship.
3. During the working stage of the nurse-client relationship, the nurse explores stressors and promotes insight.
4. During the termination stage of the nurse-client relationship, the nurse evaluates the client's progress and goal attainment.
TEST-TAKING TIP: Determine in which stage the nursing action in each answer choice occurs. There is no contact with the client in the preorientation stage of the nurse-client relationship. Knowing this eliminates Option 1. Review Table 4.1 as needed.
Content Area: Psychosocial Integrity;
Integrated Process: Nursing Process: Assessment;
Client Need: Psychosocial Integrity;
Cognitive Level: Application;
Concept: Nursing

3. ANSWER: 3
Rationale:
1. Catharsis is not an essential characteristic of a nurse-client relationship and should not be used until after a trusting relationship has developed.
2. Confrontation is not an essential characteristic of a nurse-client relationship and should not be used until after a trusting relationship has developed.
3. Genuineness refers to the nurse's ability to be open, honest, and "real" in interactions with clients. Trust cannot be established without the characteristic of genuineness; therefore, genuineness is an essential characteristic of the nurse-client relationship.
4. Giving advice is a nontherapeutic block to communication, not an essential characteristic of a nurse-client relationship. Advice should never be given because it encourages dependence and discourages self-direction.
TEST-TAKING TIP: Be aware of all of the characteristics that are essential to the development of a therapeutic nurse-client relationship.
Content Area: Psychosocial Integrity;
Integrated Process: Nursing Process: Assessment;
Client Need: Psychosocial Integrity;
Cognitive Level: Application;
Concept: Nursing

4. ANSWER: therapeutic
Rationale: A *therapeutic relationship* is an interaction between two people (usually a caregiver and a care receiver) in which input from both participants contributes to a climate of healing, growth promotion, and/or illness prevention. Therapeutic relationships are goal oriented. Ideally, the nurse and client decide together what the goal of the relationship will be.
TEST-TAKING TIP: How is a therapeutic relationship different from a social relationship? A therapeutic nurse-client relationship can be identified when interactions are noted to be client focused and goal oriented.
Content Area: Safe and Effective Care Environment: Management of Care;
Integrated Process: Nursing Process: Implementation;
Client Need: Safe and Effective Care Environment: Management of Care;
Cognitive Level: Knowledge;
Concept: Communication

5. ANSWER: 1
Rationale:
1. The nurse's primary goal during the termination phase of the nurse-client relationship should be to assist the client to evaluate goal attainment and ensure therapeutic closure.
2. The nurse's primary goal during the orientation, not termination phase of the nurse-client relationship, should be to establish trust and formulate a contract for intervention.
3. The nurse's primary goal during the preinteraction, not termination, phase of the nurse-client relationship should be to explore self-perceptions.

4. The nurse's primary goal during the working, not termination, phase of the nurse-client relationship should be to promote client change.

TEST-TAKING TIP: Review the phases of the nurse-client relationship and the specific goals of these phases. Review Table 4.1 as needed.

Content Area: Safe and Effective Care Environment: Management of Care;

Integrated Process: Nursing Process: Planning;

Client Need: Safe and Effective Care Environment: Management of Care;

Cognitive Level: Analysis;

Concept: Promoting Health

6. **ANSWER: 2**

Rationale:

1. Sympathy is the actual sharing of another's thoughts and feelings. Sympathy differs from empathy in that with empathy one experiences an objective understanding of what another is feeling rather than actually sharing those feelings. Sympathy is nontherapeutic, whereas empathy is therapeutic. There is nothing presented in the question to indicate that the nurse is employing sympathy.

2. The nurse is promoting trust by using closed-ended questions, offering finger foods, and reassuring the client. Trustworthiness is demonstrated though nursing interventions that convey a sense of warmth and caring to the client.

3. Veracity is an ethical principle that refers to one's duty to always be truthful. There is nothing presented in the question dealing with the nurse's veracity.

4. Congruency is the quality or state of agreeing. The nursing actions presented promote trust and are not focused on promoting congruency.

TEST-TAKING TIP: Using closed ended questions, offering finger foods, and reassuring the client are ways to promote trust in a client diagnosed with mania. Establishing trust is the foundation of an effective nurse-client relationship on which all interactions are based.

Content Area: Safe and Effective Care Environment: Management of Care;

Integrated Process: Nursing Process: Implementation;

Client Need: Safe and Effective Care Environment: Management of Care;

Cognitive Level: Application;

Concept: Promoting Health

7. **ANSWER: 2**

Rationale:

1. The nurse's statement, "You are feeling very depressed. I felt the same way when I lost my first baby," conveys sympathy. Sympathy implies that the nurse shares what the client is feeling through similar experiences and experiences a personal need to alleviate her own distress. The use of sympathy is nontherapeutic.

2. The nurse's statement, "I can understand you are feeling depressed. It is difficult to lose a baby. I'll sit with you," conveys empathy. With empathy one experiences an objective understanding of what another is feeling rather than actually sharing those feelings. The use of empathy is therapeutic.

3. Teaching this depressed client the five stages of grief is inappropriate at this time. The depressed client would not be receptive to learning. The nurse's role at this time would be to offer empathy.

4. Offering prn medication does not address the client's feelings of loss and depression. The nurse's role at this time would be to offer empathy.

TEST-TAKING TIP: Understand the necessity of offering self to clients who are in crisis. Empathy, unlike sympathy, is an appropriate way to connect with the client.

Content Area: Safe and Effective Care Environment: Management of Care;

Integrated Process: Nursing Process: Evaluation;

Client Need: Safe and Effective Care Environment: Management of Care;

Cognitive Level: Application;

Concept: Communication

8. **ANSWER: 3**

Rationale:

1. The preinteraction phase is when the nurse explores self-perceptions and reviews information about the perspective client.

2. The orientation phase is when the individuals first meet and is characterized by an agreement to continue to meet and work on setting client-centered goals.

3. The working phase is when nurse-client interactions are focused on behavioral change. The interaction of role-playing with a client to practice appropriate ways to deal with anger would occur in the working phase.

4. The termination phase is when the work of the relationship is reviewed and goal attainment is evaluated.

TEST-TAKING TIP: Review the phases of the nurse-client relationship and the specific interventions that are appropriate in each of these phases. Review Table 4.1 as needed.

Content Area: Safe and Effective Care Environment: Management of Care;

Integrated Process: Nursing Process: Implementation;

Client Need: Safe and Effective Care Environment: Management of Care;

Cognitive Level: Application;

Concept: Promoting Health

9. **ANSWER: 4**

Rationale:

1. Respect, not rapport, is the essential condition that is characterized in this example. Respect implies the dignity and worth of an individual regardless of his or her unacceptable behavior.

2. Empathy is the essential condition that is characterized in this example. Empathy is the ability to see beyond outward behavior and to understand the situation from the client's point of view.

3. Genuineness, not rapport, is the essential condition that is characterized in this example. Genuineness refers to the nurse's ability to be open, honest, and "real" in interactions.

4. Rapport is the essential condition that is characterized in this example. Rapport implies that the client and the nurse share a relationship based on acceptance, warmth, friendliness, common interests, a sense of trust, and a nonjudgmental attitude. The ability to truly care for and about others is the core of rapport.

TEST-TAKING TIP: First, recognize the conditions essential to development of a therapeutic relationship, then be able to distinguish the answer that demonstrates a situation that matches rapport.
Content Area: Psychosocial Integrity;
Integrated Process: Nursing Process: Assessment;
Client Need: Psychosocial Integrity;
Cognitive Level: Analysis;
Concept: Nursing

10. **ANSWER: 3**
Rationale:
Projection is the defense mechanism in which a client attributes feelings or impulses unacceptable to one's self to another person.
1. Although the nurse does not want the client to injure self or anyone else, this outcome does not address the situation presented in the question. The outcome is incorrectly written.
2. When a client expresses anger covertly rather than overtly, his or her feelings are concealed, hidden, or disguised; therefore, this outcome is inappropriate. The outcome is also incorrectly written.
3. The short-term outcome "The client will take responsibility for the dysfunctional behavior by the end of the shift" addresses the client's use of projection and is a correctly written outcome.
4. This outcome does not address the situation presented in the question and is written as a long-term, not a short-term, outcome.
TEST-TAKING TIP: Use the client information presented in the question (the use of projection) to formulate appropriate outcomes. A correctly written outcome must be client-centered, specific, realistic, and measurable and must also include a time frame. Note the term "short term" in the question. Short-term outcomes are expectations for clients during hospitalization, and long-term outcomes focus on what the client can accomplish after discharge.
Content Area: Safe and Effective Care Environment: Management of Care;
Integrated Process: Nursing Process: Planning;
Client Need: Safe and Effective Care Environment: Management of Care;
Cognitive Level: Application;
Concept: Critical Thinking

11. **ANSWER: 3**
Rationale:
1. Risk for other-directed violence R/T anger toward a family member would be important when the client is stabilized and discharged. Potential complications secondary to trauma would take precedence over this problem.
2. Although the client may have issues with body image due to head and abdominal injuries, this is not the priority nursing diagnosis. Potential complications secondary to trauma would take precedence over this problem.
3. Risk for injury R/T possible complications secondary to trauma is the priority diagnosis for this client. Because the client has experienced head and abdominal trauma, possible life-threatening internal injuries need to be ruled out.

4. Anxiety, tremors, and crying may be a problem for this client; however, it is not the priority because complications of the trauma may result in a life-threatening situation. Risk for anxiety R/T injuries AEB tremors and crying is an incorrectly written diagnosis. A "risk for" or potential nursing diagnosis should never contain an "as evidenced by" (AEB) statement.
TEST-TAKING TIP: When prioritizing a nursing diagnosis, it is necessary to focus on the client problem that needs immediate attention. Using Maslow's hierarchy of needs, this client's physiological problems would take priority over psychological problems. A correctly written nursing diagnosis must include (1) a problem statement (NANDA stem), (2) a R/T (related to) statement, and (3) an AEB (as evidenced by) statement. A correctly written "potential" or "risk for" nursing diagnosis does not include an AEB statement because the problem has not yet occurred.
Content Area: Safe and Effective Care Environment: Management of Care;
Integrated Process: Nursing Process: Analysis;
Client Need: Safe and Effective Care Environment: Management of Care;
Cognitive Level: Analysis;
Concept: Critical Thinking

12. **ANSWER: 1**
Rationale:
1. This outcome is incorrectly written because a "significant amount of weight" is not measureable. The specific amount of weight loss should be stated in the outcome.
2. This outcome is incorrectly written because there is no time frame for completion stated in the outcome.
3. This outcome is incorrectly written because it is unrealistic to expect all marital problems to be resolved in one session.
4. "The client will shower, shampoo, and shave by 8:00 a.m. tomorrow" is an example of a correctly written expected outcome. Outcomes should be measurable, realistic, client-focused goals that should translate into client behavior.
TEST-TAKING TIP: A correctly written outcome must be client-centered, specific, realistic, and must also include a time frame.
Content Area: Safe and Effective Care Environment: Management of Care;
Integrated Process: Nursing Process: Planning;
Client Need: Safe and Effective Care Environment: Management of Care;
Cognitive Level: Application;
Concept: Critical Thinking

13. **ANSWER: 1, 2, 5**
Rationale:
1. When assessing a newly admitted client, the nurse should maintain direct eye contact and avoid indirect eye contact with the client.
2. When assessing a newly admitted client, the nurse should lean forward and avoid leaning away from the client.
3. When assessing a newly admitted client, the nurse should sit squarely, facing the client.

4. When assessing a newly admitted client, the nurse should maintain an open posture with legs and arms uncrossed.

5. When assessing a newly admitted client, the nurse should be on the same level as the client and avoid standing when the client is sitting.

TEST-TAKING TIP: Use the acronym SOLER to identify facilitative skills for active listening. Sit squarely facing the client (S), observe and open posture (O), lean forward toward the client (L), establish eye contact (E), and relax (R).
Content Area: Safe and Effective Care Environment: Management of Care;
Integrated Process: Nursing Process: Implementation;
Client Need: Safe and Effective Care Environment: Management of Care;
Cognitive Level: Analysis;
Concept: Assessment

14. ANSWER: The correct order is 5, 1, 4, 3, 2
    Rationale:
    1. Analyzing a client's attitude after an assertiveness training session is a nursing intervention that occurs in the fifth step of the nursing process: evaluation.
    2. Scoring a client's alcohol withdrawal symptoms using a CIWA scale occurs in the first step of the nursing process: assessment.
    3. Facilitating an assertiveness training session occurs in the fourth step of the nursing process: implementation.
    4. Collaborating with a client to set a realistic weight loss goal would occur in the third step of the nursing process: planning.
    5. Documenting the client's problem in NANDA-I terms occurs in the second step of the nursing process: nursing diagnosis or analysis.

    TEST-TAKING TIP: Review the steps of the nursing process and the order in which they occur. Review Figure 4.1.
    Content Area: Safe and Effective Care Environment: Management of Care;
    Integrated Process: Nursing Process: Implementation;
    Client Need: Safe and Effective Care Environment: Management of Care;
    Cognitive Level: Analysis;
    Concept: Critical Thinking

15. ANSWER: 1, 3, 4, 5
    Rationale:
    1. This statement is a subjective assessment of sleep. Only the client can report sleep data.
    2. This is objective, not subjective, data related to mood assessment. Mood assessment is subjective in nature because it is only experienced by the client and cannot be objectively measured by the nurse. However, by using a mood scale rating system, the nurse can objectively evaluate this symptom.
    3. This statement is a subjective assessment of pain. If the client rated pain as 6 out of 10 on a scale rating system, the nurse would be able to objectively evaluate this symptom.
    4. This statement is a subjective assessment of mood. Mood assessment is subjective in nature because it is only experienced by the client and cannot be objectively

measured by the nurse. However, if the client rates mood on a scale rating system, the nurse would be able to objectively evaluate this symptom.
5. This statement is a subjective assessment of irritability. The symptom is subjective in nature because it is only experienced by the client and cannot be objectively measured by the nurse. However, if the client rates irritability on a scale rating system, the nurse would be able to objectively evaluate this symptom.

TEST-TAKING TIP: Objective data can be analyzed, measured, or counted. Subjective data is what the client perceives and is not perceptible or measurable by an observer.
Content Area: Psychosocial Integrity;
Integrated Process: Nursing Process: Assessment;
Client Need: Psychosocial Integrity;
Cognitive Level: Application;
Concept: Assessment

16. ANSWER: 1, 2, 4
    Rationale:
    1. The nurse would ask the client to rate his or her anxiety after administering an anxiolytic during the evaluation step of the nursing process. During the evaluation step, the nurse measures the success of interventions.
    2. The nurse would ask the client to verbalize understanding of explained unit rules during the evaluation step of the nursing process. During the evaluation step, the nurse measures the success of interventions.
    3. The nurse would ask the client to describe any thoughts of self-harm during the assessment step of the nursing process. Assessment involves collecting and analyzing data about the client that may include the following dimensions: physical, psychological, sociocultural, spiritual, cognitive, functional, developmental, economic, and lifestyle.
    4. The nurse would ask the client if the group on assertiveness skills was helpful during the evaluation step of the nursing process. During the evaluation step, the nurse measures the success of interventions.
    5. The nurse would ask the client if a prn medication would be helpful during the assessment step of the nursing process. Assessment involves collecting and analyzing data about the client that may include the following dimensions: physical, psychological, sociocultural, spiritual, cognitive, functional, developmental, economic, and lifestyle.

    TEST-TAKING TIP: Identify and differentiate between the five steps of the nursing process. Data are gathered in both the assessment and evaluation steps of the nursing process. Data are gathered before interventions in the assessment step and after interventions in the evaluation step to ascertain the client's response. Review Figure 4.1 as needed.
    Content Area: Psychosocial Integrity;
    Integrated Process: Nursing Process: Implementation;
    Client Need: Psychosocial Integrity;
    Cognitive Level: Analysis;
    Concept: Critical Thinking

17. ANSWER: 4
    Rationale:
    1. Asian/Pacific Islander Americans health concerns include hypertension, cancer, diabetes mellitus, thalassemia,

and lactose intolerance. This list does not include sickle cell disease.
2. Jewish American health concerns include Tay-Sachs disease, Gaucher's disease, familial dysautonomia, ulcerative colitis, Crohn's disease, colorectal cancer, breast and ovarian cancer. This list does not include sickle cell disease.
3. Latino Americans health concerns include heart disease, cancer, diabetes mellitus, and lactose intolerance. This list does not include sickle cell disease.
4. Arab American health concerns include sickle cell disease, thalassemia, cardiovascular disease, and cancer.
TEST-TAKING TIP: Recall biological variations of cultural groups that lead to differing health concerns. Review Table 5.4 in Chapter 5 of this text.
Content Area: Psychosocial Integrity;
Integrated Process: Nursing Process: Assessment;
Client Need: Psychosocial Integrity;
Cognitive Level: Application;
Concept: Diversity

18. **ANSWER: 2**
Rationale:
1. Jewish Americans have great respect for physicians, place emphasis on keeping the body and mind healthy, and practice preventive health care. There is nothing to indicate that they view mental illness as a social stigma.
2. Arab Americans view mental illness as a social stigma. They believe in a traditional health-care delivery system with some superstitious beliefs. Adverse outcomes are attributed to God's will.
3. Asian/Pacific Islander Americans believe in a traditional health-care delivery system. Some prefer to use folk practices (e.g., acupuncture and herbal medicine). There is nothing to indicate that they view mental illness as a social stigma.
4. Latino Americans believe in a traditional health-care delivery system. Some prefer to use a folk practitioner, called a *curandero* or *curandera*. There is nothing to indicate that they view mental illness as a social stigma.
TEST-TAKING TIP: Recall the attitudes and beliefs of various cultural groups regarding mental illness. Review Table 5.4 in Chapter 5 of this text.
Content Area: Psychosocial Integrity;
Integrated Process: Nursing Process: Assessment;
Client Need: Psychosocial Integrity;
Cognitive Level: Application;
Concept: Diversity

19. **ANSWER: 4**
Rationale:
1. Allergic reactions are physical responses. The client's behavior is not influenced by an allergy to rice, but to his adherence to Muslim dietary laws, which prohibit the ingestion of pork and pork products.
2. Vegetarianism is a personal choice. The client's behavior is not influenced by vegetarianism, but to his adherence to Muslim dietary laws, which prohibit the ingestion of pork and pork products.

3. The client is following halal, not kosher dietary laws, which forbids the consumption of pork and pork products, including ham.
4. This Muslim client is following the halal dietary laws of Islam, which forbids the consumption of pork and pork products, including ham.
TEST-TAKING TIP: It is important to understand how religious or cultural laws influence the consumption of food and drink.
Content Area: Safe and Effective Care Environment: Management of Care;
Integrated Process: Nursing Process: Evaluation;
Client Need: Safe and Effective Care Environment: Management of Care;
Cognitive Level: Analysis;
Concept: Diversity

20. **ANSWER: 1, 2, 5**
Rationale:
1. Guacher's disease is a chronic congenital disorder of lipid metabolism. This disease occurs frequently in people of Jewish extraction.
2. Familial dysautonomia is a rare hereditary disease involving the autonomic nervous system and is characterized by mental retardation. It is seen almost exclusively in Ashkenazi Jews.
3. Turner's syndrome is a genetic disorder that is not associated with any particular cultural group.
4. Spondyloschisis is a congenital fissure of one or more vertebral arches and is not associated with any particular cultural group.
5. Tay-Sachs disease is marked by neurological deterioration characterized by mental and physical retardation. The rate of occurrence in Ashkenazi Jews in the United States is estimated to be 400 per 1 million births.
TEST-TAKING TIP: Review the correlation between cultural groups and genetic diseases. Review Table 5.4 in Chapter 5 of this text.
Content Area: Psychosocial Integrity;
Integrated Process: Nursing Process: Assessment;
Client Need: Psychosocial Integrity;
Cognitive Level: Analysis;
Concept: Diversity

21. **ANSWER: 3**
Rationale: A client who recently emigrated from Italy would be considered a Western European American.
1. Western European Americans are present, not future, time oriented with a somewhat fatalistic view of the future.
2. Families in the Western European American culture tend to be large and extended, not small.
3. Western European Americans tend to be very warm and affectionate. They are family oriented and are physically expressive, using a lot of body language, including hugging and kissing.
4. In the Asian American, not Western European American, culture touching during communication may be considered unacceptable. Western European Americans tend to

be physically expressive, using a lot of body language, including hugging and kissing.

TEST-TAKING TIP: An Italian client would be included in the Western European American cultural group. Review Table 5.4 in Chapter 5 of this text.

Content Area: *Psychosocial Integrity;*
Integrated Process: *Nursing Process: Assessment;*
Client Need: *Psychosocial Integrity;*
Cognitive Level: *Analysis;*
Concept: *Diversity*

Communication

KEY TERMS

APIE (Assessment, Problem, Intervention, Evaluation)—A problem-oriented system of documentation that uses individualized flow sheets to record client care

BIRP (Behavior, Intervention, Response, Plan)—A documentation method primarily used in psychiatric settings that focuses on client behavior and response to interventions that will determine the client's plan of care

Blocks to communication—Barriers to communication between nurses and clients that hamper open communication and thereby the establishment of the nurse-client relationship

Charting by exception—A documentation method that relies on solid institutional standards of practice and procedures, allowing nurses to chart only when there has been a deviation in the care as outlined by that standard

Culture—Culture is an integrated system of learned behavior patterns that are characteristic of the members of a society and which are not a result of biological inheritance

Curandero (Curandera)—A male (female) folk healer in the Latino culture

DAR (Data, Action, Response)—A type of focus charting that may document any of the following: nursing diagnosis, current client concern or behavior, significant change in client status or behavior, significant event in the client's therapy

"Granny"—A folk practitioner in the African American culture, also known as "the old lady"

Late entry—Documentation of data entered into a client's record at a later time; the date and time the entry is being made and the date and time the care or observations actually occurred must be clearly stated

Nonverbal communication—The process of communication through sending and receiving wordless (mostly visual) cues between people

Paralanguage or vocal cues—The nonlinguistic components of speech; it consists of pitch, tone, and loudness of spoken messages; the rate of speaking; expressively placed pauses; and emphasis assigned to certain words; vocal cues greatly influence the way individuals interpret verbal messages

Personal distance—The distance between individuals who are having interactions of a personal nature, such as a close conversation; in the U.S. culture, personal distance is approximately 18 to 40 inches

Shaman—A folk practitioner in the Native American and other cultures, involved in religion and health practices

SOAPIE (Subjective data, Objective data, Assessment, Plan, Intervention, Evaluation)—A problem-oriented system of documentation that has as its basis a problem list

SOLER (Sit, Observe, Lean forward, Establish Eye contact, Relax)—An acronym that describes a system of nonverbal behaviors that facilitate attentive listening

Therapeutic communication—Communication that encourages exploration of feelings and fosters understanding of behavioral motivation; it is nonjudgmental, discourages defensiveness, and promotes trust

Therapeutic communication techniques—Technical procedures that assist the nurse with the communication process in order to interact more therapeutically with clients

Verbal communication—The use of spoken and written words to relay a message; it serves as a vehicle for expressing desires, ideas and concepts

Yin and yang—The fundamental concept of Asian health practices that represent opposite forces of energy such as negative/positive, dark/light, male/female, hot/cold, etc.

I. The Communication Process

A. Goal: to convey information, and the understanding of that information, from one person or group to another person or group (Fig. 5.1)

B. Steps
   1. The sender first develops an idea.
   2. The sender transmits a message through a channel to a receiver. (Developing a message is known as *encoding*.)
   3. The recipient receives the message.
   4. The recipient interprets the message and receives meaning. (Interpreting the message is referred to as *decoding*.)
   5. The recipient acknowledges understanding of the message through feedback.

C. **Therapeutic communication** describes an effective exchange of information, ideas and feelings to achieve desirable interpersonal relationships, which will be beneficial to a client's growth toward healthy living
   1. A professional technique centered on empathy.
   2. Practiced for the purposes of reducing stress and increasing understanding in both the caregiver and client.
   3. The need for therapeutic communication is evidence based (see Box 5.1).

MAKING THE CONNECTION

The critical factor in measuring the effectiveness of communication is common understanding. This understanding is achieved by the use of feedback. Understanding exists when all parties involved have a mutual agreement as to the information and its meaning. This is why a nurse should repeat a verbal order as it is transcribed into the client's record. Effective communication, therefore, occurs when the intended message of the sender and the interpreted message of the receiver are one and the same.

II. Types of Communication

DID YOU KNOW?

Therapeutic communication techniques are tools just like any other tool used in client care. If a nurse does not practice the use of sterile technique or how to give an injection, he or she may never become proficient and comfortable using these skills. Like any other nursing skill, it is necessary to continually practice therapeutic communication techniques to effectively facilitate any nurse-client interaction. Box 5.2 presents a guide for the effective use of therapeutic communication.

A. Verbal communication
   1. Therapeutic communication techniques.
      a. Offering self: making self available to the client. ("I'll stay with you if you'd like to talk.")
      b. Asking open-ended questions: asking neutral questions that cannot be answered by *yes* or *no* encourages the client to discuss concerns. Use *when, where, how, what.* ("What makes the pain worse?" "How are the voices you hear affecting you emotionally?")
      c. Broad openings: allow the client to take the initiative in introducing the topic. Ask specific open-ended questions. ("What would you like to discuss?")
      d. General leads: offer the client encouragement to continue. ("Go on ..."; "I see.").
      e. Verbalizing the implied: putting into words what the client has only implied or indirectly stated. (Client: "It's a waste of time to talk to my doctor." Nurse: "Do you feel like no one understands?" Client: "My family would be better off without me." Nurse: "Are you considering harming yourself?")
      f. Placing an event in time or sequence: clarifies the relationship of events in time to view them in perspective. ("When did your symptoms become worse in relationship to beginning your exercise program?" "After taking your

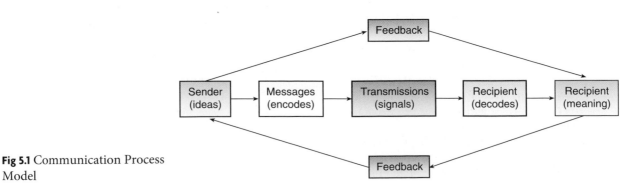

Fig 5.1 Communication Process Model

Box 5.1 The Need for Therapeutic Communication Is Evidence-Based

- Data show that many nurses do not use client-centered communication and are too task-oriented (McCabe, 2004).
- Many nurses think that talking is not part of working, and they feel a need for nurses to always look busy (Chant et. al., 2002).
- The Joint Commission emphasizes the effect that poor nurse-client communication can have on client safety, noting that "the client can also be an important source of information about potential adverse effects and hazardous conditions."

Box 5.2 The Do's of Effective Therapeutic Communication

1. Do provide/select a private, quiet, safe environment in which to hold interactions.
2. Do listen twice as much as you speak.
3. Do think of the unique situation you face before responding and consider alternatives.
4. Do acknowledge and build positive self-regard.
5. Do be simple, clear and direct in communication.
6. Do be congruent in communication.
7. Do be alert and responsive to small changes in communication.
8. Do observe all nonverbal cues in communication.
9. Do be nonjudgmental in interactions.
10. Do allow the client to proceed at his or her own pace.
11. Do accept people as they present themselves, with their strengths and weaknesses.
12. Do, through silence, provide an atmosphere for the exploration of thoughts and feelings.
13. Do remember that there is always the potential for growth and healthy living. There are no "hopeless" or "hard-core" individuals.

antidepressant, how long did it take for your mood to improve?")

g. Encouraging comparison: asking the client to compare similarities and differences in ideas, experiences, or interpersonal relationships. ("Tell me about your blood sugar levels when you were on the diet and when you were not." "Let's compare your anxiety level when you are taking your medication and when you are not.")

h. Opening remarks, or making observations: using general statements based on observations and assessments for the client to initiate discussion. ("You seemed sad after speaking with your doctor." "I noticed that you took a shower and washed your hair.")

i. Restatement: repeating the client's conversation content, typically using the same words. (Client: "I'm worried about my potential disability."

Nurse: "You're worried about your ability to function?" Client: "My father was very strict." Nurse: "Your father was very strict?")

j. Reflection: Identifying the various emotional themes in a conversation and directing these back to the client. The nurse connects feelings to verbalized content. (Client: "My husband may look at me differently after the surgery." Nurse: "You're anxious about how this surgery may affect your relationship?") (Client: "My parents are so used to my depressed moods." Nurse: "Are you feeling that you're a disappointment to your family?")

k. Focusing: guiding the client to narrow in on key concerns. Can be termed "exploring" when delving further into a subject, idea, experience, or relationship without probing. ("You've told me about your support system. Can we talk about who will assist you when you first get home from the hospital?")

l. Seeking clarification: assisting the client to put into words unclear thoughts or feelings that the nurse doesn't understand. ("Help me to understand your treatment expectations." "I'm not sure what you mean when you use the word 'scatterbrained'.")

m. Giving information: sharing with the client relevant information for his or her health care and well-being. The nurse is functioning in the role of teacher. ("I'm going to review the side effects of this new medication." "Let me tell you a few things about your diagnosis.")

n. Looking at alternatives: helping the client see options and participate in the decision-making process. ("How do you think you can best comply with your diabetic diet?" "Which do you feel is more helpful: journaling or discussing your problems with peers?")

o. Silence: allowing for a pause in the conversation that permits the nurse and client time to think about what has taken place. (No verbalization.)

p. Summarizing: highlighting the importance of a conversation by condensing what was said. Can be used to evaluate learning. ("We have reviewed the side effects of this medication, how to take it, how to store it, and how to evaluate its affect.") (See Table 5.1.)

DID YOU KNOW?
Clients seldom write letters to the CEO of the hospital to praise a nurse's "excellent technique while inserting my catheter." Letters are written to recognize the nurse that took the time to listen and encouraged open and unrestricted communication with the client.

Table 5.1 **Therapeutic Communication Techniques**

Technique	Explanation/Rationale	Examples
Using silence	Gives the client the opportunity to collect and organize thoughts, to think through a point, or to consider introducing a topic of greater concern than the one being discussed.	
Accepting	Conveys an attitude of reception and regard.	"Yes, I understand what you said." Eye contact; nodding.
Giving recognition	Acknowledging and indicating awareness; better than complimenting, which reflects the nurse's judgment.	"Hello, Mr. J. I notice that you made a ceramic ash tray in OT." "I see you made your bed."
Offering self	Making oneself available on an unconditional basis, increasing client's feelings of self-worth.	"I'll stay with you awhile." "We can eat our lunch together." "I'm interested in you."
Giving broad openings	Allows the client to take the initiative in introducing the topic; emphasizes the importance of the client's role in the interaction.	"What would you like to talk about today?" "Tell me what you are thinking."
Offering general leads	Offers the client encouragement to continue.	"Yes, I see." "Go on." "And after that?"
Placing the event in time or sequence	Clarifies the relationship of events in time so that the nurse and client can view them in perspective.	"What seemed to lead up to. . .?" "Was this before or after. . .?" "When did this happen?"
Making observations	Verbalizing what is observed or perceived. This encourages the client to recognize specific behaviors and compare perceptions with the nurse.	"You seem tense." "I notice you are pacing a lot." "You seem uncomfortable when you. . ."
Encouraging description of perceptions	Asking the client to verbalize what is being perceived; often used with clients experiencing hallucinations.	"Tell me what is happening now." "Are you hearing the voices again?" "What do the voices seem to be saying?"
Encouraging comparison	Asking the client to compare similarities and differences in ideas, experiences, or interpersonal relationships. This helps the client recognize life experiences that tend to recur as well as those aspects of life that are changeable.	"Was this something like. . .?" "How does this compare with the time when. . .?" "What was your response the last time this situation occurred?"
Restating	Repeating the main idea of what the client has said. This lets the client know whether or not an expressed statement has been understood and gives him or her the chance to continue or to clarify if necessary.	Cl: "I can't study. My mind keeps wandering." Ns: "You have trouble concentrating." Cl: "I can't take that new job. What if I can't do it?" Ns: "You're afraid you will fail in this new position."
Reflecting	Questions and feelings are referred back to the client so that they may be recognized and accepted, and so that the client may recognize that his or her point of view has value—a good technique to use when the client asks the nurse for advice.	Cl: "What do you think I should do about my wife's drinking problem?" Ns: "What do *you* think you should do?" Cl: "My sister won't help a bit toward my mother's care. I have to do it all!" Ns: "You feel angry when she doesn't help."
Focusing	Taking notice of a single idea or even a single word; works especially well with a client who is moving rapidly from one thought to another. Note: This technique is *not* therapeutic, however, with the client who is very anxious. Focusing should not be pursued until the anxiety level has subsided.	"This point seems worth looking at more closely. Perhaps you and I can discuss it together."

Table 5.1 Therapeutic Communication Techniques—cont'd

Technique	Explanation/Rationale	Examples
Exploring	Delving further into a subject, idea, experience, or relationship; especially helpful with clients who tend to remain on a superficial level of communication. However, if the client chooses not to disclose further information, the nurse should refrain from pushing or probing in an area that obviously creates discomfort.	"Please explain that situation in more detail." "Tell me more about that particular situation."
Seeking clarification and validation	Striving to explain that which is vague or incomprehensible and searching for mutual understanding. Clarifying the meaning of what has been said facilitates and increases understanding for both client and nurse.	"I'm not sure that I understand. Would you please explain?" "Tell me if my understanding agrees with yours." "Do I understand correctly that you said. . .?"
Presenting reality	When the client has a misperception of the environment, the nurse defines reality or indicates his or her perception of the situation for the client.	"I understand that the voices seem real to you, but I do not hear any voices." "There is no one else in the room but you and me."
Voicing doubt	Expressing uncertainty as to the reality of the client's perceptions; often used with clients experiencing delusional thinking.	"I understand that you believe that to be true, but I see the situation differently." "I find that hard to believe (or accept)." "That seems rather doubtful to me."
Verbalizing the implied	Putting into words what the client has only implied or said indirectly; can also be used with the client who is mute or is otherwise experiencing impaired verbal communication. This clarifies that which is *implicit* rather than *explicit*.	Cl: "It's a waste of time to be here. I can't talk to you or anyone." Ns: "Are you feeling that no one understands?" Cl: (Mute) Ns: "It must have been very difficult for you when your husband died in the fire."
Attempting to translate words into feelings	When feelings are expressed indirectly, the nurse tries to "de-symbolize" what has been said and to find clues to the underlying true feelings.	Cl: "I'm way out in the ocean." Ns: "You must be feeling very lonely right now."
Formulating a plan of action	When a client has a plan in mind for dealing with what is considered to be a stressful situation, it may serve to prevent anger or anxiety from escalating to an unmanageable level.	"What could you do to let your anger out harmlessly?" "Next time this comes up, what might you do to handle it more appropriately?"

Source: Adapted from Hays & Larson (1963).

2. Nontherapeutic blocks to communication.

On the surface, blocks to communication may sound helpful to the client, but don't be fooled. "Don't cry; everything will be alright soon" may be said to offer comfort and support, but the underlying message the client interprets is "I really would rather not hear your concerns." A nurse may resort to the use of a communication block to avoid anxiety generated by a stressful topic or situation.

a. False reassurance: Giving reassurance that is not based on the real situation, minimizing the client's concerns. ("You've got nothing to worry about.")

b. Giving advice: telling the client what to do. Focused exclusively on the nurse's experience and opinions. ("Why don't you rely on your family for financial support?" "If I were you, I would choose the residential care facility.")

c. Changing the subject: introducing an unrelated topic with the nurse taking over the direction of the discussion. (Client: "How long do people with this disease usually live?" Nurse: "Didn't you say your family was coming to visit?")

d. Being moralistic, approving, or disapproving: seeing a situation as good or bad, right or wrong. ("It is great that you made that decision.")

e. Requesting an explanation: asking the client "why" he or she has certain thoughts, feelings, or behaviors. ("Why did you stop taking your blood pressure medication?" "Tell me why you are refusing to go to group therapy?")

f. Belittling expressed feelings: statements that diminish the client's feelings, fail to recognize the client's discomfort, or ignore the uniqueness of the client's situation. ("All postop clients experience some degree of pain." "Don't worry; all schizophrenics hear voices before treatment.")

g. Making stereotyped or superficial comments: offering meaningless clichés or trite expressions. ("Time will heal." "It all happened for a reason.")

MAKING THE CONNECTION

When a nurse asks a client a "why" question, the client is forced to defend his or her behaviors or feelings. Clients may not have the insight to provide an explanation and can be intimidated and put on the defensive by the request.

h. Closed-ended questions: questions that can be answered either yes or no, thereby limiting the client's responses. ("Are you in pain?" "Are you hearing voices?") (See Table 5.2.)

Table 5.2 Nontherapeutic Communication Blocks

Block	Explanation/Rationale	Examples
Giving reassurance	Indicates to the client that there is no cause for anxiety, thereby devaluing the client's feelings; may discourage the client from further expression of feelings if he or she believes they will only be downplayed or ridiculed.	"I wouldn't worry about that If I were you." "Everything will be all right." **Better to say:** "We will work on that together."
Rejecting	Refusing to consider or showing contempt for the client's ideas or behavior. This may cause the client to discontinue interaction with the nurse for fear of further rejection.	"Let's not discuss. . ." "I don't want to hear about. . ." **Better to say:** "Let's look at that a little closer."
Approving or disapproving	Sanctioning or denouncing the client's ideas or behavior; implies that the nurse has the right to pass judgment on whether the client's ideas or behaviors are "good" or "bad," and that the client is expected to please the nurse. The nurse's acceptance of the client is then seen as conditional depending on the client's behavior.	"That's good. I'm glad that you. . ." "That's bad. I'd rather you wouldn't. . ." **Better to say:** "Let's talk about how your behavior invoked anger in the other clients at dinner."
Agreeing or disagreeing	Indicating accord with or opposition to the client's ideas or opinions; implies that the nurse has the right to pass judgment on whether the client's ideas or opinions are "right" or "wrong." Agreement prevents the client from later modifying his or her point of view without admitting error. Disagreement implies inaccuracy, provoking the need for defensiveness on the part of the client.	"That's right. I agree." "That's wrong. I disagree." "I don't believe that." **Better to say:** "Let's discuss what you feel is unfair about the new community rules."
Giving advice	Telling the client what to do or how to behave implies that the nurse knows what is best and that the client is incapable of any self-direction. It nurtures the client in the dependent role by discouraging independent thinking.	"I think you should. . ." "Why don't you. . ." **Better to say:** "What do you think you should do?" or "What do you think would be the best way to solve this problem?"
Probing	Persistent questioning of the client; pushing for answers to issues the client does not wish to discuss. This causes the client to feel used and valued only for what is shared with the nurse and places the client on the defensive.	"Tell me how your mother abused you when you were a child." "Tell me how you feel toward your mother now that she is dead." "Now tell me about. . ." **Better technique:** The nurse should be aware of the client's response and discontinue the interaction at the first sign of discomfort.

Table 5.2 Nontherapeutic Communication Blocks—cont'd		
Block	**Explanation/Rationale**	**Examples**
Defending	Attempting to protect someone or something from verbal attack. To defend what the client has criticized is to imply that he or she has no right to express ideas, opinions, or feelings. Defending does not change the client's feelings and may cause the client to think the nurse is taking sides against the client.	"No one here would lie to you." "You have a very capable physician. I'm sure he only has your best interests in mind." **Better to say:** "I will try to answer your questions and clarify some issues regarding your treatment."
Requesting an explanation	Asking the client to provide the reasons for thoughts, feelings, behavior, and events. Asking "why" a client did something or feels a certain way can be intimidating and implies that the client must defend his or her behavior or feelings.	"Why do you think that?" "Why do you feel this way?" "Why did you do that?" **Better to say:** "Describe what you were feeling just before that happened."
Indicating the existence of an external source of power	Attributing the source of thoughts, feelings, and behavior to others or to outside influences. This encourages the client to project blame for his or her thoughts or behaviors on others rather than accepting the responsibility personally.	"What makes you say that?" "What made you do that?" "What made you so angry last night?" **Better to say:** "You became angry when your brother insulted your wife."
Belittling feelings expressed	When the nurse misjudges the degree of the client's discomfort, a lack of empathy and understanding may be conveyed. The nurse may tell the client to "perk up" or "snap out of it." This causes the client to feel insignificant or unimportant. When one is experiencing discomfort, it is no relief to hear that others are or have been in similar situations.	Cl: "I have nothing to live for. I wish I were dead." Ns: "Everybody gets down in the dumps at times. I feel that way myself sometimes." **Better to say:** "You must be very upset. Tell me what you are feeling right now."
Making stereotyped comments	Clichés and trite expressions are meaningless in a nurse-client relationship. When the nurse makes empty conversation, it encourages a like response from the client.	"I'm fine, and how are you?" "Hang in there. It's for your own good." "Keep your chin up." **Better to say:** "The therapy must be difficult for you at times. How do you feel about your progress at this point?"
Using denial	Denying that a problem exists blocks discussion with the client and avoids helping the client identify and explore areas of difficulty.	Cl: "I'm nothing." Ns: "Of course you're something. Everybody is somebody." **Better to say:** "You're feeling like no one cares about you right now."
Interpreting	With this technique, the therapist seeks to make conscious that which is unconscious, to tell the client the meaning of his or her experience.	"What you really mean is. . ." "Unconsciously you're saying. . ." **Better technique:** The nurse must leave interpretation of the client's behavior to the psychiatrist. The nurse has not been prepared to perform this technique, and in attempting to do so, may endanger other nursing roles with the client.
Introducing an unrelated topic	Changing the subject causes the nurse to take over the direction of the discussion. This may occur in order to get to something that the nurse wants to discuss with the client or to get away from a topic that he or she would prefer not to discuss.	Cl: "I don't have anything to live for." Ns: "Did you have visitors this weekend?" **Better technique:** The nurse must remain open and free to hear the client and to take in all that is being conveyed, both verbally and nonverbally.

Source: Adapted from Hays & Larson (1963).

DID YOU KNOW?

When you need specific information quickly, a closed-ended question can be useful ("Are you currently considering harming yourself?"). Also when a client is experiencing pressured speech, flight of ideas, or disorganized thinking, closed-ended questions can help the client focus.

B. Nonverbal communication
   1. Facial animation.
   2. Eye contact.
   3. Occasional head nodding.
   4. Soft, firm tone of voice.
   5. Occasional smiling.
   6. Occasional hand gestures.
   7. Moderate rate of speech.
   8. Active listening (**SOLER: an acronym to assist with active listening**).
      a. S—Sit facing the client. Sends message that the nurse is listening and interested.
      b. O—Observe an Open posture.
         i. Arms and legs uncrossed
         ii. Closed posture is defensive in nature
      c. L—Lean forward toward the client.
         i. Conveys involvement in interaction
         ii. Conveys sincere effort to be attentive
      d. E—Establish Eye contact.
         i. Communicates attentiveness and involvement
         ii. Should include smiling and intermittent nodding
      e. R—Relax
         i. Communicates comfort with the client
         ii. Avoid restlessness and fidgeting (communicates discomfort) (Table 5.3)

DID YOU KNOW?

It's not what you say but how you say it! According to A. Barbour, author of *Louder Than Words: Nonverbal Communication,* the total impact of a message breaks down like this: 7% verbal (words), 38% vocal (volume, pitch, rhythm, etc.), 55% body movements (mostly facial expressions).

IV. Multicultural Considerations Related to Communication

A. Cultural factors that influence communication:
   1. Language: spoken and written word.
   2. **Paralanguage** or vocal cues: the voice quality, intonation, rhythm, and speed of speech.

Table 5.3 Summary of Facial Expressions

Facial Expression	Associated Feelings
Nose	
Nostril flare	Anger; arousal
Wrinkling up	Dislike; disgust
Lips	
Grin; smile	Happiness; contentment
Grimace	Fear; pain
Compressed	Anger; frustration
Canine-type snarl	Disgust
Pouted; frown	Unhappiness; discontented; disapproval
Pursing	Disagreement
Sneer	Contempt; disdain
Brows	
Frown	Anger; unhappiness; concentration
Raised	Surprise; enthusiasm
Tongue	
Stuck out	Dislike; disagree
Eyes	
Widened	Surprise; excitement
Narrowed; lids squeezed shut	Threat; fear
Stare	Threat
Stare/blink/look away	Dislike; disinterest
Eyes downcast; lack of eye contact	Submission; low self-esteem
Eye contact (generally intermittent, as opposed to a stare)	Self-confidence; interest

Adapted from Givens (2012b); Hughey (1990); and Simon (2005).

3. Gestures.
   a. Touch.
   b. Facial expression.
   c. Eye movements.
   d. Body posture.
4. Space.
   a. Related to the place where the communication occurs.
   b. Encompasses the concepts of territoriality, density, and distance.
      i. Intimate distance: 0 to 18 inches
      ii. **Personal distance:** 18 to 40 inches
      iii. Social distance: 4 to 12 feet
      iv. Public distance: exceeds 12 feet

Even though specific distances between people are labeled as intimate, personal, social, and public, these distances are influenced by and may be increased or decreased based on an individual's cultural background. The distance between two people who are communicating can positively or negatively affect the communication process.

    5. Time: differs in meaning and value to various cultures.
      a. Orientation.
        i. Oriented to the past: past events drive current values, relationships, and decisions
        ii. Oriented to the present: living in the here and now, basing values, relationships, and decisions on what is being currently experienced
        iii. Oriented to the future: values, relationships, and decisions are based on what might be, without possibly doing what is necessary in the present to attain future goals
      b. Some cultures, such as African and Latino Americans, are unlikely to value time or punctuality to the same degree as the dominant cultural group, which may cause them to be labeled as irresponsible.
    6. Environmental control.
      a. Perception of culturally influenced roles.
      b. The control and limitations that accompany these roles.
    7. Religion: sensitivity to religious beliefs and practices must be incorporated into the communication process.
    8. Age: communication patterns, words, acronyms, and slang vary from generation to generation.
    9. Gender: patterns of communication, both verbal and nonverbal, are influenced by the gender of the sender and the receiver.
B. Comparison of cultural phenomena in various cultural groups (see Table 5.4)

If the client receives care from a local folk healer, the folk healer should be incorporated in the communication process. Folk healers can influence both treatment adherence and nonadherence. Folk healing treatments may negatively interact with mainstream interventions.

MAKING THE CONNECTION

Although punctuality and efficiency may be a priority in one culture, a client from another culture may not place a high value on meeting scheduled appointment times. Maintaining eye contact is considered a positive assessment on a mental health examination, but clients may avoid eye contact if their cultural norms consider this behavior rude. Cultural influences must be considered when evaluating client behavior.

V. Documenting Client Care

Because of altered thinking that frequently accompanies the diagnosis of mental illness, there may be an increased risk of litigation in a psychiatric setting. For example, a client with paranoid delusions could believe that the staff is poisoning food and sue the hospital for damages. Written documentation is considered legal evidence, and every effort should be made to present accurate information.

A. Documentation requirements
  1. Promptly recorded.
  2. Dated.
  3. Clear.
  4. Concise.
  5. Legible.
  6. Signed with professional title.
B. Correcting errors in legal documentation
  1. Never obliterate a charting error.
  2. Line through incorrect information.
  3. Date, time, and initial error correction.
  4. Include explanatory note field in electronic charting.
C. Abbreviation usage
  1. Only authorized abbreviations should be used.
  2. There are many abbreviations that are unique to the mental health care setting (see Box 5.3).

The Joint Commission has published a list of "Do Not Use" abbreviations. These abbreviations, listed in Box 5.4, consistently result in significant errors because of incorrect interpretation.

DID YOU KNOW?
The documentation of client information can vary considerably from facility to facility. Documentation can be digital by the use of computerized charting systems or be handwritten in narrative form with or without the use of flow sheets. Increasing numbers of health-care institutions are moving toward the use of electronic charting.

C. Types of documentation
  1. SOAPIE.
    a. S and O (Subjective and Objective data).
    b. A (Assessment).
    c. P (Plan).
    d. I (Intervention).
    e. E (Evaluation).
  2. APIE.
    a. A (Assessment).
    b. P (Problem).
    c. I (Intervention).
    d. E (Evaluation).

Table 5.4 **Summary of Six Cultural Phenomena in Comparison of Various Cultural Groups**

Cultural Group and Countries of Origin	Communication	Space
Northern European Americans (England, Ireland, Germany, others)	National languages (although many learn English very quickly) Dialects (often regional) English More verbal than nonverbal	Territory valued Personal space: 18 inches to 3 feet Uncomfortable with personal contact and touch
African Americans (Africa, West Indian Islands, Dominican Republic, Haiti, Jamaica)	National languages Dialects (pidgin, Creole, Gullah, French, Spanish) Highly verbal and nonverbal	Close personal space Comfortable with touch
Native Americans (North America, Alaska, Aleutian Islands)	200 tribal languages recognized Comfortable with silence Direct eye contact considered rude	Large, extended space important Uncomfortable with touch
Asian/Pacific Islander Americans (Japan, China, Korea, Vietnam, Philippines, Thailand, Cambodia, Laos, Pacific Islands, others)	More than 30 languages spoken Comfortable with silence Uncomfortable with eye-to-eye contact Nonverbal connotations may be misunderstood	Large personal space Uncomfortable with touch
Latino Americans (Mexico, Spain, Cuba, Puerto Rico, other countries of Central and South America)	Spanish, with many dialects	Close personal space Lots of touching and embracing Very group oriented
Western European Americans (France, Italy, Greece)	National languages Dialects	Close personal space Lots of touching and embracing Very group oriented
Arab Americans (Algeria, Bahrain, Comoros, Djibouti, Egypt, Iraq, Jordan, Kuwait, Lebanon, Libya, Mauritania, Morocco, Oman, Palestine, Qatar, Saudi Arabia, Somalia, Sudan, Syria, Tunisia, United Arab Emirates, Yemen)	Arabic, numerous dialects English	Large personal space between members of the opposite gender outside of the family Touching common between members of same gender
Jewish Americans (Spain, Portugal, Germany, Eastern Europe)	English, Hebrew, Yiddish	Touch forbidden between opposite genders in the Orthodox tradition Closer personal space common among non-Orthodox Jews

Sources: Giger (2013); Murray, Zentner, & Yakimo (2009); Purnell & Paulanka (2008); and Spector (2009).

Social Organization	Time	Environmental Control	Biological Variations
Families: nuclear and extended Religions: Jewish and Christian Organizations: social community	Future-oriented	Most value preventive medicine and primary health care through traditional health-care delivery system Alternative methods on the increase	Health concerns: Cardiovascular disease Cancer Diabetes mellitus
Large, extended families Many female-headed households Strong religious orientation, mostly Protestant Community social organizations	Present-time oriented	Traditional health-care delivery system Some individuals prefer to use folk practitioner ("granny" or voodoo healer) Home remedies	Health concerns: Cardiovascular disease Hypertension Sickle cell disease Diabetes mellitus Lactose intolerance
Families: nuclear and extended Children taught importance of tradition Social organizations: tribe and family most important	Present-time oriented	Religion and health practices intertwined. Nontraditional healer (shaman) uses folk practices to heal Shaman may work with modern medical practitioner	Health concerns: Alcoholism Tuberculosis Accidents Diabetes mellitus Heart disease
Families: nuclear and extended Children taught importance of family loyalty and tradition Many religions: Taoism, Buddhism, Islam, Hinduism, Christianity Community social organizations	Present-time oriented Past is important and valued	Traditional health care delivery system Some prefer to use folk practices (e.g., herbal medicine, and moxibustion)	Health concerns: Hypertension Cancer Diabetes mellitus Thalassemia Lactose intolerance
Families: nuclear and large extended families Strong ties to Roman Catholicism Community social organizations	Present-time oriented	Traditional health-care delivery system Some prefer to use folk practitioner, called *curandero* or *curandera* Folk practices include "hot and cold" herbal remedies	Health concerns: Heart disease Cancer Diabetes mellitus Accidents Lactose intolerance
Families: nuclear and large extended families France and Italy: Roman Catholic Greece: Greek Orthodox	Present-time oriented	Traditional health-care delivery system Lots of home remedies and practices based on superstition	Health concerns: Heart disease Cancer Diabetes mellitus Thalassemia
Families: nuclear and extended Religion: Islam and Christianity	Past- and present- time oriented	Traditional health-care delivery system Some superstitious beliefs Authority of physician is seldom challenged or questioned Adverse outcomes are attributed to God's will Mental illness viewed as a social stigma	Health concerns: Sickle cell disease Thalassemia Cardiovascular disease Cancer
Families: nuclear and extended Community social organizations	Past-, present-, and future- time oriented	Great respect for physicians Emphasis on keeping body and mind healthy Practice preventive health care	Health concerns: Tay-Sachs disease Gaucher's disease Familial dysautonomia Ulcerative colitis Crohn's disease Colorectal cancer Breast cancer Ovarian cancer

Box 5.3 Abbreviations Commonly Used in Psychiatric Settings

Related to Diagnoses

AD	Addictive disorder
ADD	Attention-deficit disorder
ADHD	Attention deficit-hyperactivity disorder
ASD	Autism spectrum disorder
BPAD	Bipolar affective disorder
BPD	Borderline personality disorder
DID	Dissociative identity disorder
DO	disorder
FD	Factitious disorder
FNSD	Functional neurological symptom disorder
GAD	Generalized anxiety disorder
GD	Gender dysphoria
IAD	Illness anxiety disorder
IDD	Intellectual developmental disorder
MDE	Major depressive episode
NCD	Neurocognitive disorder
NDD	Neurodevelopmental disorder
OCD	Obsessive-compulsive disorder
PTSD	Post-traumatic stress disorder
R/O disorder	Rule out ex: R/O BPD (rule out borderline personality disorder)
SAFD	Schizoaffective disorder
SI disorder	Substance induced ex: SIDD (substance-induced depressive disorder)
SSD	Schizophrenia spectrum disorder
SUD	Substance use disorder
TBI	Traumatic brain injury

Related to Treatment

DOC	Department of corrections
ECT	Electroconvulsive therapy
HUD	Housing and urban development

LSW	Licensed social worker
MHA	Mental health association
MHICM	Mental health intensive case management
MSW	Master's degree in social work
NAMI	National Alliance for the Mentally Ill
OT	Occupational therapy
RCF	Residential care facility
RT	Recreational therapy
SUTC	Substance use treatment center
UR	Unit restrictions
VR	Vocational rehabilitation

Related to Assessment

AH	Auditory Hallucinations
AVH	Audio/Visual Hallucinations
CAH	Command Auditory Hallucinations
CIWA	Clinical Institute Withdrawal Assessment
DFA	Difficulty Falling Asleep
EMA	Early Morning Awakening
EPS	Extrapyramidal Symptoms
ETOH	Alcohol
FOI	Flight of Ideas
HI	Homicidal Ideation
LA	Loose associations
MNA	Middle of the night awakening
NMS	Neuroleptic malignant syndrome
SI	Suicidal ideation
TD	Tardive dyskinesia
TC	Thought content
TP	Thought process
VH	Visual hallucinations

Box 5.4 Joint Commission Official "Do Not Use" List of Abbreviations

Official "Do Not Use" List*

Do Not Use	Potential Problem	Use Instead
U (unit)	Mistaken for "0" (zero), the number "4" (four) or "cc"	Write "unit"
IU (International Unit)	Mistaken for IV (intravenous) or the number 10 (ten)	Write "International Unit"
Q.D., QD, q.d., qd (daily)	Mistaken for each other	Write "daily"
Q.O.D., QOD, q.o.d, qod (every other day)	Period after the Q mistaken for "I" and the "O" mistaken for "I"	Write "every other day"
Trailing zero (X.0 mg)†	Decimal point is missed	Write X mg
Lack of leading zero (.X mg)		Write 0.X mg
MS	Can mean morphine sulfate or magnesium sulfate	Write "morphine sulfate"
MSO4 and MgSO4	Confused for one another	Write "magnesium sulfate"

*Applies to all orders and all medication-related documentation that is handwritten (including free-text computer entry) or on preprinted forms.

†Exception: A "trailing zero" may be used only where required to demonstrate the level of precision of the value being reported, such as for laboratory results, imaging studies that report size of lesions or catheter/tube sizes. It may not be used in medication orders or other medication-related documentation.

Box 5.4 Joint Commission Official "Do Not Use" List of Abbreviations—cont'd

Additional Abbreviations, Acronyms and Symbols
(For possible future inclusion in the Official "Do Not Use" List)

Do Not Use	Potential Problem	Use Instead
> (greater than)	Misinterpreted as the number "7" (seven) or the letter "L"	Write "greater than"
< (less than)	Confused for one another	Write "less than"
Abbreviations for drug names	Misinterpreted due to similar abbreviations for multiple drugs	Write drug names in full
Apothecary units	Unfamiliar to many practitioners	Use metric units
	Confused with metric units	
@	Mistaken for the number 2" (two)	Write "at"
cc	Mistaken for U (units) when poorly written	Write "mL" or "mL" or "milliliters" ("mL" is preferred)
mcg	Mistaken for mg (milligrams) resulting in one thousand-fold overdose	Write "mcg" or "microgram"

3. **BIRP.**
    a. B (Behavior).
    b. I (Intervention).
    c. R (Response).
    d. P (Planning).
4. **DAR.**
    a. D (Data).
    b. A (Action).
    c. R (Response).
5. **Charting by exception.**
    a. Must have standards of practice and procedures in place.
    b. Only document abnormal findings.
    c. Flow sheets are used.
6. Electronic documentation.
    a. Client information is documented in digital form that is accessible to multiple providers.
    b. Provides for immediate retrieval of client information.
    c. Information can be sorted and retrieved by category.
    d. Provides links to multiple databases.
    e. Reduces errors due to illegible handwriting.

DID YOU KNOW?

Documentation of client care is classified as verbal communication. The written word is simply a replacement for the spoken word, thus the written word would qualify as "verbal" communication.

REVIEW QUESTIONS

1. A depressed client states, "I desperately want to get pregnant, but my husband is not so sure we should have children." Which response by the nurse would be an example of therapeutic communication?
   1. "Why do you think that your husband has doubts about having children?"
   2. "You still have time to convince him. I'm sure he'll change his mind."
   3. "What makes you think that your husband doesn't want children?"
   4. "Talking about this will make you anxious and increase your depression."

2. Which is an example of an open-ended question?
   1. "Did you say that your wife had a miscarriage last summer?"
   2. "Has your appetite improved since you have been admitted?"
   3. "Are you happy about being discharged today?"
   4. "How do you feel about your girlfriend's affair?"

3. During a teaching session, the nursing instructor states, "We have discussed many personality disorders. Let's concentrate on antisocial personality disorder because these individuals are so disruptive to our society." The instructor has used which communication technique?
   1. Giving information
   2. Reflection
   3. Verbalizing the implied
   4. Focusing

4. Which is an example of the therapeutic communication technique of "offering a general lead"?
   1. Client: "My wife is threatening to take sole custody of our children."
      Nurse: "I see."
   2. Client: "I need to talk to you about my divorce."
      Nurse: "Where would you like to begin?"
   3. Client: "Since the divorce I feel hollow inside."
      Nurse: "Help me understand what you mean when you say 'hollow.'"
   4. Client: "I don't think I will ever be able to marry again."
      Nurse: "You won't ever be able to marry again?"

5. Which is an example of the therapeutic communication technique of "broad opening"?
   1. Client: "I've got more problems than you can imagine."
      Nurse: "Tell me about them."
   2. Client: (Sitting quietly alone.)
      Nurse: "Is there anything you would like to talk about?"
   3. Client: "I called my mother yesterday."
      Nurse: "And?"
   4. Client: "I'm debating about whether to get a face lift."
      Nurse: "They are expensive. You should think of other ways to feel young."

6. A client on an inpatient psychiatric unit states, "I don't think I will ever be able to get into a decent relationship." The nurse responds, "You are feeling powerless about establishing relationships?" Which communication technique has the nurse employed?
   1. Restating
   2. Focusing
   3. Reflection
   4. Exploring

7. A client states, "My husband says I'm cold, but actually I think I am hot!" In an attempt to clarify the meaning of the client's statement, which nursing response is most appropriate?
   1. "In what context are you using the word 'hot'?"
   2. "Tell me more about that sensation."
   3. "I find that hard to believe."
   4. "Are you feeling rejected by your husband?"

8. A client states, "I'm worried about my potential disability." The nurse responds, "You're worried about your disability?" Which communication technique is exemplified by this exchange?
   1. Broad opening
   2. Verbalizing the implied
   3. Restating
   4. Formulating a plan of action

9. Which example of a therapeutic communication technique should the nurse use when trying to obtain general information?
   1. "You seem to be upset. Why do you feel this way?"
   2. "Are you feeling okay today?"
   3. "Let's talk about your family situation."
   4. "I hope that you are packed and ready to leave."

10. Which are correct statements related to the following nurse-client communication exchange? Client: "My mother neglected me." Nurse: "I see. Go on …" **Select all that apply.**
    1. The communication technique is classified as therapeutic.
    2. The communication technique is described as a "broad opening."
    3. The communication technique is described as "giving recognition."
    4. The communication technique is used to clarify revealed information.
    5. The communication technique is used to communicate that the nurse is listening.

11. A nursing instructor provides the following nurse-client interactions and asks a student to choose examples of "making stereotyped comments." Which student choice indicates that further instruction is needed?
    1. Client: "I'll never get over the loss of my husband."
       Nurse: "I know this is how you feel now, but time will heal."
    2. Client: "I can't believe I threw away a winning lottery ticket."
       Nurse: "I know this is upsetting, but you can't cry over spilt milk."
    3. Client: "This is the third time I didn't get what I ordered for breakfast."
       Nurse: "Did we get up on the wrong side of the bed this morning?"
    4. Client: "I don't believe my psychiatrist is being truthful with me."
       Nurse: "No one here would lie to you."

12. A client is unsure about living arrangements after discharge. The nurse states, "If I were you, I would stay at a residential care facility until you are more stable." Which client reaction is correctly matched with the communication block used by the nurse?
    1. The client is discouraged from making independent decisions.
    2. The client's concerns are minimized.
    3. The client may become defensive.
    4. The client's responses may be limited.

13. In response to the client's statement, "I feel like I'm about to jump out of my skin!" the nurse states, "Are you expecting visitors today?" The nurse has used the nontherapeutic block of

    _____   _____   _____ .

14. A nursing instructor is teaching about the use of therapeutic techniques and nontherapeutic blocks to communication. Which student statement indicates that learning has occurred?
    1. "Making an approval statement such as 'That was a great decision' is considered nontherapeutic."
    2. "The technique of 'verbalizing the implied' is considered nontherapeutic because the nurse is making an assumption."
    3. "The technique of 'suggesting collaboration' is nontherapeutic because it implies that there is collusion between the nurse and the client."
    4. "Silence is a nontherapeutic technique that should be avoided."

15. Which of the following factors can affect the communication process? **Select all that apply.**
    1. Culture
    2. Religion
    3. Age
    4. Gender
    5. Sleep patterns

16. Order the following steps of the communication process from first (1) to last (5).
    1. _____ A person receives a message.
    2. _____ A person processes a message.
    3. _____ A person sends a message.
    4. _____ A person acknowledges understanding of a message.
    5. _____ A person formulates a thought to communicate.

17. A nursing instructor is teaching about nonverbal communication. Which student statement indicates that more instruction is needed?
    1. "Maintaining eye contact is a way to nonverbally communicate."
    2. "My tone of voice can change the meaning of my verbal communication."
    3. "Charting client care is a form of nonverbal communication."
    4. "Hand gestures can enhance or detract from the communication process."

18. Which of the following statements accurately describe(s) nonverbal communication? **Select all that apply.**
    1. The majority of all communication occurs by the use of nonverbal communication.
    2. Nonverbal communication can significantly affect the communication process.
    3. Eye contact is classified as a form of nonverbal communication.
    4. Communication cannot occur without the use of nonverbal communication.
    5. A communicator can be unaware of his or her use of nonverbal communication.

19. An elderly client adheres to traditional Japanese values and practices. When communicating with this client, what fundamental health-related belief should a nurse expect to assess?
    1. The need to restore the balance of yin and yang.
    2. The need of a shaman to perform healing ceremonies.
    3. The need of a *curandero* or *curandera* to perform healing ceremonies.
    4. The need for alcohol consumption to decrease anxiety.

20. An African American client presenting in the emergency department with signs and symptoms of double pneumonia states, "I will not agree to hospital admission unless my 'granny' continues to care for me." Which would be an appropriate nursing intervention?
    1. Tell the client that "granny" is not allowed in the emergency department.
    2. Have "granny" meet the attending physician at the hospital.
    3. Tell the client that "granny's" assistance is not needed.
    4. Explain to the client that "granny" has contributed to the client's condition.

21. Religion and health practices are intertwined in the Native American culture and affect the communication process. In this culture, the medicine man (or woman) is called a(n) _____.

22. When communicating with a client of Northern European American extraction, a nurse would consider which aspect of territorial space?
    1. Touching during communication is considered unacceptable.
    2. Territory is valued and personal space is about 18 inches to 3 feet.
    3. Touch is a commonly used as a form of communication.
    4. Physical expressions include hugging and kissing.

23. During an admission assessment, the nurse discovers that an African American client is not taking medications at the prescribed times. Which of the following cultural considerations may contribute to this behavior? **Select all that apply.**
    1. The client may not value adherence to time and schedules.
    2. The client may tend to prioritize other issues over adherence to schedules.
    3. The client might follow a folk practitioner's medication schedule.
    4. The client may prefer massage, diet, and rest to mainstream medical treatment.
    5. The client will only comply with medication protocols prescribed by a shaman.

24. A nurse charts a client's output value in a narrative entry note. The nurse immediately recognizes that the value documented was in error. Which would be an appropriate nursing action to deal with this situation?
    1. Line out the entry and chart the correct value.
    2. Use provided white-out to completely obliterate the entry.
    3. Initial, date, time, line-out and correct entry with the addition of the word "error."
    4. Chart an additional "entry note" explaining the error.

25. A nurse documents a client's behavior, the interventions taken to deal with the behavior, the client's response to the interventions, and a plan to continue dealing with the behavior. This type of narrative charting is referred to as _____ charting.

REVIEW ANSWERS

1. **ANSWER: 3**
   Rationale:
   1. This is an example of "requesting an explanation," which asks the client to provide the reasons for thoughts, feeling, and behaviors and which can be an unrealistic expectation. It also may put the client on the defensive.
   2. This is an example of "giving false reassurance" by indicating to the client that there is no cause for fear or anxiety. This blocks any further interaction and expression of feelings by the client.
   3. The therapeutic technique of "exploring," along with reflective listening, draws out the client and can help the client feel valued, understood, and supported. Exploring also gives the nurse necessary assessment information to intervene appropriately.
   4. This is an example of "rejection," which shows contempt for the client's need to voice and express fears and anxiety.
   TEST-TAKING TIP: Distinguish between therapeutic and nontherapeutic communication. In this question, Options 1, 2, and 4 all are nontherapeutic communication techniques and can be eliminated immediately. A review of Table 5.1 and Table 5.2 would be helpful.
   Content Area: Safe and Effective Care Environment: Management of Care;
   Integrated Process: Nursing Process: Implementation;
   Client Need: Safe and Effective Care Environment: Management of Care;
   Cognitive Level: Application;
   Concept: Communication

2. **ANSWER: 4**
   Rationale:
   1. This is an example of a closed-ended, not open-ended, question. A closed-ended question limits client responses. The question is asked in such a way that it can be answered by one word.
   2. This is an example of a closed-ended, not open-ended, question. A closed-ended question limits client responses. The question is asked in such a way that it can be answered by one word.
   3. This is an example of a closed-ended, not open-ended, question. A closed-ended question limits client responses. The question is asked in such a way that it can be answered by one word.
   4. This is an example of an open-ended question. An open-ended question requires the client to use more than one word to answer the question. This encourages the client to provide more detailed information related to the topic being discussed.
   TEST-TAKING TIP: Remember that close-ended questions can be answered by only one word. Answer each of the questions presented in the answer choices. Option 4 is the only question that requires more than one word as an answer. A review of Table 5.1 and Table 5.2 would be helpful.
   Content Area: Safe and Effective Care Environment: Management of Care;
   Integrated Process: Nursing Process: Implementation;
   Client Need: Safe and Effective Care Environment: Management of Care;
   Cognitive Level: Application;
   Concept: Communication

3. **ANSWER: 4**
   Rationale:
   1. "Giving information" provides an individual with general data, whereas "focusing" poses a statement that helps an individual expand on a specific topic of importance. The statement presented in the question is not an example of the therapeutic technique of "giving information."
   2. "Reflection" is used when directing back what the nurse understands in regard to ideas, feelings, questions, and content. The statement presented in the question is not an example of the therapeutic technique of "reflection."
   3. "Verbalizing the implied" is used when the nurse tries to find clues to the underlying true feelings and at the same time validates an individual's statement. The statement presented in the question is not an example of the therapeutic technique of "verbalizing the implied."
   4. The instructor is using the therapeutic communication technique of "focusing" to direct the conversation to a specific topic of importance or relevance to the student.
   TEST-TAKING TIP: "Focusing" narrows communication topics, whereas "giving information" is broader in nature. Review Table 5.1 for more about these techniques.
   Content Area: Safe and Effective Care Environment: Management of Care;
   Integrated Process: Nursing Process: Implementation;
   Client Need: Safe and Effective Care Environment: Management of Care;
   Cognitive Level: Application;
   Concept: Communication

4. **ANSWER: 1**
   Rationale:
   1. The therapeutic technique of "offering a general lead" lets the client know that the nurse is engaged in the communication exchange and encourages the client to continue the communication process. The communication exchange presented is an example of the therapeutic technique of "offering a general lead."
   2. An "open-ended question" requires the client to use more than one word to answer the question. This encourages the client to provide more detailed information related to the topic being discussed. The communication exchange presented is an example of the therapeutic technique of an "open-ended question," not "offering a general lead."
   3. "Clarification" is used by a nurse to check the understanding of what has been said by the client and helps the client make his or her thoughts or feelings more explicit. The communication exchange presented is an example of the therapeutic technique of "clarification," not "offering a general lead."
   4. "Restatement" is used by a nurse to repeat to the client the main thought that the client has expressed. This lets the client know that the nurse is focused and engaged in the communication process. The communication exchange presented is an example of the therapeutic technique of "restatement," not "offering a general lead."
   TEST-TAKING TIP: When using "restatement," the nurse repeats the client's words. A "general lead" only offers the

client encouragement to continue the dialogue. Review Table 5.1 to compare these techniques.
Content Area: Safe and Effective Care Environment: Management of Care;
Integrated Process: Nursing Process: Implementation;
Client Need: Safe and Effective Care Environment: Management of Care;
Cognitive Level: Application;
Concept: Communication

5. **ANSWER: 2**
Rationale:
1. "Exploring" helps a client feel free to talk and examine issues in more depth. The communication exchange presented is an example of the therapeutic technique of "exploring," not "broad opening."
2. A "broad opening" allows the client to take the initiative in introducing the topic of conversation and emphasizes the importance of the client's role in the interaction. The communication exchange presented is an example of the therapeutic technique of "broad opening."
3. "Offering a general lead" lets the client know that the nurse is engaged in the communication exchange and encourages the client to continue the communication process. The communication exchange presented is an example of the therapeutic technique of "offering a general lead," not a "broad opening" statement.
4. The communication exchange presented is the non-therapeutic block to communication of "giving advice," not a "broad opening" statement. By telling the client what to do, the nurse takes away the client's ability to sort out options and determine the pros and cons of various choices.
TEST-TAKING TIP: Recognizing that "giving advice" is a non-therapeutic block to communication will automatically eliminate Option 4. If necessary, review communication techniques so that you will be able to recognize them in nurse-client interactions. Table 5.1 and Table 5.2 will assist with acquiring this information.
Content Area: Safe and Effective Care Environment: Management of Care;
Integrated Process: Nursing Process: Implementation;
Client Need: Safe and Effective Care Environment: Management of Care;
Cognitive Level: Application;
Concept: Communication

6. **ANSWER: 3**
Rationale:
1. The nurse uses the therapeutic technique of "restating" to provide feedback to the client. Restating lets the client know that the nurse is attentive and that the message is understood. The exchange presented is an example of "reflection," not "restating."
2. The nurse uses "focusing" to direct the conversation to a particular topic of importance or relevance to the client. The exchange presented is an example of "reflection," not "focusing."
3. "Reflection" is used when directing back what the nurse understands in regard to the client's ideas, feelings, questions, and content. Reflection is used to put the client's

feelings in the context of when or where they occur. The exchange presented is an example of "reflection."
4. The therapeutic technique of "exploring," along with reflective listening, draws out the client and can help the client feel valued, understood, and supported. Exploring also gives the nurse necessary assessment information to intervene appropriately. The exchange presented is an example of "reflection" not "exploring."
TEST-TAKING TIP: Recognize the difference between restatement and reflection. When using restatement, the nurse repeats the client's words. When using reflection, the nurse focuses on the client's underlying feelings associated with the topic of discussion. Table 5.1 gives an overview of the therapeutic communication techniques and this knowledge is needed to answer this question correctly.
Content Area: Safe and Effective Care Environment: Management of Care;
Integrated Process: Nursing Process: Implementation;
Client Need: Safe and Effective Care Environment: Management of Care;
Cognitive Level: Application;
Concept: Communication

7. **ANSWER: 1**
Rationale:
1. The therapeutic technique of "clarification" is an attempt by the nurse to check the understanding of what has been said by the client and helps the client make her thoughts or feelings more explicit. By asking for the context of the use of the word "hot," the nurse is clarifying his or her understanding of the term.
2. This is an example of "exploring," not "clarification." "Exploring" helps the client feel free to talk and examine issues in more depth.
3. This is an example of "voicing doubt," not "clarification." When using the therapeutic communication technique of "voicing doubt," the nurse expresses uncertainty as to the reality of what is being communicated.
4. This is an example of "verbalizing the implied," not "clarification." By "verbalizing the implied," the nurse puts into words what the nurse thinks the client is saying. If the implication is incorrect, it gives the client an opportunity to clarify the statement further.
TEST-TAKING TIP: Note the key word *clarify* in the question. Then choose the answer option that contains an example of the therapeutic technique of clarification. Clarification differs from exploring in that clarification is used to verify the nurse's understanding of the client's communication while exploring is used to gather further information. For comparison of these two techniques, review Table 5.1.
Content Area: Safe and Effective Care Environment: Management of Care;
Integrated Process: Nursing Process: Implementation;
Client Need: Safe and Effective Care Environment: Management of Care;
Cognitive Level: Application;
Concept: Communication

8. ANSWER: 3
Rationale:
1. A "broad opening" technique encourages the client to select topics for discussion. The example presented in the question does not reflect the communication technique of "broad opening."
2. "Verbalizing the implied" puts into words what the nurse thinks the client is saying. If the nurse's inference is incorrect, it gives the client an opportunity to clarify the statement further. The example presented in the question does not reflect the communication technique of "verbalizing the implied" because the nurse simply restated what the client said.
3. This nurse-client exchange is an example of "restating." By repeating to the client the main thought the client has expressed, the nurse has an opportunity to verify his or her understanding of the client's message. This therapeutic technique also lets the client know that the nurse is listening and wants to understand what the client is saying.
4. "Formulating a plan of action" is a therapeutic communication technique used by the nurse to assist a client in developing a plan for dealing with what is considered a stressful situation. The example presented in the question does not reflect the communication technique of "formulating a plan of action."
TEST-TAKING TIP: Recognize the difference between "restating" and "verbalizing the implied." There is no inference presented when a nurse simply restates the client's exact or similar words. For comparison of these two techniques, review Table 5.1.
Content Area: Safe and Effective Care Environment: Management of Care;
Integrated Process: Nursing Process: Implementation;
Client Need: Safe and Effective Care Environment: Management of Care;
Cognitive Level: Application;
Concept: Communication

9. ANSWER: 3
Rationale:
1. This statement is an example of the nontherapeutic block to communication of "requesting an explanation." Questions that include the word *why* can be intimidating and may be perceived as threatening. These types of questions may generate client defensiveness and hamper the nurse's ability to obtain general information.
2. This statement is a stereotyped comment and is a closed-ended nontherapeutic block to communication because it limits the client response to a "yes-or-no" answer. This communication block hampers the nurse's ability to obtain general information.
3. This nurse's statement is an example of the therapeutic communication technique of "exploring." The use of this technique enhances the nurse's ability to obtain general information.
4. This nurse's statement does not provide an opportunity for the client to share general information.
TEST-TAKING TIP: For a nurse to obtain general information from a client, the nurse must use appropriate therapeutic communication techniques. Review Tables 5.1 and 5.2 to remind yourself of the therapeutic techniques and blocks to communication.

Content Area: Safe and Effective Care Environment: Management of Care;
Integrated Process: Nursing Process: Implementation;
Client Need: Safe and Effective Care Environment: Management of Care;
Cognitive Level: Application;
Concept: Communication

10. ANSWER: 1, 5
1. The nurse is using the communication technique of "offering general leads." "Offering general leads" is a therapeutic communication technique, which is used to encourage the client to continue.
2. The communication exchange presented is an example of an "opening lead," not a "broad opening." Broad openings help the client initiate the conversation and put the client in control of the content.
3. The communication exchange presented is an example of an "opening lead," not "giving recognition." "Giving recognition" is a therapeutic communication technique that can be used by the nurse to acknowledge something that is occurring at the present moment. *Example:* "I see you've made your bed."
4. The communication exchange presented is an example of an "opening lead," not "clarification." "Clarification" is a therapeutic communication technique used by a nurse to check the understanding of what has been said by the client and helps the client make his or her thoughts or feelings more explicit.
5. The communication exchange presented is an example of the therapeutic communication technique of "offering a general lead." This technique communicates to the client that the nurse is fully present and listening.
TEST-TAKING TIP: Review Table 5.1 to familiarize yourself with therapeutic techniques to communication.
Content Area: Safe and Effective Care Environment: Management of Care;
Integrated Process: Nursing Process: Assessment;
Client Need: Safe and Effective Care Environment: Management of Care;
Cognitive Level: Application;
Concept: Communication

11. ANSWER: 4
Rationale: The nontherapeutic technique of "making stereotyped/superficial comments" offers meaningless clichés or trite expressions.
1. By stating "time will heal," the nurse is using the nontherapeutic block of "making stereotyped comments." The student choice of this example would indicate that learning has occurred.
2. By stating "You can't cry over spilt milk," the nurse is using the nontherapeutic block of "making stereotyped comments." The student choice of this example would indicate that learning has occurred.
3. By communicating that the client has "gotten up on the wrong side of the bed," the nurse is using the nontherapeutic block of "making stereotyped comments." The student choice of this example would indicate that learning has occurred.

4. This nurse-client exchange is an example of the non-therapeutic communication block of "defending," not the nontherapeutic block of "making stereotyped comments." "Defending" attempts to protect someone or something from verbal attack. It implies that the client has no right to express ideas, opinions, or feelings. The student choice of this example would indicate that the student is in need of further instruction.

TEST-TAKING TIP: Look for commonly used clichés when considering the communication block of "making stereotyped comments." Review Table 5.2 to familiarize yourself with blocks to communication.

Content Area: Safe and Effective Care Environment;
Integrated Process: Nursing Process: Implementation;
Client Need: Safe and Effective Care Environment: Management of Care;
Cognitive Level: Application;
Concept: Communication

12. **ANSWER: 1**
Rationale:
1. The nurse's statement is the nontherapeutic communication block of "giving advice." By telling the client what to do, the nurse takes away the client's ability to sort out options and determine the pros and cons of various choices. The client would be discouraged from making independent decisions.
2. A client's concerns are minimized when a nurse uses the nontherapeutic communication block of "false reassurance," not the nontherapeutic communication block of "giving advice." "False reassurance" implies that there is no cause for the client to experience fear or anxiety. This blocks any further interaction and expression of feelings and minimizes the client's concerns.
3. A client may become defensive when the nurse uses the nontherapeutic communication block of "requesting an explanation," not the nontherapeutic communication block of "giving advice." "Requesting an explanation" by the use of the word *why* can readily put a client on the defensive.
4. A client's responses may be limited when the nurse uses the nontherapeutic communication block of a "closed-ended question," not the nontherapeutic communication block of "giving advice." A "closed-ended question" is asked in such a way that it can be answered by one word.

TEST-TAKING TIP: First, identify the communication exchange in the question as the nontherapeutic block of "giving advice." Then identify the result of this block to communication.

Content Area: Safe and Effective Care Environment: Management of Care;
Integrated Process: Nursing Process: Implementation;
Client Need: Safe and Effective Care Environment: Management of Care;
Cognitive Level: Application;
Concept: Communication

13. **ANSWER: CHANGING THE SUBJECT**
Rationale: In response to the client's statement, "I feel like I'm about to jump out of my skin!" the nurse asks, "Are you expecting visitors today?" The nurse has used the nontherapeutic block of "changing the subject." "Changing the subject" puts the nurse, instead of the client, in control of the conversation in order for the nurse to avoid uncomfortable topics that the client expresses a need to discuss.

TEST-TAKING TIP: Note that the question itself eliminates the choice of any therapeutic communication technique. Review Table 5.2 for examples of blocks to communication.

Content Area: Safe and Effective Care Environment: Management of Care;
Integrated Process: Nursing Process: Implementation;
Client Need: Safe and Effective Care Environment: Management of Care;
Cognitive Level: Knowledge;
Concept: Communication

14. **ANSWER: 1**
Rationale:
1. The nontherapeutic block of "approving/disapproving" sanctions or denounces the client's ideas or behaviors. This implies that the nurse has the right to pass judgment on the client's ideas or behaviors. This student statement indicates that learning has occurred.
2. "Verbalizing the implied" puts into words what the client has only implied or said indirectly. This therapeutic technique clarifies that which is implicit rather than explicit by giving the client the opportunity to agree or disagree with the nurse's inference. This student statement indicates that further instruction is needed.
3. "Suggesting collaboration" is a therapeutic technique that the nurse uses to work together with the client for the client's benefit. This student statement indicates that further instruction is needed.
4. "Silence" is a therapeutic technique that gives the nurse and client an opportunity to collect and organize thoughts, think through a point, or consider reprioritizing subject matter. This student statement indicates that further instruction is needed.

TEST-TAKING TIP: Even though "giving approval" may sound therapeutic, this nontherapeutic communication block can create undue pressures and expectations for the client.

Content Area: Safe and Effective Care Environment: Management of Care;
Integrated Process: Nursing Process: Implementation;
Client Need: Safe and Effective Care Environment: Management of Care;
Cognitive Level: Application;
Concept: Communication

15. **ANSWER: 1, 2, 3, 4**
Rationale:
1. Communication has its roots in culture. Cultural mores, norms, ideas, and customs provide the basis for our way of thinking and can affect the communication process.
2. Religion can influence communication. Wearing of a clerical collar publicly communicates a minister's mission in life and can affect the communication process.
3. Age influences communication. An example is during adolescence when struggles to establish individual identities generate a unique pattern of communication.

4. Gender influences communication. Each culture has gender signals that are recognized as either masculine or feminine and affect the communication process.
5. In and of themselves, sleep patterns do not directly affect the communication process.
TEST-TAKING TIP: Recognize that a variety of factors influence the communication process. Culture, religion, age, and gender all have an effect on communication.
Content Area: Psychosocial Integrity;
Integrated Process: Nursing Process: Evaluation;
Client Need: Psychosocial Integrity;
Cognitive Level: Application;
Concept: Communication

16. **ANSWER: 3, 4, 2, 5, 1**
Rationale: (1) The communication process begins with the formulation of a thought to communicate. (2) Next, an individual sends a message either verbally or nonverbally. (3) Next, an individual receives the communicated message. (4) The receiver then processes the message and determines a meaning. (5) The last step of the communication process is to acknowledge an understanding of the message.
TEST-TAKING TIP: Review the steps of the communication process in Figure 5.1.
Content Area: Safe and Effective Care Environment: Management of Care;
Integrated Process: Nursing Process: Implementation;
Client Need: Safe and Effective Care Environment: Management of Care;
Cognitive Level: Analysis;
Concept: Communication

17. **ANSWER: 3**
Rationale:
1. Eye contact is a part of nonverbal communication. This student statement indicates that learning has occurred.
2. Tone of voice is a nonverbal form of communication that can change the meaning of verbal communication. This student statement indicates that learning has occurred.
3. **The documentation of client care is a form of verbal, not nonverbal, communication. This student statement indicates the need for further instruction.**
4. Hand gestures are forms of nonverbal communication and can enhance or detract from the communication process. This student statement indicates that learning has occurred.
TEST-TAKING TIP: Review examples of verbal and nonverbal communication.
Content Area: Psychosocial Integrity;
Integrated Process: Nursing Process: Evaluation;
Client Need: Psychosocial Integrity;
Cognitive Level: Application;
Concept: Communication

18. **ANSWER: 1, 2, 3, 5**
Rationale:
1. **The majority of all communication is nonverbal. According to research, only 7% of communication is verbal, and the remainder of the communication process is nonverbal.**
2. **Nonverbal communication can significantly affect the communication process. A harsh and abrasive tone**

of voice can change a positive statement to a statement that is perceived as negative.
3. Eye contact is one form of nonverbal communication. Inability to maintain eye contact can generate doubt about the truthfulness of verbalized words.
4. Communication can occur without the use of nonverbal communication. The written word, a form of verbal communication, does not include a nonverbal component.
5. A communicator can be unaware of his or her use of nonverbal communication. Nonverbal communication can occur spontaneously and without the communicator's conscious awareness.
TEST-TAKING TIP: Identify the components of nonverbal communication. Understanding that the written word is a form of verbal communication will also assist in answering this question correctly.
Content Area: Psychosocial Integrity;
Integrated Process: Nursing Process: Evaluation;
Client Need: Psychosocial Integrity;
Cognitive Level: Application;
Concept: Communication

19. **ANSWER: 1**
Rationale:
1. Restoring yin and yang is a fundamental concept of Asian health practices. Yin and yang represent opposite forces of energy.
2. In the Native American culture, not the Asian American culture, the medicine man or woman is called a shaman.
3. In the Latino American culture, not the Asian American culture, the medicine man or woman is called a *curandero* or *curandera*.
4. In the Asian American culture, the incidence of alcohol dependence is low, and therefore the need for alcohol consumption to decrease anxiety would be unlikely.
TEST-TAKING TIP: Review Table 5.4 to familiarize yourself with various cultural practices that may influence health care.
Content Area: Psychosocial Integrity;
Integrated Process: Nursing Process: Assessment;
Client Need: Psychosocial Integrity;
Cognitive Level: Application;
Concept: Diversity

20. **ANSWER: 2**
Rationale:
1. Religion and health practices are intertwined in the African American culture, and the folk practitioner, called a "granny," is part of the belief system. Refusing to allow the "granny" to be a part of the client's health care may result in the client's refusing needed treatment.
2. Respectful collaboration regarding health care for African Americans may include conferring with the folk practitioner, called a "granny." The nurse should comply with the client's request and make contact with the "granny."
3. Telling the client that "granny's" assistance is not needed shows disrespect for the client's cultural beliefs and may result in the client's refusing needed treatment.
4. Putting blame on the "granny" for the client's condition would alienate the client and undermine the client's belief system.

TEST-TAKING TIP: Clients may rely on folk healers, and these folk practitioners should be incorporated in the communication process. Review Table 5.4 to familiarize yourself with various cultural practices that may influence health care.
Content Area: Psychosocial Integrity;
Integrated Process: Nursing Process: Implementation;
Client Need: Psychosocial Integrity;
Cognitive Level: Application;
Concept: Diversity

21. **ANSWER: shaman**
Rationale: The medicine man (or woman) is called a shaman. The shaman may use a variety of methods in his or her practice of health care. Communicating with this folk healer can facilitate the client's healing progress.
TEST-TAKING TIP: Clients may rely on folk healers, and these folk practitioners should be incorporated in the communication process. Review Table 5.4 to familiarize yourself with various cultural practices that may influence health care.
Content Area: Psychosocial Integrity;
Integrated Process: Nursing Process: Evaluation;
Client Need: Psychosocial Integrity;
Cognitive Level: Knowledge;
Concept: Diversity

22. **ANSWER: 2**
Rationale:
1. Touching during communication is considered unacceptable in the Asian American, not Northern European American, culture.
2. Northern European Americans normally value territory, and personal space is about 18 inches to 3 feet.
3. Touch is commonly used as a form of communication in the Latino American, not Northern European American, culture.
4. Western European Americans, not Northern European Americans, tend to be warm and affectionate and physical expressions include hugging and kissing.
TEST-TAKING TIP: Diverse cultures have various degrees of comfort related to personal space. Review Table 5.4 to familiarize yourself with various cultural practices that may influence communication and health care.
Content Area: Safe and Effective Care Environment: Management of Care;
Integrated Process: Nursing Process: Assessment;
Client Need: Safe and Effective Care Environment: Management of Care;
Cognitive Level: Application;
Concept: Diversity

23. **ANSWER: 1, 2, 3**
1. African Americans may be unlikely to value time or punctuality to the same degree as the dominant cultural group, and this may lead to nonadherence with scheduled medications.
2. African Americans may tend to prioritize other issues over adherence to schedules. This may lead to nonadherence with scheduled medications.
3. Some African Americans may receive medical treatment from folk practitioners. This occurs mainly in the rural south. This may lead to nonadherence with scheduled medications.

4. Latino Americans, not African Americans, may prefer massage, diet, and rest to mainstream medical treatment.
5. Native Americans, not African Americans, may have their medical treatments prescribed by a medicine man (or woman) called a shaman.
TEST-TAKING TIP: Become familiar with various cultural considerations such as time orientation. Many aspects of an individual's life are influenced by whether that individual is past oriented, present oriented, or future oriented in their perception of time.
Content Area: Safe and Effective Care Environment: Management of Care;
Integrated Process: Nursing Process: Assessment;
Client Need: Safe and Effective Care Environment: Management of Care;
Cognitive Level: Application;
Concept: Diversity

24. **ANSWER: 3**
Rationale:
1. Lining out the entry and charting the correct value is an appropriate nursing action to deal with charting errors however, the nurse also needs to initial, date, and time the corrected entry.
2. Charting client care produces a legal record. Obliterating any information in this legal document is an illegal an inappropriate nursing action.
3. Initialing, dating, timing, lining out, and correcting the entry with the addition of the word "error" is an appropriate nursing action to deal with this charting error.
4. Charting an additional "late entry" note explaining the error is not needed in this situation because the nurse only replaced an incorrect value with a correct one. Furthermore, the nurse needs to initial, date, and time the corrected entry.
TEST-TAKING TIP: It is important to understand the legal ramifications of charting client care and how to appropriately correct any errors that may occur.
Content Area: Safe and Effective Care Environment: Management of Care;
Integrated Process: Nursing Process: Implementation;
Client Need: Safe and Effective Care Environment: Management of Care;
Cognitive Level: Application;
Concept: Communication

25. **ANSWER: BIRP**
Rationale: The acronym BIRP stands for the documentation of a client's **B**ehavior, nursing **I**nterventions, the client's **R**esponse, and the **P**lan to further address the behavior.
TEST-TAKING TIP: Recall the various ways that narrative charting can be organized. Note the key words in the question that form the acronym BIRP.
Content Area: Safe and Effective Care Environment: Management of Care;
Integrated Process: Nursing Process: Implementation;
Client Need: Safe and Effective Care Environment: Management of Care;
Cognitive Level: Knowledge;
Concept: Communication

Chapter 6

Legal and Ethical Considerations

KEY TERMS

Ethics—A set of concepts and principles that seek to resolve questions dealing with human morality; examples are concepts such as good and evil, right and wrong, virtue and vice, justice and crime

Ethical dilemma—A situation that arises when, on the basis of moral considerations, an appeal can be made for taking either of two opposing courses of action

Incompetence—Characterized by an inability to manage one's affairs due to mental deficiency or sometimes physical disability; being incompetent can be the basis for appointment of a guardian or conservator, after a hearing in which the party who is found to be incompetent has been interviewed by a court investigator and is present and/or represented by an attorney; this guardian is appointed to handle the incompetent person's affairs

Informed consent—Permission granted to a physician by a client to perform a therapeutic procedure before which information about the procedure has been presented to the client with adequate time given for consideration about the procedure's pros and cons

Involuntary commitment—A legal process in which an individual with symptoms of severe mental illness is court-ordered into treatment in a hospital (inpatient) or in the community (outpatient). State laws establish criteria for civil commitment. Commitment proceedings often follow a period of emergency hospitalization, during which an individual with acute psychiatric symptoms is briefly confined for evaluation; if civil commitment proceedings follow, a formal court hearing is held;

the client is entitled to legal counsel and may legally challenge a commitment order

Malpractice—The failure to render professional services that exercise a degree of skill and learning commonly applied under all circumstances in the community by the average prudent, reputable member of a profession with the result of injury, loss, or damage to the recipient of those services

Negligence—The failure to do something that a reasonable person, guided by those considerations that ordinarily regulate human affairs, would do or doing something that a prudent and reasonable person would not do

Patient Rights—Written guidelines of rights established by both the National League of Nursing and the American Hospital Association; these are not considered legal documents, but nurses and hospitals are considered responsible for upholding these patients' rights

Right—A valid, legally recognized claim or entitlement, encompassing both freedom from government interference or discriminatory treatment and the entitlement of a benefit or service; a legal right is one on which society has agreed and formalized into law

Values—Personal beliefs about the truth, beauty, or worth of a thought, object, or behavior that influence an individual's actions

Value clarification—A process of self-discovery through which people identify their personal values and their value rankings; this process increases awareness about why individuals behave in certain ways

Nurses are faced with ethical issues on a daily basis in all areas of nursing. Caring for clients diagnosed with mental illness presents the nurse with unique and complex challenges. It is especially imperative to understand the ethical and legal issues that affect nursing care for clients diagnosed with psychiatric disorders. Clients experience thought and behavior disorders that hamper them from asserting their rights. The nurse is challenged to provide safe, ethical, individualized, competent care while respecting the rights of this population of clients and the safety of others. Altered thinking can also lead to perceptions that can unjustly place a nurse at risk for litigation. In planning care, the nurse must be guided by the nurse practice act of the state in which the nurse is practicing. The nurse must also be directed by and accountable to the laws governing client rights and the public's interest, which often come into conflict.

I. Ethical Considerations

A. Ethics are moral principles that govern a person's or group's behavior
   1. Branch of philosophy dealing with values relating to human conduct, with respect to the rightness and wrongness of certain actions and to the goodness and badness of the motives and ends of such actions.
   2. "Bioethics" is the term applied to ethical principles when they refer to concepts within the scope of medicine, nursing, and allied health.
B. Values are personal beliefs about what is important and desirable
   1. **Values clarification** is a process of self-exploration through which individuals identify and rank their own personal values.
   2. Values clarification in nursing.
      a. Increases understanding about why certain choices and decisions are made over others.
      b. Increases understanding of how values affect nursing outcomes.
      c. American Nurses' Association developed a Code of Ethics for nurses.
C. Ethical theories (can be used to assess what is morally right or wrong)
   1. Utilitarianism.
      a. "Greatest happiness principle."
      b. Actions are right if they promote happiness for the majority.
      c. Actions are wrong if they promote unhappiness.
      d. Theory looks at end results of actions.
   2. Kantianism.
      a. Not the end result that makes an action right or wrong.
      b. Motivation on which action is based is a morally decisive factor.
      c. Decisions made based on respect for moral law.

   3. Christian ethics.
      a. Based on teachings of Jesus Christ.
      b. Golden rule: "Do unto others as you would have them do unto you."
      c. Treat others with respect and dignity.
   4. Natural law.
      a. Based on teachings of Thomas Aquinas.
      b. Man inherently knows (from God) the difference between good and evil.
      c. Knowledge of good and evil directs decision making.
   5. Ethical egoism.
      a. What is right or good is what is best for decision-maker.
      b. Actions are determined by decision-maker advantage.
      c. Decisions may not be best for others.
D. Ethical dilemmas
   1. Arise when there is no clear reason to choose one action over another.
   2. Choice must be made between two equally unfavorable alternatives.
   3. Reasons supporting each side can be logical and appropriate.
   4. Taking no action is considered an action taken.

🛈 Ethical dilemmas generally create a great deal of emotion. Complex situations frequently arise in caring for individuals with mental illness, and nurses are held to the highest level of legal and ethical accountability in their professional practice.

E. Model for making ethical decisions
   1. Assessment.
      a. Gather objective and subjective data about situation.
      b. Consider personal values and values of others.
   2. Problem identification (identify conflict between two or more actions).
   3. Planning.
      a. Explore benefits and consequences of each alternative.
      b. Consider principles of ethical theories.
      c. Select an alternative.
   4. Implementation.
      a. Act on decision made.
      b. Communicate decision to others.
   5. Evaluation (evaluate outcomes) (Fig. 6.1).
F. Ethical principles (guidelines that influence decision making)
   1. Autonomy.
      a. Respect for individuals as rational, autonomous agents.
      b. Respect individual's right to determine destiny.
      c. Individual must be capable of independent choice.

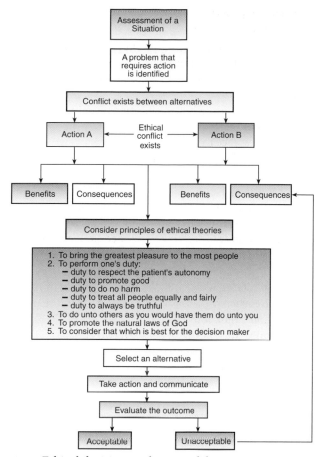

Fig 6.1 Ethical decision-making model.

d. Children and individuals who are incapacitated are incapable of making informed choices.

e. If client is a child, incapacitated, and/or incompetent, a representative is appointed to make decisions in the client's best interest.

2. Beneficence.
   a. Duty to promote good of others.
   b. Must serve individual's best interest.
   c. Advocacy is acting in another's behalf.
   d. Nurse advocate helps client fulfill needs that without assistance may go unfulfilled.

3. Nonmaleficence.
   a. Do no harm, either intentionally or unintentionally.
   b. Conflict may exist between a client's rights and what is thought best for the client.

4. Justice.
   a. Right of individuals to be treated equally regardless of race, sex, marital status, medical diagnosis, social standing, economic level, sexual orientation, or religious belief.
   b. Resources, including health care, should be distributed without respect to socioeconomic status.

5. Veracity.
   a. Duty to always be truthful.
   b. Should not intentionally deceive or mislead.

G. Ethical issues in psychiatric nursing involving **patient rights**
   1. Right to refuse treatment (medications).
      a. Consequences of medication/treatment refusal.
         i. **Involuntary commitment** (legal procedure that forces a client to stay in the hospital)
         ii. Legal competency hearing (legal procedure that appoints a guardian to make all decisions for client)
         iii. Forced discharge from facility
      b. When medications can be forced.
         i. Client is an imminent danger to self or others
            1) Must be emergent, unsafe, acute situation.
            2) Not just based on admission criteria.
         ii. Client has been deemed **incompetent** by the court
            1) Client is incapable of decision making.
            2) Guardian is appointed by court to make all decisions.
   2. Right to least restrictive treatment.
      a. Treatment based on client symptoms.
      b. Treatments on a continuum.
         i. Verbal interactions (talking the client down)
         ii. Behavioral techniques (removal from stimuli)
         iii. Chemical interventions (offered or forced medications)
         iv. Seclusion
         v. Mechanical restraints
         vi. Electroconvulsive therapy

MAKING THE CONNECTION

There are times when limitations must be placed on the principle of veracity. Withholding information from a client often does not violate the truth principle. Occasionally clients request that information be withheld. Ordinarily, respecting such requests violates no major ethical principle—not autonomy, truth, or beneficence. But clinical judgment is always required because, in some cases, even a client who requests not to be informed needs to know some truths. Not knowing may create a serious danger to self or to others, and if so, the client's request that information be withheld cannot be respected because it violates the core principles of beneficence and nonmaleficence. Clients have the **right** to know about their diagnosis, treatment, and prognosis (see Box 6.1).

Box 6.1 **Patient Self-determination Act—Patient Rights**

1. *The right to appropriate treatment and related services in a setting and under conditions that are the most supportive of such person's personal liability, and restrict such liberty only to the extent necessary consistent with such person's treatment needs, applicable requirements of law, and applicable judicial orders.*
2. *The right to an individualized, written treatment or service plan (such plan to be developed promptly after admission of such person), the right to treatment based on such plan, the right to periodic review and reassessment of treatment and related service needs, and the right to appropriate revision of such plan, including any revision necessary to provide a description of mental health services that may be needed after such person is discharged from such program or facility.*
3. *The right to ongoing participation, in a manner appropriate to a person's capabilities, in the planning of mental health services to be provided (including the right to participate in the development and periodic revision of the plan).*
4. *The right to be provided with a reasonable explanation, in terms and language appropriate to a person's condition and ability to understand, the person's general mental and physical (if appropriate) condition, the objectives of treatment, the nature and significant possible adverse effects of recommended treatment, the reasons why a particular treatment is considered appropriate, and reasons why access to certain visitors may not be appropriate, and any appropriate and available alternative treatments, services, and types of providers of mental health services.*
5. *The right not to receive a mode or course of treatment in the absence of informed, voluntary, written consent to treatment except during an emergency situation or as permitted by law when the person is being treated as a result of a court order.*
6. *The right not to participate in experimentation in the absence of informed, voluntary, written consent (includes human subject protection).*
7. *The right to freedom from restraint or seclusion, other than as a mode or course of treatment or restraint or seclusion during an emergency situation with a written order by a responsible mental health professional.*
8. *The right to a humane treatment environment that affords reasonable protection from harm and appropriate privacy with regard to personal needs.*
9. *The right to access, on request, to such person's mental health-care records.*
10. *The right, in the case of a person admitted on a residential or inpatient care basis, to converse with others privately, to have convenient and reasonable access to the telephone and mail, and to see visitors during regularly scheduled hours. (For treatment purposes, specific individuals may be excluded.)*
11. *The right to be informed promptly and in writing at the time of admission of these rights.*
12. *The right to assert grievances with respect to infringement of these rights.*
13. *The right to exercise these rights without reprisal.*
14. *The right of referral to other providers upon discharge.*

Adapted from the U.S. Code, Title 42, Section 10841, The Public Health and Welfare, 1991.

II. Legal Considerations

A. Nurse practice acts
   1. Defined within each state.
   2. General in terminology with no specific guidelines for practice.
   3. Scope of practice protected by licensure.
B. Types of law
   1. Statutory law.
      a. Enacted by legislative body.
      b. Example: nurse practice acts.
   2. Common law.
      a. Derived from decisions made in previous cases.
      b. Developed on a state basis and varies from state to state.
C. Classifications within statutory and common law
   1. Civil law (protects private and property rights).
      a. Torts.
         i. An individual has been wronged
         ii. Action has caused harm
         iii. Compensation is sought for harm suffered
            1) Intentional (touching without consent: battery).
            2) Unintentional (**malpractice** and **negligence**).
   b. Contracts.
      i. Failure to fulfill an obligation
      ii. Compensation or performance of obligation is sought
   2. Criminal law.
      a. Protection from conduct deemed injurious to public welfare.
      b. Provides punishment for such conduct.
         i. Imprisonment
         ii. Parole conditions
         iii. Loss of privilege (license)
D. Legal issues in psychiatric/mental health nursing
   1. Confidentiality and right to privacy.
      a. Protected health information (PHI) (see Box 6.2).
      b. Protected by constitutional amendments.
      c. Protected by state statues.
      d. Access to medical information available only to those involved in client's medical care.
      e. HIPAA (Health Insurance Portability and Accountability Act).
         i. Federal law
         ii. Right to access medical records
         iii. Right to have corrections to medical records made

Box 6.2 Protected Health Information (PHI): Individually Identifiable Indicators

1. *Names*
2. *Postal address information (except state), including street address, city, county, precinct, and zip code*
3. *All elements of dates (except year) for dates directly related to an individual, including birth date, admission date, discharge date, date of death; and all ages over 89 and all elements of dates (including year) indicative of such age, except that such ages and elements may be aggregated into a single category of age 90 or older*
4. *Telephone numbers*
5. *Fax numbers*
6. *E-mail addresses*
7. *Social Security numbers*
8. *Medical record numbers*
9. *Health plan beneficiary numbers*
10. *Account numbers*
11. *Certificate/license numbers*
12. *Vehicle identifiers and serial numbers, including license plate numbers*
13. *Device identifiers and serial numbers*
14. *Web Universal Resource Locators (URLs)*
15. *Internet protocol (IP) address numbers*
16. *Biometric identifiers, including finger and voice prints*
17. *Full face photographic images and any comparable images*
18. *Any other unique identifying number, characteristic, or code*

Source: U.S. Department of Health and Human Services (2003).

iv. Client decides with whom to share medical records
v. Actual document belongs to facility/therapist but information belongs to client
vi. Pertinent medical information may be released without consent in life-threatening situations
   1) Must document in client record date of disclosure
   2) Document person to whom information was disclosed
   3) Document reason for disclosure
   4) Document reason written consent could not be obtained
   5) Document specific information that was disclosed
f. Privileged communication.
   i. Professional privileges under which the professional can refuse to reveal information and communications with clients
   ii. Varies from state to state
   iii. Typically includes psychiatrists and attorneys but also may include psychologists, clergy, and nurses
g. Exceptions: duty to warn.
   i. Tarasoff ruling:
      1) Client revealed to therapist intent to kill named victim
      2) No warning given to intended victim (Tarasoff)
      3) Client killed Tarasoff
      4) Lawsuit led to ruling that mental health professionals have duty not only to client but any intended victim
      5) Confidentiality must yield if disclosure is essential to avert danger to others
      6) Guidelines for therapists to determine obligation to take protective measures
         • Assessment of threat of violence
         • Identification of intended victim
         • Ability to intervene in meaningful way to protect intended victim
2. **Informed consent.**
   a. Acts to preserve and protect an individual's autonomy in determining what will and will not happen to that person's body.
   b. Client should receive and have time to weigh the pros and cons of information regarding.
      i. Treatment
      ii. Alternatives to the treatment
      iii. Why physician feels treatment is most appropriate
      iv. Possible outcomes of treatment, other treatments, and/or no treatment
      v. Possible risks and/or adverse effects of the treatment

A health-care provider can be charged with assault and battery for providing life-sustaining treatment to a client when the client has not agreed to it. According to law, all individuals have the right to decide whether to accept or reject treatment.

   c. Conditions when treatment can be performed without informed consent.
      i. Client is mentally incompetent and treatment is necessary to preserve life or prevent harm
      ii. When lack of treatment endangers life of others
      iii. During emergency situations when client's judgment is impaired
      iv. Client is a child (consent obtained from parent or surrogate)
      v. Therapeutic privilege (withholding information from client); when physician can show that full disclosure will:
         1) Hinder or complicate necessary treatment
         2) Cause severe psychological harm
         3) Upset client to degree that rational decision making will be impossible
   d. If client has been legally determined as incompetent, consent is obtained from legal guardian.

MAKING THE CONNECTION

Difficulty implementing informed consent arises when no legal determination of competence has been made, but the client's current mental state prohibits informed decision making (e.g., psychosis, unconsciousness, inebriation). In these cases, informed consent is obtained from the nearest relative, or when time permits, the physician can ask for an emergency court appointment of a guardian. A hospital administrator may be asked to grant intervention permission if time does not permit court intervention.

    e. Agency policy defines nurse's role in obtaining informed consent.

    f. Legal liability for informed consent lies with physician.

    g. Nurse advocates for client.

      i. Knowledge: client has received adequate information on which to base decision

      ii. Competency: client has no impairment in cognition that would hamper decision making or client has a legal representative

      iii. Free will: client has given consent voluntarily without pressure or coercion

3. Restraints and seclusion.

    a. Client has legal right to freedom from restraint or seclusion except in an emergency situation.

      i. Restraints (require physician order)

        1) Only used if deemed essential to prevent harm

        2) Regulated by laws, regulations, accreditation standards, and hospital policies

        3) "Restraint" refers to any manual method or medication used to restrict a person's freedom of movement

        4) Never to be used as punishment

        5) Never to be used for convenience of staff

      ii. Seclusion (requires physician order)

        1) Physical restraint in which a client is confined alone in a room from which he or she is unable to leave

        2) Minimally furnished room with emphasis on safety and comfort

    b. The Joint Commission standards regarding seclusion and restraints:

      i. Physician order renewal guidelines (unless state law is more restrictive)

        1) Every 4 hours for adults 18 years and older

        2) Every 2 hours for children and adolescents age 9 to 17

        3) Every hour for children younger than 9 years

        4) Renewals must not exceed a 24-hour time period

      ii. Must be discontinued at the earliest possible time regardless of when order is scheduled to expire

      iii. An in-person evaluation must be conducted within 1 hour of the initiation of seclusion or restraints; an appropriately trained RN can conduct this assessment but must consult with a physician

      iv. Clients who are simultaneously restrained and secluded must be continuously monitored by trained staff either in person or through electronic equipment

      v. Staff must monitor physical and psychological well-being of client including (but not limited to) respiratory and circulatory status, skin integrity, and vital signs

🛑 When implementing restraint and seclusion, the nurse's priority is to maintain client safety for a procedure that has the potential to cause injury or death. The importance of close and careful monitoring cannot be overstated.

    c. False imprisonment.

      i. Deliberate and unauthorized confinement of a person within fixed limits by the use of verbal or physical means

      ii. If a client has been voluntarily admitted and is restrained or secluded against his or her will, the health-care worker may be charged with false imprisonment

      iii. If a client has been voluntarily admitted and becomes a danger to self or others, the initiation of seclusion and restraints would ultimately need court intervention to determine competency and/or involuntary commitment

      iv. If a client is an imminent danger to self or others, immediate restraints and seclusion may be required. Necessitates physician order and detailed documentation of this crisis situation

4. Commitment issues.

    a. Voluntary admissions.

      i. Client makes direct application to the institution for services

      ii. Should understand meaning of decision and should not have been coerced

      iii. Client may sign out of facility at any time

      iv. Upon request for discharge, if health-care professional determines client is danger to self or others, recommendation for change of admission status to involuntary may occur

    b. Involuntary commitment.

      i. Individual seeking the involuntary commitment must show probable cause why client

should be hospitalized against his or her wishes
ii. Clients in need of involuntary commitment have the right to public defense access
iii. Types of involuntary commitment
   1) Emergency commitments
      - When client is clearly and imminently a danger to self or others
      - Time limited (court hearing held within 72 hours; can vary according to state law)
      - Outcome may result in client discharge, change to involuntary status, further court hearings
   2) Mentally ill in need of treatment
      - Unable to make informed decisions regarding treatment
      - Likely to cause harm to self or others
      - Unable to fulfill basic needs for health and safety
      - Existence of mental illness alone does not justify involuntary hospitalization
      - Court hearings necessary for commitment
   3) Involuntary outpatient commitment: court order that compels client to submit to treatment on an outpatient basis based on the following eligibility criteria:
      - History of repeated decompensation requiring involuntary hospitalization
      - Without treatment, client may deteriorate to requiring inpatient commitment
      - Presence of severe and persistent mental illness and lack of insight related to illness or need for treatment
      - Risk of becoming homeless, incarcerated, violent, and/or of committing suicide
      - Existence of individualized treatment plan likely to be effective and a service provider who has agreed to provide treatment
      - If there is client nonadherence to involuntary outpatient commitment requirements, there could be another court hearing to reverse the previous ruling and the client's status could revert to inpatient involuntary commitment
   4) Gravely disabled client
      - Because of mental illness is incompetent to take care of basic personal needs
      - Not just lack of resources but inability to use resources that are available

   - A guardian, conservator, or committee will be court appointed to ensure the management of the client and his or her estate
   - Further court hearing is necessary to restore competency status
5. Nursing liability
   a. Malpractice and negligence
      i. *Negligence* is failure to exercise the standard of care that a reasonably prudent person would have exercised in a similar situation
      ii. Conduct that falls below the legally established standard
      iii. *Malpractice* is a specialized form of negligence applicable only to professionals
      iv. Liability for malpractice is based on legal precedent (decisions made in previous cases)
      v. Basic elements of a nursing malpractice lawsuit
         1) Duty to client existed based on recognized standard of care
         2) Breach of duty occurred (care not consistent with professional standard)
         3) Client was injured
         4) Injury was directly caused by breach of standard of care
   b. Types of lawsuits that occur in psychiatric nursing
      i. Breach of confidentiality
         1) Revealing aspects about client's case
         2) Revealing that client has been hospitalized
         3) Must show resulting harm
      ii. Defamation of character
         1) Shared information is detrimental to client's reputation
         2) Communication is malicious and false
         3) Libel: in writing
            - Charting that is critical or judgmental
            - Nurse must chart objectively
            - Back up statements with factual evidence
         4) Slander: oral defamation
      iii. Invasion of privacy
         1) Client searched without probable cause
         2) Must have physician's order and written rationale showing probable cause
      iv. Assault
         1) An act that results in person's fear that he or she will be touched without consent (threat)
         2) Harm need not have occurred
      v. Battery
         1) Unconsented touching of another person
         2) Treatment administered against wishes

3) Outside of an emergency situation
4) Harm need not have occurred

vi. False imprisonment
1) Confining client against his or her wishes
2) Outside of an emergency situation
3) Locking client in room
4) Taking client's clothes for purposes of detainment
5) Mechanical restraints
6) For this liability to apply, client who demands release must be competent, safe, and admitted voluntarily

c. Avoiding liability
i. Proactive nursing actions
1) Respond to client
2) Educate client

3) Comply with standard of care
4) Supervise care
5) Adhere to nursing process
6) Document carefully and completely
7) Evaluate care given

ii. Maintain good interpersonal relationships with clients
iii. Avoid defensiveness and avoidant behavior
iv. Be sensitive to client complaints
v. Attempt to meet client's emotional needs

REVIEW QUESTIONS

1. The ethical theory of _____ suggests that our actions are bound by a sense of duty. In this theory, the principle or motivation on which action is based is the morally decisive factor.

2. Which situation exemplifies a utilitarianism ethical perspective?
   1. A student refuses to cheat on a test because the resulting guilt would create an unpleasant feeling.
   2. A student refuses to cheat on a test because it is against school policy.
   3. A student refuses to cheat on a test because it would be considered a sin.
   4. A student refuses to cheat on a test because learning the material without cheating will give the student an advantage.

3. A nursing instructor is teaching about ethical dilemmas that may arise in a clinical setting. Which of the following student statements indicate that further instruction is needed? **Select all that apply.**
   1. "Within an ethical dilemma, there is evidence of both moral 'rightness' and 'wrongness' of an action."
   2. "In an ethical dilemma, there is conscious conflict regarding an individual's decision making."
   3. "In an ethical dilemma, a choice must be made between two equally favorable alternatives."
   4. "In an ethical dilemma, often the reasons supporting each side of the argument for action are illogical and inappropriate."
   5. "In most situations that involve an ethical dilemma, taking no action is considered an action taken."

4. A nurse supports a competent client's right to refuse offered medications. By doing this, which ethical principle does the nurse uphold?
   1. Nonmaleficence
   2. Beneficence
   3. Autonomy
   4. Veracity

5. Which situation exemplifies the ethical principle of beneficence?
   1. A nurse uses verbal strategies, instead of forced seclusion, to calm an agitated client.
   2. A nurse talks with a client's physician to gain permission for the client to attend an upcoming fieldtrip.
   3. A nurse encourages a client diagnosed with dementia to choose what to wear for the day.
   4. A nurse teaches a client about the chronic nature of his or her diagnosis of schizophrenia.

6. Which situation exemplifies a Christian ethics perspective?
   1. A nurse decides to work a double shift because the nurse feels needed by the staff and clients.
   2. A nurse never diverts scheduled medications because it is illegal and against hospital policy.
   3. A nurse agrees to cover an evening shift so that a coworker can attend a family reunion.
   4. A nurse volunteers to be assigned especially difficult clients because the experience will further his or her career.

7. A personal belief about what is important or desirable is defined as a _____.

8. The ethical decision-making model is used when faced with an ethical dilemma. Order the situations that exemplify the steps of this model.
   1. _____ Explore the benefits and consequences of each alternative.
   2. _____ Appraise the outcomes of the decision.
   3. _____ Identify the conflict between two or more alternative actions.
   4. _____ Consider personal values and the values of others.
   5. _____ Act on the decision made and communicate the decision to others.

9. A mentally ill client has the right to refuse treatment to the extent permitted by law. It is important for the psychiatric nurse to be aware of this ethical/legal issue. Which situation would the nurse recognize as an example of this client right of refusal?
   1. A client has expressed a desire to harm a spouse and refuses to take all medications.
   2. A client is benefiting from psychotropic medications but refuses drugs because of command hallucinations.
   3. A client who has been deemed incompetent will not take ordered medications.
   4. A client diagnosed with depression decides not to take his or her antidepressant medication.

10. Which psychiatric therapy, in relationship to the others presented, is considered least restrictive?
    1. Electroconvulsive treatment
    2. Chemical interventions
    3. Verbal rehabilitative techniques
    4. Mechanical restraints

11. Which action should the clinician take when there is reasonable certainty that a client is going to harm someone? **Select all that apply.**
    1. Assess the threat of violence toward another.
    2. Identify the person being threatened.
    3. Notify the identified victim.
    4. Notify only law enforcement authorities to protect confidentiality.
    5. Consider petitioning the court for continued commitment.

12. A nurse is attempting to administer antianxiety medication to an involuntarily committed client. The client refuses the medication, curses, and states, "I'm going to kill you." Which nursing action is most appropriate at this time?
    1. The nurse decides not to administer the medication.
    2. The nurse initiates the ordered, forced medication protocol.
    3. The nurse initiates legal action to get the client declared incompetent.
    4. The nurse teaches the client the pros and cons of medication compliance.

13. A client has been deemed a danger to self by an emergency commitment court ruling. Which might the court mandate for this client?
    1. Voluntary commitment to a locked psychiatric facility.
    2. Involuntary commitment to an outpatient mental health clinic.
    3. Declaration of incompetence with mandatory medication administration.
    4. Declaration of emergency seclusion.

14. A group of inpatient psychiatric clients on a public elevator begin discussing an out-of-control client who is now in seclusion. Which is the appropriate nursing response?
    1. "I know you are upset by the conflict on the unit. I'm glad you can talk about it."
    2. "Now you know what happens when you can't control your temper."
    3. "It is inappropriate to discuss another client's situation in public."
    4. "Let's just not talk about this now."

15. A newly employed psychiatric nurse answers the desk phone and tells the caller that he or she will be connected to the unit phone to speak to the requested client. With which legal action may the nurse be charged?
    1. Breach of confidentiality
    2. Battery
    3. Assault
    4. Defamation of character

16. The Joint Commission has established specific standards regarding the use of seclusion and restraint. Which of the following are accurate examples of these current standards? **Select all that apply.**
    1. A client who is both restrained and secluded is continuously monitored by trained staff.
    2. A physician calls in a restraint order renewal for an 18-year-old client every 6 hours.
    3. A physician calls in a restraint order renewal for a 12-year-old client every 2 hours.
    4. A physician calls in a restraint order renewal for a 6-year-old client every 1 hour.
    5. Seclusion is discontinued for an 18-year-old client at the earliest possible time regardless of when the order was scheduled to expire.

17. It has been determined that a newly admitted client is "gravely disabled." Which of the following statutes that specifically define the "gravely disabled" client would have led to this determination? **Select all that apply.**
    1. The client who, because of mental illness, cannot fulfill his or her activities of daily living.
    2. The client who, because of mental illness, is unable to provide resources to meet basic needs.
    3. The client who, because of mental illness, has been deemed a danger to self and/or others.
    4. The client who, because of mental illness, lacks the ability to make use of available resources that are needed to meet daily living requirements.
    5. The client, who because of mental illness, is having paranoid delusions about being on the FBI's most wanted list.

18. The legal "duty to warn" for protection of a third party refers to which of the following nursing obligations? **Select all that apply.**
    1. The nurse is obligated to assess a client's threat of violence toward another individual.
    2. The nurse is obligated to inform family members of the client's intent to do harm.
    3. The nurse is obligated to find out the identity of the intended victim.
    4. The nurse is obligated to report the client's intention to harm another to the psychiatrist or to other team members.
    5. The nurse is obligated to protect an intended victim in a feasible, meaningful way.

19. States have enacted laws that grant psychiatrists and attorneys the ability to refuse to reveal information about or communications with clients. This is called the doctrine of _____.

20. A nurse has been accused of defaming a client's character. Which situation and its correctly matched description could have led to this legal action?
    1. The nurse documented a critical and judgmental statement in the client's medical record: libel.
    2. The client overheard the nurse state false and malicious information about the client: invasion of privacy.
    3. Outside of an emergency situation, the nurse touched the client without the client's consent: battery.
    4. The nurse threatened the client that he or she would be touched without the client's consent: assault.

21. As part of the routine admission procedure, a nurse on a psychiatric inpatient unit searches a client. For which legal charge may this nurse be held libel?
    1. Assault
    2. Defamation of character
    3. Invasion of privacy
    4. Breach of confidentiality

REVIEW ANSWERS

1. ANSWER: Kantianism
Rationale: The ethical theory of Kantianism suggests that our actions are bound by a sense of duty. In this theory, the principle or motivation on which action is based is the morally decisive factor. Kantian-directed ethical decisions are made out of respect for moral law.
TEST-TAKING TIP: Review the principles incorporated in various ethical theories.
Content Area: Safe and Effective Care Environment: Management of Care;
Integrated Process: Nursing Process: Implementation;
Client Need: Safe and Effective Care Environment: Management of Care;
Cognitive Level: Knowledge;
Concept: Ethics

2. ANSWER 1
Rationale:
1. The basis of utilitarianism is "the greatest-happiness principle." Actions are right if they promote happiness and wrong if they produce the opposite of happiness. The unpleasant feeling the student expects to feel has prompted the action of refusing to cheat.
2. The basis of Kantianism is that ethical decisions are made out of respect for moral law. It is a moral duty to follow the law. The student in this situation is following the school policy by not cheating and is prompted to do this from a Kantian, not utilitarian, perspective.
3. Christian ethics approaches ethical decision making based on love, forgiveness, and honesty. It is focused on the teachings of Jesus Christ, who preached that to do wrong was a sin. The student's motivation not to cheat because it would be a sin is based on Christian ethics, not utilitarianism.
4. Ethical egoism approaches ethical decision making based on what is best for the individual making the decision. The student in the situation sees only his or her individual benefit from making the decision not to cheat and is prompted to do this from an ethical egoist, not utilitarian perspective.
TEST-TAKING TIP: Review the principles incorporated in various ethical theories and match the situation presented in the question with the theory it exemplifies.
Content Area: Safe and Effective Care Environment: Management of Care;
Integrated Process: Nursing Process: Assessment;
Client Need: Safe and Effective Care Environment: Management of Care;
Cognitive Level: Application;
Concept: Ethics

3. ANSWER 3, 4
Rationale:
1. Within an ethical dilemma, evidence exists to support both moral "rightness" and moral "wrongness" related to a certain action. This student statement indicates that learning has occurred.
2. In an ethical dilemma, the individual that must make the choice experiences conscious conflict regarding the decision. Ethical dilemmas generally create a great deal of emotion. This student statement indicates that learning has occurred.

3. In an ethical dilemma, a choice must be made between two equally unfavorable, not favorable, alternatives. This student statement indicates a need for further instruction.
4. An ethical dilemma arises when there is no clear reason to choose one action over another. Often the reasons supporting each side of the argument for action are logical and appropriate, not illogical and inappropriate. This student statement indicates a need for further instruction.
5. It is true that in most situations involving ethical dilemmas, taking no action is considered an action taken. This student statement indicates that learning has occurred.
TEST-TAKING TIP: Recall the concept of an ethical dilemma. The word "dilemma" would lead the test taker to eliminate Option 3 because a "favorable" choice would not pose a predicament or dilemma.
Content Area: Safe and Effective Care Environment: Management of Care;
Integrated Process: Nursing Process: Evaluation;
Client Need: Safe and Effective Care Environment: Management of Care;
Cognitive Level: Application;
Concept: Ethics

4. ANSWER 3
Rationale:
1. Nonmaleficence is the ethical principle that requires health-care providers to do no harm to their clients. The situation presented in the question is not an example of this ethical principle.
2. Beneficence is the ethical principle that refers to one's duty to benefit or promote the good of others. The situation presented in the question is not an example of this ethical principle.
3. Autonomy is the ethical principle that respects an individual's right to determine his or her destiny. This principle presumes that the client is capable of making independent choices for himself or herself. When a nurse supports a competent client's right to refuse offered medications, the nurse is implementing the ethical principle of autonomy.
4. Veracity is the ethical principle that refers to one's duty to always be truthful and not to deceive or mislead. The situation presented in the question is not an example of this ethical principle.
TEST-TAKING TIP: Review the ethical principles. These principles that a nurse should uphold during client care include autonomy, beneficence, nonmaleficence, justice, and veracity.
Content Area: Safe and Effective Care Environment: Management of Care;
Integrated Process: Nursing Process: Implementation;
Client Need: Safe and Effective Care Environment: Management of Care;
Cognitive Level: Application;
Concept: Ethics

5. ANSWER: 2
Rationale:
1. Nonmaleficence is the ethical principle that requires health-care providers to do no harm to their clients. When a nurse uses verbal strategies, instead of forced seclusion, to calm an agitated client the nurse is implementing the ethical principle of nonmaleficence, not beneficence.

2. Beneficence is the ethical principle that refers to one's duty to benefit or promote the good of others. When a nurse advocates for a client, the nurse is implementing the ethical principle of beneficence. By talking with a client's physician to gain permission for the client to attend an upcoming fieldtrip, the nurse is advocating for the client and employing the ethical principle of beneficence.

3. Autonomy is the ethical principle that respects an individual's right to determine his or her destiny. This principle presumes that individuals are capable of making independent choices for themselves. When a nurse encourages a client diagnosed with dementia to choose what to wear for the day, the nurse is implementing the ethical principle of autonomy, not beneficence.

4. Veracity is the ethical principle that refers to one's duty to always be truthful and not to deceive or mislead. When a nurse teaches a client about the chronic nature of his or her diagnosis of schizophrenia, the nurse is implementing the ethical principle of veracity, not beneficence.

TEST-TAKING TIP: Review the ethical principles. These principles that a nurse should uphold during client care include autonomy, beneficence, nonmaleficence, justice, and veracity.

Content Area: Safe and Effective Care Environment: Management of Care;
Integrated Process: Nursing Process: Implementation;
Client Need: Safe and Effective Care Environment: Management of Care;
Cognitive Level: Application;
Concept: Ethics

6. ANSWER 3

Rationale:

1. The basis of utilitarianism is "the greatest-happiness principle." Actions are right if they promote happiness and wrong if they produce the opposite of happiness. A nurse who decides to work a double shift because the nurse feels needed by the staff and clients is motivated by the good feelings of being needed by others. This action is based on the principle of utilitarianism, not Christian ethics.

2. The basis of Kantianism is that ethical decisions are made out of respect for moral law. It is a moral duty to follow the law. The nurse in this situation is following the law and hospital policy by not diverting scheduled medications and is prompted to do this from a Kantian, not Christian, ethics perspective.

3. Christian ethics approach ethical decision making based on love, forgiveness, and honesty. The basic principle is the golden rule: "Do unto others as you would have them do unto you." The decision to treat a coworker the way the nurse would want to be treated is based on Christian ethics.

4. Ethical egoism approaches ethical decision making based on what is best for the individual making the decision. The nurse in the situation sees only his or her individual career-enhancing benefit from volunteering to be assigned especially difficult clients. This action is prompted by an ethical egoism, not Christian ethics perspective.

TEST-TAKING TIP: Review the principles incorporated in various ethical theories and match the situation presented in the question with the theory it exemplifies.

Content Area: Safe and Effective Care Environment: Management of Care;
Integrated Process: Nursing Process: Assessment;
Client Need: Safe and Effective Care Environment: Management of Care;
Cognitive Level: Application;
Concept: Ethics

7. ANSWER: value

Rationale: Values are personal beliefs about what is important and desirable. Values clarification is a process of self-exploration through which individuals identify and rank their own personal values. This process increases awareness about why individuals behave in certain ways.

TEST-TAKING TIP: Recall that values are personal beliefs about the truth, beauty, or worth of thought, object, or behavior that influence an individual's actions.

Content Area: Psychosocial Integrity;
Integrated Process: Nursing Process: Assessment;
Client Need: Psychosocial Integrity;
Cognitive Level: Knowledge;
Concept: Ethics

8. ANSWERS: The correct order is: 3, 5, 2, 1, 4

Rationale:

1. Assessment: the gathering of subjective and objective data related to the situation. Personal values as well as values of others involved in the ethical dilemma are considered.

2. Problem identification: the identification of the conflict between two or more alternative actions.

3. Planning: exploring the benefits and consequences of each alternative; considering the principles of ethical theories; selecting an alternative.

4. Implementation: acting on the decision made and communicating the decision to others.

5. Evaluation: evaluating or appraising the outcomes of the decision.

TEST-TAKING TIP: Note that the steps of the ethical decision-making model closely resemble the steps of the nursing process.
Review Figure 6.1 as needed to understand the steps of the ethical decision-making model.

Content Area: Safe and Effective Care Environment: Management of Care;
Integrated Process: Nursing Process: Implementation;
Client Need: Safe and Effective Care Environment: Management of Care;
Cognitive Level: Application;
Concept: Ethics

9. ANSWER 4

Rationale:

1. The treatment team must determine that criteria have been met to force medication without client consent. One of the criteria is that the client must exhibit behavior that is dangerous to self or others. When a client, who is refusing medications, has expressed a desire to harm a spouse, the client may lose the right to refuse medications.

2. The treatment team must determine that criteria have been met to force medication without client consent. One of the criteria is that the ordered medication must have a

reasonable chance of providing help to the client. When a client is benefiting from psychotropic medications but refuses drugs due to command hallucinations, the client may lose the right to refuse medications.

3. The treatment team must determine that criteria have been met to force medication without client consent. One of the criteria is that the client must be judged incompetent to evaluate the benefits of the treatment in question. When a client who has been deemed incompetent will not take ordered medications, the client may lose the right to refuse medications.

4. The treatment team must determine that criteria have been met to force medication without client consent. When a client diagnosed with depression decides not to take his or her antidepressant medication and there is no evidence that meets criteria to allow medications to be forced without the client's consent, the client should maintain the right of medication refusal.

TEST-TAKING TIP: Review the criteria that must be met to legally force medications against a client's will.
Content Area: Safe and Effective Care Environment: Management of Care;
Integrated Process: Nursing Process: Implementation;
Client Need: Safe and Effective Care Environment: Management of Care;
Cognitive Level: Application;
Concept: Ethics

10. **ANSWER: 3**
Rationale:
1. Electroconvulsive treatment (ECT) would be considered the most restrictive psychiatric therapy in relationship to the others presented. This therapy should only be employed after all other least restrictive interventions have been attempted.
2. Chemical therapy is a restrictive intervention that should only be employed after all other least restrictive actions have been attempted.
3. Verbal rehabilitative techniques are the least restrictive interventions in relationship to the others presented. The nurse should always employ verbal strategies and "talk a client down" as a first-line intervention before enacting more restrictive therapies.
4. Mechanical restraints are restrictive interventions that should only be employed after all other least restrictive actions have been attempted.
TEST-TAKING TIP: Review the client's right to the least restrictive treatment alternative. A restrictive intervention will limit a client's ability to move freely and/or think clearly.
Content Area: Safe and Effective Care Environment: Management of Care;
Integrated Process: Nursing Process: Implementation;
Client Need: Safe and Effective Care Environment: Management of Care;
Cognitive Level: Application;
Concept: Ethics

11. **ANSWERS: 1, 2, 3, 5**
Rationale: The Tarasoff ruling states that when a clinician is reasonably certain that a client is going to harm an identified person, the therapist has the responsibility to breach the confidentiality of the relationship and warn or protect the potential victim. The courts have extended the Tarasoff duty to include all mental health-care workers.

1. It is important and necessary to assess the client's potential for violence toward others.
2. It is necessary to confirm the identification of the intended victim.
3. The Tarasoff ruling makes it mandatory to notify an identified victim.
4. The Tarasoff ruling makes it mandatory to notify an identified victim, not just law enforcement authorities. The ruling asserted that "the confidential character of patient-psychotherapist communication must yield to the extent that disclosure is essential to avert danger to others. The protective privilege ends where the public peril begins."
5. Because the client is a danger toward others, the court should be petitioned for continued involuntary commitment.

TEST-TAKING TIP: Recall the mandates of the Tarasoff ruling to choose the correct answers.
Content Area: Safe and Effective Care Environment: Management of Care;
Integrated Process: Nursing Process: Implementation;
Client Need: Safe and Effective Care Environment: Management of Care;
Cognitive Level: Application;
Concept: Safety

12. **ANSWER 2**
Rationale:
1. This client is an imminent danger to others. Not administering the medication would put the safety of the nurse and other clients in the milieu at risk.
2. Because this client is an imminent danger to others, it is the duty of the nurse to initiate a forced medication protocol to protect the nurse and other clients in the milieu. Regardless of admission status, after other least restrictive measures have failed, a hostile and/or aggressive client may lose the right to refuse medications.
3. Legal actions related to declaring this client incompetent may be a long-term solution, but they do nothing to immediately protect the nurse and other clients in the milieu.
4. This client is expressing hostility and high levels of anxiety, which precludes readiness for learning to occur. This nursing intervention also does not address safety issues.
TEST-TAKING TIP: Note that if the client is admitted involuntarily under the criterion of "danger to self or others," this does not necessarily determine the client's right to refuse medications. If the client poses an immediate threat to self or others, forced medication protocol may be initiated after obtaining the signatures of two physicians. This decision is determined not by the client's admission status but by the client's threatening behavior.
Content Area: Safe and Effective Care Environment: Management of Care;
Integrated Process: Nursing Process: Implementation;
Client Need: Safe and Effective Care Environment: Management of Care;
Cognitive Level: Application;
Concept: Nursing Roles

13. ANSWER: 2
Rationale:
1. Voluntary commitment to a locked psychiatric facility would not require a court ruling. In this case, the client would initiate admission procedures willingly. This would be inappropriate for this client, who has been deemed a danger to self.
2. Involuntary commitment to an outpatient mental health clinic is an option of the court when a client has been declared a danger to self. If the client fails to appear at regularly scheduled appointments, the client can be seized and involuntarily committed to an inpatient psychiatric unit.
3. Declaration of incompetence with mandatory medication administration may be ruled by the court but requires a hearing beyond the emergency commitment ruling.
4. Declaration of emergency seclusion is not within the scope of a court ruling. A client has to be deemed an imminent danger to self before seclusion is enacted, and the health-care team, not the court, makes this decision. The client is always given the right of least restrictive interventions.
TEST-TAKING TIP: Recall that the court has options related to involuntary commitments of clients who meet the criteria of being a danger to self or others. Either inpatient or outpatient commitment is a possible option.
Content Area: Safe and Effective Care Environment: Management of Care;
Integrated Process: Nursing Process: Implementation;
Client Need: Safe and Effective Care Environment: Management of Care;
Cognitive Level: Application;
Concept: Safety

14. ANSWER 3
Rationale:
1. In this situation, the nurse is encouraging further discussion of a client's personal information in a public setting and is disregarding the client's right to confidentiality.
2. In this situation, the nurse is participating in and contributing to divulging client confidential information and is using her position to threaten clients.
3. This statement addresses the client's right to confidentiality and sets limits on client behaviors that threaten that right.
4. This response of the nurse does not address the breach of confidentially that is occurring on the elevator. This also reflects the nontherapeutic communication technique of rejecting.
TEST-TAKING TIP: Clients have the right to expect the nurse to protect their confidentiality. Choose the answer that reflects this action by the nurse.
Content Area: Safe and Effective Care Environment: Management of Care;
Integrated Process: Nursing Process: Implementation;
Client Need: Safe and Effective Care Environment: Management of Care;
Cognitive Level: Application;
Concept: Ethics

15. ANSWER: 1
Rationale:
1. Breach of confidentiality is a common law tort that refers to disobedience of the set laws that govern the privacy of personal information. There is no indication in the question that the caller is on a "client approval list." The nurse in the question has not considered the client's right to confidentiality by allowing the caller access to the client without the client's permission. This breach of confidentiality may lead to legal action against the nurse.
2. Battery is the unconsented touching of another person. Charges can result when treatment that includes touching is administered to a client against his or her wishes and outside of an emergency situation. The nurse in the question has not committed battery.
3. Assault is an act that results in a person's genuine fear and apprehension that he or she will be touched without consent. The nurse in the question did not commit assault.
4. Defamation of character occurs when a person shares detrimental information about another. When the information is shared verbally, it is called slander. When the information is in writing, it is called libel. The nurse in the question has not defamed the character of the client.
TEST-TAKING TIP: Recall the types of lawsuits that may occur in the psychiatric setting, and be aware of the types of professional behaviors that may result in charges of malpractice.
Content Area: Safe and Effective Care Environment: Management of Care;
Integrated Process: Nursing Process: Evaluation;
Client Need: Safe and Effective Care Environment: Management of Care;
Cognitive Level: Application;
Concept: Ethics

16. ANSWERS: 1, 3, 4, 5
Rationale:
1. According to The Joint Commission standards, individuals who are simultaneously restrained and secluded must be continuously monitored by trained staff, either in person or through audio or visual equipment positioned near the individual. This is an accurate example of this current standard.
2. According to The Joint Commission standards, orders for restraint or seclusion for adults 18 years and older must be renewed every 4, not 6, hours. This example does not meet the Joint Commission standards.
3. According to The Joint Commission standards, orders for restraint or seclusion must be renewed every 2 hours for children and adolescents ages 9 to 17 years. This example meets The Joint Commission standards.
4. According to The Joint Commission standards, orders for restraint or seclusion must be renewed every 1 hour for children younger than 9 years. This example meets The Joint Commission standards.
5. The Joint Commission has established specific standards regarding the use of seclusion and restraints. The secluding or restraining of a client must be discontinued at the earliest possible time regardless of when the order is scheduled to expire. This example meets The Joint Commission standards.

TEST-TAKING TIP: Recall the current and specific standards established by the Joint Commission regarding the use of seclusion and restraints of an individual.
Content Area: Safe and Effective Care Environment: Management of Care;
Integrated Process: Nursing Process: Implementation;
Client Need: Safe and Effective Care Environment: Management of Care;
Cognitive Level: Application;
Concept: Regulations

17. **ANSWERS: 1, 4**
    Rationale:
    1. A number of states have statutes that specifically define the "gravely disabled" client. States that do not use this label similarly describe individuals who, because of mental illness, are unable to take care of basic personal needs. Therefore, the client who cannot fulfill activities of daily living because of mental illness meets the statutes that specifically define the "gravely disabled."
    2. An individual who, as the result of mental illness, is unable to provide for resources to meet basic needs does not meet the statutes that specifically define the "gravely disabled." However, a client who, because of mental illness, is unable to make use of available resources to meet basic personal needs would meet the statutes that specifically define the "gravely disabled."
    3. A client who, because of mental illness, has been deemed a danger to self and/or others may be involuntarily committed to a psychiatric facility, but there is nothing in Option 3 to indicate that the client meets the statutes that specifically define the "gravely disabled."
    4. A client who, because of mental illness, lacks the ability to make use of available resources that are needed for personal needs meets the criteria of a "gravely disabled" individual. However, a client who, because of mental illness, is unable to provide for resources for basic needs would not meet the statutes that specifically define the "gravely disabled."
    5. A client who, because of mental illness, is having paranoid delusions about being on the FBI's most wanted list may meet criteria for admission to an inpatient or outpatient facility, but there is nothing in the answer choice to indicate that the client meets the statutes that specifically define the "gravely disabled."
    TEST-TAKING TIP: Recall the statues that define the "gravely disabled" client and be able to match the situation presented in the answer choices to that statute.
    Content Area: Safe and Effective Care Environment: Management of Care;
    Integrated Process: Nursing Process: Assessment;
    Client Need: Safe and Effective Care Environment: Management of Care;
    Cognitive Level: Application;
    Concept: Regulations

18. **ANSWERS: 1, 3, 4, 5**
    Rationale:
    1. The nurse is obligated to ascertain any and all information from the client after the nurse has determined that the client poses a serious danger of violence to others.

2. The nurse is obligated to notify the psychiatrist or other team members, not the client's family, regarding the threat of violence to others.
3. The nurse is obligated to ascertain the identity of the intended victim, to the best of his or her ability.
4. The nurse is obligated to inform the psychiatrist or other team members when a client has revealed that he or she intends to do harm to another.
5. When a client poses a serious danger of violence to others, the nurse is obligated to exercise reasonable care to protect the foreseeable victim of that danger.
TEST-TAKING TIP: Recognize that once a client poses a serious danger of violence to others, the health professional is under legal obligation to prevent the client from harming others. The heath professional also must know the legalities of this obligation.
Content Area: Safe and Effective Care Environment: Management of Care;
Integrated Process: Nursing Process: Implementation;
Client Need: Safe and Effective Care Environment: Management of Care;
Cognitive Level: Application;
Concept: Ethics

19. **ANSWER: privileged communication**
    Rationale: Most states have statutes that pertain to the doctrine of privileged communication. Although the codes differ markedly from state to state, most grant certain professionals privileges under which they may refuse to reveal information about and communication with clients. In most states, this doctrine applies to psychiatrists and attorneys; in some instances, psychologists, clergy, and nurses are also included.
    TEST-TAKING TIP: Recall the doctrine of privileged communication. The word "communication" in the question should suggest the word needed to complete this "fill in the blank" question.
    Content Area: Safe and Effective Care Environment: Management of Care;
    Integrated Process: Nursing Process: Implementation;
    Client Need: Safe and Effective Care Environment: Management of Care;
    Cognitive Level: Knowledge;
    Concept: Regulations

20. **ANSWER: 1**
    Rationale:
    1. When shared information is detrimental to the client's reputation, the nurse sharing the information may be liable for defamation of character. When the information is in writing, the action is called libel. When a nurse documents a critical and judgmental statement in a client's medical record, the nurse could be sued for defamation of character by libel.
    2. When shared information is detrimental to the client's reputation, the nurse sharing the information may be liable for defamation of character. Oral defamation is called slander. When a client overhears a nurse state false and malicious information about the client, the nurse could be liable for defamation of character by slander, not invasion of privacy.

3. Battery is the unconsented touching of another person. Battery charges can result when a treatment is administered to a client against his or her wishes and outside of an emergency situation. When a nurse, outside of an emergency situation, touches the client without the client's consent, the nurse could be liable for battery, not defamation of character.

4. Assault is the act that results in a person's genuine fear and apprehension that he or she will be touched without consent. When a nurse threatens a client that he or she will be touched without consent, the nurse could be liable for assault, not defamation of character.

TEST-TAKING TIP: Review the legal terms "defamation of character," "libel," "slander," "assault," and "battery." When a question asks you to choose a statement that is correctly matched with its description, carefully read both parts of each answer option to choose the correct answer and the correct label.

Content Area: Safe and Effective Care Environment: Management of Care;
Integrated Process: Nursing Process: Evaluation;
Client Need: Safe and Effective Care Environment: Management of Care;
Cognitive Level: Analysis;
Concept: Ethics

21. **ANSWER: 3**
Rationale:
1. Assault is an act that results in a person's genuine fear and apprehension that he or she will be touched without consent. When a nurse on a psychiatric inpatient unit searches a client as part of the admission procedure, the nurse's actions would not meet the criteria for a charge of assault.

2. When shared information is detrimental to the client's reputation, the nurse sharing the information may be liable for defamation of character. When a nurse on a psychiatric inpatient unit searches a client as part of the admission procedure, the nurse's actions would not meet the criteria for a charge of defamation of character.

3. **Invasion of privacy is a charge that may result when a client is searched without probable cause. Many institutions conduct body searches on mentally ill clients as a routine intervention, especially during admission procedures. In these cases, there should be a physician's order and written rationale showing probable cause for the intervention. When a nurse on a psychiatric inpatient unit searches a client as part of the routine admission procedure, the nurse's actions could meet the criteria for a charge of invasion of privacy.**

4. Basic to the psychiatric client's hospitalization is his or her right to confidentiality and privacy. A nurse may be charged with breach of confidentiality for revealing aspects about the client's case or even for revealing that an individual has been hospitalized. When a nurse on a psychiatric inpatient unit searches a client as part of the admission procedure, the nurse's actions would not meet the criteria for a charge of breach of confidentiality.

TEST-TAKING TIP: Review the legal terms "breach of confidentiality," "invasion of privacy," "defamation of character," and "assault."

Content Area: Safe and Effective Care Environment: Management of Care;
Integrated Process: Nursing Process: Evaluation;
Client Need: Safe and Effective Care Environment: Management of Care;
Cognitive Level: Application;
Concept: Ethics

Chapter 7

Anxiety, Obsessive-Compulsive Disorder, and Related Disorders

KEY TERMS

Agoraphobia—An anxiety disorder characterized by anxiety in situations in which the sufferer perceives certain environments as dangerous or uncomfortable, often due to the environment's vast openness or crowdedness

Anxiety—Apprehension, tension, or uneasiness from anticipation of danger, the source of which is largely unknown or unrecognized; anxiety may be regarded as pathological when it interferes with social and occupational functioning, achievement of desired goals, or emotional comfort

Anxiolytics—Anxiety medications used to treat the somatic and psychological symptoms of anxiety disorders

Automatic thinking—Negative, illogical, and irrational thought processes that are activated during times of stress

Compulsions—Repetitive ritualistic behaviors the purpose of which is to prevent or reduce distress or to prevent some dreaded event or situation; the person feels driven to perform such actions in response to an obsession or according to rules that must be applied rigidly, even though the behaviors are recognized to be excessive or unreasonable

Obsessions—Recurrent and persistent thoughts, impulses, or images experienced as intrusive and stressful; recognized as being excessive and unreasonable even though they are a product of one's mind; the thought, impulse, or image cannot be expunged by logic or reasoning

Panic—A sudden overwhelming feeling of terror or impending doom; this most severe form of emotional anxiety is usually accompanied by behavioral, cognitive, and physiological signs and symptoms considered to be outside the expected range of normalcy

Phobia—Fear cued by the presence or anticipation of a specific object or situation, exposure to which almost invariably provokes an immediate anxiety response or panic attack even though the subject recognizes that the fear is excessive or unreasonable; the phobic stimulus is avoided or endured with marked distress

Secondary gains—Benefits derived from becoming the focus of attention due to an illness, such as an anxiety disorder

Thought stopping—A cognitive technique that uses a variety of strategies to help a person deliberately try to stop thinking certain thoughts

Individuals face anxiety on a daily basis. Anxiety, which provides the motivation for achievement, is a necessary force for survival. The term "anxiety" is often used interchangeably with the word "stress"; however, they are not the same. Stress, or more properly a "stressor," is an external pressure that is brought to bear on the individual. Anxiety is the subjective emotional response to that stressor.

I. Anxiety

A. *Anxiety* may be distinguished from *fear* in that the former is an emotional process, whereas fear is a cognitive one
B. Fear involves the intellectual appraisal of a threatening stimulus; anxiety involves the emotional response to that appraisal
C. Historically, anxiety disorders were viewed as purely psychological or purely biological in nature
D. Researchers have begun to focus on the interrelatedness of mind and body, and anxiety disorders provide an excellent example of this complex relationship
E. It is likely that various factors, including genetic, developmental, environmental, and psychological ones, play a role in the etiology of anxiety disorders

DID YOU KNOW?
Anxiety disorders are the most common of all psychiatric illnesses and result in considerable functional impairment and distress.

F. Anxiety disorders are more common in women than in men by two to one
G. Prevalence rates for anxiety disorders within the general population:
  1. 3% to 5% prevalence rate for generalized anxiety disorder and panic disorder.
  2. 13% prevalence rate for social anxiety disorder.
  3. 25% prevalence rate for phobias.
  4. 2% to 3% prevalence rate for obsessive-compulsive disorder (OCD).
H. Research data suggest a familial predisposition to anxiety disorders

II. Normal Versus Abnormal Anxiety

A. Anxiety is usually considered a normal reaction to a realistic danger or threat to biological integrity or self-concept
B. Normal anxiety dissipates when the danger or threat is no longer present
C. The normality of the anxiety experienced in response to a stressor is defined by societal and cultural standards
D. Criteria can be used to determine whether an individual's anxious response falls outside normal limits:
  1. It is out of proportion to the situation that is creating it.

  2. The anxiety interferes with social, occupational, or other important areas of functioning.

III. Anxiety Issues in the Elderly

A. Some anxiety disorders appear for the first time after age 60
B. The autonomic nervous system is more fragile in older persons
C. The response to a major stressor is often quite intense
D. In older adults, symptoms of anxiety and depression often accompany each other, making it difficult to determine which disorder is dominant

IV. Sleep Disorders in the Elderly

A. Sleep disturbances affect 50% of people age 65 and older who live at home and 66% of those who live in long-term care facilities
B. Common causes of sleep disturbances:
  1. Aging decreases the ability to sleep ("sleep decay")
  2. Increased prevalence of sleep apnea.
  3. Depression.
  4. Dementia.
  5. Anxiety.
  6. Pain.
  7. Impaired mobility.
  8. Medications.
  9. Psychosocial factors.
    a. Loneliness.
    b. Inactivity.
    c. Boredom.
C. Sleep aids used for the elderly:
  1. Sedative-hypnotics.
  2. Anxiolytics.
  3. Nonpharmacological approaches.
  4. Changes in aging associated with metabolism and elimination must be considered when maintenance medications are administered for chronic insomnia.

Ⓘ Caution should be taken in administering antianxiety drugs to elderly clients because of their decreased hepatic and renal functioning.

V. Treatment Modalities for Anxiety

DID YOU KNOW?
Treatment of anxiety and related disorders includes individual psychotherapy, cognitive therapy, behavior therapy (including implosion therapy, systematic desensitization, and habit-reversal therapy), and psychopharmacology.

A. Therapies
1. Individual psychotherapy.
   a. Decreases client's anxiety by discussing situation with a concerned, empathetic therapist.
   b. Helps clients understand the hypothesized unconscious meaning of the anxiety.
   c. Helps clients understand the symbolism of the avoided situation.
   d. Helps clients understand the need to repress impulses.
   e. Focuses on helping clients understand the **secondary gains** that may be achieved from the symptoms exhibited.
   f. May provide client with psychoeducational information.
2. Cognitive therapy.
   a. The cognitive model is based on how individuals respond in stressful situations to their subjective cognitive appraisal of the event.
   b. Impaired cognition can contribute to anxiety and related disorders when the individual's appraisals are chronically negative.
   c. Automatic negative appraisals provoke self-doubts, negative evaluations, and negative predictions.
   d. Cognitive therapy assists the individual to reduce anxiety responses by altering cognitive distortions.
   e. Anxiety can be the result of exaggerated, **automatic thinking.**
   f. Cognitive therapy is brief and time limited
      i. Usually lasting from 5 to 20 sessions
      ii. Discourages the client's dependency on the therapist
      iii. Encourages the client's self-sufficiency
   g. Treatment consists of encouraging the client to face frightening situations.
   h. Encourages the client to view frightening situations realistically and to talk about them.
   i. Collaborative effort between client and therapist.
   j. Assists client to become aware of thoughts and to examine thoughts for cognitive distortions.
   k. Teaches client to substitute more balanced thoughts and develop new patterns of thinking.
   l. Therapy is structured and orderly.
   m. Focuses on solving current problems.
   n. Homework assignments provide an experimental, problem-solving approach to overcoming long-held anxieties.
3. Behavior therapy.
   a. Habit-reversal therapy (HRT).
      i. A system of positive and negative reinforcements to modify behaviors
         1) Attempts to extinguish unwanted behaviors

2) Increases awareness of the behavior
3) Identifies times of occurrence
4) Substitutes a more adaptive coping strategy
5) Used in the treatment of trichotillomania
   b. Systematic desensitization.
      i. Based on behavioral conditioning principles
      ii. Client is gradually exposed to a phobic stimulus, either in a real or imagined situation
         1) *Reciprocal inhibition* is the restriction of anxiety before the effort of reducing avoidance behavior
         2) Relaxation is antagonistic to anxiety; individuals cannot be anxious and relaxed at the same time
      iii. Systematic desensitization with reciprocal inhibition involves two main elements:
         1) Training in relaxation techniques (e.g., progressive relaxation, mental imagery, tense and relax, meditation)
         2) Progressive exposure to a hierarchy of fear stimuli while in the relaxed state
      iv. Used in the treatment of clients with phobic disorders
      v. Modifies the stereotyped behavior of clients with OCD
   c. Implosion therapy (flooding).
      i. A therapeutic process in which the client must imagine situations or participate in real-life situations that he or she finds extremely frightening, for a prolonged period of time
      ii. Relaxation training is not a part of this technique
      iii. Therapist "floods" the client with vivid details concerning situations that trigger anxiety
      iv. Therapy continues until a topic no longer elicits inappropriate anxiety
      v. Used for the treatment of phobic disorders
B. Psychopharmacology
1. Antianxiety agents or **anxiolytics.**
   a. Antianxiety medications, except buspirone, depress the central nervous system (CNS).
   b. Used for short-term treatment of anxiety.
   c. Potentiate the effects of the powerful inhibitory neurotransmitter, GABA, producing a calming effect.
   d. Contraindicated in individuals with known hypersensitivity to any of the drugs within the classification.

🛑 Central nervous system (CNS) depressants, like anxiolytics, should not be taken in combination with other CNS depressants, such as alcohol. The combined effect can decrease respirations and increase the risk of apnea and possible death.

e. Contraindicated in pregnancy and lactation, narrow-angle glaucoma, shock, and coma.

f. Caution is advised when administering these drugs to elderly or debilitated clients and clients with hepatic or renal dysfunction. (The dosage usually has to be decreased.)

g. Caution is advised with individuals who have a history of drug abuse or addiction.
   i. Tolerance and dependence can develop with continued use
   ii. Withdrawal symptoms can be life threatening
   iii. Not to be discontinued abruptly; must be tapered off the medication

h. Caution is advised when individuals are depressed or suicidal. In depressed clients, CNS depressants can exacerbate symptoms.

i. Increased effects of antianxiety agents can occur when taken concomitantly with alcohol, barbiturates, narcotics, antipsychotics, antidepressants, antihistamines, neuromuscular blocking agents, cimetidine, or disulfiram.

j. Increased effects can also occur with herbal depressants (e.g., kava, valerian).

k. Decreased effects can be noted with nicotine and caffeine use.

l. Buspirone, because it does not depress the CNS, is often the drug of choice when treating anxiety for client with addiction problems.

2. Antidepressants.
   a. Several antidepressants are effective as major antianxiety agents.
   b. Used for long-term treatment of anxiety.
   c. Selective serotonin reuptake inhibitors (SSRIs) are the treatment of choice because they have fewer side effects than tricyclics.

3. Antihypertensive agents.
   a. Beta blockers and alpha 2-receptor agonists have been used to decrease anxiety symptoms.
   b. These antihypertensive medications have an effect on somatic manifestations of anxiety (palpitations, tremors).
   c. Less effect on psychic component of anxiety.

MAKING THE CONNECTION

Researchers investigate predisposing factors to anxiety disorders from various theoretical perspectives and create theories of origin. This aids in the formulation of a correct diagnostic assessment and the development of appropriate interventions.

VI. Types of Anxiety Disorders

A. Theories of origin
   1. Psychoanalytic theory.
      a. Inability of ego to intervene in id and superego conflicts.
      b. Ego development delayed due to:
         i. Unsatisfactory parent-child relationship
         ii. Conditional love
         iii. Provisional gratification
      c. Overuse or ineffective use of ego defense mechanisms.
      d. Freud believed phobias came from faulty processing of the Oedipal/Electra complex.
         i. Incestuous feelings and fear of retribution from the same-gender parent results in repression and displacement onto a safe and neutral phobic stimulus.
         ii. Unconscious fears expressed in a symbolic manner prevent confrontation of real fear.
      e. Individuals diagnosed with OCD:
         i. Have weak, underdeveloped egos and regress to an earlier stage of development
         ii. Use the ego defenses of isolation, undoing, displacement, and reaction formation
         iii. Regression and overuse of defenses produce obsessions and compulsions
   2. Cognitive theory.
      a. Faulty, distorted, or counterproductive thinking patterns.
      b. Leads to disturbances in feelings and behaviors.
      c. Anxiety due to dysfunctional appraisal of situations.
         i. Negative self-statements
         ii. Irrational beliefs
      d. Loss of ability to reason out the problem.
      e. Avoidance behaviors used to prevent anxiety reactions lead to phobias.
         i. "Locus of control" can be internal or external (Fig. 7.1)
         ii. With external locus of control, anxiety is attributed to an external source leading to a phobia
         iii. With internal locus of control, anxiety is attributed to a stressor leading to problem solving
   3. Biological theory.
      a. Temperament and innate fears are inherited characteristics.
      b. They influence reactions to stressful situations and may predispose an individual to phobic responses.
      c. Genetics.
         i. Research shows gene variant
         ii. Twin studies indicate familial predisposition

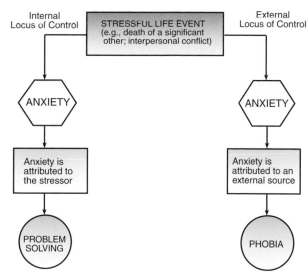

Fig 7.1 Locus of control as a variable in the etiology of phobias.

  iii. Trichotillomania has been associated with OCD among first-degree relatives
 d. Neuroanatomical.
  i. Emotional states affected by lower brain centers
   1) Limbic system
   2) Thalamus
   3) Hypothalamus
   4) Reticular formation
 e. Structural brain imaging indicates temporal lobe pathology.
 f. Trichotillomania anomalies.
  i. Structural brain abnormalities
  ii. Alterations in serotonin and endogenous opioid systems
 g. OCD anomalies.
  i. Abnormal metabolic rates in the brain
  ii. Neuroendocrine imbalances
  iii. Abnormal serotonin levels noted in both OCD and body dysmorphic disorder (BDD)
4. Learning theory.
 a. Classical conditioning: a stressful stimulus produces an "unconditioned" response.
 b. A harmless object alone can trigger a "conditioned" response of fear after being continually paired with a stressful stimulus.
 c. Direct learning or "modeling" can produce a phobic response.
 d. Obsessive-compulsive behavior is a conditioned response to a traumatic event.
 e. Individuals learn to avoid the anxiety-producing situation either passively or actively.
 f. Active avoidance includes behavior patterns that provide relief from anxiety and discomfort, such as obsessions and compulsions.

5. Psychosocial influences related to trichotillomania.
 a. One-fourth of cases are related to stressful situations.
 b. Can result from dysfunctional mother-child relationship, fear of abandonment, recent object loss.
 c. May be associated with body dysmorphic disorder and childhood abuse.
B. Panic disorder
 1. Nursing process: assessment.
  a. Characterized by recurrent panic attacks.
   i. Unpredictable onset
   ii. Organic factors must be ruled out
   iii. Symptoms occur unexpectedly
    1) Do not occur immediately before or after exposure to something that generates anxiety (phobia)
    2) Not triggered by the person being the focus of attention (social anxiety disorder)
   iv. Intense apprehension, fear, terror
   v. Feelings of impending doom
   vi. Intense physical discomfort
   vii. Usually last minutes
   viii. Apprehension may occur between attacks
   ix. Depression is common
  b. Required criteria for diagnosis (at least four must be present):
   i. Palpitations, pounding heart, or accelerated heart rate
   ii. Sweating
   iii. Trembling or shaking
   iv. Sensations of shortness of breath or smothering
   v. Feelings of choking
   vi. Chest pain or discomfort
   vii. Nausea or abdominal distress
   viii. Feeling dizzy, unsteady, lightheaded, or faint
   ix. Chills or heat sensations
   x. Paresthesias (numbness or tingling sensations)
   xi. Derealization (feelings of unreality) or depersonalization (feelings of being detached from oneself)
   xii. Fear of losing control or going crazy
   xiii. Fear of dying
  c. Age of onset: late 20s.
  d. Frequency and severity of attacks vary widely.
  e. May have remissions and exacerbations.
 2. Nursing process: diagnosis (analysis)—nursing diagnoses for clients with anxiety, OCD, and related disorders are formulated from the data gathered during the assessment phase and with background knowledge regarding predisposing factors to the disorder. Table 7.1 presents a list of

Table 7.1 Assigning Nursing Diagnoses to Behaviors Commonly Associated With Anxiety, Obsessive-Compulsive Disorder, and Related Disorders

Behaviors	Nursing Diagnosis
Palpitations, trembling, sweating, chest pain, shortness of breath, fear of going crazy, fear of dying (*panic disorder*); excessive worry, difficulty concentrating, sleep disturbance (*generalized anxiety disorder*)	**Panic anxiety**
Verbal expressions of having no control over life situation; nonparticipation in decision making related to own care or life situation; expressions of doubt regarding role performance (*panic and generalized anxiety disorders*)	**Powerlessness**
Behavior directed toward avoidance of a feared object or situation (*phobic disorder*)	**Fear**
Stays at home alone, afraid to venture out alone (*agoraphobia*)	**Social isolation**
Ritualistic behavior; obsessive thoughts, inability to meet basic needs; severe level of anxiety (*obsessive-compulsive disorder [OCD]*)	**Ineffective coping**
Inability to fulfill usual patterns of responsibility because of need to perform rituals (*OCD*)	**Ineffective role performance**
Preoccupation with imagined defect; verbalizations that are out of proportion to any actual physical abnormality that may exist; numerous visits to plastic surgeons or dermatologists seeking relief (*body dysmorphic disorder*)	**Disturbed body image**
Repetitive and impulsive pulling out of one's hair (*hair-pulling disorder [trichotillomania]*)	**Ineffective impulse control**

client behaviors and the NANDA nursing diagnoses that correspond to those behaviors, which may be used in planning care.

3. Nursing process: planning.
   a. Short-term outcome: client will verbalize ways to interrupt escalating anxiety within 1 week.
   b. Long-term outcome: by discharge from treatment, the client will be able to recognize onset of symptoms and be able to intervene before reaching panic level.
4. Nursing process: implementation.
   a. Stay with the client and offer reassurance of safety and security. Do not leave the client alone during a panic attack.
   b. Maintain a calm, nonthreatening, matter-of-fact approach.

DID YOU KNOW?

Anxiety is contagious and may be transferred from staff to client or vice versa. Clients develop a feeling of security in the presence of a calm staff person.

   c. Use simple words and brief messages, spoken calmly and clearly.
   d. Decrease environmental stimuli (dim lighting, few people, simple decor).

DID YOU KNOW?

In an intensely anxious situation, a client is unable to comprehend anything but the most elemental communication. Because of a lack of concentration and focus, this is not the time to attempt any client teaching.

   e. Administer ordered tranquilizing medication and assess for effectiveness and side effects.

   f. After decreased level of anxiety, explore reasons for occurrence.
   g. After decreased level of anxiety, teach signs and symptoms of escalating anxiety and ways to interrupt anxiety progression.
      i. Relaxation techniques, such as deep-breathing exercises and meditation
      ii. Physical exercise, such as brisk walks and jogging

🛑 During extreme anxiety, hyperventilation causes decreased carbon dioxide (CO_2) levels, which may result in symptoms of lightheadedness, rapid heart rate, shortness of breath, numbness or tingling in hands or feet, and syncope. Possible client injury then becomes a nursing safety priority. Have the client breathe 6 to 12 times into a small paper bag. This should reverse this condition, bring CO_2 back to normal levels, and reduce distressing symptoms. This technique is not recommended for clients diagnosed with coronary or respiratory disorders, such as coronary artery disease, asthma, or chronic obstructive pulmonary disease (COPD).

5. Nursing process: evaluation—Suggested questions used in the evaluation process are presented later in this outline.
6. Psychopharmacology.
   a. Anxiolytics.
      i. Alprazolam, lorazepam, and clonazepam are effective with panic disorder
      ii. Risks include dependence and life-threatening withdrawal symptoms
   b. Antidepressants.
      i. SSRIs, serotonin and norepinephrine reuptake inhibitors (SNRIs), and buspirone are first-line choices of treatment for panic disorders

ii. Paroxetine, fluoxetine, and sertraline have been approved by the U.S. Food and Drug Administration (FDA) for panic disorder
   1) SSRIs must be titrated slowly
   2) With sensitivity to SSRIs, overstimulation may occur
iii. The tricyclics clomipramine and imipramine have been used with success with panic disorder
iv. High doses of tricyclics needed for panic disorder response can lead to severe side effects

c. Antihypertensive agents.
   i. Propranolol has potent effects on somatic symptoms of anxiety, but it is not the first line of treatment for panic disorder
   ii. Clonidine has limited usefulness in long-term treatment of panic disorder because of development of tolerance

C. Generalized anxiety disorder (GAD)
1. Nursing process: assessment.
   a. Characterized by persistent, unrealistic, and excessive anxiety and worry.
   b. Symptoms must have occurred more days than not for at least 3 months.
   c. Symptoms cannot be attributed to specific organic factors, such as caffeine intoxication or hyperthyroidism.
   d. Symptoms cause clinically significant distress or impairment in social, occupational, or other important areas of functioning.
   e. Anxiety is associated with muscle tension, restlessness, or feeling keyed up or on edge.
   f. Avoidance of activities with possible negative outcomes.
   g. Considerable time and effort preparing for activities with possible negative outcomes.
   h. Procrastination in behavior or decision making.
   i. Repeatedly seeking reassurance.
   j. May begin in childhood or adolescence; onset is not uncommon after age 20.
   k. Depressive symptoms are common.
   l. Numerous somatic complaints may also be present.
   m. Tends to be chronic, with frequent stress-related exacerbations and fluctuations in the course of the illness.
2. Nursing process: diagnosis (analysis)—Table 7.1 presents a list of client behaviors and the NANDA nursing diagnoses that correspond to those behaviors, which may be used in planning care.
3. Nursing process: planning.
   a. Short-term goal: client will be able to identify sources of anxiety by (time frame to be determined according to client situation).

b. Long-term goal: by time of discharge from treatment, client will be able to function effectively in role performance.
4. Nursing process: implementation.
   a. Stay with the client and assure him or her that the nurse can offer assistance.
   b. Speak slowing and calmly.
   c. Use short, simple sentences and give brief directions.
   d. Provide quiet environment to decrease stimuli.
   e. Administer ordered anxiolytic medications if necessary.
   f. Encourage client to discuss precipitating events and to link behaviors to feelings.
   g. Employ cognitive therapy.
   h. Anxiety results from dysfunctional situation appraisal.
   i. Anxiety results from automatic thinking.
   j. Challenge illogical thinking.
   k. Assist client to identify what has relieved anxiety in the past.
   l. Assist client to reframe anxiety-provoking situations in ways that are manageable.
5. Nursing process: evaluation—suggested questions used in the evaluation process are presented later in this outline.
6. Psychopharmacology.
   a. Anxiolytics.
      i. Benzodiazepines have been used with success in the treatment of GAD
      ii. Can be prescribed on an as-needed basis
      iii. Buspirone is effective in about 60% to 80% of clients with generalized anxiety disorder
         1) Disadvantage: a 10- to 14-day delay in alleviating symptoms
         2) Advantage: lack of physical dependence and tolerance
         3) Drug of choice in the treatment of GAD
   b. Antidepressants.
      i. The use of antidepressants for GAD is still being investigated
      ii. Some success has been reported with the tricyclic imipramine and with the SSRIs
      iii. FDA has approved paroxetine, escitalopram, duloxetine, and extended-release venlafaxine in the treatment of GAD

D. Specific phobias
1. Nursing process: assessment.
   a. A specific phobia is identified by fear of specific objects or situations that could conceivably cause harm (e.g., snakes).
   b. Reactions to such objects or situations are excessive, unreasonable, and inappropriate.
   c. Irrational fear restricts the individual's activities and interferes with his or her daily living.

d. The phobic person may be no more (or less) anxious than anyone else until exposed to the phobic object or situation.
e. Exposure to the phobic stimulus produces overwhelming symptoms of panic.
   i. Palpitations
   ii. Sweating
   iii. Dizziness
   iv. Difficulty breathing
f. Symptoms can occur by merely thinking about the phobic stimulus.
g. Client recognizes that fear is excessive or unreasonable.
h. Powerless to change.
i. Phobias may begin at almost any age.
   i. Beginning in childhood, symptoms often disappear without treatment
   ii. Beginning or persisting into adulthood, symptoms usually require assistance with therapy
j. Diagnosed more often in women than in men.
k. Individuals seldom seek treatment unless the phobia interferes with ability to function.
l. Specific phobias have been classified according to the phobic stimulus. A list of some of the more common ones appears in Table 7.2.

DID YOU KNOW?

Anyone with a little knowledge of Greek or Latin can produce a phobia classification by adding the suffix *–phobia* to the Greek or Latin word that described the feared object or situation.

2. Nursing process: diagnosis (analysis)—Table 7.1 presents a list of client behaviors and the NANDA nursing diagnoses that correspond to those behaviors, which may be used in planning care.
3. Nursing process: planning.
   a. Short-term goal: client will discuss the phobic object with the health-care provider by (time frame to be determined according to client situation).
   b. Long-term goal: by time of discharge from treatment, client will be able to function in presence of phobic object without experiencing panic anxiety.
4. Nursing process: implementation.
   a. Reassure client that he or she is safe.
   b. Explore client's perception of the threat to physical integrity or to self-concept.
   c. Discuss reality of the situation.
   d. Assist with recognition of what can be changed and what cannot.
   e. Assist client to replace maladaptive coping strategies with adaptive ones.
   f. If client elects to work on elimination of the fear, techniques of desensitization or implosion therapy may be employed.

Table 7.2 Classifications of Specific Phobias

Classification	Fear
Acrophobia	Height
Ailurophobia	Cats
Algophobia	Pain
Anthophobia	Flowers
Anthropophobia	People
Aquaphobia	Water
Arachnophobia	Spiders
Astraphobia	Lightning
Belonephobia	Needles
Brontophobia	Thunder
Claustrophobia	Closed spaces
Cynophobia	Dogs
Dementophobia	Insanity
Equinophobia	Horses
Gamophobia	Marriage
Herpetophobia	Lizards, reptiles
Homophobia	Homosexuality
Murophobia	Mice
Mysophobia	Dirt, germs, contamination
Numerophobia	Numbers
Nyctophobia	Darkness
Ochophobia	Riding in a car
Ophidiophobia	Snakes
Pyrophobia	Fire
Scoleciphobia	Worms
Siderodromophobia	Railroads or train travel
Taphophobia	Being buried alive
Thanatophobia	Death
Trichophobia	Hair
Triskaidekaphobia	The number 13
Xenophobia	Strangers
Zoophobia	Animals

MAKING THE CONNECTION

It is important to understand the client's perception of the phobic object or situation to assist with the desensitization process. The client must accept the reality of the situation (aspects that cannot change) before the work of reducing the fear can progress.

g. Encourage client to explore underlying feelings that may be contributing to irrational fears and to face them rather than suppress them.
5. Evaluation: suggested questions used in the evaluation process are presented later in this outline.
6. Psychopharmacology: specific phobias are generally not treated with medication unless panic attacks accompany the phobia.

E. Agoraphobia
1. Nursing process: assessment.
   a. Fear of being in open spaces.
   b. True fear is being separated from a source of security.
   c. Onset of symptoms most commonly occurs in the 20s and 30s and persists for many years.
   d. More common in women than in men.
   e. Impairment can be severe.
   f. The individual may be unable to leave his or her home without being accompanied by a friend or relative.
   g. Panic attacks are common.
2. Nursing process: diagnosis (analysis)—Table 7.1 presents a list of client behaviors and the NANDA nursing diagnoses that correspond to those behaviors, which may be used in planning care.
3. Nursing process: planning.
   a. Short-term goal: client will discuss the situation with the health-care provider within (time frame to be determined according to client situation).
   b. Long-term goal: by time of discharge from treatment, client will be able to function even if separated from a source of security.
4. Nursing process: implementation—nursing actions related to agoraphobia are similar to those used with specific phobias.
5. Nursing process: evaluation—suggested questions used in the evaluation process are presented later in this outline.
6. Psychopharmacology: the tricyclic imipramine and the monoamine oxidase inhibitor (MAOI) phenelzine have been effective in diminishing symptoms of agoraphobia.

F. Social anxiety disorder (social phobia)
1. Nursing process: assessment.
   a. Excessive fear of situations in which a person might do something embarrassing or be evaluated negatively by others.
   b. Client has extreme concerns about being exposed to scrutiny by others.
   c. Fears social or performance situations in which embarrassment may occur.
   d. In some instances, the fear may be quite defined.
   e. In other cases, the social phobia may involve general social situations.
   f. Exposure to the phobic situation usually results in feelings of panic anxiety, with sweating, tachycardia, and dyspnea.
   g. Onset of symptoms often begins in late childhood or early adolescence and runs a chronic, sometimes lifelong, course.
   h. More common in women than in men.
   i. Impairment interferes with social or occupational functioning or causes marked distress.

3. Nursing process: diagnosis (analysis)—Table 7.1 presents a list of client behaviors and the NANDA nursing diagnoses that correspond to those behaviors, which may be used in planning care.
4. Nursing process: planning.
   a. Short-term goal: client will participate in group therapy on a daily basis.
   b. Long-term goal: client will participate in scheduled family reunion during Fourth of July holiday.
5. Nursing process: implementation.
   a. Early in treatment, accompany client to group sessions.
   b. Encourage client to list personal strengths.
   c. Role-play social interactions.
   d. Assist client to identify social supports.
   e. Provide positive feedback for attempts at socialization.
   f. Explore cognitive distortions and negative thinking.
6. Nursing process: evaluation—suggested questions used in the evaluation process are presented later in this outline.
7. Psychopharmacology.
   a. Anxiolytics.
      i. Benzodiazepines have been successful in the treatment of social anxiety disorder (social phobia)
      ii. Alprazolam and clonazepam reduce symptoms of social anxiety
         1) Well tolerated
         2) Rapid onset of action
         3) They have potential for abuse and dependence
         4) Therefore, not considered first-line choice of treatment
   b. Antidepressants.
      i. The tricyclic imipramine and the monoamine oxidase inhibitor (MAOI) phenelzine have been effective in diminishing symptoms of social anxiety disorder
      ii. SSRIs are first-line treatment for social anxiety disorder
      iii. Paroxetine and sertraline have been FDA approved for this purpose
G. Anxiety disorder due to another medical condition
1. Nursing process: assessment.
   a. The symptoms associated with these disorders are a direct physiological consequence of another medical condition.
   b. Symptoms are due to the direct physiological effects of intoxication or withdrawal from a substance.

c. A number of medical conditions have been associated with the development of anxiety symptoms.
  i. Cardiac conditions
    1) Myocardial infarction
    2) Congestive heart failure
    3) Mitral valve prolapse
  ii. Endocrine conditions
    1) Hypoglycemia
    2) Hypo- or hyperthyroidism
    3) Pheochromocytoma
  iii. Respiratory conditions
    1) Chronic obstructive pulmonary disease (COPD)
    2) Hyperventilation
  iv. Neurological conditions
    1) Complex partial seizures
    2) Neoplasms
    3) Encephalitis
d. The diagnosis of substance-induced anxiety disorder is made when anxiety symptoms are in excess of those usually associated with the intoxication or withdrawal syndrome.
e. To substantiate the diagnosis, evidence of intoxication or withdrawal must be available from:
  i. History
  ii. Physical examination
  iii. Laboratory findings
f. Substance-induced anxiety disorder may be associated with use of the following substances:
  i. Alcohol
  ii. Amphetamines
  iii. Cocaine
  iv. Hallucinogens
  v. Sedatives
  vi. Hypnotics
  vii. Anxiolytics
  viii. Caffeine
  ix. Cannabis

H. Obsessive-compulsive disorder (OCD)
1. Nursing process: assessment.
  a. **Obsessions**, **compulsions**, or both must be present
  b. An *obsession* is a persistent or recurring idea or feeling that causes emotional distress or that interferes with effective living.
  c. A *compulsion* is a repetitive stereotyped act performed to relieve fear connected with obsession. If denied, causes uneasiness.
  d. Severity of symptoms must be significant enough to cause distress or impairment in social, occupational, or other important areas of functioning.
  e. Individual recognizes that the behavior is excessive or unreasonable.
  f. Individual is compelled to continue the act because it provides feelings of relief from discomfort.
  g. Common compulsions include:
    i. Hand washing
    ii. Ordering
    iii. Checking
    iv. Praying
    v. Counting
    vi. Repeating words silently
  h. Equally common among men and women.
  i. Single people are affected more often than married people.
  j. May begin in childhood but more often begins in adolescence or early adulthood.
  k. Chronic course.
  l. May be complicated by depression or substance abuse.
2. Nursing process: diagnosis (analysis)—Table 7.1 presents a list of client behaviors and the NANDA nursing diagnoses that correspond to those behaviors, which may be used in planning care.
3. Nursing process: planning.
  a. Short-term goal: within 1 week, the client will decrease participation in ritualistic behavior by half.
  b. Long-term goal: by time of discharge from treatment, client will demonstrate ability to cope effectively without resorting to ritualistic behaviors.
4. Nursing process: implementation.
  a. Assist client to determine types of situations that increase anxiety and result in ritualistic behaviors.
  b. In the beginning of treatment, allow plenty of time for rituals.

🛑 Early in treatment, it is important to allow a client diagnosed with OCD to continue ritualistic behaviors. These rituals are a defense against overwhelming anxiety that will manifest without the protective behavior. After treatment, anxiety levels are monitored, and rituals can be limited as anxiety levels decrease.

  c. Do not be judgmental or verbalize disapproval of the behavior.
  d. Assist client in exploring the meaning and purpose of the behavior.
  e. Early in treatment, provide structured schedule of activities, including adequate time for completion of rituals.

DID YOU KNOW?
Structure provides a feeling of security for the anxious client.

  f. Later in treatment, gradually begin to limit amount of time allotted for ritualistic behavior.

g. Give positive reinforcement for nonritualistic behaviors.

h. Teach client techniques to interrupt obsessive thoughts and ritualistic behaviors:

   i. Thought stopping

   ii. Relaxation

   iii. Physical exercise

5. Nursing process: evaluation—suggested questions used in the evaluation process are presented later in this outline.

6. Psychopharmacology.

  a. Antidepressants.

    i. The SSRIs fluoxetine, paroxetine, sertraline, and fluvoxamine have been approved by the FDA for the treatment of OCD

    ii. May require higher doses than what is effective for treating depression

    iii. Common, often transient, side effects include:

     1) Sleep disturbances

     2) Headache

     3) Restlessness

     4) Fewer side effects than tricyclics

    iv. FDA approved the tricyclic antidepressant clomipramine in the treatment of OCD

    v. Tricyclic side effects may make them less desirable than SSRIs

I. Body dysmorphic disorder (BDD)

1. Nursing process: assessment.

  a. Exaggerated belief that the body is deformed or defective in some specific way.

  b. Most common complaints:

    i. Imagined or slight flaws of the face or head

    ii. Wrinkles or scars

    iii. Shape of the nose

    iv. Excessive facial hair

    v. Facial asymmetry

    vi. Some aspect of the ears, eyes, mouth, lips, or teeth

    vii. In some instances, a true defect is present

     1) Significance of the defect is unrealistically exaggerated

     2) Concern is grossly excessive

    viii. May have symptoms of depression

    ix. Obsessive-compulsive personality characteristics are common

    x. Social and occupational impairment may occur

    xi. To correct imagined defects, numerous visits to plastic surgeons and dermatologists are common

    xii. May undergo unnecessary surgical procedures

    xiii. Closely associated with delusional thinking

    xiv. Must be differentiated from delusional disorder, somatic type

     1) In delusional disorder, somatic type, a client has a delusional belief that a body part is grossly deformed and distorted

     2) In BDD the client is not delusional and is able to acknowledge that his or her concerns are exaggerated

    xv. Common to have traits associated with schizoid, obsessive-compulsive, and narcissistic personality disorders

2. Nursing process: diagnosis (analysis)—Table 7.1 presents a list of client behaviors and the NANDA nursing diagnoses that correspond to those behaviors, which may be used in planning care.

3. Nursing process: planning.

  a. Short-term goal: client will verbalize understanding that changes in bodily structure or function are exaggerated out of proportion to the change that actually exists. (Time frame for this goal must be determined according to individual client's situation.)

  b. Long-term goal: client will verbalize perception of own body that is realistic to actual structure or function by time of discharge from treatment.

4. Nursing process: implementation.

  a. Assess client's perception of his or her body image.

  b. Recognize that this image is real to the client

  c. Assist the client to see that his or her body image is distorted or that it is out of proportion in relation to the significance of an actual physical anomaly.

DID YOU KNOW?

Recognition that a misperception exists is necessary before the client diagnosed with BDD can accept reality and reduce the significance of the imagined defect.

  d. Encourage verbalization of fears and anxieties associated with identified stressful life situations.

  e. Discuss alternative adaptive coping strategies.

  f. Involve client in activities that reinforce a positive sense of self, not based on appearance.

DID YOU KNOW?

When the client is able to develop self-satisfaction based on accomplishments and unconditional acceptance, the significance of the imagined defect or minor physical anomaly will diminish.

  g. Make referrals to support groups of individuals with similar histories.

5. Evaluation: Suggested questions used in the evaluation process are presented later in this outline.

6. Psychopharmacology: clomipramine (Anafranil) and fluoxetine (Prozac) have been shown to reduce symptoms in more than 50% of clients with BDD.
J. Trichotillomania (hair-pulling disorder)
   1. Nursing process: assessment.
      a. The recurrent pulling out of one's own hair that results in noticeable hair loss .
      b. Must rule out **alopecia.**

DID YOU KNOW?
Alopecia is the absence of hair or hair loss that may result from serious illness, drugs, endocrine disorders, dermatitis, hereditary factors, radiation, or physiological changes during aging.

      c. The impulse to pull out hair is preceded by an increasing sense of tension.
      d. Pulling out the hair results in a sense of release or gratification.
      e. Most common sites for hair pulling:
         i. Scalp
         ii. Eyebrows
         iii. Eyelashes
         iv. May occur in any area of the body on which hair grows
      f. Hair loss often found on the opposite side of the body from the dominant hand.
      g. Pain is seldom reported.
      h. Tingling and pruritus are not uncommon.
      i. Comorbid psychiatric disorders:
         i. Mood disorders
         ii. Eating disorders
         iii. Anxiety disorders
         iv. Substance abuse disorders
         v. Personality disorders
            1) Histrionic
            2) Borderline
            3) Obsessive-compulsive
      j. Begins in childhood and may be accompanied by nail biting, head banging, scratching, biting, or other acts of self-mutilation.
      k. Rare phenomenon.
      l. Occurs more often in women than in men.
      m. Affects 1% to 4% of adolescents and college students.

DID YOU KNOW?
Dermatillomania, or excoriation disorder, is an impulse control disorder characterized by the repeated urge to pick at one's own skin, often to the extent that damage is caused.

   2. Nursing process: diagnosis (Analysis)—Table 7.1 presents a list of client behaviors and the NANDA nursing diagnoses that correspond to those behaviors, which may be used in planning care.

   3. Nursing process: planning.
      a. Short-term goal: client will verbalize adaptive ways to cope with stress by means other than pulling out own hair by (time dimension to be individually determined).
      b. Long-term goal: client will be able to demonstrate adaptive coping strategies in response to stress and a discontinuation of hair pulling behavior by (time dimension to be individually determined).
   4. Nursing process: implementation.
      a. Support client in his or her effort to stop hair pulling. Offer hope that it is possible to discontinue the behavior.
      b. Convey a nonjudgmental attitude.
      c. Avoid criticism of the behavior.
      d. Assist client with habit reversal training (HRT). Three components of HRT include:
         i. Awareness training: assist client to be aware of times when the hair-pulling most often occurs
         ii. Competing response training:
            1) Client learns to substitute an alternate response for the urge to pull hair
            2) Suggest that the individual ball up his/her hands into fists, tightening arm muscles, and "locking" his/her arms to make hair pulling impossible at that moment
         iii. Social support: encourage family members to participate and to offer positive feedback during HRT
      e. When hair pulling is anticipated, suggest that client hold something (a ball, paperweight, or other item) in his or her dominant hand.
      f. Practice stress management techniques:
         i. Deep breathing
         ii. Meditation
         iii. Stretching
         iv. Physical exercise
         v. Listening to soft music
      g. Offer support and encouragement when setbacks occur.
      h. Encourage client to persevere when change does not occur as quickly as expected.
   5. Evaluation: suggested questions used in the evaluation process are presented later in this outline.
   6. Psychopharmacology.
      a. Chlorpromazine, amitriptyline, and lithium carbonate have been tried in the treatment of hair-pulling disorder, with moderate result.
      b. Recent success with SSRIs augmented with pimozide.
      c. One recent study showed olanzapine to be a safe and effective treatment for hair-pulling disorder.

K. Evaluation (the following types of questions can be used to reassess whether nursing actions have been successful in achieving the objectives of care for various anxiety disorders).
  1. Can the client recognize signs and symptoms of escalating anxiety?
  2. Can the client use skills learned to interrupt the escalating anxiety before it reaches the panic level?
  3. Can the client demonstrate the activities most appropriate for him or her that can be used to maintain anxiety at a manageable level (e.g., relaxation techniques; physical exercise)?
  4. Can the client maintain anxiety at a manageable level without medication?
  5. Can the client verbalize a long-term plan for preventing panic anxiety in the face of a stressful situation?
  6. Can the client resume usual patterns of responsibility?
  7. Can the client discuss the phobic object or situation without becoming anxious?
  8. Can the client function in the presence of the phobic object or situation without experiencing panic anxiety?
  9. Can the client with OCD refrain from performing rituals when anxiety level rises?
  10. Can the client with OCD demonstrate substitute behaviors to maintain anxiety at a manageable level?
  11. Does the client with OCD recognize the relationship between escalating anxiety and the dependence on ritualistic behaviors for relief?
  12. Can the client with trichotillomania refrain from hair-pulling?
  13. Can the client with trichotillomania successfully substitute a more adaptive behavior when urges to pull hair occur?
  14. Does the client with body dysmorphic disorder verbalize a realistic perception and satisfactory acceptance of personal appearance?

L. Anxiety assessment scales
  1. Used to measure severity of anxiety symptoms.
      a. Clinician administered.
          i. Hamilton Anxiety Rating Scale (Box 7.1)
          ii. Consists of 14 items and measures both psychic and somatic anxiety symptoms
      b. Self-administered, self-rating scales.
          i. Beck Anxiety Inventory
          ii. Zung Self-Rated Anxiety Scale

Box 7.1 Hamilton Anxiety Rating Scale (HAM-A)

Below are descriptions of symptoms commonly associated with anxiety. Assign the client the rating between 0 and 4 (for each of the 14 items) that best describes the extent to which he/she has these symptoms.

0 = Not present; 1 = Mild; 2 = Moderate; 3 = Severe; 4 = Very severe

Rating

1. **Anxious mood** _____ Worries, anticipation of the worst, fearful anticipation, irritability
2. **Tension** _____ Feelings of tension, fatigability, startle response, moved to tears easily, trembling, feelings of restlessness, inability to relax
3. **Fears** _____ Of dark, of strangers, of being left alone, of animals, of traffic, of crowds
4. **Insomnia** _____ Difficulty in falling asleep, broken sleep, unsatisfying sleep and fatigue on waking, dreams, nightmares, night terrors
5. **Intellectual** _____ Difficulty in concentration, poor memory
6. **Depressed mood** _____ Loss of interest, lack of pleasure in hobbies, depression, early waking, diurnal swing
7. **Somatic (muscular)** _____ Pains and aches, twitching, stiffness, myoclonic jerks, grinding of teeth, unsteady voice, increased muscular tone
8. **Somatic (sensory)** _____ Tinnitus, blurred vision, hot/cold flushes, feelings of weakness, tingling sensation
9. **Cardiovascular symptoms** _____ Tachycardia, palpitations, pain in chest, throbbing of vessels, feeling faint
10. **Respiratory symptoms** _____ Pressure or constriction in chest, choking feelings, sighing, dyspnea
11. **Gastrointestinal symptoms** _____ Difficulty swallowing, flatulence, abdominal pain and fullness, burning sensations, nausea/vomiting, borborygmi, diarrhea, constipation, weight loss
12. **Genitourinary symptoms** _____ Urinary frequency, urinary urgency, amenorrhea, menorrhagia, loss of libido, premature ejaculation, impotence
13. **Autonomic symptoms** _____ Dry mouth, flushing, pallor, tendency to sweat, giddiness, tension headache
14. **Behavior at interview** _____ Fidgeting, restlessness or pacing, tremor of hands, furrowed brow, strained face, sighing or rapid respiration, facial pallor, swallowing, clearing throat

Client's Total Score _____

SCORING:
14 – 17 = Mild Anxiety
18 – 24 = Moderate Anxiety
25 – 30 = Severe Anxiety

The HAM-A is in the public domain.
Source: Hamilton, M. (1959). The assessment of anxiety states by rating. *British Journal of Medical Psychology, 32*: 50-55.

REVIEW QUESTIONS

1. Which interaction is an example of dialogue that would be used in the context of behavioral therapy?
   1. *Client:* "I can't stop pulling out my eyelashes when I'm stressed." *Nurse:* "When you get this urge, try locking your arms to make eyelash pulling impossible."
   2. *Client:* "I was punished frequently by my mother, and now I can't do anything right." *Nurse:* "Tell me about your feelings of anger."
   3. *Client:* "I see no benefit in my going to group therapy." *Nurse:* "Group therapy offers you an opportunity to appropriately interact with others."
   4. *Client:* "My stupid doctor hates me, so he revoked my pass." *Nurse:* "What is it that makes you think the doctor hates you?"

2. In the context of cognitive therapy, anxiety is described as being the result of exaggerated, _____ thinking.

3. Which symptoms should a nurse recognize that differentiate a client diagnosed with body dysmorphic disorder (BDD) from a client diagnosed with a delusional disorder-somatic type?
   1. Clients diagnosed with BDD experience the delusional belief that the body is deformed or defective in some specific way, and clients diagnosed with delusional disorder do not.
   2. Clients diagnosed with delusional disorder experience the exaggerated belief that the body is deformed or defective in some specific way, and clients diagnosed with BDD do not.
   3. Clients diagnosed with BDD are able to acknowledge that their concerns are exaggerated, and clients diagnosed with delusional disorder cannot.
   4. Clients diagnosed with delusional disorder are able to acknowledge that their concerns are exaggerated, and clients diagnosed with BDD cannot.

4. A home health nurse has been assigned a client diagnosed with agoraphobia. Which of the following symptoms would the nurse expect to assess? **Select all that apply.**
   1. Fear of standing in a line.
   2. Fear of authoritative figures.
   3. Fear of being outside of the home alone.
   4. Fear of traveling in a car.
   5. Fear of loud noises.

5. A client is experiencing a panic attack. The client states, "I'm losing control. I feel like I'm going crazy." Which nursing intervention takes priority?
   1. Stay with the client and offer support.
   2. Distract the client by redirecting to physical activities.
   3. Teach the etiology and management of panic disorders.
   4. Encourage the client to express feelings.

6. A nursing student experiencing acute test anxiety is prescribed propranolol (Inderal). What is the rationale for this treatment?
   1. Inderal is a mood stabilizer that will decrease situational anxiety.
   2. Inderal is an antihypertensive medication. Question this order.
   3. Inderal has potent effects on the somatic manifestations of anxiety.
   4. Inderal is an anxiolytic used specifically for generalized anxiety.

7. A client has a history of excessive fear of lightening. What is the term that a nurse would chart to document this specific phobia?
   1. Cynophobia
   2. Murophobia
   3. Pyrophobia
   4. Astraphobia

8. A client with a history of generalized anxiety disorder presents with restlessness, irritability, a blood pressure of 140/90 mm Hg, a pulse rate of 96, and respirations of 20. On the basis of these assessed data, which assumption would be correct?
   1. The client is exhibiting signs of an exacerbation of generalized anxiety disorder.
   2. The client's signs and symptoms are due to an underlying medical condition.
   3. A physical examination is needed to determine the etiology of the client's symptoms.
   4. The client's anxiolytic dosage needs to be increased.

9. A client newly admitted to an inpatient psychiatric unit is diagnosed with obsessive-compulsive disorder. Which correctly stated nursing diagnosis takes priority?
   1. Anxiety R/T regression of ego development AEB ritualistic behaviors
   2. Powerlessness R/T ritualistic behaviors AEB statements of lack of control
   3. Fear R/T a traumatic event AEB stimulus avoidance
   4. Social isolation R/T increased levels of anxiety AEB not attending groups

10. A client diagnosed with generalized anxiety disorder has a nursing diagnosis of panic anxiety R/T altered perceptions. Which short-term outcome is most appropriate for this client?
    1. The client will be able to intervene before reaching panic levels of anxiety by discharge.
    2. The client will verbalize decreased levels of anxiety by day 2.
    3. The client will address life situations by using effective problem solving.
    4. The client will voluntarily participate in group therapy activities by discharge.

11. A nursing instructor is teaching about anxiety issues in the elderly. Which student statement indicates that learning has occurred?
    1. "Anxiety disorders do not manifest themselves after age 50."
    2. "There are fewer sleep disturbances noted in the elderly population."
    3. "The response to a major stressor in the elderly is diminished."
    4. "In the elderly, anxiety and depression symptoms often accompany each other."

12. Which of the following is an example of normal anxiety? **Select all that apply.**
    1. A mother experiences dread when she discovers evidence that her teenage daughter has missed two menstrual periods.
    2. Long after a minor car accident, a man continues to experience tachycardia on revisiting the scene of the accident.
    3. To help decrease her fear, an elderly woman attends daily Mass and prays the rosary for her grandson, who is on active duty in the army.
    4. A police officer has to apply for a leave of absence because of the feelings experienced after a near fatal car chase.
    5. An individual who recently lost a parent due to a long chronic illness now cannot leave the home.

13. Recurrent and persistent thoughts, impulses, or images experienced as intrusive and stressful can be referred to as a/an _____.

14. An 82 year-old client is prescribed lorazepam (Ativan) for sleep disturbances. Which of the following reasons would cause the nurse to question the physician's order? **Select all that apply.**
    1. After age 70, lorazepam is no longer effective.
    2. The age of the client could indicate a decrease in hepatic and renal functioning.
    3. Metabolic changes in the elderly may affect appropriate absorption of the drug.
    4. There is a higher incidence of allergies to hypnotic medications in the elderly.
    5. Elimination issues may cause drug accumulation in an elderly client's system.

15. A nursing instructor is grading a matching test related to various types of therapy used for anxiety disorders. Which fact has the student correctly matched with the appropriate therapy?
    1. Relaxation training is not a part of this technique: *Systematic desensitization with reciprocal inhibition*
    2. Progressive exposure to a hierarchy of fear stimuli while in a relaxed state: *habit-reversal therapy*
    3. Client must participate in real-life situations that he or she finds extremely frightening, for a prolonged period of time: *implosion therapy*
    4. Attempts to extinguish unwanted behavior by a system of positive and negative reinforcements: *flooding*

16. Which medication would be a first-line consideration in the treatment of anxiety for a client actively abusing alcohol?
    1. Buspirone (BuSpar)
    2. Alprazolam (Xanax)
    3. Chlordiazepoxide (Librium)
    4. Clonazepam (Klonopin)

17. A client who is being treated for an anxiety disorder with clonazepam (Klonopin) complains that the medication seems ineffective. To correctly assess the client, which of the following questions should the nurse ask? **Select all that apply.**
    1. Are you a smoker?
    2. How long have you been taking the drug?
    3. How much coffee do you drink?
    4. Do you have any kidney problems?
    5. Do you take the herbal supplement valerian?

18. A nurse is planning to teach a client diagnosed with agoraphobia about this disorder. Which fact should the nurse include in the teaching plan?
    1. The origin of agoraphobia is the lack of control over life situations.
    2. The origin of agoraphobia is a change in body functioning resulting from inner conflict.
    3. The origin of agoraphobia is the true fear of being separated from a source of security.
    4. The origin of agoraphobia is the direct physiological effect of a substance.

19. A psychiatrist ordered habit reversal therapy (HRT) for a client diagnosed with hair-pulling behavior. After several weeks of treatment, which of the following client behaviors would the nurse expect? **Select all that apply.**
    1. The client is attempting to extinguish unwanted behavior.
    2. The client is becoming less aware of the behavior.
    3. The client can identify times of hair-pulling occurrence.
    4. The client has substituted a more adaptive coping strategy.
    5. The client understands that hair-pulling behaviors are genetic in nature.

20. A client refuses to accept a promotion because his job would require crossing a high bridge daily. How should a nurse explain to the client's wife the root of this fear from a learning theory perspective?
    1. Unresolved intrapsychic conflicts resulted in projected anxiety.
    2. A distorted and unrealistic appraisal of the situation resulted in the avoidance.
    3. His mother's extreme fear of heights contributed to his current fear.
    4. The client's high norepinephrine levels resulted in distorted thinking.

21. An instructor is teaching about phobias and the different treatments used to decrease fear driven anxiety. Which of the following student statements about implosion therapy (flooding) indicates that learning has occurred? **Select all that apply.**
    1. "A client must imagine or participate in extremely frightening situations for a prolonged period of time."
    2. "A client must participate in relaxation training to decrease the onset of a panic attack."
    3. "A client is flooded with soothing music and images of cloud formations when triggers to anxiety are presented."
    4. "The client continues implosion therapy (flooding) until the stimulus no longer elicits anxiety."
    5. "The client learns to be anxious and relaxed at the same time while being exposed to the anxiety provoking triggers."

22. A client diagnosed with obsessive-compulsive disorder (OCD) has an obsession with dirt and germs and has a continual compulsion to spray all surfaces with a disinfectant. How would the nurse explain this client's action?
    1. The compulsion to spray disinfectant reduces bacterial growth.
    2. The compulsion to spray disinfectant relieves the client's anxiety.
    3. The compulsion to spray disinfectant encourages ego integrity.
    4. The compulsion to spray disinfectant increases the client's self-esteem.

1. ANSWER: 1
Rationale:
1. Behavioral therapy includes habit-reversal therapy (HRT), systematic desensitization, and implosion therapy (flooding). In HRT the client substitutes an incompatible behavior (locking arms) in an effort to extinguish the undesirable behavior (eyelash pulling).
2. Intrapersonal, not behavioral, therapy includes exploring how situations during developmental stages affect current emotions.
3. Interpersonal, not behavioral, therapy deals with faulty patterns of relating to others and encourages interactions with others to develop the self-system.
4. Cognitive, not behavioral, therapy is a type of therapy in which the client is taught to control thought distortions that are considered to be a factor in the development and maintenance of emotional disorders.
TEST-TAKING TIP: Determine which type of therapy each answer choice represents. Compare the therapy to the dialogue presented and choose the answer that reflects behavioral therapy.
Content Area: Safe and Effective Care Environment: Management of Care;
Integrated Process: Nursing Process: Implementation;
Client Need: Safe and Effective Care Environment: Management of Care;
Cognitive Level: Application;
Concept: Nursing

2. ANSWER: automatic
Rationale: In the context of cognitive therapy, anxiety is described as being the result of exaggerated, automatic thinking. Cognitive therapy strives to assist the individual to reduce anxiety responses by altering cognitive distortions.
TEST-TAKING TIP: Note the key term "cognitive therapy" in the question stem. Recall the concepts of cognitive therapy.
Content Area: Safe and Effective Care Environment: Management of Care;
Integrated Process: Nursing Process: Implementation;
Client Need: Safe and Effective Care Environment: Management of Care;
Cognitive Level: Knowledge;
Concept: Stress

3. ANSWER: 3
Rationale:
1. Clients diagnosed with delusional disorder somatic type, not BDD, experience the delusional belief that the body is deformed or defective in some specific way. Clients diagnosed with BDD are not delusional and are able to acknowledge that concerns are exaggerated.
2. Clients diagnosed with BDD, not delusional disorder somatic type, experience the exaggerated belief that the body is deformed or defective in some specific way. Clients diagnosed with a delusional disorder are delusional in their belief that the body is deformed or defective.
3. Clients diagnosed with BDD are able to acknowledge that concerns are exaggerated, whereas clients diagnosed with delusional disorder somatic type cannot.

4. Clients diagnosed with BDD are able to acknowledge that concerns are exaggerated and clients diagnosed with delusional disorder somatic type cannot.
TEST-TAKING TIP: Recall the differences between clients diagnosed with BDD and clients diagnosed with delusional disorder somatic type. Delusional thinking is a form of psychosis. The client is out of touch with reality. In BDD, reality testing is maintained.
Content Area: Psychosocial Integrity;
Integrated Process: Nursing Process: Evaluation;
Client Need: Psychosocial Integrity;
Cognitive Level: Application;
Concept: Assessment

4. ANSWERS: 1, 3, 4
Rationale: Symptom requirements for the diagnosis of agoraphobia include a marked fear or anxiety about at least one situation from two or more of the following five groups of situations: Public transportation (e.g., traveling in automobiles, buses, trains, shops, or planes); open spaces (e.g., parking lots, market places, or bridges); being in shops, theaters, or cinemas; standing in line or being in a crowd; and being outside of the home alone in other situations.
1. Symptom requirements for the diagnosis of agoraphobia include the fear of standing in line.
2. Symptom requirements for the diagnosis of agoraphobia do not include the fear of authoritative figures.
3. Symptom requirements for the diagnosis of agoraphobia include the fear of being outside of the home alone.
4. Symptom requirements for the diagnosis of agoraphobia include the fear of traveling in a car.
5. Symptom requirements for the diagnosis of agoraphobia do not include the fear of loud noises.
TEST-TAKING TIP: Review the symptom requirements for the diagnosis of agoraphobia.
Content Area: Psychosocial Integrity;
Integrated Process: Nursing Process: Assessment;
Client Need: Psychosocial Integrity;
Cognitive Level: Comprehension;
Concept: Assessment

5. ANSWER: 1
Rationale:
1. During a panic attack, the client is experiencing extreme levels of anxiety. The symptoms experienced may mimic life-threatening physiological symptoms such as chest pain and feelings of suffocation and/or impending doom. Clients need reassurance that these symptoms are psychologically and not physiologically based. It is a priority to be present for the client and offer this support.
2. Distracting the client by redirecting to physical activities may increase, rather than decrease, anxiety levels. A more appropriate approach would be to decrease environmental stimuli while staying with the client and offering support.
3. Educating a client about the etiology and management of panic disorders is important. However, because of decreased attention span and inability to concentrate, this discussion is neither appropriate nor effective when anxiety is at a panic level.
4. Encouraging the expression of feelings when a client is experiencing panic levels of anxiety would only increase the

client's anxiety. The client's anxiety needs to decrease to a mild or moderate level before the nurse encourages the client to express feelings.

TEST-TAKING TIP: Note the key word "priority" in the question stem. Any of the nursing interventions might be helpful at some point. However, which one takes priority *during* a client's panic attack?
Content Area: Safe and Effective Care Environment: Management of Care;
Integrated Process: Nursing Process: Implementation;
Client Need: Safe and Effective Care Environment: Management of Care;
Cognitive Level: Application;
Concept: Critical Thinking

6. **ANSWER: 3**
Rationale:
1. Inderal is an antihypertensive beta blocker, not a mood stabilizer. Inderal can be used in the treatment of acute situational anxiety.
2. Inderal is an antihypertensive medication, but because it can be effective in the treatment of the somatic manifestations of acute situational anxiety, there is no need to question this order.
3. **Research studies show that Inderal is effective in decreasing anxiety symptoms. It has potent effects on the somatic manifestations of anxiety such as palpitations and tremors but has less dramatic effects on the psychic components of anxiety. It is most effective in the treatment of acute situational anxiety, such as performance anxiety and/or test anxiety.**
4. Inderal is an antihypertensive beta blocker, not an anxiolytic. Inderal can be used specifically for acute situational anxiety, not generalized anxiety.

TEST-TAKING TIP: Recall that Inderal is an antihypertensive beta blocker that can be used to treat anxiety.
Content Area: Safe and Effective Care Environment: Management of Care;
Integrated Process: Nursing Process: Implementation;
Client Need: Safe and Effective Care Environment: Management of Care;
Cognitive Level: Application;
Concept: Medication

7. **ANSWER: 4**
Rationale:
1. The nurse should determine that an excessive fear of dogs is identified as cynophobia and document accordingly. Astraphobia is fear of lightening.
2. The nurse should determine that an excessive fear of mice is identified as murophobia and document accordingly. Astraphobia is fear of lightening.
3. The nurse should determine that an excessive fear of fire is identified as pyrophobia and document accordingly. Astraphobia is fear of lightening
4. **The nurse should determine that an excessive fear of lightening is identified as astraphobia and document accordingly.**

TEST-TAKING TIP: Use any knowledge you have of Greek or Latin to figure out the meaning of a phobia classification. Review Table 7.1 as needed.

Content Area: Psychosocial Integrity;
Integrated Process: Nursing Process: Assessment;
Client Need: Psychosocial Integrity;
Cognitive Level: Comprehension;
Concept: Stress

8. **ANSWER: 3**
Rationale:
1. Although the client may be exhibiting signs and symptoms of an exacerbation of generalized anxiety disorder, the nurse cannot assume this to be true before a thorough physical assessment is done.
2. Although the client may be experiencing an underlying medical condition that is causing the anxiety, the nurse cannot assume this to be true before a thorough physical assessment is done.
3. **Physical problems should be ruled out before determining a psychological cause for this client's symptoms.**
4. Although the client may need an anxiolytic dosage increase, the nurse cannot assume this to be true before a thorough physical assessment is done.

TEST-TAKING TIP: Remember that although a client may have a history of a psychiatric illness, a complete, thorough physical assessment must be done before assuming exhibited symptoms are related to a psychiatric disorder.
Content Area: Safe and Effective Care Environment: Management of Care;
Integrated Process: Nursing Process: Assessment;
Client Need: Safe and Effective Care Environment: Management of Care;
Cognitive Level: Application;
Concept: Stress

9. **ANSWER: 1**
Rationale:
1. **Anxiety is the underlying cause of the diagnosis of obsessive-compulsive disorder (OCD); therefore, anxiety R/T regression of ego development is the priority nursing diagnosis for the client newly admitted for the treatment of this disorder.**
2. Powerlessness R/T ritualistic behaviors is an appropriate nursing diagnosis for a client diagnosed with OCD; however, for the client to begin working on feelings of powerlessness, interventions must be geared toward initially decreasing the level of anxiety.
3. Fear R/T a traumatic event AEB stimulus avoidance would be an appropriate nursing diagnosis for a client diagnosed with posttraumatic stress disorder (PTSD), not for a client diagnosed with OCD.
4. Social isolation R/T increased levels of anxiety is an appropriate diagnosis for a client diagnosed with OCD; however, interventions must be geared toward decreasing anxiety before the client can work on developing social skills.

TEST-TAKING TIP: Note the key word "priority" in the question stem. Consider which client problem would need to be addressed before any other problem can be explored. When anxiety is decreased, social isolation should improve, and feelings about powerlessness can be expressed. Therefore, anxiety is the priority diagnosis.
Content Area: Psychosocial Integrity;
Integrated Process: Nursing Process: Assessment;

Client Need: Psychosocial Integrity;
Cognitive Level: Application;
Concept: Critical Thinking

10. **ANSWER: 1**
Rationale:
1. The client's ability to intervene before reaching panic levels of anxiety by discharge is measurable, relates to the stated nursing diagnosis, has a time frame, and is an appropriate short-term outcome for this client.
2. The "verbalization of decreased levels of anxiety" in this outcome is neither specific nor measurable. Instead of a general "decrease" in anxiety, the use of an anxiety scale would make this outcome measurable.
3. The client's addressing life situations by using effective problem-solving methods relates to the stated nursing diagnosis; however, it does not have a time frame, and it is not measurable.
4. The client's ability to participate voluntarily in group therapy activities is a short-term outcome; however, this outcome does not relate to the stated nursing diagnosis.
TEST-TAKING TIP: When evaluating outcomes, make sure that the outcome is specific to the client's need, is realistic, is measurable, and contains a reasonable time frame. If any of these components is missing, the outcome is incorrectly written and can be eliminated.
Content Area: Safe and Effective Care Environment: Management of Care;
Integrated Process: Nursing Process: Planning;
Client Need: Safe and Effective Care Environment: Management of Care;
Cognitive Level: Application;
Concept: Critical Thinking

11. **ANSWER: 4**
Rationale:
1. Some anxiety disorders appear for the first time after age 60. This student statement indicates that further instruction is needed.
2. Sleep disturbances are very common in the aging individual. This student statement indicates that further instruction is needed.
3. The response to a major stressor is often quite intense, not diminished, in the elderly. This student statement indicates that further instruction is needed.
4. In older adults, symptoms of anxiety and depression often accompany each other, making it difficult to determine which disorder is dominant. This student statement indicates that learning has occurred.
TEST-TAKING TIP: Recall the anxiety issues that may occur in the elderly client.
Content Area: Psychosocial Integrity;
Integrated Process: Nursing Process: Evaluation;
Client Need: Psychosocial Integrity;
Cognitive Level: Application;
Concept: Stress

12. **ANSWERS: 1, 3**
Rationale:
1. When a mother experiences dread after discovering that her teenage daughter has missed two periods, the
mother is experiencing a normal anxiety reaction. Anxiety is usually considered a normal reaction to a realistic danger or threat to biological integrity or self-concept.
2. When a man continues to experience tachycardia on revisiting the scene of the accident long after the collision, the man is experiencing abnormal levels of anxiety. Normal anxiety should dissipate when the danger or threat is no longer present.
3. An elderly woman who decreases her fear by praying daily for her grandson is experiencing a normal anxiety reaction. The normality of the anxiety experienced in response to a stressor is defined by societal and cultural standards.
4. When a police officer has to apply for a leave of absence because of the feelings experienced after a near fatal car chase, the officer is experiencing an abnormal anxiety reaction. When anxiety interferes with social, occupational, or other important areas of functioning, it can be determined to be an abnormal reaction.
5. When an individual who recently lost a parent due to a long chronic illness, cannot leave the home, the individual is experiencing an abnormal anxiety reaction. This anxiety response is out of proportion to the situation that has created it.
TEST-TAKING TIP: Review the criteria for abnormal and normal anxiety.
Content Area: Psychosocial Integrity;
Integrated Process: Nursing Process: Evaluation;
Client Need: Psychosocial Integrity;
Cognitive Level: Application;
Concept: Stress

13. **ANSWER: obsession**
Rationale: An obsession is recognized as being excessive and unreasonable even though the obsession is a product of one's mind. The thought, impulse, or image cannot be expunged by logic or reasoning.
TEST-TAKING TIP: Recall the meaning of the word *obsession* and how it differs from *compulsion*.
Content Area: Safe and Effective Care Environment: Management of Care;
Integrated Process: Nursing Process: Evaluation;
Client Need: Safe and Effective Care Environment: Management of Care;
Cognitive Level: Knowledge;
Concept: Stress

14. **ANSWERS: 2, 3, 5**
Rationale: Lorazepam (Ativan) is an antianxiety medication and can be used to treat insomnia.
1. There is no indication that the effectiveness of lorazepam is decreased with age.
2. Caution should be taken in administering antianxiety drugs to elderly clients due to decreased hepatic and renal functioning.
3. Changes in aging associated with metabolism must be considered when maintenance medications are administered for chronic insomnia.
4. Ativan is an antianxiety medication, not a hypnotic medication. All clients should be monitored for medication allergies.

5. Changes in aging associated with elimination must be considered when maintenance medications are administered for chronic insomnia.
TEST-TAKING TIP: Recall that Ativan is an antianxiety medication. The aging process affects the absorption, metabolism, and elimination of all medications.
Content Area: Safe and Effective Care Environment: Management of Care;
Integrated Process: Nursing Process: Implementation;
Client Need: Safe and Effective Care Environment: Management of Care;
Cognitive Level: Application;
Concept: Medication

15. **ANSWER: 3**
Rationale:
1. *Systematic desensitization with reciprocal inhibition* involves two main elements: training in relaxation techniques (e.g., progressive relaxation, mental imagery, tense and relax, meditation) and progressive exposure to a hierarchy of fear stimuli while in the relaxed state.
2. Progressive exposure to a hierarchy of fear stimuli while in a relaxed state is part of systematic desensitization with reciprocal inhibition, not *habit-reversal therapy.*
3. Implosion therapy, or flooding, is a therapeutic process in which the client must imagine situations or participate in real-life situations that he or she finds extremely frightening for a prolonged period of time.
4. Attempts to extinguish unwanted behavior by a system of positive and negative reinforcements is part of habit-reversal therapy, not *flooding.*
TEST-TAKING TIP: Review the various therapies used to treat anxiety.
Content Area: Safe and Effective Care Environment: Management of Care;
Integrated Process: Nursing Process: Evaluation;
Client Need: Safe and Effective Care Environment: Management of Care;
Cognitive Level: Application;
Concept: Stress

16. **ANSWER: 1**
Rationale:
1. Buspirone is often the drug of choice when treating anxiety for clients with addiction problems because it does not depress the central nervous system (CNS) nor cause withdrawal symptoms.
2. Because of tolerance potential leading to dependence, caution is required when using antianxiety agents such as alprazolam to treat individuals who have a history of drug abuse or addiction. This medication suppresses the central nervous system and causes withdrawal symptoms.
3. Because of tolerance potential leading to dependence, caution is required when using antianxiety agents such as chlordiazepoxide to treat individuals who have a history of drug abuse or addiction. This medication suppresses the central nervous system and causes withdrawal symptoms.
4. Because of tolerance potential leading to dependence, caution is required when using antianxiety agents such as clonazepam to treat individuals who have a history of drug abuse or addiction. This medication suppresses the central nervous system and causes withdrawal symptoms.

TEST-TAKING TIP: Recall that buspirone is not classified as a benzodiazepine, is not a CNS depressant, and does not put the client at risk for addiction.
Content Area: Safe and Effective Care Environment: Management of Care;
Integrated Process: Nursing Process: Assessment;
Client Need: Safe and Effective Care Environment: Management of Care;
Cognitive Level: Application;
Concept: Medication

17. **ANSWERS: 1, 3**
Rationale: Clonazepam (Klonopin) is classified as a benzodiazepine.
1. Decreased effects of benzodiazepines can be noted with cigarette smoking. Asking this question would help the nurse accurately assess what might contribute to the ineffectiveness of the medication.
2. Unlike buspirone (BuSpar), clonazepam (Klonopin) is a quick-acting benzodiazepine. This question would not help the nurse accurately assess what might contribute to the ineffectiveness of the medication.
3. Decreased effects of benzodiazepines can be noted with caffeine consumption. Asking this question would help the nurse accurately assess what might contribute to the ineffectiveness of the medication.
4. Caution should be taken in administering benzodiazepines to clients with hepatic or renal dysfunction. The drug can build up in the client's system causing increased, rather than decreased, effects.
5. Increased, not decreased, effects of benzodiazepines can occur when the drug is ingested with herbal depressants (e.g., kava; valerian).
TEST-TAKING TIP: Recall that clonazepam is classified as a benzodiazepine. All information related to that class of medication applies.
Content Area: Safe and Effective Care Environment: Management of Care;
Integrated Process: Nursing Process: Implementation;
Client Need: Safe and Effective Care Environment: Management of Care;
Cognitive Level: Application;
Concept: Medication

18. **ANSWER: 3**
Rationale:
1. The origin of agoraphobia is the true fear of being separated from a source of security, not the lack of control over life situations.
2. The origin of agoraphobia is the true fear of being separated from a source of security, not a change in body functioning resulting from inner conflict.
3. Agoraphobia is characterized by the fear of being in places or situations from which escape might be difficult or embarrassing, although the basis of the true fear is being separated from a source of security.
4. The origin of agoraphobia is the true fear of being separated from a source of security, not the direct physiological effect of a substance.
TEST-TAKING TIP: Recall the origin of the disorder of agoraphobia.

Content Area: Psychosocial Integrity;
Integrated Process: Nursing Process: Implementation;
Client Need: Psychosocial Integrity;
Cognitive Level: Application;
Concept: Nursing Roles

19. **ANSWERS: 1, 3, 4**
Rationale: HRT includes a system of positive and negative reinforcements in an effort to modify hair-pulling behaviors.
1. After several weeks of treatment, the nurse would expect the client to attempt to extinguish the unwanted behavior of hair pulling.
2. After several weeks of treatment, the nurse would expect the client to become more, not less, aware of the hair-pulling behavior.
3. After several weeks of treatment, the nurse would expect the client to be able to identify times of occurrence and gain insight into the hair-pulling behavior etiology.
4. After several weeks of treatment, the nurse would expect the client to substitute a more adaptive coping strategy than that of the maladaptive coping strategy of hair pulling.
5. Hair-pulling behavior is not genetic in nature.
TEST-TAKING TIP: Review the behavioral therapy of HRT.
Content Area: Safe and Effective Care Environment: Management of Care;
Integrated Process: Nursing Process: Evaluation;
Client Need: Safe and Effective Care Environment: Management of Care;
Cognitive Level: Application;
Concept: Stress

20. **ANSWER: 3**
Rationale:
1. The nurse should explain that from a psychoanalytic, not a learning, perspective, the client's unresolved intrapsychic conflicts resulted in projected anxiety.
2. The nurse should explain that from a cognitive, not a learning, perspective, the client is experiencing a distorted and unrealistic appraisal of the situation. Fear is the result of faulty cognitions or anxiety-inducing self-instructions.
3. The nurse should explain that from a learning perspective, the client's mother's extreme fear of heights contributed to his current fear. Phobias may be acquired by direct learning or imitation (modeling; e.g., a mother who exhibits fear toward an object will provide a model for the child, who may also develop a phobia of the same object).
4. The nurse should explain that from a biological, not a learning, perspective, the client's high norepinephrine levels resulted in distorted thinking. Norepinephrine is known to mediate arousal, and it causes hyperarousal and anxiety.
TEST-TAKING TIP: Recall the various theories of origin of anxiety disorders and match the theory with the situations presented in the answer choices.
Content Area: Safe and Effective Care Environment: Management of Care;
Integrated Process: Nursing Process: Implementation;
Client Need: Safe and Effective Care Environment: Management of Care;
Cognitive Level: Application;
Concept: Stress

21. **ANSWERS: 1, 4**
Rationale:
1. Implosion therapy (flooding) is a therapeutic process in which the client must imagine or participate in real-life situations that he or she finds extremely frightening, for a long period of time. This student's statement indicates that learning has occurred.
2. Implosion therapy (flooding) is a therapeutic process in which relaxation-training techniques are not used. This student's statement indicates that further instruction is needed.
3. Implosion therapy (flooding) is a therapeutic process in which a client is flooded with vivid details that trigger anxiety, not flooded with soothing music and images of soft clouds. This student's statement indicates that further instruction is needed.
4. Implosion therapy (flooding) is a therapeutic process in which the client continues the therapy until the stimulus no longer elicits anxiety. This student's statement indicates that learning has occurred.
5. It is impossible for individuals to be anxious and relaxed at the same time. This student's statement indicates that further instruction is needed.
TEST-TAKING TIP: Review the information about implosion therapy (flooding). You can immediately eliminate Option 5 because an individual can never be relaxed and anxious at the same time.
Content Area: Safe and Effective Care Environment: Management of Care;
Integrated Process: Nursing Process: Evaluation;
Client Need: Safe and Effective Care Environment: Management of Care;
Cognitive Level: Application;
Concept: Stress

22. **ANSWER: 2**
Rationale:
1. The nurse attributes this client's action to relieving anxiety, not to reducing bacterial growth.
2. The nurse attributes this client's action to an effort to relieve the client's anxiety. The client recognizes that the behavior is excessive and unreasonable, but because of the feeling of relief from the anxiety that it promotes, the client is compelled to continue the act. Common compulsions include hand washing, ordering, checking, praying, counting, and repeating words silently.
3. The nurse attributes this client's action to relieving anxiety, not to encouraging ego integrity.
4. The nurse attributes this client's action to relieving anxiety, not to increasing client's self-esteem.
TEST-TAKING TIP: Recall that obsessions are recurrent thoughts, and compulsions are the actions taken to relieve the anxiety that the thoughts produce.
Content Area: Safe and Effective Care Environment: Management of Care;
Integrated Process: Nursing Process: Evaluation;
Client Need: Safe and Effective Care Environment: Management of Care;
Cognitive Level: Application;
Concept: Stress

CASE STUDY: Putting it All Together

Addy was 10 years old when her younger brother died from scarlet fever. His illness caused the family to be quarantined to avoid the spread of the disease. Now, at 35 years of age, Addy lives with her parents and is being counseled by a psychiatric nurse practitioner (PNP), Gavin. She has an extreme fear of dirt and germs and tells Gavin, "The filthy world is a dangerous place and that is why I'm hoping you can help me." Gavin notes that Addy's affect is apprehensive and her eye contact is minimal. She fidgets constantly and continually washes her hands and disinfects surfaces with antibacterial wipes. Addy claims that she rarely has contact with people other than her immediate family, and she cannot maintain employment because of her debilitating fears. Gavin has explored the predisposing factors that may have contributed to Addy's unrealistic and unjustified fears. Gavin is exploring various behavioral techniques to help Addy cope more effectively and is considering prescribing antianxiety medications.

1. Based on the client's symptoms and actions, what medical diagnosis would Gavin assign to Addy?
2. What term would correctly describe Addy's fear?
3. What are Addy's subjective symptoms that would lead to the determination of this diagnosis?
4. What are Addy's objective symptoms that would lead to the determination of this diagnosis?
5. What predisposing factors may have led to Addy's disorder?
6. List the behavioral techniques Gavin might employ to treat Addy.
7. What classification of medications might Gavin prescribe for the short-term treatment of Addy's symptoms?
8. What classification of medications might Gavin prescribe for the long-term treatment of Addy's symptoms?
9. What NANDA nursing diagnosis would address Addy's current problem?
10. On the basis of this nursing diagnosis, what short-term outcome would be appropriate for Addy?
11. On the basis of this nursing diagnosis, what long-term outcome would be appropriate for Addy?
12. List the nursing interventions (actions) that will assist Addy in successfully meeting these outcomes.
13. List the questions that should be asked to determine the success of the nursing interventions.

Trauma- and Stressor-Related Disorders

Acute stress disorder (ASD)—Precipitating traumatic events and symptomatology are similar to post-traumatic stress disorder, but in ASD, the symptoms are time limited, up to 1 month after the trauma; by definition, if the symptoms last longer than 1 month, the diagnosis would be PTSD

Adjustment disorder—Characterized by a maladaptive reaction to an identifiable stressor or stressors that results in the development of clinically significant emotional or behavioral symptoms

Crisis—A sudden event in one's life that disturbs homeostasis, during which usual coping mechanisms cannot resolve the problem

Crisis intervention—A problem-solving activity for correcting or preventing the continuation of an emergency, especially one caused by psychological distress

Disaster—A natural or manmade occurrence that overwhelms the resources of an individual or community and increases the need for emergency evacuation and medical services

Eye movement desensitization and reprocessing (EMDR)—A treatment for post-traumatic stress disorder and other conditions in which a person recalls a disturbing memory while looking to the left or right, or listening to sounds, or attending to tactile stimulation

Post-traumatic stress disorder (PTSD)—A reaction to an extreme trauma, which is likely to cause pervasive distress to almost anyone, such as natural or manmade disasters, combat, serious accidents, witnessing the violent death of others, being the victim of torture, terrorism, rape, or other crimes

Prodromal syndrome—A syndrome of symptoms that often precedes the onset of aggressive or violent behavior; these symptoms include anxiety and tension, verbal abuse and profanity, and increasing hyperactivity

Stress—Mental, emotional, or physical strain experienced by an individual in response to stimuli from the external or internal environment

Trauma—An extremely distressing experience that causes severe emotional shock and may have long-lasting psychological effects

Triage—The screening and classification of causalities to make optimal use of treatment resources and to maximize the survival and welfare of clients

The concept of post-trauma response is not new. It has been described by terms such as shell shock, battle fatigue, accident neurosis, and post-traumatic neurosis. This chapter focuses on disorders that occur following exposure to an identifiable stressor or an extreme traumatic event. In the *DSM-5* (American Psychiatric Association, 2013), the diagnoses of **post-traumatic stress disorder** (PTSD), **acute stress disorder,** and **adjustment disorder** are combined into a single chapter titled "Trauma- and Stressor-Related Disorders."

I. Comparison of Post-Traumatic Stress Disorder (PTSD) and Adjustment Disorder (AD)

A. The trauma that precedes PTSD is an event that is outside the range of usual human experience, such as rape, war, physical attack, torture, or natural or manmade disasters

B. Stress reactions due to "normal" daily events (e.g., divorce, failure, rejection) are classified as adjustment disorders

C. Less than 10% of trauma victims develop PTSD

D. Adjustment disorders are probably quite common

E. Both PTSD and AD are more common in women than in men

F. AD is common in:
  1. Unmarried persons.
  2. Younger people.

G. AD can occur at any age, from childhood to senescence

H. PTSD can occur in adults, adolescents, and children older than 6 years

II. Predisposing Factors to Trauma-Related Disorders

A. Psychosocial theory:
  1. Variability of stress response includes characteristics that relate to:
    a. The traumatic experience:
      i. Severity and duration of the stressor
        1) In adjustment disorders, continuous stressors over an extended period of time are more likely than sudden-shock stressors to precipitate maladaptive functioning
      ii. Extent of anticipatory preparation for the event
      iii. Exposure to death of others
      iv. Risk of personal injury or death
      v. Amount of control over recurrence
      vi. Location where the trauma was experienced
    b. The individual's response:
      i. Degree of ego strength
      ii. Effectiveness of coping resources
      iii. Presence of preexisting psychopathology
      iv. Outcomes of previous experiences with stress/trauma
      v. Behavioral tendencies (temperament)
      vi. Current psychosocial developmental stage
      vii. Demographic factors (e.g., age, socioeconomic status, education)
    c. The recovery environment:
      i. Availability of social supports
      ii. The cohesiveness and protectiveness of family and friends
      iii. The attitudes of society regarding the experience
      iv. Cultural and religious support groups
      v. Personal and general economic conditions
      vi. Occupational and recreational opportunities

DID YOU KNOW?

In research with Vietnam veterans, it was shown that the best predictors of PTSD were the severity of the stressor and the degree of psychosocial isolation in the recovery environment.

  2. Adjustment disorder is a maladaptive response to stress caused by:
    a. Early childhood trauma.
    b. Increased dependency.
    c. Retarded ego development.
  3. Birth characteristics (temperament) can contribute to an individual's response to stress.
  4. Adjustment disorder may be precipitated by a specific, meaningful stressor related to a point of vulnerability in an individual of otherwise adequate ego strength.
  5. Response to stress leading to adjustment disorders may be influenced by:
    a. Developmental maturity.
    b. Timing of the stressor.
    c. Available support.
    d. Adequate coping strategies.
  6. AD may be related to dysfunctional grieving.
    a. May be fixated in a particular stage of grief (e.g., denial, anger).
    b. Inadequate defense mechanisms to complete the grieving process.

B. Learning theory
  1. In PTSD, the individual learns that avoidance behaviors and psychic numbing decrease emotional pain.
  2. Behavioral disturbances, such as drug or alcohol abuse, anger, and aggression, are learned maladaptive ways to reduce emotional pain.

C. Cognitive theory
  1. Considers the cognitive appraisal of an event.
  2. Focuses on assumptions that an individual makes about the world:
    a. The world is benevolent and a source of joy.
    b. The world is meaningful and controllable.
    c. The self is worthy (i.e., lovable, good, and competent).
  3. Individual is vulnerable to trauma-related disorders when fundamental beliefs are invalidated by a trauma that cannot be comprehended.
  4. A sense of helplessness and hopelessness prevail.

D. Biological theory
  1. Individuals who have experienced previous trauma are more likely to develop PTSD symptoms after another stressful life event.
  2. This suggests that an endogenous opioid peptide response may have occurred.
  3. Opioid psychoactive properties include:
    a. Tranquilizing action.
    b. Reduction of rage/aggression.

c. Reduction of paranoia.

d. Reduction of feelings of inadequacy.

e. Antidepressant action.

4. When the stressor terminates, the individual may experience opioid withdrawal, the symptoms of which bear strong resemblance to those of PTSD.

5. Evidence suggests that biological dysregulation of the opioid, glutamatergic, noradrenergic, serotonergic, and neuroendocrine pathways are involved in the pathophysiology of PTSD.

6. Chronic disorders, such as neurocognitive disorders or intellectual development disorders, can impair the ability of an individual to adapt to stress, causing increased vulnerability to adjustment disorder.

7. Genetic factors may influence individual risks for maladaptive response to stress.

III. Post-Traumatic Stress Disorder (PTSD)

A. Nursing process: assessment

1. Individual experiences extreme trauma.

a. Natural or manmade disasters.

b. Combat.

c. Serious accidents.

d. Witnessing the violent death of others.

e. Being a victim of torture.

f. Terrorism.

g. Rape.

h. Crime.

2. Experiences do not usually include:

a. Uncomplicated bereavement.

b. Marital conflict.

c. Chronic illness.

3. Likely to cause pervasive distress to anyone.

4. May experience the trauma alone or in the presence of others.

5. Characteristic symptoms:

a. Reexperiencing the traumatic event.

b. A sustained high level of anxiety or arousal.

c. A general numbing of responsiveness.

d. Isolation and avoidance behaviors interfere with interpersonal relatedness.

e. Intrusive recollections or nightmares of the event.

f. Dissociative reactions (e.g., flashbacks) in which the individual feels or acts as if the traumatic events were recurring.

g. Inability to remember certain aspects of the trauma.

h. Persistent and exaggerated negative beliefs or expectations about oneself, others, or the world.

i. Can experience depressive symptoms severe enough to warrant a diagnosis of a depressive disorder.

j. Painful guilt feelings about surviving when others did not (survivor's guilt).

k. Substance abuse.

l. Anger and aggressive behavior.

m. Full symptom picture must be present for more than 1 month.

n. Causes significant interference with social, occupational, and other areas of functioning.

🛑 Following a trauma, individuals are at high risk for physical injury because of a disruption in ability to concentrate and problem solve combined with lack of sufficient sleep.

o. Symptoms may begin within the first 3 months after the trauma, or there may be a delay of several months or even years.

B. Nursing process: diagnosis (analysis)

1. Post-trauma syndrome R/T traumatic event AEB flashbacks, nightmares, and psychological numbness.

2. Complicated grieving R/T self image change due to trauma and perceived losses incurred after the event AEB uncontrolled anger and survivor guilt.

C. Nursing process: planning

1. Short-term goal: client will demonstrate ability to discuss emotional reactions to traumatic situation by discharge.

2. Long-term goal: client will renew significant relationships and establish meaningful goals for the future (within time frame specific to individual).

D. Nursing process: implementation

1. Accept client; establish trust; be consistent; keep all promises; convey acceptance; spend time with client.

🛑 A post-trauma client may be suspicious of others in his or her environment. Respect client's wishes regarding interaction with others, especially individuals of the opposite sex if the trauma was rape.

2. Assess client's stage in grief process.

3. Assess impact of trauma on ability to perform roles.

4. Assess for self-destructive ideas or behavior.

5. Assess for maladaptive coping (e.g., substance abuse).

6. Stay with client during flashbacks.

7. Encourage client to talk about the trauma when he or she is ready.

a. Provide a nonthreatening, private environment.

b. Include a significant other if the client wishes.

c. Acknowledge and validate client's feelings as they are expressed.

8. Discuss coping strategies.

9. Assist client in comprehending the trauma and how it will be assimilated into his or her persona.

10. Acknowledge feelings of guilt or self-blame.

E. Nursing process: evaluation: the following questions can be used to evaluate the client's response to the

---

MAKING THE CONNECTION

Various types of traumas elicit different responses in clients (e.g., human-engendered traumas often generate a greater degree of humiliation and guilt in victims than trauma associated with natural disasters). The debriefing process is the first step in the progression toward resolution. Resolution of the post-trauma response is largely dependent on the effectiveness of the coping strategies employed.

implementation of nursing actions focused on assisting the client diagnosed with PTSD to achieve stated outcomes.

1. Can the client discuss the traumatic event without experiencing panic anxiety?
2. Does the client voluntarily discuss the traumatic event?
3. Can the client discuss changes that have occurred in his or her life because of the traumatic event?
4. Does the client have "flashbacks"?
5. Can the client sleep without medication?
6. Does the client have nightmares?
7. Has the client learned new, adaptive coping strategies for assistance with recovery?
8. Can the client demonstrate successful use of these new coping strategies in times of stress?
9. Can the client verbalize stages of grief and the normal behaviors associated with each?
10. Can the client recognize his or her own position in the grieving process?
11. Is guilt being alleviated?
12. Has the client maintained or regained satisfactory relationships with significant others?
13. Can the client look to the future with optimism?
14. Does the client attend a regular support group for victims of similar traumatic experiences?
15. Does the client have a plan of action for dealing with symptoms, if they return?

IV. Acute Stress Disorder (ASD)

A. Similar to PTSD
B. Similar precipitating traumatic events and symptomatology
C. Symptoms are time limited, up to 1 month after the trauma
D. If the symptoms last longer than 1 month, the diagnosis would be PTSD

V. Adjustment Disorders (AD)

Sadock and Sadock (2007) report that adjustment disorders are one of the most common psychiatric diagnoses for

disorders of patients hospitalized for medical and surgical problems. In one study, 5% of people admitted to a hospital over a 3-year period were classified as having an adjustment disorder (p. 786).

A. Nursing process: assessment
 1. A maladaptive reaction to an identifiable stressor or stressors.
 2. Results in the development of clinically significant emotional or behavioral symptoms.
 3. Response occurs within 3 months after onset of the stressor.
 4. Response has persisted for **no longer than 6 months** after the stressor or its consequences have ended.
 5. Impairment occurs in social and occupational functioning.
 6. Client exhibits symptoms that are in excess of an expected reaction to the stressor.
B. Clinical presentations of AD
 1. AD with depressed mood.
   a. Most commonly diagnosed.
   b. Predominant mood disturbance.
   c. Less pronounced than major depressive episode.
   d. Symptoms exceed normative response to stressor.
     i. Depressed mood
     ii. Tearfulness
     iii. Hopelessness
 2. AD with anxiety
   a. Predominant manifestation is anxiety.
   b. Must differentiate from anxiety disorder (see Chapter 7).
   c. Symptoms:
     i. Nervousness
     ii. Worry
     iii. Jitteriness
 3. AD with mixed anxiety and depressed mood.
   a. Predominant features a combination of disturbances of mood and anxiety.
   b. Depression, feelings of hopelessness and sadness.
   c. Nervousness, worry, jitteriness.
   d. More intense than what would be expected as a normative response.
 4. AD with disturbance of conduct.
   a. Characterized by conduct in which there is violation of the rights of others.
   b. Violation of major age-appropriate societal norms and rules.
   c. Must differentiate from conduct disorder or antisocial personality disorder (see Chapter 13).
   d. Symptoms may include:
     i. Truancy
     ii. Vandalism
     iii. Reckless driving

iv. Fighting

v. Defaulting on legal responsibilities

5. AD with mixed disturbance of emotions and conduct

a. Predominant features of this category include both emotional disturbances:

i. Anxiety

ii. Depression

b. And disturbances of conduct:

i. Violation of the rights of others

ii. Violation of major age-appropriate societal norms and rules

1) Truancy

2) Vandalism

3) Fighting

6. AD unspecified: when the maladaptive reaction is not consistent with any of the other categories.

C. Nursing process: diagnosis (analysis)

1. Complicated grieving R/T loss of any concept of value to the individual AEB interference with life functioning, developmental regression, or somatic complaints.

2. Anxiety (severe) R/T situational crisis AEB restlessness and increased helplessness.

D. Nursing process: planning

1. Major Goals:

a. Relieve symptoms associated with stressor.

b. Enhance coping with stressors that cannot be reduced or removed.

c. Establish support systems that maximize adaptation.

2. Short-term goal: client will verbalize acceptable behaviors associated with each stage of the grief process by discharge.

3. Long-term goal: client will demonstrate ability for adequate occupational and social functioning (within time frame specific to individual).

E. Nursing process: implementation

1. Develop a trusting relationship.

2. Assess client's stage of grief.

3. Encourage client to express anger.

🛑 The initial expression of anger by the client may be displaced on the nurse or therapist. Do not become defensive but attempt to help the client explore angry feelings so that they may be directed toward the intended object or person. Anger is a normal stage in the grieving process and, if not released in an appropriate manner, may be turned inward on the self, leading to pathological depression.

4. Encourage large motor activities to release tension.

5. Help client correct misperceptions about the loss.

6. Assist client with problem solving.

7. Assess client's spiritual needs.

8. Role-play to practice potential stressful situations.

9. After anxiety has decreased, explain stages of grief.

MAKING THE CONNECTION

It is important for the nurse to assist the client to give up an idealized perception and be able to accept both positive and negative aspects about the painful life change before the grief process can be successfully completed. With support and sensitivity, point out the reality of the situation in areas where misrepresentations are expressed.

F. Nursing process: evaluation—the following questions can be used to evaluate the client's response to the implementation of nursing actions focused on assisting the client diagnosed with an adjustment disorder to achieve stated outcomes

1. Does the client verbalize understanding of the grief process and his or her position in the process?

2. Does the client recognize his or her adaptive and maladaptive behaviors associated with the grief response?

3. Does the client demonstrate evidence of progression along the grief response?

4. Can the client accomplish activities of daily living independently?

5. Does the client demonstrate the ability to perform occupational and social activities adequately?

6. Does the client discuss the change in health status and modification of the lifestyle it will affect?

7. Does the client demonstrate acceptance of the modification?

8. Can the client participate in decision making and problem solving for his or her future?

9. Does the client set realistic goals for the future?

10. Does the client demonstrate new adaptive coping strategies for dealing with the change in lifestyle?

11. Can the client verbalize available resources to whom he or she may go for support or assistance should it be necessary?

VI. Treatment Modalities for Trauma- and Stressor-Related Disorders

A. Individual psychotherapy

1. Most common treatment for AD.

2. Allows client to examine the stressor that is causing the problem.

3. Assists client to possibly assign personal meaning to the stressor.

4. Assists client to confront unresolved issues that may be exacerbating this crisis.

5. Clarifies links between the current stressor and past experience.

6. Assists with the development of more adaptive coping strategies.

B. Cognitive therapy
1. Strives to help the client diagnosed with post-traumatic stress disorder or acute stress disorder to recognize and modify trauma-related thoughts and beliefs.
2. Modifies the relationships between thoughts and feelings.
3. Identifies and challenges inaccurate or extreme automatic negative thoughts.
4. Goal of therapy:
   a. To replace negative thoughts with more accurate and less distressing thoughts.
   b. To cope more effectively with feelings such as anger, guilt, and fear.
   c. To regain hope and optimism about safety, trust, power and control, esteem, and intimacy.

C. Prolonged exposure therapy
1. A type of behavioral therapy similar to implosion therapy or flooding.
2. The client is exposed to repeated and prolonged mental recounting of the traumatic experience.
3. Exposure involves systematic confrontation, within safe limits, of trauma-related situations that are feared and avoided.
4. Has four main parts:
   a. Education about the treatment.
   b. Breathing retraining for relaxation.
   c. Imagined exposure through repeated discussion about the trauma with a therapist.
   d. Exposure to real-world situations related to the trauma.

D. Group/family therapy
1. Advocated for clients with PTSD.
2. Emphasizes sharing their experiences with empathetic peers.
3. Emphasizes talking about problems in social adaptation.
4. Emphasizes discussing options for managing aggression toward others.
5. The identification, support, and hopefulness of peer settings can facilitate therapeutic change.
6. Family therapy for clients diagnosed with adjustment disorders:
   a. Maladaptive response is viewed as symptomatic of a dysfunctional family system.
   b. All family members are included in the therapy.
   c. Goal of treatment is to improve family functioning.
   d. Emphasis is placed on communication, family rules, and interaction patterns among the family members.
7. Self-help groups for clients diagnosed with ADs:
   a. Clients may consider and compare their responses to individuals with similar life experiences.

   b. Members benefit from learning that they are not alone in their painful experiences.
   c. Hope is derived from knowing that others have survived and even grown from similar experiences.
   d. Members of the group exchange advice, share coping strategies, and provide support and encouragement for each other.

E. Behavior therapy
1. Goal of behavior therapy is to replace ineffective response patterns with adaptive ones.
2. Ineffective responses are identified.
3. Strategies to alter maladaptive response patterns:
   a. Carefully designed reinforcement schedules.
   b. Role modeling.
   c. Coaching.
   d. Effective in an inpatient setting where behavior and its consequences are more readily controlled.

F. Eye movement desensitization and reprocessing (EMDR)
1. Psychotherapy that involves rapid eye movements while processing painful emotions.
2. Empirically validated for trauma-related disorders such as PTSD and acute stress disorder.
3. Contraindicated in clients with:
   a. Neurological impairments (e.g., seizure disorders).
   b. Suicidal ideations.
   c. Psychosis.
   d. Severe dissociative disorders.
   e. Unstable substance abuse.
   f. Detached retina.
   g. Glaucoma.
4. Some individuals report rapid results.
5. Research indicates that 5 to 12 sessions are required to achieve lasting effects.
6. EMDR encompasses an eight-phase process:
   a. Phase 1: History and treatment planning.
      i. Therapist takes thorough history and develops treatment plan
      ii. Client is not required to discuss the traumatic event unless he or she chooses to do so

---

MAKING THE CONNECTION

The EMDR process: while concentrating on a particular emotion or physical sensation surrounding the traumatic event, the client is asked to focus his or her eye movements on the therapist's fingers as the therapist moves them from left to right and back again. The goal is to relieve the anxiety associated with the trauma so that the original event can be examined from a more detached perspective.

iii. Emphasis is placed on the emotions and physical sensations surrounding the traumatic event

b. Phase 2: Preparation.

   i. Therapist teaches the client certain self-care techniques (e.g., relaxation techniques)

   ii. It is important for the client to develop a sense of trust in the therapist

c. Phase 3: Assessment.

   i. Therapist asks the client to identify a specific scene from the event identified in Phase 1

   ii. Client directed to express a negative self-belief associated with the memory (e.g., "I am bad" or "I'm in danger")

   iii. Client directed to identify a self-statement that he or she would *rather* believe (e.g., "I am good" or "I'm safe now")

   iv. Client rates the validity of each of the statements on the Validity of Cognition (VOC) scale from (1 − *completely false*) to (7 = *completely true*)

   v. Client ranks the disturbing emotions on the Subjective Units of Disturbance (SUD) scale from (0 = *not disturbing at all*) to (10 = *worst feeling ever had*)

d. Phase 4: Desensitization.

   i. Client concentrates on negative beliefs and disturbing emotions associated with the event while focusing vision on the back-and-forth motion of the therapist's finger

   ii. After each set of rapid eye movements, the therapist reassesses the level of disturbance associated with the feelings, images, and beliefs

   iii. Process continues until the distress level is reduced to zero or 1 on the SUD scale

e. Phase 5: Installation.

   i. Client gives attention to identified positive belief to replace the negative belief associated with the trauma while simultaneously visually tracking the therapist's finger

   ii. After each set of rapid eye movements, the client is asked to rate the positive belief on the VOC scale

   iii. Goal is to strengthen the positive belief or self-statement until it is accepted as completely true (VOC score of 7)

f. Phase 6: Body scan.

   i. Client identifies any residual body tension

   ii. Positive self-beliefs must be believed on more than just an intellectual level

   iii. Phase 6 is not complete until the client can think about the traumatic event without experiencing bodily tension

g. Phase 7: Closure.

   i. Ensures that client leaves each session feeling better than he or she felt at the beginning

   ii. Therapist directs the client through a variety of self-calming relaxation techniques to help him or her regain emotional equilibrium

   iii. Client is briefed about what to expect between sessions because disturbing images, thoughts, and emotions may arise between therapy sessions

   iv. Therapist instructs the client to record these experiences in a journal so that they may be used as targets for processing in future therapy sessions

h. Phase 8: Reevaluation.

   i. Begins each new therapy session

   ii. Therapist assesses whether the positive changes have been maintained

   iii. Therapist determines whether previous target areas need reprocessing

   iv. Therapist identifies any new target areas that need attention

G. Psychopharmacology

1. Antidepressants.

a. Selective serotonin reuptake inhibitors (SSRIs) are first-line treatment of choice for PTSD due to their efficacy, tolerability, and safety ratings.

b. Paroxetine (Paxil) and sertraline (Zoloft) have been approved by the Food and Drug Administration for PTSD.

c. Tricyclic antidepressants such as amitriptyline (Elavil) and imipramine (Tofranil) have been effective in the treatment of PTSD.

d. Monoamine oxidase (MAO) inhibitors such as phenelzine (Nardil) have been effective in the treatment of PTSD.

e. Trazodone (Desyrel), a heterocyclic, has been effective in the treatment of PTSD.

2. Anxiolytics.

a. Alprazolam (Xanax) is used for its antidepressant and antipanic effects for clients diagnosed with PTSD.

b. Other benzodiazepines have also been used, despite the absence of controlled studies.

c. Addictive properties make benzodiazepines less desirable than other medications.

d. Buspirone (BuSpar), which has serotonergic properties similar to the SSRIs, may also be useful for PTSD.

3. Antihypertensives: the beta blocker propranolol (Inderal) and alpha$_2$-receptor agonist clonidine (Catapres) have been successful in alleviating some of the symptoms associated with PTSD.

a. Marked reductions in nightmares and intrusive recollections.

b. Decreased hypervigilance and insomnia.

c. Decreased startle responses, and angry outbursts.

4. Other medications.

a. Carbamazepine (Tegretol) , valproic acid (Depakote), and lithium carbonate (Lithobid) have been used with clients diagnosed with PTSD to alleviate symptoms of:

i. Intrusive recollections

ii. Flashbacks

iii. Nightmares

iv. Impulsivity

v. Irritability

vi. Violent behavior

b. Little positive evidence exists concerning the use of antipsychotics in PTSD.

c. Antipsychotics should be reserved for the short-term control of severe aggression and agitation.

5. Psychopharmacology use with AD.

a. AD is not commonly treated with medications.

i. Effects of medications may be temporary and mask the real problem, interfering with the possibility of finding a more permanent solution

ii. Psychoactive drugs carry the potential for physiological and psychological dependence

b. Antianxiety or antidepressant medication may be used for symptoms of anxiety or depression.

c. Antianxiety or antidepressant medications are only adjuncts to psychotherapy to help clients cope and should not be primary therapy.

VII. Crisis Intervention

A. Characteristics of a crisis

1. Any stressful situation can precipitate a crisis.

2. Precipitated by specific identifiable events.

3. Crisis occurs in all individuals at one time or another.

4. Personal by nature. What may be considered a crisis situation by one individual may not be so for another.

5. Acute, not chronic, and will be resolved in one way or another within a brief period.

6. Disequilibrium can result, requiring problem-solving skills that are often diminished by the level of anxiety.

7. Not necessarily equated with psychopathology.

8. Contains the potential for psychological growth or deterioration.

B. Assessment

1. Feel helpless to change.

2. Do not believe resources available to deal with the precipitating stressor.

3. Level of anxiety rises.

a. Becomes overwhelmed and nonfunctional.

b. Thoughts become obsessional.

MAKING THE CONNECTION

Lengthy psychological interpretations are not appropriate for crisis intervention. It is a time for doing what is needed to help the individual get relief and for calling into action all the people and other resources required to do so. The goal of crisis intervention is the resolution of an immediate crisis. Its focus is on the restoration of the individual to his or her precrisis level of functioning or possibly to a higher level of functioning.

---

c. All behavior is aimed at relief of the anxiety being experienced.

d. May affect physical and psychological well-being.

C. Factors affecting crisis response

1. The individual's perception of the event.

a. If perceived realistically, more likely to draw on adequate resources to restore equilibrium.

b. If perception is distorted, attempts at problem-solving can be ineffective, and restoration of equilibrium goes unresolved.

2. The availability of situational supports. Without adequate situational supports, an individual is most likely to feel overwhelmed and alone.

3. The availability of adequate coping mechanisms.

a. Individuals draw on behavioral strategies that have in the past been successful.

b. If these coping strategies work, a crisis may be averted.

c. If not, disequilibrium may continue and tension and anxiety increase.

D. Types of crises

1. Dispositional crises: an acute response to an external situational stressor.

2. Crises of anticipated life transitions: normal life-cycle transitions that may be anticipated but over which the individual may feel a lack of control.

3. Crises resulting from traumatic stress: crises precipitated by unexpected external stressors over which the individual has little or no control and from which he or she feels emotionally overwhelmed and defeated.

4. Maturational/developmental crises: crises that occur in response to situations that trigger emotions related to unresolved conflicts in one's life. These crisis are of internal origin and reflect underlying developmental issues that involve dependency, value conflicts, sexual identity, control, and capacity for emotional intimacy.

5. Crises reflecting psychopathology: emotional crises in which preexisting psychopathology has been instrumental in precipitating the crisis or in which psychopathology significantly impairs or

complicates adaptive resolution. Examples of psychopathology that may precipitate crises include borderline personality disorder, severe neuroses, other personality disorders, and schizophrenia.

6. Psychiatric emergencies: crisis situations in which general functioning has been severely impaired and the individual rendered incompetent or unable to assume personal responsibility. Examples include acutely suicidal individuals, drug overdoses, reactions to hallucinogenic drugs, acute psychoses, uncontrollable anger, and alcohol intoxication.

E. Role of the nurse in crisis intervention
   1. Assessment.
      a. Ask for description of event that precipitated crisis.
      b. Determine when it occurred.
      c. Assess the individual's physical and mental status.
      d. Determine whether stressor has been previously experienced. If so, what method of coping was used?
      e. If previous coping methods were tried, what was the result?
      f. If new coping methods were tried, what was the result?
      g. Assess suicide or homicide potential, plan, and means.
      h. Assess potential for violent behaviors.

DID YOU KNOW?

The Brøset Violence Checklist (BVC) is a quick, simple, and reliable checklist that can be used as a risk assessment for potential violence. Testing has shown 63% accuracy for prediction of violence at a score of 2 and higher (Box 8.1).

   i. Assess the adequacy of support systems.
   j. Determine level of precrisis functioning and ability to problem solve.
   k. Assess the individual's perception of personal strengths and limitations.
   l. Assess the individual's use of substances.

   2. Nursing diagnosis (analysis).
      a. Ineffective coping.
      b. Anxiety (severe to panic).
      c. Disturbed thought processes.
      d. Risk for self- or other-directed violence.
      e. Rape-trauma syndrome.
      f. Post-trauma syndrome.
      g. Fear.

   3. Planning.
      a. Consider type of crisis.
      b. Consider individual's strengths and available resources for support.
      c. Goals are established for crisis resolution and a return to, or increase in, the precrisis level of functioning.

Box 8.1 The Brøset Violence Checklist

Behaviors	Score (Score 1 point for each behavior observed. At a score of ≥2, begin deescalation techniques.)
Confusion	
Irritability	
Boisterousness	
Physical threats	
Verbal threats	
Attacks on objects	
TOTAL SCORE	

Deescalation techniques:

Calm voice	Walk outdoors or fresh air
Helpful attitude	Reduction in demands
Identify consequences	Group participation
Open hands and nonthreatening posture	Relaxation techniques
Allow phone call	Express concern
Offer food or drink	Verbal redirection and limit setting
Reduce stimulation and loud noise	Time-out, quiet time, open seclusion
Decrease waiting times and request refusals	Offer prn medication
Distract with a more positive activity (e.g., soft music or a quiet room)	

If deescalation techniques fail:
1. *Suggest prn medications*
2. *Time-out or unlocked seclusion, which can progress to locked seclusion*

Source: Almvik, Woods, & Rasmussen (2000). Deescalation techniques reprinted with permission from Barbara Barnes, Milwaukee County Behavioral Health Division.

4. Implementation.
   a. Crisis intervention takes place in both inpatient and outpatient settings.

DID YOU KNOW?

Crises can occur on an inpatient unit. Prevention is the key in the management of aggressive or violent behavior. The individual who becomes violent usually feels an underlying helplessness. Three factors that have been identified as important considerations in assessing for potential violence include a past history of violence, the client's diagnosis, and the current exhibited behavior. Diagnoses that have a strong association with violent behavior are schizophrenia, major depression, bipolar disorder, and substance use disorders. Substance abuse in addition to mental illness compounds the increased risk of violence. Dementia and antisocial, borderline, and intermittent explosive personality disorders have also been associated with a risk for violent behavior.

   b. The goal of crisis intervention is the resolution of an immediate crisis.

c. Use a reality-oriented approach. The focus of the problem is on the here and now.

d. Remain with the individual who is experiencing panic anxiety.

e. Establish a rapid working relationship by showing unconditional acceptance, by active listening, and by attending to immediate needs.

f. Discourage lengthy explanations or rationalizations of the situation; promote an atmosphere for verbalization of true feelings.

g. Set firm limits on aggressive, destructive behaviors. Establish at the outset what is acceptable and what is not, and maintain consistency.

🛑 Escalating aggressive behaviors that are characterized by anxiety and tension, verbal abuse, profanity, and increasing hyperactivity can be described as a "**prodromal syndrome.**" Most assaultive behavior is preceded by a period of increasing hyperactivity. Behaviors associated with the prodromal syndrome should be considered emergent and demand immediate attention. These behaviors include rigid posture; clenched fists and jaws; grim, defiant affect; talking in a rapid, raised voice; arguing and demanding; using profanity and threatening verbalizations; agitation and pacing; and pounding and slamming.

h. Clarify the problem. The nurse does this by describing his or her perception of the problem and comparing it with the individual's perception of the problem.

i. Help the individual determine what he or she believes precipitated the crisis.

j. Acknowledge feelings of anger, guilt, helplessness, and powerlessness, without giving positive feedback for these feelings.

k. Guide the individual through a problem-solving process that facilitates movement toward positive life change.

l. Help the individual confront the source of the problem that is creating the crisis response.

m. Encourage the individual to discuss realistic changes he or she would like to make.

n. Encourage exploration of feelings and ways of adaptively coping with aspects that cannot be changed.

o. Discuss alternative strategies for creating realistic changes.

p. Weigh benefits and consequences of each alternative.

q. Assist the individual to select alternative coping strategies that will help alleviate future crisis situations.

5. Evaluation: reassessment to determine whether outcomes have been met.

a. Have positive behavioral changes occurred?

b. Has the individual developed more adaptive coping strategies, and have they been effective?

c. Has the individual grown from the experience by gaining insight into his or her responses to crisis situations?

d. Does the individual believe that he or she could respond with healthy adaptation in future stressful situations to prevent crisis development?

e. Can the individual describe a plan of action for dealing with stressors similar to the one that precipitated this crisis?

F. Disaster nursing: a **disaster** event overwhelms local resources and threatens the function and safety of the community

1. Potential cause of property devastation or loss of life.

2. Victims left with a damaged sense of safety and well-being, and varying degrees of emotional trauma.

3. Children are particularly vulnerable.
   a. Lack life experiences.
   b. Lack coping skills.

4. Emotional effects may show up immediately or appear weeks or months later.

5. Psychological and behavioral responses to a disaster.
   a. Adult response similar to symptoms of PTSD.
   b. Preschool children experience separation anxiety, regressive behaviors, nightmares, and hyperactive or withdrawn behaviors.
   c. Older children may have difficulty concentrating, somatic complaints, sleep disturbances, and concerns about safety.
   d. Adolescents' responses are often similar to those of adults.

6. Nursing assessments related to disaster.
   a. Assess the client for serious injury or resolution of injuries (**triage**).
   b. Assess for infections with focus on prevention.
   c. Assess ability to maintain anxiety at manageable level.
   d. Assess ability to demonstrate appropriate problem-solving skills.
   e. Assess ability to discuss beliefs about spiritual issues.
   f. Assess ability to deal with emotional reactions in an individually appropriate manner.
   g. Assess physical symptoms associated with the disaster (e.g., pain, nightmares, flashbacks, fatigue).
   h. Assess factors affecting the community's ability to meet its own demands or needs.
   i. Assess activities initiated to improve community functioning.
   j. Assess for establishment of a plan to deal with future contingencies related to the disaster.

REVIEW QUESTIONS

1. A 13-year-old client's father has recently been deployed to a war zone. The client is constantly tearful and exhibits truancy, vandalism, and aggression. The pediatric nurse practitioner should identify this behavior with which adjustment disorder (AD)?
   1. An AD with anxiety
   2. An AD with disturbance of conduct
   3. An AD with mixed disturbance of emotions and conduct
   4. An AD unspecified

2. After a spouse dies, a client is diagnosed with adjustment disorder (AD) with depressed mood. Symptoms include chronic migraines, feelings of hopelessness, social isolation, and self-care deficit. Which appropriate client outcome should a nurse assign?
   1. By discharge, client will no longer use impulsive behaviors to cope with stress.
   2. By discharge, client will accomplish activities of daily living independently.
   3. By discharge, client will be able to delay gratification to cope with stress.
   4. By discharge, client will verbalize a positive body image.

3. A student nurse is reviewing a client's record. Which of the following events could have precipitated the client's diagnosis of post-traumatic stress disorder (PTSD)? **Select all that apply.**
   1. Witnessing the violent death of a brother
   2. Being diagnosed with diabetes mellitus
   3. Experiencing marital discord for several years
   4. Being raped at age 13
   5. Losing a mother to cancer

4. A client who is a veteran of a recent military conflict is being assessed by a nurse for post-traumatic stress disorder (PTSD). Which of the following client symptoms would support this diagnosis? **Select all that apply.**
   1. The client has experienced symptoms of the disorder for 2 weeks.
   2. The client fears a physical integrity threat to self.
   3. The client feels detached and estranged from others.
   4. The client experiences fear and helplessness.
   5. The client is lethargic and somnolent.

5. A nurse would recognize which as a goal of behavior therapy for a client diagnosed with adjustment disorder (AD) and in what setting would this therapy be most effective?
   1. To clarify links between the current stressor and past experiences; outpatient setting
   2. To replace ineffective response patterns with more adaptive ones; inpatient setting
   3. To derive hope from sharing with others similar life experiences; outpatient setting
   4. To resolve the immediate crisis and restore the client's adaptive functioning; inpatient setting

6. Which of the following clients would be a candidate for eye movement desensitization and reprocessing (EMDR)? **Select all that apply.**
   1. A client diagnosed with epilepsy
   2. A client with active suicidal ideations
   3. A client experiencing visual hallucinations
   4. A client diagnosed with acute stress disorder (ASD)
   5. A client diagnosed with post-traumatic stress disorder (PTSD)

7. A nurse would recognize which of the following medications as appropriate treatment for a client diagnosed with post-traumatic stress disorder (PTSD)? **Select all that apply.**
   1. Fluoxetine (Prozac)
   2. Alprazolam (Xanax)
   3. Propranolol (Inderal)
   4. Lithium carbonate (Lithobid)
   5. Ziprasidone (Geodon)

8. After years of infertility, a woman delivers a stillborn infant. She is tearful, trembling, and screams at the nurse, "My baby is crying. Bring him to me now!" Which is the priority nursing diagnosis for this client?
   1. Deficient knowledge R/T situational crisis
   2. Ineffective denial R/T loss of infant AEB client's statement demanding infant
   3. Risk for self-directed violence R/T hopelessness
   4. Postpartum depression R/T loss of infant

9. Order the following eight-phase process used in eye movement desensitization and reprocessing (EMDR).
   1. _____ Body scan
   2. _____ Desensitization
   3. _____ Closure
   4. _____ Preparation
   5. _____ History and treatment planning
   6. _____ Reevaluation
   7. _____ Installation
   8. _____ Assessment

10. A nurse has charted a client's score of 7 on the Validity of Cognition (VOC) scale after an eye movement desensitization and reprocessing (EMDR) treatment. Which client statement led to this documentation?
    1. "When I remember the accident, it is the worse feeling I have ever had."
    2. "My statement that *I am a good person* is completely false."
    3. "My statement that *I am a good father* is completely true."
    4. "The memories of fighting in the war are hardly upsetting anymore."

11. In an outpatient clinic, a nurse is caring for a client diagnosed with an adjustment disorder. When evaluating psychopharmacological treatment, which of the following should the nurse consider? **Select all that apply.**
    1. Antipsychotic medications are the first line of treatment for adjustment disorders.
    2. When treating adjustment disorders, medications are commonly prescribed for the symptoms of depression and anxiety.
    3. Adjustment disorders are not commonly treated with medications because they may mask the underlying problem.
    4. Adjustment disorders are not commonly treated with anxiolytic medications because they carry the potential for dependence.
    5. Anxiolytic medications are considered the primary therapy for adjustment disorders.

12. Which nursing action is inappropriate during a crisis situation?
    1. Taking an active role in problem solving and making decisions for the client
    2. Guiding the client to appropriate resources
    3. Encouraging independent thinking to promote insight
    4. Creating a highly structured environment for the client

13. A nurse has charted a client's score of 4 on the Subjective Units of Disturbance (SUD) scale after an eye movement desensitization and reprocessing (EMDR) treatment. Which client statement led to this documentation?
    1. "When I remember the fire, it's the worse feeling I have ever had."
    2. "When I remember the fire, it makes me sad, but grateful to be alive."
    3. "When I remember the fire, it's hard for me to understand the devastation."
    4. "When I remember the fire, it's over, and I don't dwell on it."

14. When an individual is exposed to massive trauma, which of the following variables should the nurse consider important when evaluating his or her response to the traumatic experience? **Select all that apply.**
    1. Degree of ego strength
    2. Birth order
    3. Behavioral tendencies (temperament)
    4. Presence of preexisting psychopathology
    5. Demographic factors

15. Years ago a client overcame a stress response to a severe traumatic event. Recently, after a minor auto accident, this client was hospitalized with a diagnosis of post-traumatic stress disorder (PTSD). Which theory would explain this phenomenon?
    1. Biological theory
    2. Cognitive theory
    3. Psychosocial theory
    4. Learning theory

16. An instructor is teaching about *dispositional crises.* Which student statement indicates that learning has occurred?
    1. "*Dispositional crisis* occurs when normal life-cycle transitions are anticipated, but the individual may feel a lack of control."
    2. "*Dispositional crisis* occurs when an individual has little control and feels emotionally overwhelmed by an unexpected external stressor."
    3. "*Dispositional crisis* occurs when an individual has an acute response to an external situation."
    4. "*Dispositional crisis* occurs in response to situations that trigger emotions related to unresolved conflicts in one's life."

17. Which situation would a nurse evaluate as an example of a *maturational/developmental crisis*?
    1. A client with dependency and severe attachment problems suffers frequent panic attacks after the sudden death of her mother.
    2. Dominated by her father since childhood, a client becomes severely hyperactive and violent whenever her husband is directive and demanding.
    3. A woman is overwhelmed after the birth of her first child and begins to complain to a health-care practitioner of numerous physical symptoms.
    4. After being passed over for the rank of major for the second time, an Air Force pilot comes home and becomes physically violent with his wife and children.

18. In the context of disaster nursing, _____ _____ is the screening and classification of casualties to make optimal use of treatment resources and to maximize the survival and welfare of clients.

19. Which psychological and behavioral responses to a disaster situation would the nurse expect to observe in a preschool child?
    1. Symptoms similar to those of post-traumatic stress disorder (PTSD)
    2. Regressive, hyperactive, or withdrawn behaviors and nightmares
    3. Difficulty concentrating and sleep disturbances
    4. Psychic numbing, weight loss, and alopecia

20. A newly admitted client on an inpatient unit verbally abuses the staff, uses profanity, and paces in the common room. How would the nurse document this client's behavior syndrome?
    1. "Post-traumatic stress syndrome"
    2. "Borderline personality disorder syndrome"
    3. "Prodromal syndrome"
    4. "Adjustment disorder with anxiety syndrome"

21. A nurse has used the Brøset Violence Checklist (BVC) to evaluate an inpatient client's risk for violent behavior. The client scored a 3. Which of the following interventions should the nurse initially employ? **Select all that apply.**
    1. Place client in ordered unlocked seclusion
    2. Verbally redirect the client and set limits
    3. Maintain an authoritative stance
    4. Reduce stimulation and loud noise
    5. Offer prn medications

REVIEW ANSWERS

1. **ANSWER: 3**
   Rationale:
   1. An adjustment disorder with anxiety denotes a maladaptive response to a stressor in which the predominant manifestation is anxiety. The symptoms presented in the question indicate that the client is experiencing an adjustment disorder with mixed disturbance of emotions and conduct, not an adjustment disorder with anxiety.
   2. An adjustment disorder with disturbance of conduct is characterized by conduct in which there is violation of the rights of others or of major age-appropriate societal norms and rules. The symptoms presented in the question indicate that the client is experiencing an adjustment disorder with mixed disturbance of emotions and conduct, not an adjustment disorder with disturbance of conduct.
   3. The predominant features of an adjustment disorder with mixed disturbance of emotions and conduct include symptoms of anxiety or depression as well as behaviors that include violations of rights of others, truancy, vandalism, and fighting. The client's tearfulness together with truancy, vandalism, and aggression indicate a diagnosis of adjustment disorder with mixed disturbance of emotions and conduct.
   4. An adjustment disorder unspecified subtype is used when the maladaptive reaction is not consistent with any of the other categories. The symptoms presented in the question are consistent with a diagnosis of adjustment disorder with mixed disturbance of emotions and conduct.
   TEST-TAKING TIP: Review the various categories of adjustment disorders and be able to match the clinical presentation in the question with the appropriate category.
   Content Area: Psychosocial Integrity;
   Integrated Process: Nursing Process: Assessment;
   Client Need: Psychosocial Integrity;
   Cognitive Level: Application;
   Concept: Stress

2. **ANSWER: 2**
   Rationale:
   1. Impulsive behaviors are symptoms of impulse control, not adjustment disorders.
   2. Assigning an outcome of independent self-care will direct nursing interventions toward encouraging the client to meet self-care needs.
   3. The inability to delay gratification is a symptom of impulse control, not adjustment disorders.
   4. There is no evidence presented in the question indicating that the client has a body image distortion.
   TEST-TAKING TIP: First, check to see whether the outcome is written correctly and then match the appropriate outcome to the client symptoms presented in the question.
   Content Area: Psychosocial Integrity;
   Integrated Process: Nursing Process: Planning;
   Client Need: Psychosocial Integrity;
   Cognitive Level: Application;
   Concept: Critical Thinking

3. **ANSWERS: 1, 4**
   Rationale: PTSD is a reaction to an extreme trauma such as natural or manmade disasters, combat, serious accidents, witnessing the violent death of others, being a victim of torture, terrorism, rape, or other crimes.
   1. PTSD is a reaction to an extreme trauma such as witnessing the violent death of the client's brother.
   2. PTSD is not related to common experiences such as chronic illness.
   3. PTSD is not related to common experiences such as marital conflict.
   4. PTSD is a reaction to an extreme trauma such as rape.
   5. PTSD is not related to common experiences such as uncomplicated grieving such as losing a mother to cancer.
   TEST-TAKING TIP: First, differentiate between the types of stressors that would lead to a post-trauma reaction and those that would not. Look for extreme trauma that would precipitate a diagnosis of PTSD.
   Content Area: Psychosocial Integrity;
   Integrated Process: Nursing Process: Evaluation;
   Client Need: Psychosocial Integrity;
   Cognitive Level: Application;
   Concept: Stress

4. **ANSWERS: 2, 3, 4**
   Rationale:
   1. The full symptom picture of PTSD must be present for more than 1 month, not 2 weeks, and cause significant interference with social, occupational, and other areas of functioning.
   2. The nurse should determine that a client who fears a physical integrity threat to self would meet the criteria for the diagnosis of PTSD.
   3. The nurse should determine that a client who experiences detachment and estrangement from others would meet the criteria for a diagnosis of PTSD.
   4. The nurse should determine that a client who feels intense fear and helplessness would meet the criteria for a diagnosis of PTSD.
   5. Characteristic symptoms of PTSD include reexperiencing the traumatic event, a sustained high level of arousal, and a general numbing of responsiveness, but not lethargy and somnolence.
   TEST-TAKING TIP: Review the criteria for the diagnosis of PTSD and match the symptoms presented to these criteria.
   Content Area: Psychosocial Integrity;
   Integrated Process: Nursing Process: Assessment;
   Client Need: Psychosocial Integrity;
   Cognitive Level: Application;
   Concept: Stress

5. **ANSWER: 2**
   Rationale:
   1. The goal of psychotherapy, not behavior therapy, is to clarify links between the current stressor and past experiences.
   2. The goal of behavior therapy is to replace ineffective response patterns with more adaptive ones. This occurs most effectively in an inpatient setting.
   3. The goal of self-help groups, not behavior therapy, is to derive hope from sharing with others similar life experiences.
   4. The goal of crisis intervention, not behavior therapy, is to resolve the immediate crisis and restore adaptive functioning.
   TEST-TAKING TIP: Note the words "response patterns" in Option 2. This should lead the test taker to recognize this as a behavioral therapy goal.

Content Area: Safe and Effective Care Environment: Management of Care;
Integrated Process: Nursing Process: Planning;
Client Need: Safe and Effective Care Environment: Management of Care;
Cognitive Level: Application;
Concept: Nursing

6. **ANSWERS: 4, 5**
   Rationale:
   1. EMDR is contraindicated in clients who have neurological impairments such as seizure disorders.
   2. EMDR is contraindicated in clients experiencing suicidal ideations.
   3. EMDR is contraindicated in clients experiencing psychosis, unstable substance use disorder, severe dissociative disorders, and detached retina.
   4. EMDR has been used for depression, adjustment disorder, phobias, addictions, generalized anxiety disorder, and panic disorder. It has been empirically validated for trauma-related disorders, such as acute stress disorder.
   5. EMDR has been empirically validated for trauma-related disorders such as PTSD.
   TEST-TAKING TIP: Review in which circumstances EMDR is the treatment of choice and under which circumstances it is contraindicated.
   Content Area: Safe and Effective Care Environment: Management of Care;
   Integrated Process: Nursing Process: Evaluation;
   Client Need: Safe and Effective Care Environment: Management of Care;
   Cognitive Level: Application;
   Concept: Stress

7. **ANSWERS: 1, 2, 3, 4**
   Rationale:
   1. Antidepressants, especially SSRIs such as fluoxetine, are now considered the first-line treatment for PTSD.
   2. Benzodiazepines, such as alprazolam, are used short-term for antidepressant and antipanic effects, even though there is an absence of controlled studies demonstrating their efficacy.
   3. Beta blockers, such as propranolol, alleviate some of the PTSD symptoms.
   4. Lithium has been reported to alleviate symptoms of intrusive recollections, flashbacks, nightmares, impulsivity, irritability, and violent behavior in clients diagnosed with PTSD.
   5. Little positive evidence exists for the use of antipsychotics such as ziprasidone in the treatment of PTSD. Some researchers believe that these drugs should be reserved for the short-term control of severe aggression and agitation.
   TEST-TAKING TIP: Review the various classifications of medications that may be used in the treatment of PTSD.
   Content Area: Safe and Effective Care Environment: Management of Care;
   Integrated Process: Nursing Process: Evaluation;
   Client Need: Safe and Effective Care Environment: Management of Care;
   Cognitive Level: Application;
   Concept: Medication

8. **ANSWER: 2**
   Rationale:
   1. The nursing diagnosis of *Deficient knowledge* is defined as the absence or deficiency of cognitive information related to a specific topic. The information presented in the question indicates that the client does not meet the criteria for this nursing diagnosis because the client may know that her infant is deceased but is in denial of this fact. Furthermore, this nursing diagnosis is incorrectly written because it does not contain an "as evidenced by" statement.
   2. The priority nursing diagnosis for this client is *ineffective denial*, which is the conscious or unconscious attempt to disavow the knowledge or meaning of an event to reduce anxiety and/or fear, leading to the detriment of health. The information presented in the question, especially the client's statement, indicates that the client meets the criteria for this correctly written nursing diagnosis.
   3. The nursing diagnosis of *Risk for self-directed violence* is defined as the risk for behaviors in which an individual demonstrates that he or she can be physically, emotionally, and/or sexually harmful to self. There is no information presented in the question that indicates that the client is at risk for self-harm.
   4. Postpartum depression is a medical and not nursing diagnosis. Medical diagnoses are never used in the formulation of a nursing diagnosis.
   TEST-TAKING TIP: Match the assessment information in the question to the appropriate nursing diagnosis. Always check that the nursing diagnoses presented are formulated correctly.
   Content Area: Safe and Effective Care Environment: Management of Care;
   Integrated Process: Nursing Process: Diagnosis (Analysis);
   Client Need: Safe and Effective Care Environment: Management of Care;
   Cognitive Level: Analysis;
   Concept: Critical Thinking

9. **ANSWERS: 6, 4, 7, 2, 1, 8, 5, 3**
   Rationale:
   Phase 1: History and treatment planning. In the first phase, the therapist takes a thorough history and develops a treatment plan. The client problem and current symptoms are discussed. The client is not required to discuss the traumatic event in detail. Emphasis is placed on the emotions and physical sensations surrounding the traumatic event.
   Phase 2: Preparation. The therapist teaches the client certain self-care techniques (e.g., relaxation techniques) for dealing with emotional disturbances that may arise during or between sessions.
   Phase 3: Assessment. The client identifies a specific scene from the target event that best represents the memory. The client then expresses a negative self-belief associated with the memory (e.g., "I am bad") and identifies a self-statement that he or she would *rather* believe (e.g., "I am good"). The client then rates the validity of each of the statements on a Validity of Cognition scale and ranks the disturbing emotions on a zero to 10 Subjective Units of Disturbance scale.
   Phase 4: Desensitization. The client gives attention to the negative beliefs and disturbing emotions associated with the traumatic event while focusing his or her vision on the

back-and-forth motion of the therapist's finger. All personal feelings and physical reactions are noted and after the treatment, the level of disturbance is reassessed. This desensitization process continues until the distress level is reduced to 0 or 1.

Phase 5: Installation. The client gives attention to the positive belief that he or she has identified to replace the negative belief associated with the trauma. This is accomplished while simultaneously visually tracking the therapist's finger. The goal is to strengthen the positive belief or self-statement until it is accepted as completely true.

Phase 6: Body scan. After the positive belief is strengthened, the client concentrates on any lingering physical sensations. While focusing on the traumatic event, the client identifies any areas of the body where residual tension is experienced. Phase 6 is not complete until the client is able to think about or discuss the traumatic event without experiencing bodily tension.

Phase 7: Closure. Closure ensures that the client leaves each session feeling better than he or she felt at the beginning. Self-calming relaxation techniques are used to help the client regain emotional equilibrium. The therapist teaches the client how to deal with disturbing images, thoughts, and emotions that may occur between sessions.

Phase 8: Reevaluation. Reevaluation begins each new therapy session. The therapist assesses whether the positive changes have been maintained, determines whether previous target areas need reprocessing, and identifies any new target areas that need attention.

TEST-TAKING TIP: Review the chronological order of the phases of EMDR. Although assessment is usually the first phase of any treatment, in EMDR it follows the *History and treatment planning* and *Preparation* phases.
Content Area: Safe and Effective Care Environment: Management of Care;
Integrated Process: Nursing Process: Implementation;
Client Need: Safe and Effective Care Environment: Management of Care;
Cognitive Level: Analysis;
Concept: Stress

10. **ANSWER: 3**
Rationale: The VOC is the Validity of Cognition scale. Using this scale the client can rank his or her self-assessment as *completely false* (1) to *completely true* (7). The SUD is the Subjective Units of Disturbance scale. Using this scale the client can rank his or her disturbing emotions as *not disturbing at all* (0) to *worst feeling ever* (10).
1. On the basis of this client statement, the nurse would use the SUD, not the VOC scale, to document this client's disturbing emotions as 10.
2. On the basis of this client statement, the nurse would use the VOC scale to document this client's self-assessment as a 1, not a 7.
3. **On the basis of this client statement, the nurse would use the VOC scale to document this client's self-assessment as 7.**
4. On the basis of this client statement, the nurse would use the SUD, not the VOC scale, to document this client's disturbing emotions as 0.

TEST-TAKING TIP: Review the differences between the VOC and SUD scales. Note the word "Validity" and look for a statement that is true and valid and therefore rated high on the VOC scale.
Content Area: Safe and Effective Care Environment: Management of Care;
Integrated Process: Nursing Process: Implementation;
Client Need: Safe and Effective Care Environment: Management of Care;
Cognitive Level: Application;
Concept: Stress

11. **ANSWERS: 2, 3, 4**
Rationale:
1. Adjustment disorders are not commonly treated with medications. Antipsychotic medications are not used in the treatment of adjustment disorders.
2. **When a client diagnosed with adjustment disorder has symptoms of anxiety or depression, the physician may prescribe antianxiety or antidepressant medication. These medications are considered only adjuncts to psychotherapy and should not be given as the primary therapy.**
3. **An adjustment disorder is not commonly treated with medications because their effect may be temporary and may only mask the real problem, interfering with the possibility of finding a more permanent solution.**
4. **An adjustment disorder is not commonly treated with anxiolytic medications because these drugs carry the potential for physiological and psychological dependence.**
5. Adjustment disorders are not commonly treated with medications. Anxiolytic medications may be prescribed for anxiety symptoms but are considered only adjuncts to psychotherapy and should not be given as the primary therapy.

TEST-TAKING TIP: Remember that adjustment disorders are not commonly treated with medications.
Content Area: Safe and Effective Care Environment: Management of Care;
Integrated Process: Nursing Process: Evaluation;
Client Need: Safe and Effective Care Environment: Management of Care;
Cognitive Level: Application;
Concept: Assessment

12. **ANSWER: 3**
Rationale:
1. Because of increased anxiety, the individual in crisis is unable to problem solve, so the nurse must take an active role in problem solving and make decisions for the client.
2. Because of increased anxiety, the individual in crisis is unable to problem solve, so he or she requires guidance and support from the nurse to help mobilize the resources needed to resolve the crisis.
3. **Because of increased anxiety, the individual in crisis is unable to problem solve, so the nurse must take an active role in problem solving and decision making for the client. It would be inappropriate for the nurse to encourage independent thinking to promote insight.**
4. Crisis intervention is short term and relies heavily on orderly problem-solving techniques and a highly structured environment. This structured environment provides the client with security as adaptive functioning is restored.

TEST-TAKING TIP: Recognize that during crisis, nursing actions change from a supportive to a directive role.
Content Area: Safe and Effective Care Environment: Management of Care;
Integrated Process: Nursing Process: Implementation;
Client Need: Safe and Effective Care Environment: Management of Care;
Cognitive Level: Application;
Concept: Stress

13. **ANSWER: 2**
Rationale: Using the SUD, the client is asked to rank his or her disturbing emotions on a 0 to 10 scale (with 0 meaning the disturbance is not disturbing at all and 10 meaning it is the worst feeling he or she has ever had).
1. On the basis of this client statement, the nurse would use the SUD scale to document this client's disturbing emotions as 10.
2. On the basis of this client statement, the nurse would use the SUD scale to document this client's disturbing emotions as 4.
3. On the basis of this client statement, the nurse would use the SUD scale to document this client's disturbing emotions as 8.
4. On the basis of this client statement, the nurse would use the SUD scale to document this client's disturbing emotions as 0.
TEST-TAKING TIP: Remember that the Subjective Units of Disturbance scale is used to rank disturbing emotions.
Content Area: Safe and Effective Care Environment: Management of Care;
Integrated Process: Nursing Process: Implementation;
Client Need: Safe and Effective Care Environment: Management of Care;
Cognitive Level: Application;
Concept: Stress

14. **ANSWERS: 1, 3, 4, 5**
Rationale:
1. A nurse should consider the individual's degree of ego strength when evaluating his or her response to a traumatic experience.
2. Birth order is not used in evaluating an individual's response to a traumatic experience.
3. A nurse should consider the individual's behavioral tendencies when evaluating his or her response to a traumatic experience.
4. A nurse should consider the individual's preexisting psychopathology when evaluating his or her response to a traumatic experience.
5. A nurse should consider the individual's demographic factors (e.g., age, socioeconomic status, education) when evaluating his or her response to a traumatic experience.
TEST-TAKING TIP: Know the variables that are considered important in determining an individual's response to a traumatic experience. These variables include characteristics that relate to (1) the traumatic experience, (2) the individual, and (3) the recovery environment.
Content Area: Safe and Effective Care Environment: Management of Care;

Integrated Process: Nursing Process: Evaluation;
Client Need: Safe and Effective Care Environment: Management of Care;
Cognitive Level: Application;
Concept: Trauma

15. **ANSWER: 1**
Rationale:
1. Biological theorists suggest that an individual who has experienced previous trauma is more likely to develop symptoms after a stressful life event. These individuals with previous traumatic experiences may be more likely to become exposed to future traumas because they can be inclined to reactivate the behaviors associated with the original trauma. Biological theory supports a type of "addiction to trauma."
2. Cognitive theorists take into consideration the individual's cognitive appraisal of an event and focus on assumptions that an individual makes about the world. The situation presented in the question does not reflect the principles of cognitive theory.
3. Psychosocial theorists explain the development of trauma-related disorders based on an individual's response to variables, which include characteristics that relate to (1) the traumatic experience, (2) the individual, and (3) the recovery environment. The situation presented in the question does not reflect the principles of psychosocial theory.
4. Learning theorists view negative reinforcement as behavior that leads to a reduction in an aversive experience, thereby reinforcing and resulting in repetition of the behavior. The situation presented in the question does not reflect the principles of learning theory.
TEST-TAKING TIP: Know that only biological theorists believe that an individual who has experienced previous trauma is more likely to develop symptoms after a subsequent stressful life event. Their hypothesis supports a type of "addiction to the trauma."
Content Area: Psychosocial Integrity;
Integrated Process: Nursing Process: Assessment;
Client Need: Psychosocial Integrity;
Cognitive Level: Application;
Concept: Evidenced-based Practice

16. **ANSWER: 3**
Rationale:
1. *Crises of anticipated life transitions,* not *dispositional crisis,* occur when normal life-cycle transitions are anticipated, and the individual may feel a lack of control. This student's statement indicates that further instruction is needed.
2. *Crises resulting from traumatic stress,* not *dispositional crisis,* occur when an individual has little control and feels emotionally overwhelmed by an unexpected external stressor. This student's statement indicates that further instruction is needed.
3. *Dispositional crisis* occurs when an individual has an acute response to an external situation, such as when an individual experiences a traumatic stressor and violently displaces it on to another person. This student's statement indicates that learning has occurred.

4. *Maturational/development crises,* not *dispositional crisis,* occur in response to situations that trigger emotions related to unresolved conflicts in one's life. This student's statement indicates that further instruction is needed.

TEST-TAKING TIP: Review the six classes of emotional crises and be able to match a situation to the appropriate crisis type.

Content Area: Psychosocial Integrity;
Integrated Process: Nursing Process: Evaluation;
Client Need: Psychosocial Integrity;
Cognitive Level: Application;
Concept: Stress

17. ANSWER: 2

Rationale:

1. A *crisis reflecting psychopathology* is an emotional crisis in which preexisting psychopathology has been instrumental in precipitating the crisis. The situation presented in the answer choice is reflective of a *crisis reflecting psychopathology,* not a *maturational/developmental crisis.*

2. A *maturational/developmental crisis* occurs in response to situations that trigger emotions related to unresolved conflicts in one's life. The situation presented in the answer choice is reflective of a *maturational/developmental crisis.*

3. A *crisis of anticipated life transitions* is related to normal life-cycle transitions that may be anticipated but over which the individual may feel a lack of control. The situation presented in the answer choice is reflective of a *crisis of anticipated life transitions,* not a *maturational/developmental crisis.*

4. A *dispositional crisis* is an acute response to an external situational stressor. The situation presented in the answer choice is reflective of a *dispositional crisis,* not a *maturational/developmental crisis.*

TEST-TAKING TIP: Review the six classes of emotional crises and be able to match a situation to the appropriate crisis type.

Content Area: Psychosocial Integrity;
Integrated Process: Nursing Process: Evaluation;
Client Need: Psychosocial Integrity;
Cognitive Level: Application;
Concept: Stress

18. ANSWER: triage

Rationale: Triage is the screening and classification of casualties to make optimal use of treatment resources and to maximize the survival and welfare of clients. Triage is used by the nurse in a disaster situation to provide appropriate and efficient client care.

TEST-TAKING TIP: Review the key words at the beginning of the chapter.

Content Area: Safe and Effective Care Environment: Management of Care;
Integrated Process: Nursing Process: Assessment;
Client Need: Safe and Effective Care Environment: Management of Care;
Cognitive Level: Knowledge;
Concept: Trauma

19. ANSWER: 2

Rationale:

1. Adults, not preschool children, respond to a disaster situation with similar symptoms to those of post-traumatic stress disorder (PTSD).

2. Preschool children experience separation anxiety, regressive behaviors, nightmares, and hyperactive or withdrawn behaviors as a response to a disaster situation.

3. Older children, not preschool children, may have difficulty concentrating, somatic complaints, sleep disturbances, and concerns about safety as a response to a disaster situation.

4. Psychic numbing, weight loss and alopecia are not typical responses to a disaster situation by a preschool child.

TEST-TAKING TIP: Review how various age groups psychologically and behaviorally respond to a disaster.

Content Area: Psychosocial Integrity;
Integrated Process: Nursing Process: Assessment;
Client Need: Psychosocial Integrity;
Cognitive Level: Application;
Concept: Trauma

20. ANSWER: 3

Rationale:

1. Post-traumatic stress disorder (PTSD) is a reaction to an extreme trauma such as natural or manmade disasters, combat, serious accidents, witnessing the violent death of others, being a victim of torture, terrorism, rape, or other crimes. This disorder is not referred to as a syndrome.

2. Borderline personality disorder is characterized by a pattern of intense and chaotic relationships, with affective instability and fluctuating attitudes toward other people. This disorder is not referred to as a syndrome.

3. Escalating aggressive behaviors that are characterized by anxiety and tension, verbal abuse, profanity, and increasing hyperactivity can be described as a "prodromal syndrome"

4. An adjustment disorder with anxiety denotes a maladaptive response to a stressor in which the predominant manifestation is anxiety. This disorder is not referred to as a syndrome.

TEST-TAKING TIP: Review the key words at the beginning of the chapter.

Content Area: Safe and Effective Care Environment: Management of Care;
Integrated Process: Nursing Process: Evaluation;
Client Need: Safe and Effective Care Environment: Management of Care;
Cognitive Level: Application;
Concept: Stress

21. ANSWERS: 2, 4, 5

Rationale:

1. A score of 2 or higher on the BVC is an indication to begin deescalation techniques. Only if deescalation techniques fail should the nurse consider placing the client in ordered unlocked seclusion.

2. A score of 2 or higher on the BVC is an indication to begin deescalation techniques such as verbal redirection and limit setting.

3. A score of 2 or higher on the BVC is an indication to begin deescalation techniques such as maintaining open hands and a nonthreatening posture, not an authoritative stance.

4. A score of 2 or higher on the BVC is an indication to begin deescalation techniques such as reducing stimulation and loud noise.

5. A score of 2 or higher on the BVC is an indication to begin deescalation techniques such as offering prn medications. If deescalation techniques fail, the nurse should suggest prn medications.

TEST-TAKING TIP: See Box 8.1 to review the Brøset Violence Checklist.
Content Area: Safe and Effective Care Environment: Management of Care;
Integrated Process: Nursing Process: Implementation;
Client Need: Safe and Effective Care Environment: Management of Care;
Cognitive Level: Application;
Concept: Violence

CASE STUDY: Putting it All Together

Bobby is 43 years old, married, and the father of two teenagers. He responded to a three-alarm fire in which two of his fellow firefighters perished. Bobby has been admitted to a psychiatric inpatient facility after developing numerous psychological symptoms. He suffers from frequent nightmares from which he awakens in a cold sweat with heart palpitations. Bobby's affect is flat. He exhibits hypervigilant behavior as evidenced by eyes that dart constantly around the milieu. He spends much of his time pacing and wringing his hands. He also complains of feeling emotionally detached from family since the distressing fire event. After 1 week of therapy with a psychiatric nurse practitioner (PNP) Willie, Bobby is finally able to verbally express thoughts and feelings. He confides in Willie, saying, "I'm always terrified that if I let my guard down, my family will burn up in a fire that I could have prevented. I'm only comfortable when we're all home, the family has demonstrated fire drill safety, and the smoke alarms have been checked and rechecked. My wife has become angry with my demands, and my children are becoming belligerent." Bobby states that all he wants is to feel normal again, become congenial with his family, and return to work. Willie has explored the predisposing factors that have led up to Bobby's fears, the various techniques that may help Bobby with his recovery, and psychopharmacological interventions that might assist in relieving his symptoms.

1. On the basis of Bobby's symptoms and actions, what medical diagnosis would Willie assign to Bobby?
2. What are Bobby's subjective symptoms that would lead to the determination of this diagnosis?
3. What are Bobby's objective symptoms that would lead to the determination of this diagnosis?
4. List the psychological treatments the PNP might employ to treat the symptoms of Bobby's disorder.
5. What medications might Willie prescribe to relieve Bobby's symptoms?
6. What NANDA nursing diagnosis would be appropriate for Bobby?
7. On the basis of this nursing diagnosis, what short-term outcome would be appropriate for Bobby?
8. On the basis of this nursing diagnosis, what long-term outcome would be appropriate for Bobby?
9. List the nursing interventions (actions) that will assist Bobby in successfully achieving these outcomes.
10. List the questions that should be answered in determining the success of the nursing actions.

Chapter 9

Substance Use and Addictive Disorders

KEY TERMS

Alcoholics Anonymous—An international fellowship of men and women who have or have had a drinking problem; it is nonprofessional, self-supporting, multiracial, apolitical, and available almost everywhere; there are no age or education requirements, and membership is open to anyone who wants to do something about his or her drinking problem

Ascites—The buildup of fluid in the space between the lining of the abdomen and abdominal organs; it results from high pressure in the blood vessels of the liver (portal hypertension) and low levels of serum albumin; liver damage due to alcoholism can result in ascites

Addiction—A compulsive or chronic requirement; the need is so strong that, if left unfulfilled, it will generate distress (either physical or psychological)

Blackout—An alcoholic blackout is amnesia for the events of any part of a drinking episode without loss of consciousness; it is characterized by memory impairment during intoxication in the relative absence of other skill deficits

Codependency—Dependence on the needs of, or control by, another; often involves placing a lower priority on one's own needs while being excessively preoccupied with the needs of others; codependency can occur in any type of relationship, including family, work, friendship, and also romantic, peer, or community relationships

Detoxification—The gradual withdrawal of an abused substance in a controlled environment

Dual diagnosis—A term used to describe people with mental illness who have coexisting problems with drugs and/or alcohol

Gambling disorder—Behavior that includes an urge to continuously gamble despite harmful negative consequences or a desire to stop

Intoxication—A physical and mental state of exhilaration and emotional frenzy or lethargy and stupor

Substance-induced disorder—The immediate effects of substance use, called intoxication, and the immediate effects of discontinuing a substance, called substance withdrawal; also included as substance-induced disorders are delirium, neurocognitive disorder (NCD), psychosis, bipolar disorder, depressive disorder, obsessive-compulsive disorder (OCD), anxiety disorder, sexual dysfunction, and sleep disorders

Substance use disorder—A disorder characterized by a pattern of continued pathological use of a medication, nonmedically indicated drug, or toxin that results in repeated adverse social consequences related to drug use, such as failure to meet work, family, or school obligations, interpersonal conflicts, or legal problems

Substitution therapy—During alcohol detoxification, the substitution of cross-tolerant drugs that have effects similar to the effects of alcohol to prevent alcohol withdrawal

Tolerance—A reduced sensitivity to alcohol or other substances which requires that higher quantities of alcohol or other substances be consumed in order to achieve the same effects as before tolerance was established

Withdrawal—The physiological and mental readjustment that accompanies the discontinuation of an addictive substance

Substance addiction is a significant health problem worldwide. Because of this prevalence, nurses will frequently be faced with caring for clients suffering from these disorders. Therefore, the nurse must be knowledgeable regarding the various substances abused and the symptoms clients experience during intoxication and/or withdrawal. Substance addiction is often hidden and denied by the client, so the nurse must be vigilant in assessing for the signs and symptoms that may indicate life-threatening complications. Substance-related disorders are composed of two groups: the substance-use disorders (addiction) and the substance-induced disorders (intoxication, withdrawal, delirium, neurocognitive disorder (NCD), psychosis, bipolar disorder, depressive disorder, obsessive-compulsive disorder (OCD), anxiety disorder, sexual dysfunction, and sleep disorders).

I. Definitions

A. Substance use disorder
1. Substance use interferes with ability to fulfill role obligations at work, school, or home.
2. Attempts to cut down or control substance use fails, and use continues to increase.
3. Intense craving for substance.
4. Excessive time spent in procurement and recovery from substance use.
5. Use causes dysfunctional interpersonal relationships and social isolation.
6. Impairment results in risky behaviors.
7. Despite awareness of physical or psychological problems, use continues.
8. **Addiction** is evident when:
   a. Tolerance develops (amount required to achieve the desired effect continues to increase).
   b. Withdrawal occurs (attempts to discontinue use of substance causes symptoms, specific to the substance).
B. Substance-induced disorders
1. Substance **intoxication.**
   a. Development of a reversible syndrome of symptoms after excessive use of a substance.
      i. Symptoms are drug-specific, occurring during or shortly after ingestion
      ii. Direct effect on the central nervous system (CNS)
      iii. Disruption in physical and psychological functioning
      iv. Disturbed judgment results in maladaptive behavior
      v. Impaired social and occupational functioning
2. Substance **withdrawal.**
   a. Occurs with abrupt reduction or discontinuation of substance used regularly over prolonged period of time.

   b. Syndrome includes clinically significant physical signs and symptoms.
   c. Psychological changes such as disturbances in thinking, feeling, and behavior.

II. Predisposing Factors

There is no single theory that can adequately explain the etiology.

A. Biological factors
1. Genetics.
   a. Hereditary factors implicated.
   b. Heredity apparent with alcoholism, but less so with other substances.
   c. Children of alcoholics are four times more likely than other children to become alcoholics.
   d. Monozygotic twins have higher rate for concordance of alcoholism than dizygotic twins.
   e. Biological offspring of alcoholic parents have a significantly greater incidence of alcoholism than offspring of nonalcoholic parents, whether the child was reared by the biological parents or by nonalcoholic adoptive parents.
2. Biochemical factors.
   a. Alcohol may produce morphine-like substances in the brain.
   b. Substances are formed by the reaction of biologically active amines (e.g., dopamine, serotonin) with products of alcohol metabolism.
B. Psychological factors
1. Developmental influences.
   a. A punitive superego and fixation at the oral stage of psychosexual development contributes to substance-related disorders.
   b. Individuals with punitive superegos turn to substances to diminish unconscious anxiety and increase feelings of power and self-worth.
2. Personality factors.
   a. Personality traits associated with addictive behavior.
      i. Low self-esteem
      ii. Frequent depression
      iii. Passivity
      iv. Inability to relax
      v. Inability to defer gratification
      vi. Inability to communicate effectively
   b. Associated with antisocial personality disorder and depressive response styles.
      i. Antisocial personality type cannot anticipate aversive behavioral consequences
      ii. Depressive personality type treats dysphoric symptoms with substance use. Relief provides positive reinforcement that leads to abuse

C. Sociocultural factors
1. Social learning.
   a. Modeling, imitation, and identification during childhood influences behavior.
   b. Parents provide a model for substance use.
   c. Peers are influential, especially for first-time users.
   d. Modeling may continue once the individual enters the workforce.
2. Conditioning.
   a. Pleasurable experiences encourage repeated use.
   b. Reinforcing properties of addictive drugs "condition" the individual to seek out repeated use.
3. Cultural and ethnic influences.
   a. Culture helps to establish patterns of substance use by:
      i. Molding attitudes
      ii. Cultural acceptance
      iii. Availability of the substance
   b. High incidence of alcohol addiction in the Native American culture.
      i. Twice the alcohol-attributable deaths than that of the U.S. general population
      ii. Possible reasons:
         1) Physical cause (difficulty metabolizing alcohol)
         2) Parental modeling
         3) Unemployment and poverty
         4) Loss of traditional religion
   c. Alcohol addiction is higher among northern than southern Europeans.
   d. Alcohol addiction among Asians is low (possible genetic intolerance).

III. Alcohol Use Disorder

A. Profile of the substance
1. Alcohol is a natural substance formed by the reaction of fermenting sugar with yeast spores.
2. Its abbreviation is ETOH (ethyl alcohol).
3. ETOH, a CNS depressant, results in behavioral and mood changes.
4. Effects of ETOH on the CNS are proportional to blood alcohol concentration.

MAKING THE CONNECTION

The average-sized drink, regardless of beverage, contains a similar amount of ETOH. Twelve ounces of beer, 3 to 5 ounces of wine, or a cocktail with 1 ounce of whiskey all contain approximately 0.5 ounces of ETOH. If consumed at the same rate, they all would have an equal effect on the body.

5. A blood ETOH level of 0.08% is considered legal intoxication in most states.
6. The body burns ETOH at the rate of about 0.5 ounces per hour.
7. Slowly consuming one average-sized drink per hour should not cause behavioral changes.
8. Other factors that influence the effects of ETOH:
   a. Individual's size.
   b. Full or empty stomach.
   c. Emotional stress or fatigue.

B. Patterns of use
1. Enhances the flavor of food.
2. Encourages relaxation and conviviality at social gatherings.
3. Promotes a feeling of celebration at special occasions.
4. Wine used as part of sacred ritual in some religious ceremonies.
5. Major ingredient in some over-the-counter and prescription drugs.

DID YOU KNOW?

Alcohol can be harmless and enjoyable—sometimes even beneficial—if it is used responsibly and in moderation. Like any other mind-altering drug, however, alcohol has the potential for abuse. Indeed, it is the most widely abused drug in the United States today.

6. Alcoholism is the nation's number one health problem.
7. Alcoholism is the third leading cause of preventable death in the United States.
8. ETOH is a factor in more than half of all homicides, suicides, and traffic accidents.
9. Incidents of domestic violence are commonly alcohol related.
10. Heavy drinking contributes to heart disease, cancer, and stroke.

C. Patterns of ETOH use progression
1. Phase I: the prealcoholic phase.
   a. Used to relieve everyday stress and tensions.
   b. **Tolerance** develops (amount required to achieve the desired effect increases steadily).
2. Phase II: the early alcoholic phase.
   a. Begins with **blackouts**—brief periods of amnesia that occur during or immediately after a period of drinking.
   b. Alcohol no longer pleasurable but required.
   c. Common behaviors include:
      i. Sneaking drinks or secret drinking
      ii. Preoccupation with drinking and maintaining ETOH supply
      iii. Rapid gulping of drinks and further blackouts
      iv. Feelings of guilt and becoming defensive about drinking
      v. Excessive use of denial and rationalization

3. Phase III: the crucial phase.
   a. Loss of control and marked physiological addiction.
   b. Inability to choose whether or not to drink.
   c. Binge drinking, lasting from a few hours to several weeks.
   d. Episodes are characterized by sickness, loss of consciousness, squalor, and degradation.
   e. Individual is extremely ill.
   f. Anger and aggression are common manifestations.
   g. Drinking is the total focus; willing to risk losing everything in an effort to maintain the addiction.
   h. Experiences may include the loss of job, marriage, family, friends, and self-respect.
4. Phase IV: the chronic phase.
   a. Characterized by emotional and physical disintegration.
   b. Usually more intoxicated than sober.
   c. Profound helplessness and self-pity.
   d. Impairment in reality testing may result in psychosis.
   e. Life-threatening physical manifestations in every body system.
   f. ETOH withdrawal results in hallucinations, tremors, convulsions, severe agitation, and panic.

🛑 During the chronic phase of drinking progression, depression and ideas of suicide are not uncommon.

D. Effects on the body
1. A general, nonselective, reversible depression of the CNS.
2. About 20% of ETOH is absorbed immediately into bloodstream through stomach wall.
3. Alcohol does not have to be digested.
4. Alcohol immediately slows down or depresses brain activity.
5. After consumption, ETOH is found in all body tissues, organs, and secretions.
6. Rapidity of absorption is influenced by various factors.
   a. Delayed when sipped, rather than gulped.
   b. Delayed when stomach contains food, rather than empty.
   c. Delayed when drink is wine or beer, rather than distilled, "hard" liquor.

E. Physiological impairments due to chronic abuse
1. Peripheral neuropathy.
   a. Nerve damage (pain, burning, tingling of extremities).
   b. Direct result of deficiencies in the B vitamins, particularly thiamine.

DID YOU KNOW?
Nutritional deficiencies are common in chronic alcoholics because of insufficient intake of nutrients as well as the toxic effect of alcohol that results in malabsorption of nutrients.

   c. Reversible with abstinence and restoration of nutritional deficiencies.
   d. Without interventions, permanent muscle wasting and paralysis can occur.
2. Alcoholic myopathy.
   a. Result of B vitamin deficiency.
   b. May be an acute or chronic condition.
   c. Acute: individual experiences:
      i. Sudden onset of muscle pain, swelling, and weakness
      ii. Reddish tinge in the urine caused by myoglobin, a muscle breakdown by-product
      iii. A rapid rise in muscle enzymes
         1) Creatine phosphokinase (CPK)
         2) Lactate dehydrogenase (LDH)
         3) Aldolase, and aspartate aminotransferase (AST)
   d. Chronic: individual experiences:
      i. Gradual wasting and weakness in skeletal muscles
      ii. Pain and tenderness are absent
      iii. Elevated muscle enzymes are absent
   e. Improvement observed with ETOH abstinence, nutritious diet with vitamin supplements.
3. Wernicke's encephalopathy.
   a. Most serious form of thiamine deficiency.
   b. Symptoms include:
      i. Paralysis of the ocular muscles
      ii. Diplopia
      iii. Ataxia
      iv. Somnolence
      v. Stupor
   c. If thiamine replacement therapy is not undertaken quickly, death will ensue.
4. Korsakoff's psychosis.
   a. Syndrome of confusion, recent memory loss, and confabulation.
   b. Encountered when recovering from Wernicke's encephalopathy.
   c. When the two disorders are considered together they are called "Wernicke-Korsakoff syndrome."
   d. Treatment is with parenteral or oral thiamine replacement.
5. Alcoholic cardiomyopathy.
   a. Lipids accumulate in myocardial cells, resulting in enlarged and weakened heart leading to congestive heart failure or arrhythmias.

b. Symptoms include:
  i. Decreased exercise tolerance
  ii. Tachycardia
  iii. Dyspnea
  iv. Edema
  v. Palpitations
  vi. Nonproductive cough
  vii. Elevation of the enzymes CPK, AST, alanine aminotransferase (ALT), and LDH
  viii. Electrocardiogram changes
c. Treatment is total, permanent abstinence from alcohol.
d. Congestive heart failure is treated with rest, oxygen, digitalization, sodium restriction, and diuretics.

6. Esophagitis.
  a. Esophageal inflammation and pain.
  b. Toxic effects of alcohol on the esophageal mucosa.
  c. Related to frequent vomiting associated with alcohol abuse.

7. Gastritis.
  a. Inflammation of the stomach lining.
  b. Epigastric distress, nausea, vomiting, and distention.
  c. Alcohol breaks down the stomach's protective mucosal barrier, allowing hydrochloric acid to erode the stomach wall.
  d. Damage to blood vessels may result in hemorrhage.

8. Pancreatitis.
  a. Categorized as either "acute" or "chronic."
  b. Acute pancreatitis usually occurs 1 or 2 days after an alcohol binge.
  c. Symptoms include:
    i. Constant, severe epigastric pain
    ii. Nausea and vomiting
    iii. Abdominal distention
  d. Chronic pancreatitis leads to pancreatic insufficiency, resulting in malnutrition, weight loss, and diabetes mellitus.

9. Alcoholic hepatitis.
  a. Inflammation of liver.
  b. Clinical manifestations include:
    i. Enlarged and tender liver
    ii. Nausea and vomiting
    iii. Lethargy
    iv. Anorexia
    v. Elevated white blood cell count
    vi. Fever
    vii. Jaundice
    viii. Ascites and weight loss evident in more severe cases
    ix. Severe cases can lead to cirrhosis or hepatic encephalopathy

c. Can experience complete recovery with treatment (strict abstinence from alcohol, proper nutrition, and rest).

10. Cirrhosis of the liver.
  a. End-stage of alcoholic liver disease caused by any chronic injury to the liver including long-term alcohol abuse.
  b. Widespread destruction of liver cells, which are replaced by fibrous (scar) tissue.
  c. Clinical manifestations include:
    i. Nausea and vomiting
    ii. Anorexia
    iii. Weight loss
    iv. Abdominal pain
    v. Jaundice
    vi. Edema
    vii. Anemia
    viii. Blood coagulation abnormalities
  d. Treatment includes:
    i. Abstention from alcohol
    ii. Correction of malnutrition
    iii. Supportive care to prevent complications
  e. Complications include:
    i. Portal hypertension: defective blood flow through the cirrhotic liver, resulting in elevated blood pressure
    ii. **Ascites:** excessive amount of serous fluid accumulates in the abdominal cavity, occurs in response to portal hypertension. The increased pressure results in the seepage of fluid from the surface of the liver into the abdominal cavity
    iii. Esophageal varices: veins in the esophagus that become distended because of excessive pressure from defective blood flow through the cirrhotic liver. As this pressure increases, these varicosities can rupture, resulting in hemorrhage and sometimes death
    iv. Hepatic encephalopathy
      1) Occurs in response to the inability of the diseased liver to convert ammonia to urea for excretion. The continued rise in serum ammonia results in:
        • Progressively impaired mental functioning
        • Apathy
        • Euphoria or depression
        • Sleep disturbance
        • Increasing confusion
        • Progression to coma and eventual death.
      2) Treatment requires complete abstention from alcohol, temporary elimination of protein from the diet, and reduction of

intestinal ammonia using neomycin or lactulose
11. Leukopenia.
    a. The production, function, and movement of the white blood cells are impaired.
    b. Places the individual at high risk for infectious diseases.
12. Thrombocytopenia.
    a. Platelet production and survival is impaired.
    b. At risk for hemorrhage.
    c. Abstinence from alcohol rapidly reverses this deficiency.
13. Sexual dysfunction.
    a. Alcohol interferes with the normal production and maintenance of female and male hormones.
    b. For women, this can mean changes in the menstrual cycles and a decrease or loss of ability to become pregnant.
    c. For men, the decreased hormone levels result in a diminished libido, decreased sexual performance, and impaired fertility.
14. Fetal alcohol syndrome.

DID YOU KNOW?
Fetal alcohol syndrome is the most common preventable cause of mental retardation in the United States.

    a. The most common fetal alcohol spectrum disorder (FASD) caused by prenatal exposure to alcohol.
    b. Any alcohol consumption during any stage of pregnancy can damage a fetus.
    c. FAS symptoms include:
        i) Physical, mental, behavioral, and/or learning disabilities
        ii) Problems with memory, attention span, communication, vision, hearing, or a combination of these

IV. Alcohol Intoxication

A. Symptoms are listed in Table 9.1
B. Usually occurs at blood alcohol levels between 100 and 200 mg/dL
C. Death has been reported at levels ranging from 400 to 700 mg/dL

V. Alcohol Withdrawal

Rebound stimulation of the CNS after long-term depression due to effects of alcohol.
A. Within 4 to 12 hours of cessation of or reduction in heavy and prolonged (several days or longer) alcohol use
B. Symptoms are listed in Table 9.1

C. A complicated withdrawal syndrome may progress to "alcohol withdrawal delirium"
1. Onset of delirium is usually on the second or third day after cessation of, or reduction in prolonged, heavy alcohol use.
2. Characterized by a disturbance in attention and awareness and a change in cognition that develops rapidly.
3. Symptoms include:
    a. Seizure activity.
    b. Difficulty sustaining and shifting attention.
    c. Extreme distractibility.
    d. Disorganized thinking.
    e. Rambling, irrelevant, pressured, and incoherent speech.
    f. Impaired reasoning.
    g. Impaired goal-directed behavior.
    h. Disorientation to time and place.
    i. Impairment of recent memory.
    j. Misperceptions of environment that include hallucinations and illusions.
    k. Disturbances in sleep-wake cycle.

🛈 Once a client has experienced a complicated withdrawal (alcohol withdrawal delirium), the incidence of a reoccurrence is high. Previous seizures "kindle" the CNS, putting the client at high risk for future seizure activity. It is important for the nurse to assess the client's history of previous withdrawal experiences.

VI. Sedative, Hypnotic, or Anxiolytic Use Disorder

A. Profile of the substance
1. The sedative/hypnotic compounds are drugs of diverse chemical structures that are all capable of inducing varying degrees of CNS depression.
    a. Tranquilizing relief of anxiety.
    b. Anesthesia.
    c. Coma.
    d. Death.
2. Categories:
    a. Barbiturates.
    b. Nonbarbiturate hypnotics.
    c. Antianxiety agents.
3. Principles that apply to CNS depressants.
    a. Effects are additive with one another and with the behavioral state of the user.

🛈 In combination with each other or in combination with alcohol, the depressive effects of CNS depressants are compounded. Depression or physical fatigue may cause an exaggerated response to a dose of the drug that would only slightly affect a person in a normal or excited state. These factors can lead to unintentional overdose.

    b. CNS depressants are capable of producing physiological addiction.
      i. When taken for a prolonged duration, a period of CNS hyperexcitability occurs on withdrawal of the drug
      ii. The response can be quite severe, even leading to convulsions and death
    c. CNS depressants are capable of producing psychological addiction.
      i. May generate within the individual a psychic drive for periodic or continuous administration of the drug
      ii. Seeks to achieve a maximum level of functioning or feeling of well-being
    d. Cross-tolerance and cross-dependence may exist between various CNS depressants.
      i. Cross-tolerance is exhibited when one drug results in a lessened response to another drug
      ii. Cross-dependence is a condition in which one drug can prevent withdrawal symptoms associated with physical addiction to a different drug

B. Effects on the body
  1. The sedative/hypnotic compounds induce a general depressant effect.
  2. They depress the activity of the brain, nerves, muscles, and heart tissue.
  3. Physiological effects.
    a. Sleep and dreaming.
      i. Use decreases sleep time spent in dreaming
      ii. Rebound insomnia and increased dreaming (termed "REM rebound") are not uncommon with abrupt withdrawal from long-term use of these drugs as sleeping aids
    b. Respiratory function.
      i. Inhibits the reticular activating system, resulting in respiratory depression
      ii. Additive effects occur with concurrent use of other CNS depressants, effecting a life-threatening situation
    c. Cardiovascular function.
      i. Hypotension may be a problem with large doses
      ii. High dosages of barbiturates may result in decreased cardiac output, decreased cerebral blood flow, and direct impairment of myocardial contractility
    d. Renal function.
      i. In doses high enough to produce anesthesia, barbiturates may suppress urine function
      ii. No effect on kidneys at usual sedative/hypnotic dosage

    a. Hepatic function.
      i. The barbiturates may produce jaundice with doses large enough to produce acute intoxication
      ii. Barbiturates stimulate the production of liver enzymes, resulting in decreased plasma levels of barbiturates and other drugs metabolized in the liver
      iii. Preexisting liver disease may predispose an individual to additional liver damage
    a. Body temperature.
      i. High doses of barbiturates can greatly decrease body temperature
      ii. Normal dosages do not effect body temperature
    b. Sexual functioning.
      i. There is an initial increase in libido, presumably from the primary disinhibitory effects of the drug
      ii. A decrease in the ability to maintain an erection follows

VII. Sedative, Hypnotic, or Anxiolytic Intoxication

A. Sedative/hypnotic intoxication is the presence of clinically significant maladaptive behavioral or psychological changes that develop during, or shortly after, use of one of these substances
B. Symptoms are listed in Table 9.1
C. "Club drugs" in this category include gamma hydroxybutyric acid (GHB) and flunitrazepam (Rohypnol)

DID YOU KNOW?

The drugs gamma hydroxybutyric acid (GHB) and flunitrazepam (Rohypnol) produce a state of disinhibition, excitement, drunkenness, and amnesia. They have been implicated as "date rape" drugs. They produce anterograde amnesia, rendering the victim unable to remember events experienced while under their influence.

VIII. Sedative, Hypnotic, or Anxiolytic Withdrawal

A. Onset of the symptoms depends on the drug
  1. Short-acting sedative/hypnotics (e.g., alprazolam, lorazepam).
    a. Symptoms may begin between 12 and 24 hours after the last dose.
    b. Peak between 24 and 72 hours.
    c. Subside in 5 to 10 days.
  2. Substances with longer half-lives (e.g., diazepam, phenobarbital, chlordiazepoxide).
    a. Symptoms may begin within 2 to 7 days.

b. Peak on the fifth to eighth day.

c. Subside in 10 to 16 days.

3. High dosages for prolonged periods can produce severe withdrawal.

4. Withdrawal symptoms have been reported with moderate dosages taken over a relatively short duration.

5. Symptoms are listed in Table 9.1.

IX. Stimulant Use Disorder

A. Profile of the substance

1. CNS stimulants induce behavioral stimulation and psychomotor agitation.

2. Caffeine-related disorders and tobacco-related disorders are categorized as distinct diagnoses.

3. Groups within the stimulant category are classified according to similarities in mechanism of action.

   a. Psychomotor stimulants induce stimulation by augmentation or potentiation of the neurotransmitters norepinephrine, epinephrine, or dopamine.

   b. General cellular stimulants (caffeine and nicotine) exert their action directly on cellular activity.

4. Two most prevalent, available, and widely used stimulants are caffeine and nicotine.

   a. Caffeine is a common ingredient in coffee, tea, colas, and chocolate.

   b. Nicotine is the primary psychoactive substance found in tobacco products.

5. The more potent stimulants, because of their potential for physiological addiction, are under regulation by the Controlled Substances Act.

6. These controlled stimulants are available for therapeutic purposes by prescription only; however, they are widely distributed illegally.

   a. Methamphetamine "Crystal Meth."

   b. "Bath salts."

B. Patterns of use

1. Because of their pleasurable effects, CNS stimulants have a high abuse potential.

2. With continued use, the pleasurable effects diminish, and there is a corresponding increase in dysphoric effects.

3. The amount consumed usually increases over time as tolerance develops.

4. Chronic users tend to rely on CNS stimulants to feel more powerful, more confident, and more decisive.

5. Pattern can develop of taking "uppers" in the morning and "downers," such as alcohol or sleeping pills, at night.

6. The average American consumes two cups of coffee (about 200 mg of caffeine) per day.

7. At a level of 500 to 600 mg of daily caffeine consumption, symptoms of anxiety, insomnia, and depression are not uncommon.

8. Caffeine dependence and withdrawal can occur.

9. Next to caffeine, nicotine is the most widely used psychoactive substance in the United States.

10. Because of public health reports on the effects of smoking, the percentage of total smokers has declined.

11. More than $96 billion a year of the direct health-care costs in the United States go to treat tobacco-related illnesses.

DID YOU KNOW?

Since 1964, when the results of the first public health report on smoking were issued, the percentage of total smokers has been on the decline. However, the percentage of women and teenage smokers has declined more slowly than that of adult men. The Centers for Disease Control and Prevention (2011c) reports that an estimated 443,000 people die annually because of tobacco use or exposure to second-hand smoke.

C. Effects on the body

1. The CNS stimulants are a group of pharmacological agents that are capable of exciting the entire nervous system.

2. CNS effects:

   a. Stimulation results in tremor, restlessness, anorexia, insomnia, agitation, and increased motor activity.

   b. Amphetamines, nonamphetamine stimulants, and cocaine produce increased alertness, decrease in fatigue, elation and euphoria, and subjective feelings of greater mental agility and muscular power.

   c. Chronic use may result in compulsive behavior, paranoia, hallucinations, and aggressive behavior.

3. Cardiovascular/pulmonary effects.

   a. Amphetamines can induce increased systolic and diastolic blood pressure, increased heart rate, and cardiac arrhythmias.

   b. Stimulants relax bronchial smooth muscle.

   c. Cocaine intoxication produces a rise in myocardial demand for oxygen and an increase in heart rate.

   d. Severe vasoconstriction may occur and can result in myocardial infarction, ventricular fibrillation, and sudden death.

   e. Inhaled cocaine can cause pulmonary hemorrhage, chronic bronchiolitis, and pneumonia.

   f. Nasal rhinitis is a result of chronic cocaine snorting.

g. Caffeine ingestion can result in increased heart rate, palpitations, extrasystoles, and cardiac arrhythmias.

h. Caffeine induces dilation of pulmonary and general systemic blood vessels and constriction of cerebral blood vessels.

i. Nicotine stimulates the sympathetic nervous system, resulting in an increase in heart rate, blood pressure, and cardiac contractility, thereby increasing myocardial oxygen consumption and demand for blood flow.

j. Contractions of gastric smooth muscle associated with hunger are inhibited, thereby producing a mild anorectic effect.

4. Gastrointestinal (GI) and renal effects.

a. A decrease in GI tract motility commonly results in constipation.

b. Contraction of the bladder sphincter makes urination difficult.

c. Caffeine exerts a diuretic effect on the kidneys.

d. Nicotine stimulates the hypothalamus to release antidiuretic hormone, reducing the excretion of urine.

e. Because nicotine increases the tone and activity of the bowel, it may occasionally cause diarrhea.

f. Most CNS stimulants induce a small rise in metabolic rate and various degrees of anorexia.

g. Amphetamines and cocaine can cause a rise in body temperature.

5. Sexual functioning.

a. CNS stimulants apparently promote the coital urge in both men and women.

b. Some men may experience sexual dysfunction with the use of stimulants.

c. For the majority of individuals, these drugs exert a powerful aphrodisiac effect.

X. Stimulant Intoxication

A. Amphetamine and cocaine intoxication typically produce:

1. Euphoria or affective blunting.
2. Changes in sociability.
3. Hypervigilance.
4. Interpersonal sensitivity.
5. Anxiety, tension, or anger.
6. Stereotyped behaviors.
7. Chest pain.
8. Cardiac arrhythmias.
9. Confusion.
10. Seizures.
11. Dyskinesias.
12. Dystonias.
13. Coma.

14. Weight loss.
15. Psychomotor agitation or retardation.
16. Muscular weakness.
17. Respiratory depression.
18. Other symptoms are listed in Table 9.1.

B. Symptoms of caffeine intoxication are listed in Table 9.1

XI. Stimulant Withdrawal

A. Cessation or reduction of amphetamine (or cocaine) use may lead to a withdrawal syndrome often referred to as a "crash"

B. Symptoms include:
1. Fatigue and depression.
2. Nightmares.
3. Headache.
4. Profuse sweating.
5. Muscle cramps.
6. Hunger.
7. Symptoms peak in 2 to 4 days.
8. Intense dysphoria can occur, peaking between 48 and 72 hours after the last dose of the stimulant.
9. Other symptoms are listed in Table 9.1.

C. A withdrawal syndrome can occur with abrupt cessation of caffeine intake after a prolonged daily use of the substance

D. Symptoms begin within 24 hours after last consumption

E. Caffeine withdrawal symptoms include:
1. Headache.
2. Fatigue.
3. Drowsiness.
4. Dysphoric mood.
5. Irritability.
6. Difficulty concentrating.

F. Nicotine withdrawal symptoms are listed in Table 9.1

XII. Inhalant Use Disorder

A. Profile of the substance
1. Induced by inhaling the aliphatic and aromatic hydrocarbons found in substances such as fuels, solvents, adhesives, aerosol propellants, and paint thinners.
2. Examples: gasoline, varnish remover, lighter fluid, airplane glue, rubber cement, cleaning fluid, spray paint, shoe conditioner, and typewriter correction fluid.

B. Patterns of use
1. Inhalant substances are readily available, legal, and inexpensive.
2. Making inhalants a drug of choice for poor people, children, and young adults.

DID YOU KNOW?

Methods of use of inhalants include "huffing," a procedure in which a rag soaked with the substance is applied to the mouth and nose and the vapors breathed in. Another common method is called "bagging," in which the substance is placed in a paper or plastic bag and inhaled from the bag by the user. The substance may also be inhaled directly from the container or sprayed in the mouth or nose.

    3. Tolerance to inhalants has been reported with heavy use.

    4. A mild withdrawal syndrome does not appear to be clinically significant.

C. Effects on the body

    1. Inhalants are absorbed through the lungs and reach the CNS rapidly.

    2. Inhalants generally act as CNS depressants.

    3. The effects are brief, lasting from several minutes to a few hours, depending on the specific substance and amount consumed.

    4. CNS effects.

       a. Neurological damage, such as ataxia, peripheral and sensorimotor neuropathy, speech problems, and tremor, can occur.

       b. With heavy inhalant use, symptoms include:

         i. Ototoxicity

         ii. Encephalopathy

         iii. Parkinsonism

         iv. Damage to the protective sheath around certain nerve fibers in the brain and peripheral nervous system

    5. Respiratory effects.

       a. Coughing, wheezing, dyspnea, emphysema, and/or pneumonia.

       b. Increased airway resistance due to inflammation of the passages.

       c. Death can occur due to suffocation.

    6. GI effects.

       a. Symptoms include:

         i. Abdominal pain

         ii. Nausea and vomiting

         iii. A rash around the individual's nose and mouth

         iv. Unusual breath odors

         v. Liver toxicity with long-term use

    7. Renal system effects.

       a. Acute and chronic renal failure and hepatorenal syndrome.

       b. Renal toxicity from toluene exposure.

         i. Renal tubular acidosis

         ii. Hypokalemia

         iii. Hypophosphatemia

         iv. Hyperchloremia

         v. Azotemia

         vi. Sterile pyuria

         vii. Hematuria

         viii. Proteinuria

XIII. Inhalant Intoxication

A. Clinically significant behavioral or psychological changes that develop during or shortly after exposure to inhalants

B. Symptoms are similar to alcohol intoxication and are listed in Table 9.1

XIV. Opioid Use Disorder

A. Profile of the substance

    1. A group of compounds that includes opium, opium derivatives, and synthetic substitutes.

    2. Opioids exert both a sedative and an analgesic effect.

    3. Medical uses: relief of pain, the treatment of diarrhea, and cough relief.

    4. Have addictive qualities:

       a. Can induce tolerance.

       b. Can induce physiological and psychological addiction.

    5. Desensitizes an individual to both psychological and physiological pain.

    6. Induces a sense of euphoria.

    7. Induces lethargy and indifference to the environment.

    8. Methods of administration include oral, snorting, smoking, and by subcutaneous, intramuscular, and intravenous injection.

B. Patterns of use

    1. Development of opioid addiction may follow one of two behavior patterns.

       a. Individual has obtained the drug by prescription for the relief of a medical problem. Abuse and addiction occur when the individual increases the amount and frequency of use to treat symptoms.

       b. Individuals who use the drugs for recreational purposes and obtain them from illegal sources.

         i. Opioids may be used alone to induce euphoric effects

         ii. In combination with stimulants or other drugs to enhance the euphoria or to counteract the depressant effects of the opioid

         iii. Tolerance develops, and addiction occurs

         iv. Individual procures substance by any means to support habit

C. Effects on the body

    1. Classified as "narcotic analgesics."

    2. Exert their major effects primarily on the CNS, the eyes, and the GI tract.

3. Chronic morphine use or acute morphine toxicity is manifested by:
   a. Sedation.
   b. Chronic constipation.
   c. Decreased respiratory rate.
   d. Pinpoint pupils.
   e. Intensity of symptoms is dose dependent.
4. CNS effects.
   a. Symptoms include:
      i. Euphoria
      ii. Mood changes
      iii. Mental clouding
      iv. Drowsiness
      v. Pain reduction
      vi. Pupillary constriction (stimulation of the oculomotor nerve)
      vii. Respiratory depression (depression of the respiratory centers)
      viii. Antitussive response (suppression of the cough center)
      ix. Nausea and vomiting (stimulation of the centers within the medulla)
5. GI effects.
   a. Both stomach and intestinal tone are increased.
   b. Peristaltic activity of the intestines is diminished.
   c. Decrease in the movement of food through the GI tract (therapeutic effect in the treatment of severe diarrhea).
   d. Constipation, and even fecal impaction, may be a serious problem for the chronic opioid user.
6. Cardiovascular effects.
   a. Minimal effect on the action of the heart.
   b. Morphine is used extensively to relieve pulmonary edema and the pain of myocardial infarction.
   c. At high doses, opioids induce hypotension, which may be caused by direct action on the heart or by opioid-induced histamine release.
7. Sexual functioning.
   a. Decreased sexual function and diminished libido.
   b. Retarded ejaculation, impotence, and orgasm failure (in both men and women).
   c. Sexual side effects from opioids influenced by dosage.

XV. Opioid Intoxication

A. Clinically significant maladaptive behavioral or psychological changes that develop during, or shortly after, opioid use
B. Symptoms are listed in Table 9.1

🛑 Severe opioid intoxication can lead to respiratory depression, coma, and death.

XVI. Opioid Withdrawal

A. Symptoms that develop after cessation of, or reduction in, heavy and prolonged use of an opiate or related substance
B. Symptoms are listed in Table 9.1
C. With short-acting drugs such as heroin:
   1. Withdrawal symptoms occur within 6 to 8 hours after the last dose.
   2. Peak within 1 to 3 days.
   3. Gradually subside over a period of 5 to 10 days.
D. With longer-acting drugs such as methadone:
   1. Withdrawal symptoms begin within 1 to 3 days after the last dose.
   2. Peaks between days 4 and 6.
   3. Complete in 14 to 21 days.
E. With ultra-short-acting meperidine:
   1. Withdrawal symptoms begin quickly.
   2. Peaks in 8 to 12 hours.
   3. Complete in 4 to 5 days.

XVII. Hallucinogen Use Disorder

A. Profile of the substance
   1. Distorts perception of reality.
   2. Alters sensory perception and induces hallucinations.
   3. Manifestations have been likened to a psychotic break.
   4. Clients diagnosed with schizophrenia experience auditory hallucinations.
   5. Substance-induced hallucinations are usually visual.
   6. "Flashback" is a spontaneous reoccurrence of hallucinogenic state without drug ingestion.
   7. Can occur months after the drug was last taken.
   8. Recurrent use produces tolerance, leading users to higher dosages.
   9. No physical addiction is detectable when drug is withdrawn.
   10. Recurrent use can induce a psychological addiction.
   11. The effects of hallucinogens are highly unpredictable with each use.
B. Patterns of use
   1. Use is usually episodic.
   2. Cognitive and perceptual abilities are markedly affected.
   3. User must set aside time from normal activities for indulging in consequences.
   4. Lysergic acid diethylamide (LSD) does not lead to physical addiction or withdrawal symptoms.

DID YOU KNOW?

Tolerance to LSD does develop quickly and to a high degree. An individual who uses LSD repeatedly for a period of 3 to 4 days may develop complete tolerance to the drug. Recovery from the tolerance also occurs rapidly (in 4–7 days), so that the individual is able to achieve the desired effect from the drug repeatedly and often.

5. Phencyclidine hydrochloride (PCP) is usually taken episodically in binges that can last for several days.
6. Physical addiction does not occur with PCP.
7. Psychological addiction characterized by craving for the drug has been reported in chronic users.
8. Tolerance to PCP develops quickly with frequent use.
9. Psilocybin is an ingredient of the *Psilocybe* mushroom.
10. Ingestion produces a similar effect to LSD but with a shorter duration.
11. Mescaline is the only hallucinogenic compound used legally for religious purposes by the Native American Church of the United States.
12. Mescaline does not produce physical nor psychological addiction.
13. Tolerance to mescaline can develop quickly with frequent use.
14. 3,4-methylene-dioxyamphetamine (MDMA), or ecstasy, is a synthetic drug with both stimulant and hallucinogenic qualities.
15. Ecstasy has a chemical structure similar to methamphetamine and mescaline.

DID YOU KNOW?

Because of ecstasy's growing popularity, the demand for this drug has led to the sale of tablets and capsules that are not pure MDMA. Many of these tablets contain drugs such as methamphetamine, PCP, amphetamine, ketamine, and *p*-methoxyamphetamine (PMA), a stimulant with hallucinogenic properties, making these mixed tablets more toxic than pure MDMA. This practice has increased the dangers associated with MDMA use.

C. Effects on the body
1. Effects of various hallucinogens are highly unpredictable.
2. Effects may be related to dosage, mental state, and the use environment.
3. Symptoms include:
   a. Nausea and vomiting.
   b. Chills.
   c. Pupil dilation.
   d. Increased pulse, blood pressure, and temperature.
   e. Mild dizziness.
   f. Trembling.
   g. Loss of appetite.
   h. Insomnia.
   i. Sweating.
   j. A slowing of respirations.
   k. Elevation in blood sugar.
   l. Heightened response to color, texture, and sounds.
   m. Heightened body awareness.
   n. Distortion of vision.
   o. Sense of slowing of time.
   p. All feelings magnified: love, lust, hate, joy, anger, pain, terror, despair.
   q. Fear of losing control.
   r. Paranoia, panic.
   s. Euphoria, bliss.
   t. Projection of self into dreamlike images.
   u. Serenity, peace.
   v. Depersonalization.
   w. Derealization.
   x. Increased libido.
4. Two types of toxic reactions.
   a. Panic reaction, or "bad trip." Symptoms include:
      i. Intense level of anxiety, fear, and stimulation
      ii. Hallucinations
      iii. Fears of going insane
      iv. Paranoia and acute psychosis
   b. Flashbacks: transient, spontaneous repetition of a previous hallucinogenic-induced experience that occurs in the absence of the substance.

XVIII. Hallucinogen Intoxication

A. Symptoms develop during, or shortly after hallucinogen use
B. Symptoms include:
1. Marked anxiety or depression.
2. Ideas of reference (delusional thinking that all activity within one's environment is "referred to" [about] one's self).
3. Fear of losing one's mind.
4. Paranoid ideation.
5. Impaired judgment.
6. Intensification of perceptions.
7. Depersonalization.
8. Derealization.
9. Illusions.
10. Hallucinations.
11. Synesthesias (subjective sensations of a sense other than the one being stimulated).
12. Other symptoms are listed in Table 9.1.

DID YOU KNOW?

Because hallucinogens are sympathomimetics, they can cause tachycardia, hypertension, sweating, blurred vision, pupillary dilation, and tremors.

C. Symptoms of PCP intoxication are unpredictable

D. Symptoms are dose related and are listed in Table 9.1

E. Symptoms of ketamine intoxication appear similar to those of PCP

F. General effects of ecstasy include increased heart rate, blood pressure, and body temperature; dehydration; confusion; insomnia; and paranoia

G. Overdose of Ecstasy can result in:

1. Panic attacks.
2. Hallucinations.
3. Severe hyperthermia.
4. Dehydration.
5. Seizures.

🛑 Overdose of ecstasy can lead to respiratory depression, coma, and death. Death can also occur from kidney or cardiovascular failure.

XIX. Cannabis Use Disorder

A. Profile of the substance

1. Cannabis is second to alcohol as most widely abused drug in the United States.
2. The major psychoactive ingredient of this class of substances is delta-9-tetrahydrocannabinol (THC).
3. Marijuana, the most prevalent type of cannabis preparation, is composed of the dried leaves, stems, and flowers of the plant.
4. Hashish is a more potent concentrate of the resin derived from the flowering tops of the plant.
5. Cannabis products are smoked in the form of loosely rolled cigarettes.
6. Cannabis can also be taken orally when it is prepared in food.

DID YOU KNOW?

About two to three times the amount of cannabis must be ingested orally to equal the potency of that obtained by the inhalation of its smoke.

7. At moderate dosages, cannabis drugs produce effects resembling alcohol and other CNS depressants.
8. Psychological addiction can occur.
9. Tolerance can develop.
10. Withdrawal symptoms can occur when use is discontinued.

B. Patterns of use

1. Marijuana is the most commonly used illicit drug.
2. Cannabis is incorrectly regarded as a substance of low abuse potential.
3. Tolerance does occur with chronic use.

4. As tolerance develops, physical addiction also occurs.
5. Results in a withdrawal syndrome upon cessation of drug use.

C. Effects on the body

1. Cardiovascular effects.
   a. Induces tachycardia.
   b. Induces orthostatic hypotension.
2. Respiratory effects.
   a. Marijuana produces a greater amount of "tar" than its equivalent weight in tobacco.

🛑 Because of the method through which marijuana is smoked—that is, the smoke is held in the lungs for as long as possible to achieve the desired effect—larger amounts of tar are deposited in the lungs, promoting deleterious effects to the lungs. Cannabis smoke contains more carcinogens than tobacco smoke; therefore, lung damage and cancer are real risks for heavy users.

   b. Initial reaction to marijuana is bronchodilation, facilitating respiratory function.
   c. Chronic use results in obstructive airway disorders.
   d. Frequent marijuana users often have laryngitis, bronchitis, cough, and hoarseness.
3. Reproductive effects.
   a. Heavy use may decrease sperm count, motility, and structure.
   b. Heavy use may suppress ovulation, disrupt menstrual cycles, and alter hormone levels.
4. CNS effects.
   a. Symptoms include:
      i. Euphoria
      ii. Relaxed inhibitions
      iii. Disorientation
      iv. Depersonalization
      v. Relaxation
      vi. Tremors
      vii. Muscle rigidity
      viii. Conjunctival redness
      ix. At higher doses symptoms include:
         1) Impairment in judgment of time and distance
         2) Impairment in recent memory
         3) Impairment in learning ability
      vii. Toxic effects are characterized by panic reactions
      viii. Very heavy usage can precipitate acute psychosis that is self-limited and short-lived once drug is removed
      ix. Heavy long-term cannabis use is associated with "amotivational syndrome"
         1) Preoccupation with substance use
         2) Symptoms include lethargy, apathy, social and personal deterioration, and lack of motivation

5. Sexual functioning.
   a. Enhances sexual experience in both men and women.
   b. Intensified sensory awareness and subjective slowness of time perception increase sexual satisfaction.

XX. Cannabis Intoxication

A. Evidenced by the presence of clinically significant behavioral or psychological changes that develop during, or shortly after, use
B. Symptoms are listed in Table 9.1
C. Effects are additive to those of alcohol, which is commonly used in combination with cannabis

XXI. Cannabis Withdrawal

A. Symptoms occur on cessation of heavy prolonged use
B. Symptoms occur within a week after cessation of use
C. Symptoms are listed in Table 9.1

MAKING THE CONNECTION

Table 9.1 summarizes the symptoms associated with the syndromes of intoxication and withdrawal from various substances.

Table 9.1 **Summary of Symptoms Associated With the Syndromes of Intoxication and Withdrawal**

Class of Drugs	Intoxication	Withdrawal	Comments
Alcohol	Aggressiveness, impaired judgment, impaired attention, irritability, euphoria, depression, emotional lability, slurred speech, incoordination, unsteady gait, nystagmus, flushed face	Tremors, nausea/vomiting, malaise, weakness, tachycardia, sweating, elevated blood pressure, anxiety, depressed mood, irritability, hallucinations, headache, insomnia, seizures	Alcohol withdrawal begins within 4–6 hr after last drink. May progress to delirium tremens on second or third day. Use of Librium or Serax is common for substitution therapy.
Amphetamines and related substances	Fighting, grandiosity, hypervigilance, psychomotor agitation, impaired judgment, tachycardia, pupillary dilation, elevated blood pressure, perspiration or chills, nausea and vomiting	Anxiety, depressed mood, irritability, craving for the substance, fatigue, insomnia or hypersomnia, psychomotor agitation, paranoid and suicidal ideation	Withdrawal symptoms usually peak within 2–4 days, although depression and irritability may persist for months. Antidepressants may be used.
Caffeine	Restlessness, nervousness, excitement, insomnia, flushed face, diuresis, gastrointestinal complaints, muscle twitching, rambling flow of thought and speech, cardiac arrhythmia, periods of inexhaustibility, psychomotor agitation	Headache	Caffeine is contained in coffee, tea, colas, cocoa, chocolate, some over-the-counter analgesics, "cold" preparations, and stimulants.
Cannabis	Euphoria, anxiety, suspiciousness, sensation of slowed time, impaired judgment, social withdrawal, tachycardia, conjunctival redness, increased appetite, hallucinations	Restlessness, irritability, insomnia, loss of appetite, depressed mood, tremors, fever, chills, headache, stomach pain	Intoxication occurs immediately and lasts about 3 hours. Oral ingestion is more slowly absorbed and has longer-lasting effects.
Cocaine	Euphoria, fighting, grandiosity, hypervigilance, psychomotor agitation, impaired judgment, tachycardia, elevated blood pressure, pupillary dilation, perspiration or chills, nausea/vomiting, hallucinations, delirium	Depression, anxiety, irritability, fatigue, insomnia or hypersomnia, psychomotor agitation, paranoid or suicidal ideation, apathy, social withdrawal	Large doses of the drug can result in convulsions or death from cardiac arrhythmias or respiratory paralysis.
Inhalants	Belligerence, assaultiveness, apathy, impaired judgment, dizziness, nystagmus, slurred speech, unsteady gait, lethargy, depressed reflexes, tremor, blurred vision, stupor or coma, euphoria, irritation around eyes, throat, and nose		Intoxication occurs within 5 minutes of inhalation. Symptoms last 60–90 minutes. Large doses can result in death from central nervous system depression or cardiac arrhythmia.

Table 9.1 Summary of Symptoms Associated With the Syndromes of Intoxication and Withdrawal—cont'd

Class of Drugs	Intoxication	Withdrawal	Comments
Nicotine		Craving for the drug, irritability, anger, frustration, anxiety, difficulty concentrating, restlessness, decreased heart rate, increased appetite, weight gain, tremor, headaches, insomnia	Symptoms of withdrawal begin within 24 hours of last drug use and decrease in intensity over days, weeks, or sometimes longer.
Opioids	Euphoria, lethargy, somnolence, apathy, dysphoria, impaired judgment, pupillary constriction, drowsiness, slurred speech, constipation, nausea, decreased respiratory rate and blood pressure	Craving for the drug, nausea/vomiting, muscle aches, lacrimation or rhinorrhea, pupillary dilation, piloerection or sweating, diarrhea, yawning, fever, insomnia	Withdrawal symptoms appear within 6–8 hours after last dose, reach a peak in the second or third day, and subside in 5–10 days. Times are shorter with meperidine and longer with methadone.
Phencyclidine and related substances	Belligerence, assaultiveness, impulsiveness, psychomotor agitation, impaired judgment, nystagmus, increased heart rate and blood pressure, diminished pain response, ataxia, dysarthria, muscle rigidity, seizures, hyperacusis, delirium		Delirium can occur within 24 hours after use of phencyclidine, or may occur up to a week after recovery from an overdose of the drug.
Sedatives, hypnotics, and anxiolytics	Disinhibition of sexual or aggressive impulses, mood lability, impaired judgment, slurred speech, incoordination, unsteady gait, impairment in attention or memory disorientation, confusion	Nausea/vomiting, malaise, weakness, tachycardia, sweating, anxiety, irritability, orthostatic hypotension, tremor, insomnia, seizures	Withdrawal may progress to delirium, usually within 1 week of last use. Long-acting barbiturates or benzodiazepines may be used in withdrawal substitution therapy.

XXII. Nursing Process

A. Assessment
1. Nurses must fully understand and accept their own attitudes and feelings about substance abuse or they cannot be empathetic toward clients' problems.
2. Clients in recovery need to know they are accepted for themselves, regardless of past behaviors.
3. Nurses must be able to separate the client from the behavior and to accept that individual with unconditional positive regard.

B. Assessment tools
1. Box 9.1 presents a drug history and assessment that could be used in conjunction with the general biopsychosocial assessment.
2. The Clinical Institute Withdrawal Assessment of Alcohol Scale, Revised (CIWA-Ar; Box 9.2) assesses risk and severity of withdrawal from alcohol.
3. Michigan Alcoholism Screening Test and the CAGE Questionnaire are used to determine whether an individual has a problem with substances.

4. The CAGE Questionnaire is a simple four-question screening assessment tool to quickly determine substance use problems.

C. Dual diagnosis
1. A secondary alcoholism problem in addition to a psychiatric problem.
2. Most dual-diagnosis programs take a more supportive and less confrontational approach.
3. Psychodynamic therapy examines how psychiatric disorders and substance abuse reinforce each other and presents ways to break the cycle.
4. Cognitive and behavioral therapies train clients to monitor moods and thought patterns that lead to substance abuse.
5. Clients with dual diagnosis often resist attending 12-step programs and do better in groups designed for people with psychiatric disorders.

D. Nursing diagnosis
1. The individual who abuses or is dependent on substances undoubtedly has many unmet physical and emotional needs.
2. Table 9.2 presents a list of client behaviors and the NANDA nursing diagnoses that correspond to those behaviors, which may be used in planning care for the client with a substance use disorder.

Box 9.1 Drug History and Assessment

1. *When you were growing up, did anyone in your family drink alcohol or take other kinds of drugs?*
2. *If so, how did the substance use affect the family situation?*
3. *When did you have your first drink/drugs?*
4. *How long have you been drinking/taking drugs on a regular basis?*
5. *What is your pattern of substance use?*
   a. *When do you use substances?*
   b. *What do you use?*
   c. *How much do you use?*
   d. *Where are you and with whom when you use substances?*
6. *When did you have your last drink/drug? What was it, and how much did you consume?*
7. *Does using the substance(s) cause problems for you? Describe. Include family, friends, job, school, other.*
8. *Have you ever experienced injury as a result of substance use?*
9. *Have you ever been arrested or incarcerated for drinking/using drugs?*
10. *Have you ever tried to stop drinking/using drugs? If so, what was the result? Did you experience any physical symptoms, such as tremors, headache, insomnia, sweating, or seizures?*
11. *Have you ever experienced loss of memory for times when you have been drinking/using drugs?*
12. *Describe a typical day in your life.*
13. *Are there any changes you would like to make in your life? If so, what?*
14. *What plans or ideas do you have for seeing that these changes occur?*

Box 9.2 Clinical Institute Withdrawal Assessment of Alcohol Scale, Revised (CIWA-Ar)

Patient: **Date:**   **Time:**

Pulse or heart rate, taken for one minute:

Nausea and Vomiting—Ask "Do you feel sick to your stomach? Have you vomited?" Observation.
0 no nausea and no vomiting
1 mild nausea with no vomiting
2
3
4 intermittent nausea with dry heaves
5
6
7 constant nausea, frequent dry heaves and vomiting

Tremor—Arms extended and fingers spread apart. Observation.
0 no tremor
1 not visible, but can be felt fingertip to fingertip
2
3
4 moderate, with patient's arms extended
5
6
7 severe, even with arms not extended

Paroxysmal Sweats—Observation.
0 no sweat visible
1 barely perceptible sweating, palms moist
2
3
4 beads of sweat obvious on forehead
5
6
7 drenching sweats

Blood pressure:

Tactile Disturbances—Ask "Have you any itching, pins and needles sensations, any burning, any numbness, or do you feel bugs crawling on or under your skin?" Observation.
0 none
1 very mild itching, pins and needles, burning or numbness
2 mild itching, pins and needles, burning or numbness
3 moderate itching, pins and needles, burning or numbness
4 moderately severe hallucinations
5 severe hallucinations
6 extremely severe hallucinations
7 continuous hallucinations

Auditory Disturbances—Ask "Are you more aware of sounds around you? Are they harsh? Do they frighten you? Are you hearing anything that is disturbing to you? Are you hearing things you know are not there?" Observation.
0 not present
1 very mild harshness or ability to frighten
2 mild harshness or ability to frighten
3 moderate harshness or ability to frighten
4 moderately severe hallucinations
5 severe hallucinations
6 extremely severe hallucinations
7 continuous hallucinations

Visual Disturbances—Ask "Does the light appear to be too bright? Is its color different? Does it hurt your eyes? Are you seeing anything that is disturbing to you? Are you seeing things you know are not there?" Observation.
0 not present
1 very mild sensitivity
2 mild sensitivity
3 moderate sensitivity
4 moderately severe hallucinations
5 severe hallucinations
6 extremely severe hallucinations
7 continuous hallucinations

Box 9.2 Clinical Institute Withdrawal Assessment of Alcohol Scale, Revised (CIWA-Ar)—cont'd

Anxiety—Ask "Do you feel nervous?" Observation.
0 no anxiety, at ease
1 mild anxious
2
3
4 moderately anxious, or guarded, so anxiety is inferred
5
6
7 equivalent to acute panic states as seen in severe delirium or acute schizophrenic reactions

Agitation—Observation.
0 normal activity
1 somewhat more than normal activity
2
3
4 moderately fidgety and restless
5
6
7 paces back and forth during most of the interview, or constantly thrashes about

The CIWA-Ar is not copyrighted and may be reproduced freely. This assessment for monitoring withdrawal symp- toms requires approximately 5 minutes to administer. The maximum score is 67 (see instrument). Patients scoring less than 10 do not usually need additional medication for withdrawal.

Headache, Fullness in Head—Ask "Does your head feel different? Does it feel like there is a band around your head?" Do not rate for dizziness or lightheadedness. Otherwise, rate severity.
0 not present
1 very mild
2 mild
3 moderate
4 moderately severe
5 severe
6 very severe
7 extremely severe

Orientation and Clouding of Sensorium—Ask "What day is this? Where are you? Who am I?"
0 oriented and can do serial additions
1 cannot do serial additions or is uncertain about date
2 disoriented for date by no more than 2 calendar days
3 disoriented for date by more than 2 calendar days
4 disoriented for place/or person

Total CIWA-Ar Score _____

Rater's Initials _____
Maximum Possible Score: 67

Source: Sullivan et al (1989). Assessment of alcohol withdrawal: The revised Clinical Institute Withdrawal Assessment for Alcohol scale (CIWA-Ar). British Journal of Addiction (84), 1353–1357.

Table 9.2 Assigning Nursing Diagnoses to Behaviors Commonly Associated With Substance-Related Disorders

Behaviors	Nursing Diagnosis
Makes statements such as, "I don't have a problem with (substance). I can quit any time I want to." Delays seeking assistance; does not perceive problems related to use of substances; minimizes use of substances; unable to admit impact of disease on life pattern	**Ineffective denial**
Abuse of chemical agents; destructive behavior toward others and self; inability to meet basic needs; inability to meet role expectations; risk taking	**Ineffective coping**
Loss of weight, pale conjunctiva and mucous membranes, decreased skin turgor, electrolyte imbalance, anemia, drinks alcohol instead of eating	**Imbalanced nutrition: less than body requirements/ deficient fluid volume**
Risk factors: malnutrition, altered immune condition, failing to avoid exposure to pathogens	**Risk for infection**
Criticizes self and others, self-destructive behavior (abuse of substances as a coping mechanism), dysfunctional family background	**Chronic low self-esteem**
Denies that substance is harmful; continues to use substance in light of obvious consequences	**Deficient knowledge**
For the client withdrawing from CNS depressants: Risk factors: CNS agitation (tremors, elevated blood pressure, nausea and vomiting, hallucinations, illusions, tachycardia, anxiety, seizures)	**Risk for injury**
For the client withdrawing from CNS stimulants: Risk factors: Intense feelings of lassitude and depression; "crashing," suicidal ideation	**Risk for suicide**

E. Planning: the following outcomes may be assigned when planning care for the client experiencing a substance use disorder
By discharge, the client will:
1. Exhibit no evidence of physical injury.
2. Not have harmed self or others.
3. Accept responsibility for own behaviors.
4. Acknowledge association between personal problems and use of substance(s).
5. Demonstrate more adaptive coping mechanisms that can be used in stressful situations (instead of taking substances).
6. Show no signs or symptoms of infection or malnutrition.
7. Exhibit evidence of increased self-worth by attempting new projects without fear of failure.
8. Demonstrate less defensive behavior toward others.
9. Verbalize importance of abstaining from use of substances in order to maintain optimal wellness.

F. Implementation
1. A long-term process, often beginning with detoxification and progressing to total abstinence.
2. Major treatment objectives.
   a. **Detoxification.**
      i. Provide a safe and supportive environment for the detoxification process
      ii. Administer **substitution therapy** as ordered
   b. Intermediate care.
      i. Provide explanations of physical symptoms
      ii. Promote understanding and identify the causes of substance dependency
      iii. Provide education and assistance to client and family
   c. Rehabilitation.
      i. Encourage continued participation in long-term treatment
      ii. Promote participation in outpatient support system (e.g., Alcoholics Anonymous)
      iii. Assist client to identify alternate sources of satisfaction
      iv. Provide support for health promotion and maintenance
3. Other nursing actions.
   a. Accept client unconditionally.
   b. Identify ways in which use of alcohol has contributed to maladaptive behaviors.
   c. Do not allow client to blame others for behaviors associated with alcohol abuse.
   d. Set limits on manipulative behavior.
   e. Practice alternative, more adaptive, coping strategies.
   f. Give positive feedback for delaying gratification and using adaptive coping strategies.

g. Consult dietitian.
h. Monitor intake and output and daily weights.
i. Monitor protein intake of client with impaired liver function.
j. Restrict sodium intake to minimize fluid retention.
k. Provide small frequent feedings of nonirritating foods.
l. Assess client's level of knowledge and readiness to learn.
m. Include significant others in teaching.
n. Provide information about physical effects of alcohol on body.
o. Teach about possibility of using disulfiram (Antabuse).

G. Evaluation: evaluation of the nursing actions for the client with a substance use disorder may be facilitated by gathering information using the following types of questions:
1. Has detoxification occurred without complications?
2. Is the client still in denial?
3. Does the client accept responsibility for his or her own behavior? Has he or she acknowledged a personal problem with substances?
4. Has a correlation been made between personal problems and the use of substances?
5. Does the client still make excuses or blame others for use of substances?
6. Has the client remained substance-free during hospitalization?
7. Does the client cooperate with treatment?
8. Does the client refrain from manipulative behavior and violation of limits?
9. Is the client able to verbalize alternative adaptive coping strategies to substitute for substance use? Has the use of these strategies been demonstrated? Does positive reinforcement encourage repetition of these adaptive behaviors?
10. Has nutritional status been restored? Does the client consume a diet adequate for his or her size and level of activity? Is the client able to discuss the importance of adequate nutrition?
11. Has the client remained free of infection during hospitalization?
12. Is the client able to verbalize the effects of substance abuse on the body?
13. Does the client verbalize that he or she wants to recover and lead a life free of substances?

XXIII. Chemically Impaired Nurse

A. Ten to 15% of nurses suffer from substance use
B. Alcohol is the most widely abused drug, followed closely by narcotics

C. Clues for recognizing substance impairment in nurses
   1. High absenteeism if the person's source is outside the work area.
   2. Rarely miss work if the substance source is at work.
   3. Increase in "wasting" of drugs.
   4. Higher incidences of incorrect narcotic counts.
   5. Higher record of signing out drugs than other nurses.
   6. Poor concentration.
   7. Difficulty meeting deadlines.
   8. Inappropriate responses.
   9. Poor memory or recall.
   10. Problems with relationships.
   11. Irritability.
   12. Mood swings.
   13. Tendency to isolate.
   14. Elaborate excuses for behavior.
   15. Unkempt appearance.
   16. Impaired motor coordination.
   17. Slurred speech.
   18. Flushed face.
   19. Inconsistent job performance.
   20. Frequent use of the restroom.
   21. Frequently medicates other nurses' clients.
   22. Client complaints of inadequate pain control.
   23. Discrepancies in documentation.
D. Interventions with chemically impaired nurse
   1. Keep careful, objective records.
   2. Confrontation will undoubtedly result in hostility and denial.
   3. Confrontation always in the presence of a supervisor or other nurse.
   4. Offer assistance in seeking treatment.
   5. A state board may deny, suspend, or revoke a license based on a report of chemical abuse by a nurse.
   6. State nurses' associations have developed peer assistance programs for impaired nurses.
   7. Peer assistance programs help nurses recognize their impairment, obtain treatment, and regain accountability within their profession.
   8. When safe to return to practice, the nurse may be closely monitored for several years and random drug screenings may be required.
   9. The nurse may be required to practice under specifically circumscribed conditions for a designated period of time.

XXIV. Codependency

A. Dysfunctional behaviors that are evident among members of the family of a chemically dependent person

B. Codependent persons may come from families that harbor secrets of physical or emotional abuse, other cruelties, or pathological conditions
C. They may experience unmet needs for autonomy and self-esteem
D. They may experience a profound sense of powerlessness
E. They are able to achieve a sense of control by fulfilling the needs of others
F. The codependent person's personal identity is relinquished and boundaries are blurred
G. Traits associated with codependency:
   1. Confusion about his or her own identity.
   2. Derives self-worth from that of the partner, whose feelings and behaviors determine how the codependent should feel and behave.
   3. To feel good, partner must be happy and behave in appropriate ways.
   4. Feels responsible for *making* partner happy.
   5. Home life is fraught with stress.
   6. Ego boundaries are weak.
   7. Behaviors often enmeshed with those of the pathological partner.
   8. Denial that problems exist is common.
   9. Feelings are kept in control.
   10. Anxiety may result in stress-related illnesses or compulsive behaviors such as eating, spending, working, or use of substances.

DID YOU KNOW?

Individuals who are codependent have a long history of focusing thoughts and behavior on other people. They are "people pleasers" and will do almost anything to get the approval of others. They outwardly appear very competent but actually feel quite needy, helpless, or perhaps nothing at all. They often have experienced abuse or emotional neglect as a child. They are outwardly focused toward others and know very little about how to direct their own lives from their own sense of self.

   11. Codependent nurses have a need to be in control.
   12. These nurses strive for an unrealistic level of achievement.
   13. Their self-worth comes from being needed and of maintaining control.
   14. They nurture the dependence of others and accept the responsibility for the happiness and contentment of others.
   15. They rarely express their true feelings and do what is necessary to preserve harmony and maintain control.
   16. They are at high risk for physical and emotional burn out.

DID YOU KNOW?

Many health-care workers who are reared in homes with a chemically dependent person or in an otherwise dysfunctional family are at risk for having any unresolved codependent tendencies activated. Nurses who as children assumed the "fixer" role in their dysfunctional families of origin may attempt to resume that role in their caregiving professions. They are attracted to a profession in which they are needed, but they nurture feelings of resentment for receiving so little in return.

H. Stages in the recovery process of the codependent personality
1. Stage I: the survival stage.
   a. Begin to let go of the denial that problems exist or that their personal capabilities are unlimited.
   b. May be a very emotional and painful period.
2. Stage II: the reidentification stage.
   a. Accept the label of "codependent" and take responsibility for their own dysfunctional behavior.
   b. Enter reidentification only after being convinced that it is more painful not to.
   c. Accept their limitations and are ready to face the issues of codependence.
3. Stage III: the core issues stage.
   a. Face reality that relationships can't be managed by force of will.
   b. Each partner must be independent and autonomous.
   c. Goal is to detach from control of those things that are beyond the individual's power to control.
4. Stage IV: the reintegration stage.
   a. Self-acceptance and willingness to change.
   b. Relinquish the power *over others* that was not rightfully theirs but reclaim the *personal* power that they do possess.
   c. Control is achieved through self-discipline and self-confidence.

XXV. Treatment Modalities for Substance-Related Disorders

A. Alcoholics Anonymous (AA)
1. Major self-help, peer-support organization for the treatment of alcoholism.
2. Purpose is to help members stay sober.
3. Requirement for membership is a desire on the part of the alcoholic person to stop drinking.
4. AA accepts alcoholism as an illness and promotes total abstinence as the only cure.
5. When sobriety has been achieved, members are expected to help other alcoholic persons.

6. The 12 Steps that embody the philosophy of AA provide specific guidelines on how to attain and maintain sobriety (see Box 9.3).

DID YOU KNOW?

Al-Anon is an addiction self-help group that provides support for families of alcoholics. Alateen is a group focused on adolescent children of alcoholics. Both organizations share the philosophical and organizational structure of Alcoholics Anonymous.

B. Pharmacotherapy
1. Disulfiram (Antabuse).
   a. A deterrent to drinking.
   b. Clients must be assessed before beginning disulfiram therapy.
      i. Medical screening
      ii. Written informed consent required
      iii. Must have no cognitive deficits
      iv. Contraindicated for clients who are at high risk for alcohol ingestion
      v. Contraindicated for psychotic clients and clients with severe cardiac, renal, or hepatic disease
   c. Ingestion of alcohol while disulfiram is in the body results in a syndrome of symptoms that produces discomfort.
   d. Can result in death if the blood alcohol level is high.
   e. Reaction varies according to the sensitivity of the individual and the amount of alcohol ingested.
   f. Inhibits the enzyme aldehyde dehydrogenase, thereby blocking the oxidation of alcohol at the stage when acetaldehyde is converted to acetate.
   g. Results in an accumulation of acetaldehyde in the blood, producing symptoms associated with the disulfiram-alcohol reaction.
   h. Reaction can occur within 5 to 10 minutes of ingestion of alcohol.
   i. Mild reactions can occur at blood alcohol levels as low as 5 to 10 mg/dL.
   j. Symptoms are fully developed at a blood level of approximately 50 mg/dL.
      i. Flushed skin
      ii. Throbbing in the head and neck
      iii. Respiratory difficulty
      iv. Dizziness
      v. Nausea and vomiting
      vi. Sweating
      vii. Hyperventilation
      viii. Tachycardia
      ix. Hypotension
      x. Weakness
      xi. Blurred vision
      xii. Confusion

Box 9.3 Alcoholics Anonymous

The Twelve Steps	The Twelve Traditions
1. *We admitted we were powerless over alcohol—that our lives have become unmanageable.*	1. *Our common welfare should come first; personal recovery depends on AA unity.*
2. *Came to believe that a Power greater than ourselves could restore us to sanity.*	2. *For our group purpose there is but one ultimate authority—a loving God as He may express Himself in our group conscience. Our leaders are but trusted servants; they do not govern.*
3. *Made a decision to turn our will and our lives over to the care of God as we understood Him.*	3. *The one requirement for AA membership is a desire to stop drinking.*
4. *Made a searching and fearless moral inventory of ourselves.*	4. *Each group should be autonomous except in matters affecting other groups or AA as a whole.*
5. *Admitted to God, to ourselves, and to another human being the exact nature of our wrongs.*	5. *Each group has but one primary purpose—to carry its message to the alcoholic who still suffers.*
6. *Were entirely ready to have God remove all these defects of character.*	6. *An AA group ought never endorse, finance, or lend the AA name to any related facility or outside enterprise, lest problems of money, property, and prestige divert us from our primary purpose.*
7. *Humbly asked Him to remove our shortcomings.*	7. *Every AA group ought to be fully self-supporting, declining outside contributions.*
8. *Made a list of all persons we had harmed and became willing to make amends to them all.*	8. *Alcoholics Anonymous should remain forever nonprofessional, but our service centers may employ special workers.*
9. *Made direct amends to such people wherever possible except when to do so would injure them or others.*	9. *Alcoholics Anonymous, as such, ought never be organized; but we may create service boards of committees directly responsible to those they serve.*
10. *Continued to take personal inventory and when we were wrong promptly admitted it.*	10. *Alcoholics Anonymous has no opinion on outside issues; hence, the Alcoholics Anonymous name ought never be drawn into public controversy.*
11. *Sought through prayer and meditation to improve our conscious contact with God as we understood Him, praying only for knowledge of His will for us and the power to carry that out.*	11. *Our public relations policy is based on attraction rather than promotion; we need always maintain personal anonymity at the level of press, radio, and films.*
12. *Having had a spiritual awakening as the result of these steps, we tried to carry this message to alcoholics and to practice these principles in all our affairs.*	12. *Anonymity is the spiritual foundation of all our traditions, ever reminding us to place principles before personalities.*

k. With a blood alcohol level of approximately 125 to 150 mg/dL, severe reactions can occur.
  i. Respiratory depression
  ii. Cardiovascular collapse
  iii. Arrhythmias
  iv. Myocardial infarction
  v. Acute congestive heart failure
  vi. Unconsciousness
  vii. Convulsions
  viii. Death
l. Abstinence from alcohol is necessary for at least 12 hours before disulfiram administration.
m. Sensitivity to alcohol may last for as long as 2 weeks. Consuming alcohol or alcohol-containing substances during this 2-week period could result in the disulfiram–alcohol reaction.

n. Client needs to be aware of the large number of alcohol-containing substances that, if ingested or even rubbed on the skin, are capable of producing symptoms.
  i. Liquid cough and cold preparations
  ii. Vanilla extract
  iii. Aftershave lotions
  iv. Colognes
  v. Mouthwash
  vi. Nail polish removers
  vii. Isopropyl alcohol
o. Must read labels carefully
p. Must inform any doctor, dentist, or other health care professional that he or she is taking disulfiram.
q. Must carry a card explaining participation in disulfiram therapy, possible consequences of

---

MAKING THE CONNECTION

When a client is prescribed disulfiram, nursing assessment and teaching are critical to the client's care. The nurse must first determine whether the client has intact cognitive functioning. The client must be able to recognize possible unintended exposure to alcohol and understand the negative effectives this exposure will have. Teaching about unlikely products that might contain alcohol is necessary for the client to be able to avoid these substances.

the therapy, and symptoms that may indicate an emergency situation.

2. Naltrexone (Revia).
   a. Narcotic antagonist.
   b. Approved by the U.S. Food and Drug Administration (FDA) for alcohol addiction.
   c. Affects pleasure receptors in the brain.
   d. Oral form of nalmefene (Revex).
3. Selective serotonin reuptake inhibitors (SSRIs): success was observed in moderate versus heavy drinkers.
4. Acamprosate (Campral).
   a. Indicated for the maintenance of abstinence.
   b. Mechanism of action not completely understood.
   c. Must achieve alcohol abstinence before treatment.

C. Counseling
1. Goal-directed.
2. Length of the counseling may vary from weeks to years.
3. Focus:
   a. Current reality.
   b. Development of a working treatment relationship.
   c. Strengthening ego assets.
4. Effective counselor traits.
   a. Warm, kind, and nonjudgmental.
   b. Able to set limits firmly.
   c. Demonstrates insight, respect, genuineness, concreteness, and empathy.
5. Phases of counseling.
   a. Assessment phase.
      i. Collect data
      ii. Determine whether problem exists
      iii. Determine functioning impairment
   b. Working phase.
      i. Work on acceptance of the fact that the use of substances causes significant problems
      ii. Work on awareness of inability to prevent substance use from occurring
      iii. Client states a desire to make changes

      iv. Strength of the denial system determined
      v. Individual works to gain self-control and abstinence
      vi. Once the problem has been identified and sobriety is achieved, the client must have a concrete and workable plan for getting through the early weeks of abstinence
      vii. Anticipatory guidance through role-play helps the individual practice how he or she will respond when substances are readily obtainable and the impulse to partake is strong
6. Counseling often includes the family or specific family members.
7. Referrals are often made to self-help groups:
   a. AA
   b. Al-Anon
   c. Nar-Anon
   d. Alateen
   e. Families Anonymous
   f. Adult Children of Alcoholics

D. Group therapy
1. Share experiences with others with similar problems.
2. Able to "see themselves in others."
3. Confront their defenses about giving up the substance.
4. Gives opportunity for directly communicating needs and feelings.
5. Task-oriented education groups:
   a. Presents material associated with substance abuse and its effects on the person's life.
   b. Topics taught:
      i. Assertiveness techniques
      ii. Relaxation training
      iii. Adaptive ways of coping
      iv. How to deal with problems that may have arisen or were exacerbated by the former substance use
      v. Ways to improve quality of life
      vi. Ways to function effectively without substances

E. Psychopharmacology for substance intoxication and substance withdrawal
1. Substitution therapy may be required to reduce the life-threatening effects of intoxication or withdrawal from some substances.
2. The severity of the withdrawal syndrome depends on:
   a. Particular drug used.
   b. How long it has been used.
   c. Dose used.
   d. Rate at which the drug is eliminated from the body.

3. Alcohol.
   a. Benzodiazepines are the most widely used group of drugs for substitution therapy.
   b. Chlordiazepoxide (Librium), oxazepam (Serax), lorazepam (Ativan), and diazepam (Valium) are the most commonly used agents.
   c. In clients with liver disease, longer-acting agents (chlordiazepoxide, diazepam) should be avoided, and the shorter-acting benzodiazepines (lorazepam, oxazepam) should be used.
   d. Anticonvulsant medication (e.g., carbamazepine, valproic acid, or gabapentin) may be used for management of withdrawal seizures.
   e. Repeated episodes of withdrawal appear to "kindle" even more serious withdrawal episodes, including the production of withdrawal seizures that can result in brain damage.
   f. Multivitamin therapy, in combination with daily injections or oral administration of thiamine, is common protocol.
   g. Deficient thiamine is common in chronic alcoholics. Replacement therapy prevents neuropathy, confusion, and encephalopathy.
4. Opioids.
   a. Drugs in the opioid classification include opium, morphine, codeine, heroin, hydromorphone, oxycodone, and hydrocodone. Synthetic opiate-like narcotic analgesics include meperidine, methadone, pentazocine, and fentanyl.
   b. With short-acting drugs, such as heroin, withdrawal symptoms occur within 6 to 8 hours after the last dose, peak within 1 to 3 days, and gradually subside over a period of 5 to 7 days.
   c. With longer-acting drugs, such as methadone, withdrawal symptoms begin within 1 to 3 days after the last dose, peak between days 4 and 6, and are complete in 14 to 21 days.
   d. Withdrawal from the ultrashort-acting meperidine begins quickly, reaches a peak in 8 to 12 hours, and is complete in 4 to 5 days.
   e. Opioid intoxication is treated with narcotic antagonists such as naloxone (Narcan), naltrexone (Revia), or nalmefene (Revex).
   f. Withdrawal therapy includes rest, adequate nutritional support, and methadone substitution.
   g. The FDA approved the drug buprenorphine for treating opiate addiction.
   h. Buprenorphine is less powerful than methadone but is considered to be somewhat safer and causes fewer side effects.
   i. Clonidine (Catapres) is used to suppress opiate withdrawal symptoms.
   j. As monotherapy, clonidine is not as effective as substitution with methadone, but it is nonaddicting and serves effectively as a bridge to enable the client to stay opiate free long enough to facilitate termination of methadone maintenance.
5. Depressants.
   a. Substitution therapy for CNS depressant withdrawal (particularly barbiturates) is most commonly achieved with the long-acting barbiturate phenobarbital (Luminal).
   b. Long-acting benzodiazepines are used for substitution therapy when the abused substance is a nonbarbiturate CNS depressant.
6. Stimulants.
   a. Treatment of stimulant intoxication usually begins with minor tranquilizers such as chlordiazepoxide and progresses to major tranquilizers such as haloperidol (Haldol).
   b. Antipsychotics should be administered with caution because they lower seizure threshold.
   c. Repeated seizures are treated with intravenous diazepam.
   d. Withdrawal from CNS stimulants is not the medical emergency observed with CNS depressants.
   e. Treatment is aimed at reducing drug craving and managing severe depression.
   f. Suicide precautions may need to be instituted.
   g. Antidepressant therapy may help in treating depressive symptoms.
   h. Desipramine has been successful with symptoms of cocaine withdrawal and abstinence.
7. Hallucinogens and cannabinols.
   a. Substitution therapy is not required.
   b. With adverse reactions, such as anxiety or panic, benzodiazepines (e.g., diazepam or chlordiazepoxide) may be prescribed.
   c. Psychotic reactions may be treated with antipsychotic medications.

XXVI. Non-Substance Addictions: Gambling Disorder

A. Persistent and recurrent problematic gambling behavior
B. The preoccupation with and impulse to gamble intensifies when the individual is under stress
C. Physical sensation of restlessness and anticipation that can only be relieved by placing a bet
D. As the need to gamble increases, the individual is forced to obtain money by any means available, including illegal actions
E. Family relationships disrupted
F. Impairment in occupational functioning
G. Runs a chronic course, with periods of waxing and waning dependent on periods of stress

H. More common in men than women

I. Narcissistic personality characteristics and impulse control problems are common

J. High rates of personality disorders (e.g., obsessive-compulsive, avoidant, schizotypal, and paranoid)

K. Predisposing factors:

1. Common genetic vulnerability for pathological gambling and alcohol addiction in men.
2. Abnormalities in the serotonergic, noradrenergic, and dopaminergic neurotransmitter systems.
3. Alterations in electroencephalographic patterns.
4. Loss of a parent by death, separation, divorce, or desertion before the child is 15 years of age.
5. Inappropriate parental discipline (absence, inconsistency, or harshness).
6. Exposure to and availability of gambling activities for the adolescent.
7. Family emphasis on material and financial symbols.
8. Lack of family emphasis on saving, planning, and budgeting.

L. Treatment modalities

1. Gamblers deny that they have a problem, making treatment difficult.
2. Most only seek treatment due to legal difficulties, family pressures, or other psychiatric complaints
3. Behavior therapy, cognitive therapy, and psychoanalysis have been used.
4. The SSRIs and clomipramine are used in the treatment of pathological gambling as a form of obsessive-compulsive disorder.
5. Lithium, carbamazepine, and naltrexone are effective.
6. Most effective treatment is Gamblers Anonymous.
   a. Treatment is based on peer pressure, public confession, and the availability of other reformed gamblers to help individuals resist the urge to gamble.
   b. Gam-Anon (for family and spouses of compulsive gamblers) and Gam-a-Teen (for adolescent children of compulsive gamblers) are sources of treatment.

REVIEW QUESTIONS

1. When teaching a client diagnosed with alcohol use disorder about nutritional needs, which nutritional concept should the nurse emphasize?
   1. Eat a high-protein, low-carbohydrate diet to promote lean body mass.
   2. Increase sodium-rich foods to increase iodine levels.
   3. Take a multivitamin supplement that includes thiamine and folic acid.
   4. Restrict fluid intake to decrease renal load.

2. A client with no history of complicated withdrawal syndrome presents in the emergency department exhibiting signs of alcohol withdrawal, including complaints of right upper quadrant pain. Which medication would be most appropriate to treat this client's immediate problem?
   1. Valproic acid (Depakene)
   2. Thiamine (B$_1$)
   3. Chlordiazepoxide (Librium)
   4. Lorazepam (Ativan)

3. A client who is going through alcohol detoxification states, "I see bugs crawling on the wall." Which is the best nursing response?
   1. "I'll remove the bugs from the wall."
   2. "You are confused because of your alcohol addiction."
   3. "There are no bugs on the wall. I'll stay with you until you feel less anxious."
   4. "You are hallucinating. You do not see any bugs on the wall."

4. A client is being discharged from an alcohol use disorder treatment program. The client's wife states, "I'm so afraid that when my husband leaves here, he'll relapse. How can I deal with this?" Which nursing statement would be most appropriate?
   1. "Many family members of clients diagnosed with alcohol use disorder find the Al-Anon support group helpful."
   2. "You should try going out with him to monitor him and prevent his drinking."
   3. "Just make sure he doesn't drink while at home. If you find hidden bottles, you must empty them immediately."
   4. "Tell your husband that if he drinks again, you will leave him."

5. Substance _____ is defined as the development of a reversible syndrome of symptoms after excessive use of a substance.

6. According to Jellinek's model of progression, order the symptoms that occur in the four phases through which an alcoholic's pattern of drinking progresses.
   1. _____ Client experiences loss of control, and physiological dependence is evident.
   2. _____ Client experiences emotional and physical disintegration.
   3. _____ Client uses alcohol to relieve everyday stress and tensions of life.
   4. _____ Client experiences "blackouts" and brief periods of amnesia.

7. A nursing coworker notices that a fellow staff nurse has come to work smelling of alcohol. Which of the following further assessment data would lead the coworker to report the staff nurse as possibly impaired? **Select all that apply.**
   1. The staff nurse is inconsistent in job performance.
   2. The staff nurse has had recent problems in relationships.
   3. The staff nurse has poor concentration.
   4. The staff nurse isolates self.
   5. The staff nurse rarely is absent from work.

8. An employee health nurse is about to meet with a client diagnosed with a gambling disorder. Which of the following personality traits is the nurse likely to assess? **Select all that apply.**
   1. Traits of narcissistic personality disorder
   2. Obsessive-compulsive traits
   3. Paranoid traits
   4. Traits of schizoid personality disorder
   5. Passive-aggressive traits

9. A client diagnosed with a gambling disorder asks the nurse about medications that may be ordered by the client's physician to treat this disorder. The nurse would give the client information on which medications?
   1. Paroxetine (Paxil) and loxapine (Loxitane)
   2. Clomipramine (Anafranil) and fluvoxamine (Luvox)
   3. Lithium carbonate (Lithobid) and risperidone (Risperdal)
   4. Carbamazepine (Tegretol) and aripiprazole (Abilify)

10. A client has a 6-month history of heavy drinking and is brought to the emergency department by family members, who report that the client's last drink was 3 hours ago. It is now 1:00 a.m. When should a nurse expect the client to begin experiencing withdrawal symptoms?
    1. Between 2 a.m. and 4 a.m.
    2. Shortly after a 24-hour period
    3. At the beginning of the third day
    4. Withdrawal is individualized and cannot be predicted

11. From a biochemical perspective, what factor is implicated in the predisposition to the abuse of substances?
    1. Children whose parents are alcoholics are four times more likely to be alcoholics than other children.
    2. Animal tests show that injections of the morphine-like substance that is produced by alcohol results in addicted test animals.
    3. Fixation in the oral stage of psychosocial development can be the cause of substance use disorders.
    4. Depressive response cycles and antisocial personality disorders are associated with substance use disorders.

12. A client with a long history of alcohol use disorder comes to the emergency department with shortness of breath and an enlarged abdomen. Which complication of alcoholism is this client experiencing, and what is the probable cause?
    1. Malnutrition resulting from thiamine deficiency
    2. Ascites resulting from cirrhosis of the liver
    3. Enlarged liver resulting from alcoholic hepatitis
    4. Gastritis resulting from inflammation of the stomach lining

13. Which is the priority nursing diagnosis for a client experiencing cocaine intoxication?
    1. Risk for altered cardiac perfusion
    2. Chronic low self-esteem
    3. Ineffective denial
    4. Dysfunctional grieving

14. A client has been attending Alcoholics Anonymous (AA) meetings as part of the recovery process. Which client statement would indicate a realistic view of AA's goal for client recovery?
    1. "I really am glad the professional leader of this group is working with me."
    2. "If I wasn't monitored by my sponsor, I wouldn't be able to maintain sobriety."
    3. "I realize that drinking hurts my family. AA meetings will promote my sobriety."
    4. "I have lost my job and may not be able to afford attending AA meetings."

15. Which of the following client symptoms would indicate evidence of substance addiction? **Select all that apply.**
    1. The client needs more of the substance to achieve the previously attained result.
    2. The client drinks more than two drinks per day.
    3. The client attempts to discontinue the use of the substance and symptoms occur.
    4. The client has used both cocaine and anxiolytics within the same week.
    5. The client has received a DUI.

16. Which of the following situations would a nurse recognize as influencing a client's response to the ingestion of alcohol? **Select all that apply.**
    1. The client is participating in muscle-building exercises and has gained 20 pounds.
    2. The client has been extremely busy and has skipped breakfast and lunch.
    3. The client has worked a double shift, getting off work at 11:00 p.m.
    4. The client is a woman on a business trip.
    5. The client is a male bartender.

17. Which nursing intervention relates to intermediate care for a client recovering from alcohol use disorder?
    1. Administering substitution therapy as ordered
    2. Promoting understanding and identifying the causes of substance dependency
    3. Promoting participation in outpatient support systems
    4. Assisting clients to identify alternative sources of satisfaction

18. A nursing instructor is teaching about stimulant use disorder. Which of the following student statements indicate that more instruction is needed? **Select all that apply.**
    1. "The two most prevalent, available, and widely used stimulants are caffeine and nicotine."
    2. "The more potent stimulants are under regulation by the Controlled Substances Act."
    3. "With continued use, the pleasurable effects of stimulants increase."
    4. "Caffeine and nicotine exert their action by augmentation of neurotransmitters."
    5. "CNS stimulants induce behavioral stimulation and psychomotor agitation."

19. A client's father asks the nurse how the doctors determined that his child's hallucinations were substance induced rather than from a diagnosis of schizophrenia. Which is the best nursing response?
1. Hallucinations experienced with schizophrenia are usually black and white, and substance induced hallucinations are usually colorful.
2. Substance-induced hallucinations are usually black and white, and hallucinations experienced with schizophrenia are usually colorful.
3. Clients experiencing substance-induced hallucinations experience auditory hallucinations, and those diagnosed with schizophrenia experience visual hallucinations.
4. Clients diagnosed with schizophrenia experience auditory hallucinations, and substance-induced hallucinations are usually visual.

20. A nursing instructor is teaching about cannabis use disorder. Which of the following student statements indicate that more instruction is needed? **Select all that apply.**
1. "Marijuana is composed of the flowering tops of the cannabis plant."
2. "Hashish is derived from dried leaves, stems, and flowers of the cannabis plant."
3. "Cannabis is second to alcohol as most widely abused drug in the United States."
4. "Cannabis is correctly regarded as a substance of low abuse potential."
5. "Withdrawal symptoms can occur when the use of cannabis is discontinued."

REVIEW ANSWERS

1. ANSWER: 3
Rationale:
1. The diet for clients diagnosed with alcohol use disorder should include both high protein and high carbohydrate foods. Taking in high-protein foods without a balance of carbohydrates can have a negative effect on the renal system.
2. Compromised iodine levels are not usually an issue for clients diagnosed with alcohol use disorder.
3. Vitamin B deficiencies contribute to the nervous system disorders seen in alcohol use disorder. Supplements of these vitamins are important to prevent complications. It is important that vitamin supplements include both thiamine (B$_1$) and folic acid.
4. Alcohol acts as a diuretic. Therefore, increased, not restricted, fluid intake is necessary to prevent dehydration.
TEST-TAKING TIP: Review the nutritional needs of clients diagnosed with alcohol use disorder.
Content Area: Safe and Effective Care Environment: Management of Care;
Integrated Process: Nursing Process: Implementation;
Client Need: Safe and Effective Care Environment: Management of Care;
Cognitive Level: Analysis;
Concept: Nutrition

2. ANSWER: 4
Rationale:
1. Valproic acid is used for management of seizures and may be used in conjunction with central nervous system (CNS) depressants to treat alcohol withdrawal syndrome. It should be used cautiously in clients who suffer from hepatic disease. Because this client has no history of complicated withdrawal and may have some liver involvement as indicated by right upper quadrant pain, it would not be the most appropriate drug to treat this client's alcohol withdrawal syndrome symptoms.
2. Because clients diagnosed with alcoholism suffer from marked dietary and vitamin deficiencies, thiamine is given to prevent complications. Thiamine is not used to treat the symptoms of alcohol withdrawal syndrome.
3. Librium is a CNS depressant that is extensively used for the treatment of alcohol withdrawal symptoms. It should be used cautiously in clients who suffer from hepatic disease because it has an extended half-life of as high as 30 hours. Because this client may have some liver involvement as indicated by right upper quadrant pain, it would not be the most appropriate drug to treat this client's symptoms of alcohol withdrawal syndrome.
4. Ativan is a CNS depressant that is extensively used for the treatment of alcohol withdrawal syndrome symptoms. Ativan has a relatively short half-life of 10 to 16 hours. Because this client may have some liver involvement as indicated by right upper quadrant pain, Ativan would be the most appropriate drug to treat this client's alcohol withdrawal syndrome symptoms.
TEST-TAKING TIP: Note the client is experiencing alcohol withdrawal. You would suspect liver involvement due to complaints of right upper quadrant pain. The correct answer would be a drug that would treat alcohol withdrawal syndrome symptoms without further compromising a damaged liver.
Content Area: Safe and Effective Care Environment: Management of Care;
Integrated Process: Nursing Process: Evaluation;
Client Need: Safe and Effective Care Environment: Management of Care;
Cognitive Level: Application;
Concept: Medication

3. ANSWER 3
Rationale:
1. This statement reinforces the hallucination. The client needs to be presented with objective reality.
2. This response presents reality but does not address the client's visual hallucinations.
3. This statement presents objective reality and may help decrease the client's anxiety by the nurse's therapeutic offering of self.
4. This response rejects the client's statement and is confrontational. During a visual hallucination, the client does see things that others do not see, but there is no basis in reality for this perception.
TEST-TAKING TIP: Understand that during a hallucination, the nurse should present objective reality. Hallucinations are frightening, so the nurse should remain with the client and communicate support.
Content Area: Safe and Effective Care Environment: Management of Care;
Integrated Process: Nursing Process: Implementation;
Client Need: Safe and Effective Care Environment: Management of Care;
Cognitive Level: Application;
Concept: Addiction

4. ANSWER: 1
Rationale:
1. This therapeutic response addresses the wife's concerns by giving information about Al-Anon. Al-Anon is a nonprofit organization that provides group support for the family and close friends of clients diagnosed with alcohol use disorder.
2. This is an inappropriate, nontherapeutic nursing response that gives incorrect advice. A client diagnosed with alcohol use disorder must be responsible for his or her continued sobriety.
3. This inappropriate, nontherapeutic nursing response gives advice and encourages codependent behavior.
4. This inappropriate, nontherapeutic nursing response gives advice and encourages the ineffective use of threats.
TEST-TAKING TIP: Look for an appropriate therapeutic communication technique that does not encourage codependent behavior.
Content Area: Safe and Effective Care Environment: Management of Care;
Integrated Process: Nursing Process: Implementation;
Client Need: Safe and Effective Care Environment: Management of Care;

Cognitive Level: Application;
Concept: Addiction

5. ANSWER: intoxication
Rationale: "Intoxication" is defined as "the development of a reversible syndrome of symptoms following excessive use of a substance." The symptoms are drug-specific and occur during or shortly after the ingestion of the substance.
TEST-TAKING TIP: Review the Key Words to find this definition.
Content Area: Psychosocial Integrity;
Integrated Process: Nursing Process: Assessment;
Client Need: Psychosocial Integrity;
Cognitive Level: Knowledge;
Concept: Addiction

6. ANSWER: The correct order is 3, 4, 1, 2
Rationale: Jellinek outlines four phases through which the alcoholic's pattern of drinking progresses. Some variability among individuals is to be expected within this model of progression.
1. Prealcoholic phase (characterized by the use of alcohol to relieve the everyday stress and tensions of life).
2. Early alcoholic phase (begins with "blackouts," brief periods of amnesia that occur during or immediately after a period of drinking).
3. Crucial phase (the individual loses control, and physiological dependence is clearly evident).
4. Chronic phase (characterized by emotional and physical disintegration. The individual is usually intoxicated more than sober).
TEST-TAKING TIP: Review Jellinek's model of drinking progression.
Content Area: Safe and Effective Care Environment: Management of Care;
Integrated Process: Nursing Process: Evaluation;
Client Need: Safe and Effective Care Environment: Management of Care;
Cognitive Level: Analysis;
Concept: Addiction

7. ANSWERS: 1, 2, 3, 4
Rationale: A number of clues for recognizing substance impairment in nurses have been identified. They are not easy to detect and will vary according to the substance being used. There may be high absenteeism if the person's source is outside the work area, or the individual may rarely miss work if the substance source is at work. Some other possible signs are irritability, mood swings, elaborate excuses for behavior, unkempt appearance, impaired motor coordination, slurred speech, flushed face, and frequent use of the restroom.
1. A possible sign of substance impairment is inconsistent job performance.
2. A possible sign of substance impairment is problems with relationships.
3. A possible sign of substance impairment is poor concentration, memory, or recall.
4. A possible sign of substance impairment is a tendency to isolate self.

5. A possible sign of substance impairment is high absenteeism, especially if the person's source, in this case alcohol, is outside the work area.
TEST-TAKING TIP: Review clues for recognizing substance impairment in nurses.
Content Area: Safe and Effective Care Environment: Management of Care;
Integrated Process: Nursing Process: Assessment;
Client Need: Safe and Effective Care Environment: Management of Care;
Cognitive Level: Application;
Concept: Assessment

8. ANSWERS: 1, 2, 3
Rationale:
1. Evidence points to the common existence of narcissistic personality characteristics and impulse control problems in pathological gamblers.
2. High rates of obsessive-compulsive traits are noted in pathological gamblers.
3. High rates of paranoid traits are noted in pathological gamblers.
4. Schizoid traits are not typically observed in this disorder.
5. Passive-aggressive traits are not typically observed in this disorder.
TEST-TAKING TIP: Review the personality traits that are associated with the diagnosis of a gambling disorder.
Content Area: Safe and Effective Care Environment: Management of Care;
Integrated Process: Nursing Process: Assessment;
Client Need: Safe and Effective Care Environment: Management of Care;
Cognitive Level: Application;
Concept: Assessment

9. ANSWER: 2
Rationale:
1. The SSRIs, such as Paxil, have been used successfully in the treatment of pathological gambling: but antipsychotic medications, such as loxapine, are not treatments of choice for this disorder.
2. Clomipramine has been used successfully in the treatment of pathological gambling as a form of obsessive-compulsive disorder, and the SSRIs, such as fluvoxamine, have also been used successfully in the treatment of this disorder.
3. Lithium carbonate has been shown to be effective in the treatment of pathological gambling, but antipsychotic medications, such as risperidone, are not treatments of choice for this disorder.
4. Carbamazepine has been shown to be effective in the treatment of pathological gambling, but antipsychotic medications, such as aripiprazole, are not treatments of choice for this disorder.
TEST-TAKING TIP: Review the medications used in the treatment of pathological gambling disorder.
Content Area: Safe and Effective Care Environment: Management of Care;
Integrated Process: Nursing Process: Implementation;

Client Need: *Safe and Effective Care Environment:*
Management of Care;
Cognitive Level: *Application;*
Concept: *Medication*

10. ANSWER: 1
    Rationale:
    **1. Symptoms of alcohol withdrawal usually occur within
    4 to 6 hours of cessation of or reduction in heavy and
    prolonged alcohol use. The nurse should expect that the
    client will begin experiencing withdrawal symptoms
    from alcohol between 2 a.m. and 4 a.m.**
    2. Symptoms of alcohol withdrawal usually occur within 4
    to 6 hours, not after a 24-hour period, of cessation of or re-
    duction in heavy and prolonged alcohol use.
    3. Symptoms of alcohol withdrawal usually occur within
    4 to 6 hours, not after a 36-hour period, of cessation of or
    reduction in heavy and prolonged alcohol use.
    4. Withdrawal from alcohol can be predicted to usually
    occur within 4 to 6 hours of cessation of or reduction in
    heavy and prolonged alcohol use.
    TEST-TAKING TIP: Review Table 9.1 for information related
    to the timing of alcohol withdrawal symptoms.
    Content Area: *Safe and Effective Care Environment:*
    Management of Care;
    Integrated Process: *Nursing Process: Assessment;*
    Client Need: *Safe and Effective Care Environment:*
    Management of Care;
    Cognitive Level: *Analysis;*
    Concept: *Addiction*

11. ANSWER: 2
    1. This statement of substance use disorder causation is
    from a genetic, not biochemical, perspective.
    **2. This true statement of substance use disorder causa-
    tion is from a biochemical perspective.**
    3. This statement of substance use disorder causation is
    from a developmental, not biochemical, perspective.
    4. This statement of substance use disorder causation is
    from a personality type, not biochemical, perspective.
    TEST-TAKING TIP: The "morphine-like substance" presented
    in the answer choice should be a clue to the biochemical
    nature of this perspective.
    Content Area: *Psychosocial Integrity;*
    Integrated Process: *Nursing Process: Assessment;*
    Client Need: *Psychosocial Integrity;*
    Cognitive Level: *Application;*
    Concept: *Addiction*

12. ANSWER: 2
    Rationale:
    1. Clients with long histories of alcohol use disorder often
    experience malnutrition because they get calories from
    alcohol rather than nutritious foods. This malnutrition
    is due to overall deficits in nutritional intake, not just
    thiamine. This client does not present with signs and
    symptoms of malnutrition.
    **2. Ascites is a condition in which an excessive amount of
    serous fluid accumulates in the abdominal cavity, result-
    ing in a protuberant abdomen. This condition occurs in
    response to portal hypertension caused by cirrhosis of**

the liver resulting from alcohol use disorder. Increased
pressure results in the seepage of fluid from the surface
of the liver into the abdominal cavity. Pressure of the enlarged abdomen on the diaphragm can cause shortness
of breath.
3. An enlarged liver would not manifest as an enlarged abdomen. Anatomically, the liver is located in the right upper
quadrant of the abdomen and, if enlarged, can be palpated.
Hepatitis can cause liver enlargement, but ascites resulting
from cirrhosis of the liver is this client's presenting
problem.
4. Gastritis resulting from inflammation of the stomach
lining is often a complication of alcohol use disorder. The
effects of alcohol on the stomach include inflammation of
the stomach lining characterized by epigastric distress,
nausea, vomiting, and distention. The client in the question is not complaining of gastric distress. Distention of
the abdomen resulting from gastritis would not be significant enough to cause shortness of breath.
TEST-TAKING TIP: Review the various physical complications of chronic alcohol use disorder. Read all symptoms
presented in the question carefully to choose the complication that reflects the symptoms described.
Content Area: *Safe and Effective Care Environment:*
Management of Care;
Integrated Process: *Nursing Process: Assessment;*
Client Need: *Safe and Effective Care Environment:*
Management of Care;
Cognitive Level: *Application;*
Concept: *Addiction*

13. ANSWER: 1
    Rationale:
    **1. Central nervous system stimulants, such as cocaine,
    can induce increased systolic and diastolic blood pres-
    sure, increased heart rate, and cardiac arrhythmias.
    Cocaine intoxication also typically produces an increase
    in myocardial demand for oxygen. These effects on the
    heart put a client experiencing cocaine intoxication at
    risk for altered cardiac perfusion.**
    2. Chronic low self-esteem is long-standing negative self-
    evaluation and feelings about self or self-capabilities. This
    may be an appropriate diagnosis for a client experiencing
    cocaine use disorder, not intoxication. Compared with the
    other diagnoses presented, it would not take priority.
    3. Ineffective denial is the conscious or unconscious at-
    tempt to disavow knowledge or meaning of an event to
    reduce anxiety or fear, leading to the detriment of health.
    This may be an appropriate diagnosis for a client experi-
    encing cocaine use disorder, not intoxication. Compared
    with the other diagnoses presented, it would not take
    priority.
    4. Dysfunctional grieving is the extended, unsuccessful use
    of intellectual and emotional responses by which individu-
    als attempt to work through the process of modifying
    self-concept based on the perception of loss. Loss typically
    accompanies substance use disorder, but there is no indi-
    cation of behaviors that support the nursing diagnosis in
    the question. Also the nurse must prioritize the client's
    potential for injury related to cocaine intoxication.

TEST-TAKING TIP: Remember to always prioritize client safety. Only Option 1 could cause the client to be physically injured.
Content Area: Safe and Effective Care Environment: Management of Care;
Integrated Process: Nursing Process: Diagnosis;
Client Need: Safe and Effective Care Environment: Management of Care;
Cognitive Level: Application;
Concept: Critical Thinking

14. **ANSWER: 3**
    Rationale:
    1. AA is a self-help group that is not led by professionals.
    2. AA encourages self-determination; therefore, AA sponsors encourage but do not monitor members.
    3. Recognition of and motivation to maintain sobriety is the goal of Alcoholics Anonymous. The client is verbalizing recognition of problems with alcohol use and realizes that a support group will enhance chances of recovery and sobriety.
    4. There is no charge for AA meeting attendance. It is a free, community-based, self-help group available to anyone who needs assistance with recovery from alcohol use disorder.
    TEST-TAKING TIP: Review Box 9.3 to understand the goals of AA.
    Content Area: Safe and Effective Care Environment: Management of Care;
    Integrated Process: Nursing Process: Evaluation;
    Client Need: Safe and Effective Care Environment: Management of Care;
    Cognitive Level: Application;
    Concept: Promoting Health

15. **ANSWERS: 1, 3**
    Rationale:
    1. When a client needs more of the substance to achieve the previously attained result, the client is experiencing tolerance. Tolerance is evidence of substance addiction.
    2. Drinking more than two drinks a day is not necessarily evidence of substance addiction.
    3. When a client attempts to discontinue the use of the substance and symptoms occur, the client is experiencing withdrawal. Withdrawal is evidence of substance addiction.
    4. Using both cocaine and anxiolytics within the same week is not necessarily evidence of substance addiction.
    5. Receiving a DUI is not necessarily evidence of substance addiction.
    TEST-TAKING TIP: Remember that tolerance and withdrawal are cardinal signs of substance addiction.
    Content Area: Safe and Effective Care Environment: Management of Care;
    Integrated Process: Nursing Process: Assessment;
    Client Need: Safe and Effective Care Environment: Management of Care;
    Cognitive Level: Application;
    Concept: Addiction

16. **ANSWERS: 1, 2, 3**
    Rationale: Various factors affect an individual's response to the ingestion of alcohol.
    1. An individual's size and body mass will affect how an individual responds to the ingestion of alcohol.
    2. Having a full or empty stomach will affect how an individual responds to the ingestion of alcohol.
    3. Emotional stress and fatigue will affect how an individual responds to the ingestion of alcohol.
    4. Going on a business trip may provide a setting to encourage alcohol intake but would not affect how the individual would respond to any alcohol ingested. Also, gender does not affect an individual's response to ingested alcohol.
    5. Being a bartender may provide a setting to encourage alcohol intake but would not affect how the individual would respond to any alcohol ingested. Also, gender does not affect an individual's response to ingested alcohol.
    TEST-TAKING TIP: Review the factors that affect how an individual responds to alcohol ingestion.
    Content Area: Safe and Effective Care Environment: Management of Care;
    Integrated Process: Nursing Process: Evaluation;
    Client Need: Safe and Effective Care Environment: Management of Care;
    Cognitive Level: Application;
    Concept: Assessment

17. **ANSWER: 2**
    Rationale:
    1. Administering substitution therapy as ordered is a nursing intervention during the alcohol detoxification process, not during intermediate care.
    2. Promoting understanding and identifying the causes of substance dependency is a nursing intervention during intermediate care.
    3. Promoting participation in outpatient support systems is a nursing intervention during rehabilitative, not intermediate care.
    4. Assisting clients to identify alternative sources of satisfaction is a nursing intervention during rehabilitation not intermediate care.
    TEST-TAKING TIP: Review the stages of recovery from alcohol use disorder. The focus of this question is intermediate care.
    Content Area: Safe and Effective Care Environment: Management of Care;
    Integrated Process: Nursing Process: Implementation;
    Client Need: Safe and Effective Care Environment: Management of Care;
    Cognitive Level: Application;
    Concept: Nursing

18. **ANSWERS: 3, 4**
    Rationale:
    1. The two most prevalent, available, and widely used stimulants are caffeine and nicotine. Caffeine is a common ingredient in coffee, tea, colas, and chocolate. Nicotine is the primary psychoactive substance found in tobacco products. This student statement indicates that learning has occurred.

2. The more potent stimulants, because of their potential for physiological addiction, are under regulation by the Controlled Substances Act. This student statement indicates that learning has occurred.

3. With continued use, the pleasurable effects of stimulants diminish, rather than increase, and there is a corresponding increase in dysphoric effects. This student statement indicates a need for further instruction.

4. General cellular stimulants (caffeine and nicotine) exert their action directly on cellular activity, not by augmentation of neurotransmitters. This student statement indicates a need for further instruction.

5. CNS stimulants do induce behavioral stimulation and psychomotor agitation. This student statement indicates that learning has occurred.

TEST-TAKING TIP: Review information about stimulant use disorder. When answering a "need for further instruction" type question, look for incorrect answers.
Content Area: Safe and Effective Care Environment: Management of Care;
Integrated Process: Nursing Process: Evaluation;
Client Need: Safe and Effective Care Environment: Management of Care;
Cognitive Level: Application;
Concept: Nursing Roles

19. **ANSWER: 4**
Rationale:
1. Hallucinations are false sensory perceptions that can vary in content and color from person to person.
2. Hallucinations are false sensory perceptions that can vary in content and color from person to person.
3. Clients experiencing substance-induced hallucinations experience auditory hallucinations, and those diagnosed with schizophrenia experience visual hallucinations.
4. Clients diagnosed with schizophrenia experience auditory hallucinations, and substance-induced hallucinations are usually visual. This distinction helps to differentiate substance-induced hallucinations from the hallucinations of schizophrenia.

TEST-TAKING TIP: Review information about hallucinogenic use disorder.
Content Area: Safe and Effective Care Environment: Management of Care;
Integrated Process: Nursing Process: Implementation;
Client Need: Safe and Effective Care Environment: Management of Care;
Cognitive Level: Application;
Concept: Nursing Roles

20. **ANSWERS: 1, 2, 4**
Rationale:
1. Marijuana, the most prevalent type of cannabis plant preparation, is composed of the dried leaves, stems, and flowers of the plant, not just the flowering tops. This student statement indicates a need for further instruction.
2. Hashish is a more potent concentrate of the resin derived from the flowering tops of the plant, not the dried leaves, stems, and flowers. This student statement indicates a need for further instruction.
3. Cannabis is second to alcohol as the most widely abused drug in the US. This student statement indicates that learning has occurred.
4. Cannabis is incorrectly, not correctly, regarded as a substance of low abuse potential. This student statement indicates a need for further instruction.
5. Withdrawal symptoms can occur when the use of cannabis is discontinued. This student statement indicates that learning has occurred.

TEST-TAKING TIP: Review information about cannabis use disorder.
Content Area: Safe and Effective Care Environment: Management of Care;
Integrated Process: Nursing Process: Evaluation;
Client Need: Safe and Effective Care Environment: Management of Care;
Cognitive Level: Application;
Concept: Addiction

CASE STUDY: Putting it All Together

Steve, a 40-year-old house painter, was hospitalized after running his car into a stone wall. He was charged with driving under the influence (DUI) because of a blood alcohol level of 0.08%. After stabilization, Steve was transferred to a drug and alcohol rehabilitation center, where he was successfully detoxed without complications. Steve's history reveals long-term, heavy alcohol use and a long rap sheet including extortion, domestic violence, delinquent child support, and two previous DUIs. During an interview with his psychiatric nurse practitioner (PNP) Cathy, Steve states that his father was an alcoholic and beat his mother. He blames the accident on a run-in with his overcritical boss that precipitated a drinking binge. Steve becomes tearful and says, "I know you can help me with some of these problems. I can tell you're a good person. I have a family who will go hungry if I don't get out of here quickly and go back to work. If you can loan me $200 and get me discharged, I will pay you back, and I'll always be there for you." Cathy asks, "Have you ever been intoxicated or had a problem with the law?" Steve becomes indignant and adamantly replies, "Never! I'm a God-fearing man who's depressed and down on his luck." The PNP looks Steve in the eye and says, "Steve, you have serious, life-threatening problems, none of which involves a quick discharge or getting back to your job. Besides that, you are court ordered to this treatment center. Are you open to exploring these problems with me?" Steve looks down at his feet and reluctantly agrees.

1. The PNP would document which tentative medical diagnoses for Steve?
2. What predisposing factors may have contributed to Steve's diagnosis?
3. What subjective symptoms lead the PNP to this diagnosis?
4. What objective symptoms lead the PNP to this diagnosis?
5. What therapy might the PNP use in Steve's recovery process?
6. Which NANDA nursing diagnosis would be appropriate for Steve?
7. What short-term outcome would be appropriate for Steve?
8. What long-term outcome would be appropriate for Steve?
9. List the nursing interventions (actions) that will assist Cathy to meet these outcomes.
10. List the questions that would determine whether the nursing actions are successful.
11. List the complications that might result from Steve's diagnosis.
12. Which defense mechanism is Steve employing?
13. Which personality trait is Steve exhibiting?
14. What classification of medications could be used to treat Steve?

Chapter 10

Schizophrenia Spectrum and Other Psychotic Disorders

Associative looseness—Sometimes called loose associations, a thinking process characterized by speech in which ideas shift from one unrelated subject to another; the individual is unaware that the topics are not connected

Catatonia—A condition marked by changes in muscle tone or activity typically associated with schizophrenia; two distinct sets of symptoms are characteristic of this condition: in catatonic stupor, the individual experiences a deficit of motor (movement) activity that can render him or her motionless; catatonic excitement, or excessive movement, can be associated with violent behavior directed toward oneself or others

Circumstantiality—In speaking, the *delay* of an individual to reach the point of a communication, owing to unnecessary and tedious details

Delusion—A rigid system of beliefs with which a person is preoccupied and to which the person firmly holds, despite the logical absurdity of the beliefs and a lack of supporting evidence

Hallucination—The experience of perceiving objects or events that do not have an external source, such as hearing one's name called by a voice that no one else seems to hear

Illusion—A mental impression derived from misinterpretation of an actual sensory stimulus

Magical thinking—An irrational belief that one can bring about a circumstance or event by thinking about it or wishing for it; magical thinking is normal in preschool children, and it can also occur in schizophrenia

Negative symptoms—Symptoms of schizophrenia characterized by the absence or elimination of certain behaviors; three such negative symptoms are affective flattening, poverty of speech, and loss of will or initiative

Paranoia—A condition characterized by an elaborate, overly suspicious system of thinking; in schizophrenia, paranoia is characterized by persecutory delusions and hallucinations of a threatening nature

Positive symptoms—Symptoms of schizophrenia that are characterized by the production or presence of behaviors that are grossly abnormal or excessive, including hallucinations and thought-process disorder; positive symptoms can be subdivided into psychotic and disorganized symptoms

Psychosis—A severe mental condition in which there is disorganization of the personality, deterioration in social functioning, and loss of contact with or distortion of reality; there may be evidence of hallucinations and delusional thinking; psychosis can occur with or without the presence of organic impairment

Religiosity—Excessive demonstration of or obsession with religious ideas and behavior

Tangentiality—The inability to get to the point of a story; the speaker introduces many unrelated topics, until the original topic of discussion is lost

Word Salad—A group of words that are put together ("tossed") in a random fashion without any logical connection

Perhaps no psychological disorder is more crippling than schizophrenia. Characteristically, disturbances in thought processes, perception, and affect invariably result in a severe deterioration of social and occupational functioning. Schizophrenia probably does not have a single cause but results from a variable combination of genetic predisposition, biochemical dysfunction, physiological factors, and psychosocial stress. There is not now and probably never will be a single treatment that cures the disorder. Instead, effective treatment requires a comprehensive, multidisciplinary effort, including pharmacotherapy and various forms of psychosocial care, such as living skills and social skills training, rehabilitation and recovery, and family therapy. With comprehensive treatment, clients diagnosed with schizophrenia or other psychotic disorders can lead meaningful, productive lives.

🛑 Potential for suicide is a major concern among clients diagnosed with schizophrenia. About one-third of people with schizophrenia attempt suicide, and about 1 in 10 die of the act. Studies have shown that 40% to 55% of individuals with schizophrenia report suicidal ideations.

I. Nature of the Disorder

A. Disturbances in thought processes, perception, and affect
B. Deterioration of social and occupational functioning
C. Prevalence is about 1% in the general population
D. When symptoms occur
  1. Generally appear in late adolescence or early adulthood.
  2. May occur in middle or late adult life.
  3. Symptoms occurring before age 17 suggest *early-onset schizophrenia*.
  4. Symptoms occurring before age 13 (which is very rare) suggest *very early-onset schizophrenia*.
E. Pattern of development
  1. Phase I: premorbid phase.
    a. Characterized by social maladjustment, social withdrawal, irritability, and antagonistic thoughts and behavior.
    b. Shy and withdrawn, poor peer relationships, do poorly in school, and demonstrate antisocial behavior.
    c. May exhibit schizoid or schizotypal personalities.
    d. Characterized as quiet, passive, and introverted children, with few friends.
  2. Phase II: prodromal phase.
    a. Begins with a change from premorbid functioning and extends until the onset of frank psychotic symptoms.
    b. Can be as brief as a few weeks or months.

  c. Average length is two to 5 years.
  d. Substantial functional impairment.
  e. May experience sleep disturbance, anxiety, irritability, depressed mood, poor concentration, fatigue, and behavioral deficits such as deterioration in role functioning and social withdrawal.
  f. Positive symptoms such as perceptual abnormalities, ideas of reference, and suspiciousness develop late in the prodromal phase heralding the imminent onset of psychosis.
  g. Early recognition can lead to early onset of treatment.
  3. Phase III: schizophrenia.
    a. Psychotic symptoms are prominent.
    b. The presence of delusions, hallucinations, disorganized speech.
    c. May include grossly abnormal psychomotor behavior, including catatonia.
    d. May include negative symptoms (e.g., diminished emotional expression or avolition).
    e. Functioning (e.g., school, work, interpersonal relations, self-care) is markedly below the level achieved before the onset of symptoms.
    f. Symptoms last for at least 6 months.
    g. Depressive or bipolar disorder with psychotic features and schizoaffective disorder must be ruled out.
    h. Symptoms are not due to the direct physiological effects of a substance (e.g., an abused drug, a medication) or a general medical condition.
  4. Phase IV: residual phase.
    a. Symptoms of the acute stage are either absent or no longer prominent.
    b. Negative symptoms may remain.
    c. Flat affect and impairment in role functioning are common.
    d. Residual impairment often increases between episodes of active psychosis.
F. Prognosis: complete return to full premorbid functioning is not common

DID YOU KNOW?

The factors associated with positive outcomes for clients diagnosed with schizophrenia are good premorbid functioning, a later age of onset, and female gender. Also associated with positive outcomes is abrupt onset of symptoms with an obvious precipitating factor (as opposed to gradual, insidious onset of symptoms). An associated mood disturbance, rapid resolution of active-phase symptoms, minimal residual symptoms, absence of structural brain abnormalities, normal neurological functioning, and no family history of schizophrenia also contribute to a positive outcome.

II. Predisposing Factors

A. Cause uncertain

B. No single factor can be implicated in the etiology

C. Results from a combination of influences including biological, psychological, and environmental factors

🛑 Early conceptualizations of the cause of schizophrenia focused on family relationship factors, probably due to the absence of information related to a biological connection. These early theories implicated poor parent-child relationships and dysfunctional family systems as the cause of schizophrenia, but they no longer hold any credibility. It is important to recognize that relatives may blame themselves and feel guilt related to a family member's diagnosis based on this false information.

D. Biological influences
  1. Genetic vulnerability.
     a. Siblings of someone diagnosed with schizophrenia have a 10% risk of developing the disorder.
     b. Offspring with one parent who has schizophrenia have a 5% to 6% chance of developing the disorder.
     c. How schizophrenia is inherited is uncertain.
     d. No definitive biological marker has as yet been found.
     e. The rate of schizophrenia among monozygotic twins is four times that of dizygotic twins and approximately 50 times that of the general population.
     f. Identical twins reared apart have the same rate of development of the illness as do those reared together.
     g. Adopted children who were born to mothers with schizophrenia were more likely to develop the illness than those born to mothers without schizophrenia.
     h. Children born to nonschizophrenic parents, but reared by parents afflicted with the illness, do not seem to suffer more often from schizophrenia.
  2. Biochemical influences.
     a. Attributed to abnormal brain biochemistry.
     b. Dopamine hypothesis.
        i. Increased dopamine receptor sensitivity, OR
        ii. Too many dopamine receptors, OR
        iii. A combination of these mechanisms
        iv. Research, response to antipsychotic drugs, and autopsy results all support this hypothesis
     c. Other biochemical hypotheses.
        i. Abnormalities in the neurotransmitters norepinephrine, serotonin, acetylcholine, and gamma-aminobutyric acid
        ii. Abnormalities in neuroregulators, such as prostaglandins and endorphins
        iii. Recent research has implicated the neurotransmitter glutamate
  3. Physiological influences.
     a. Viral infections.
        i. High incidence of schizophrenia after prenatal exposure to influenza
        ii. Seasonality of birth consistent with viral infection
     b. Anatomical abnormalities.
        i. Ventricular enlargement (most consistent finding)
           a) Poor premorbid functioning
           b) Negative symptoms
           c) Poor response to treatment
           d) Cognitive impairment
        ii. Sulci enlargement
        iii. Cerebellar atrophy
        iv. Decreased cerebral and intracranial size

DID YOU KNOW?

Physical conditions, such as epilepsy (particularly temporal lobe), Huntington's disease, birth trauma, head injury in adulthood, alcohol abuse, cerebral tumor (particularly in the limbic system), cerebrovascular accidents, systemic lupus erythematosus, myxedema, parkinsonism, and Wilson's disease have been related to the diagnosis of schizophrenia.

E. Environmental influences
  1. Sociocultural factors.
     a. Greater numbers from the lower socioeconomic classes.
     b. Conditions associated with living in poverty.
        i. Congested housing
        ii. Inadequate nutrition
        iii. Absence of prenatal care
        iv. Few resources for dealing with stressful situations
        v. Feelings of hopelessness
     c. Social conditions could be consequence rather than cause of schizophrenia.
  2. Stressful life events.
     a. No scientific evidence to indicate that stress causes schizophrenia.
     b. Stress may contribute to the severity and course of the illness.
     c. Extreme stress can precipitate psychotic episodes.
     d. May precipitate symptoms in an individual who possesses a genetic vulnerability.
     e. May exacerbate symptoms and increase rates of relapse.

DID YOU KNOW?

No single theory or hypothesis has been postulated that substantiates a clear-cut explanation for the disease. The most current theory seems to be that schizophrenia is a biologically based disease, the onset of which is influenced by factors within the environment (either internal or external).

III. Types of Schizophrenia and Other Psychotic Disorders

A. General information
1. Schizophrenia is a spectrum of psychotic disorders whose psychopathology varies from least to most severe.
2. The level, number, and duration of psychotic signs and symptoms defines the severity of the disorder.
3. Less severe or time-limited conditions should be eliminated before assigning the diagnosis of more severe psychotic disorders.
4. The beginning of the schizophrenic spectrum begins with schizotypal personality disorder (covered in Chapter 13).

B. Delusional disorder

DID YOU KNOW?

A **delusion** is a belief that is not based on objective reality. The client truly believes the delusion; presenting reality and arguing the validity of the thought will not change the client's belief. The delusion can also be termed a "fixed delusion" because of the rigid nature of the belief system. An appropriate nursing intervention is to distract the client from perseverating on the delusion.

1. Characterized by the presence of delusions lasting at least 1 month.
2. Hallucinations are not prominent, and behavior is not bizarre.
3. The subtype of delusional disorder is based on the predominant delusional theme.
   a. Erotomania type.
      i. Believes that someone, usually of a higher status, is in love with him or her
      ii. Feelings may be hidden, or client may pursue object of his or her affection
   b. Grandiose type.
      i. Have irrational ideas regarding their own worth, talent, knowledge, or power
      ii. May believe that they have a special relationship with a famous person or even assume the identity of a famous person
      iii. When of a religious nature may lead to assumption of the identity of a deity or religious leader
   c. Jealous type.
      i. Centers on the idea that the person's sexual partner is unfaithful
      ii. The idea is irrational and without cause
   d. Persecutory type.
      i. Most common type
      ii. Believe they are being persecuted or malevolently treated
      iii. Frequent themes include being plotted against, cheated or defrauded, followed and spied on, poisoned, or drugged
   e. Somatic type: believe they have some type of general medical condition.
   f. Mixed type: delusions are prominent, but no single theme is predominant.

C. Brief psychotic disorder
1. Sudden onset of psychotic symptoms that may or may not be preceded by a severe psychosocial stressor.
2. Symptoms last at least 1 day but less than 1 month.
3. Full return to the premorbid level of functioning.
4. Experiences emotional turmoil or confusion.
5. Evidence of impaired reality testing.
   a. Incoherent speech.
   b. Delusions.
   c. Hallucinations.
   d. Bizarre behavior.
   e. Disorientation.
6. Susceptible if preexisting personality disorder exists (most commonly, histrionic, narcissistic, paranoid, schizotypal, and borderline personality disorders).
7. May have catatonic features.

D. Substance/medication-induced psychotic disorder
1. Hallucinations and delusions are found to be directly attributable to substance intoxication or withdrawal.
2. Symptoms occur but are more excessive and severe than those usually associated with intoxication or withdrawal.
3. Medical history, physical examination, or laboratory findings provide evidence of the use of a substance.
4. Catatonic features may be present.

E. Psychotic disorder associated with another medical condition
1. Hallucinations and delusions can be directly attributed to a general medical condition.
2. Cannot occur during delirium.
3. See Table 10.1 for a list of medical conditions that may cause psychotic symptoms.

F. Catatonic disorder due to another medical condition
1. Catatonic symptoms are evidenced from medical history, physical examination, or laboratory findings to be directly attributable to the physiological consequences of a general medical condition.

Table 10.1	General Medical Conditions That May Cause Psychotic Symptoms

Acute intermittent porphyria
Cerebrovascular disease
CNS infections
CNS trauma
Deafness
Fluid or electrolyte imbalances
Hepatic disease
Herpes encephalitis
Huntington's disease
Hypoadrenocorticism
Hypo- or hyperparathyroidism
Hypo- or hyperthyroidism
Metabolic conditions (e.g., hypoxia, hypercarbia, hypoglycemia)
Migraine headache
Neoplasms
Neurosyphilis
Normal pressure hydrocephalus
Renal disease
Systemic lupus erythematosus
Temporal lobe epilepsy
Vitamin deficiency (e.g., B$_{12}$)
Wilson's disease

CNS, central nervous system.
Sources: American Psychiatric Association (2013); Black & Andreasen (2011); Sadock & Sadock (2007).

2. Types of medical conditions include:
   i. Metabolic disorders (e.g., hepatic encephalopathy, hypo- and hyperthyroidism, hypo- and hyperadrenalism, and vitamin B$_{12}$ deficiency)
   ii. Neurological conditions (e.g., epilepsy, tumors, cerebrovascular disease, head trauma, and encephalitis)

DID YOU KNOW?

Catatonia is a syndrome seen most frequently in schizophrenia, characterized by muscular rigidity and mental stupor, sometimes alternating with great excitement and confusion.

G. Schizophreniform disorder
   1. Features are identical to those of schizophrenia, with the exception that the duration, including prodromal, active, and residual phases, is at least 1 month but less than 6 months.
   2. Diagnosis is changed to schizophrenia if clinical picture persists beyond 6 months.
   3. Catatonic features may also be present.
   4. Good prognosis when:
      i. Affect is not blunted or flat
      ii. Rapid onset of psychotic symptoms from the time the unusual behavior is noticed

iii. Premorbid social and occupational functioning was satisfactory
H. Schizoaffective disorder
   1. Schizophrenic behaviors present with strong symptoms associated with mood disorders (depression or mania).
   2. Presence of hallucinations and/or delusions that occur for at least 2 weeks in the absence of a major mood episode.
   3. Mood disorder symptoms must be evident majority of time.
   4. Catatonic features may be present.
   5. Prognosis is generally better than that for other schizophrenic disorders but worse than that for mood disorders alone.

IV. Nursing Process: Assessment

A. Symptoms associated with the active phase of schizophrenia
B. Assessment may be a complex process, based on information gathered from a number of sources
C. Clients in an acute episode of their illness are seldom able to make a significant contribution to their history
D. Data may be obtained from family members, old records, or from other individuals who have been in a position to report on the progression of the client's behavior
E. Symptoms are commonly described as positive or negative
F. Most clients exhibit a mixture of both types of symptoms
G. See Box 10.1 for lists of both types of symptoms
H. Positive Symptoms
   1. Positive symptoms reflect an alteration or distortion of normal mental functions.
   2. Positive symptoms are associated with normal brain structures and relatively good responses to treatment.
   3. Thought content.
      a. Delusions are false personal beliefs inconsistent with the person's intelligence or cultural background.
      b. Continues to have the belief despite obvious proof that it is false or irrational.
         i. Delusions of persecution: feeling threatened and the belief that others intend harm or persecution
         ii. Delusions of grandeur: an exaggerated feeling of importance, power, knowledge, or identity
         iii. Delusions of reference: a belief that all events within the environment refer to the client

Box 10.1 Positive and Negative Symptoms of Schizophrenia

Positive Symptoms	Negative Symptoms
Content of Thought	**Affect**
Delusions	Inappropriate affect
Religiosity	Bland or flat affect
Paranoia	Apathy
Magical thinking	**Volition**
Form of Thought	Inability to initiate goal-directed activity
Associative looseness	Emotional ambivalence
Neologisms	Deteriorated appearance
Concrete thinking	
Clang associations	**Impaired Interpersonal**
Word salad	**Functioning and Relationship**
Circumstantiality	**to the External World**
Tangentiality	Impaired social interaction
Mutism	Social isolation
Perseveration	**Psychomotor Behavior**
Perception	Anergia
Hallucinations	Waxy flexibility
Illusions	Posturing
Sense of Self	Pacing and rocking
Echolalia	**Associated Features**
Echopraxia	Anhedonia
Identification and imitation	Regression
Depersonalization	

DID YOU KNOW?

Ideas of reference are less rigid than delusions of reference. An example of an idea of reference is irrationally assuming that, when in the presence of others, one is the object of their discussion or ridicule.

      iv. Delusions of control or influence: the belief that certain objects or persons have control over behavior

      v. Somatic delusion: a false idea about the functioning of the body

      vi. Nihilistic delusion: a false idea that the self, a part of the self, others, or the world is nonexistent

   c. **Religiosity.**

      i. An excessive demonstration of or obsession with religious ideas and behavior

      ii. Difficult to assess due to varied religious beliefs and commitments

   d. **Paranoia:** extreme suspiciousness of others and of their actions or perceived intentions.

   e. **Magical thinking.**

      i. Belief that personal thoughts or behaviors have control over specific situations or people

      ii. Common and normal in developing children

4. Thought form.

   a. Associative looseness.

      i. Speech in which ideas shift from one unrelated subject to another

      ii. Unaware that the topics are unconnected

      iii. If severe, speech may be incoherent

   b. Neologisms.

      i. Invention of new words that are meaningless to others but have symbolic meaning to the psychotic person

      ii. New meanings can also be assigned to existing words

   c. Concrete thinking.

      i. A literal interpretation of the environment, represents a regression to an earlier level of cognitive development

      ii. It is difficult for the client to think abstractly

DID YOU KNOW?

Expecting a client diagnosed with schizophrenia to interpret abstract sayings is unrealistic. Such a client would have great difficulty describing the abstract meaning of sayings such as "I'm climbing the walls" or "It's raining cats and dogs."

   d. Clang associations.

      i. Choice of words governed by sounds

      ii. Often take the form of rhyming

   e. Word salad.

      i. A group of words that are put together randomly

      ii. Words without any logical connection

   f. Circumstantiality.

      i. Unnecessary and tedious details delaying reaching the point of a communication

      ii. Needs to be constantly redirected to stay on track

   g. Tangentiality.

      i. Differs from circumstantiality in that the client never really gets to the point of the communication

      ii. Unrelated topics are introduced, and the focus of the original discussion is lost

   h. Mutism: an individual's inability or refusal to speak.

   i. Perseveration: persistently repeats the same word or idea in response to different questions.

5. Perception.

   a. **Hallucinations:** false sensory perceptions not associated with real external stimuli, involving any of the five senses. These perceptions are typically negative and disturbing in nature.

      i. Auditory

         a) The most common type of hallucination

         b) False perceptions of sound

         c) Most commonly voices

         d) May report clicks, rushing noises, music, and other noises

---

MAKING THE CONNECTION

When caring for a client experiencing hallucinations, it is critical to appreciate that the client is actually perceiving sensations not based in reality. Recognize that hallucinations are frightening and communicate an appreciation of the client's emotional reaction to the situation. Next, do not try to convince the client that he or she is not experiencing the hallucination but calmly present the objective reality. Then, redirect the client away from the altered sensory perception.

🛑 Command auditory hallucinations are voices that direct the client to say and/or do things. Asking the client what the voices are saying, without reinforcing the hallucination, enables the nurse to assess potentially dangerous situations. This is critical to the client's safety and the safety of others.

    ii. Visual
      1) False visual perceptions
      2) May consist of formed images, such as people, or of unformed images, such as flashes of light
    iii. Tactile
      1) False perceptions of the sense of touch
      2) Formication (a specific tactile hallucination): the sensation that something is crawling on or under the skin
    iv. Gustatory
      1) False perception of taste
      2) Described as unpleasant
    v. Olfactory
      1) False perceptions of the sense of smell
      2) Described as unpleasant
  b. **Illusions:** misperceptions or misinterpretations of real external stimuli.
6. Sense of self:
  a. Describes the uniqueness and individuality a person feels.
  b. Extremely weak ego boundaries lead to a lack of feeling of uniqueness.
  c. Confusion regarding identity.
  d. Echolalia.
    i. Repetition of words
    ii. An attempt to identify with the person speaking
  e. Echopraxia: purposelessly imitates movements made by others.
  f. Identification and imitation.
    i. Identification is an ego defense that occurs on an unconscious level
    ii. Imitation is an ego defense that occurs on a conscious level
    iii. Difficulty knowing where their ego boundaries end and another's begin
    iv. Behavior takes on the form of others

  g. Depersonalization: unstable self-identity may lead to feelings of unreality (e.g., feeling that one's extremities have changed in size; or a sense of seeing oneself from a distance).
I. **Negative symptoms**
  1. Reflect a diminution or loss of normal functions.

DID YOU KNOW?
Negative symptoms, functions that are missing, are the most difficult to treat and respond less well to antipsychotic medications. They are most debilitating because they render the client inert and unmotivated.

  2. Affect.
    a. Behavior associated with an individual's feeling state or emotional tone.
    b. Inappropriate affect: emotional tone is incongruent with circumstances.
    c. Bland affect: very weak emotional tone.
    d. Flat affect: void of emotional tone.
    e. Apathy: indifference to or disinterest in the environment.
  3. Impaired volition.
    a. Inability to initiate goal-directed activity (e.g., inadequate interest, motivation, or ability to choose a logical course of action).
    b. Emotional ambivalence.
      i. Coexistence of opposite emotions toward the same object, person, or situation
      ii. Interferes with the client's ability to make even a simple decision
    c. Deteriorated appearance.
      i. Neglected grooming and self-care activities
      ii. Appears disheveled and untidy
      iii. May need to be reminded of the need for personal hygiene
  4. Interpersonal function and relationship to the external world.
    a. Functioning reflected in social isolation.
    b. Emotional detachment.
    c. Lack of regard for social convention.
    d. Impaired social interaction:
      i. May cling to others and intrude on personal space
      ii. May exhibit unacceptable social and cultural behaviors
    e. Social isolation: focus inward on themselves and exclude the external environment.
  5. Psychomotor behavior.
    a. Anergia: a deficiency of energy; lacks sufficient energy to carry out activities of daily living or to interact with others.
    b. Waxy flexibility:
      i. Client allows body parts to be placed in bizarre or uncomfortable positions

ii. Once placed in position, the body part remains in that position for long periods, regardless of discomfort

🛑 A client experiencing waxy flexibility is in need of nursing care. Keeping a body part motionless for long periods of time can affect circulation and muscle strength and can cause muscle cramping. Range of motion exercises, if permitted by the client, can lessen or prevent these problems.

   c. Posturing: the voluntary assumption of inappropriate or bizarre postures.
   d. Pacing and rocking.
     i. Pacing back and forth
     ii. Body rocking (usually while sitting)
6. Associated features.
   a. Anhedonia.
     i. Inability to experience pleasure
     ii. Compels some clients to attempt suicide

b. Regression.
   i. The retreat to an earlier level of development
   ii. A primary defense mechanism of schizophrenia
   iii. A dysfunctional attempt to reduce anxiety
   iv. The basis for many of the behaviors associated with schizophrenia

V. Nursing Process: Diagnosis (Analysis)

Table 10.2 presents a list of client behaviors and the NANDA nursing diagnoses that correspond to those behaviors, which may be used in planning care for the client with a psychotic disorder.

Table 10.2 Assigning Nursing Diagnoses to Behaviors Commonly Associated With Psychotic Disorders

BEHAVIORS	NURSING DIAGNOSES
Impaired communication (inappropriate responses), disordered thought sequencing, rapid mood swings, poor concentration, disorientation, stops talking in midsentence, tilts head to side as if listening	Disturbed sensory perception*
Delusional thinking; inability to concentrate; impaired volition; inability to problem solve, engage in abstract thought, or conceptualize; extreme suspiciousness of others; inaccurate interpretation of the environment	Disturbed thought processes*
Withdrawal, sad dull affect, need-fear dilemma, preoccupation with own thoughts, expression of feelings of rejection or of aloneness imposed by others, uncommunicative, seeks to be alone	Social isolation
Risk factors: aggressive body language (e.g., clenching fists and jaw, pacing, threatening stance), verbal aggression, catatonic excitement, command hallucinations, rage reactions, history of violence, overt and aggressive acts, goal-directed destruction of objects in the environment, self-destructive behavior, or active aggressive suicidal acts	Risk for violence: self- or other-directed
Loose association of ideas, neologisms, word salad, clang associations, echolalia, verbalizations that reflect concrete thinking, poor eye contact, difficulty expressing thoughts verbally, inappropriate verbalization	Impaired verbal communication
Difficulty carrying out tasks associated with hygiene, dressing, grooming, eating, and toileting	Self-care deficit
Neglectful care of client in regard to basic human needs or illness treatment, extreme denial or prolonged overconcern regarding client's illness, depression, hostility and aggression	Disabled family coping
Inability to take responsibility for meeting basic health practices, history of lack of health-seeking behavior, lack of expressed interest in improving health behaviors, demonstrated lack of knowledge regarding basic health practices	Ineffective health maintenance
Unsafe, unclean, disorderly home environment, household members express difficulty in maintaining their home in a safe and comfortable condition	Impaired home maintenance

*These diagnoses have been resigned from the NANDA-I list of approved diagnoses. They are used in this instance because they are most compatible with the identified behaviors.

VI. Nursing Process: Planning

The following outcomes may be developed to guide the care of a client diagnosed with schizophrenia. **The client will:**

A. Not harm self or others
B. Demonstrate an ability to relate satisfactorily with others
C. Perceive self realistically
D. Demonstrate the ability to perceive the environment correctly
E. Recognize that false ideas occur at times of increased anxiety
F. Be able to differentiate between delusional thinking and reality
G. Be able to define and test reality with reduction in hallucinations
H. Recognize that auditory hallucinations are a result of his or her illness
I. Demonstrate ways to interrupt hallucinations
J. Maintain anxiety at a manageable level
K. Demonstrate the ability to trust others
L. Use appropriate verbal communication in interactions with others
M. Perform self-care activities independently

VII. Nursing Process: Implementation

A. Interventions for client's actively hallucinating
  1. Observe client for signs of hallucinations (listening pose, laughing or talking to self, stopping in midsentence).
  2. Avoid touching the client without warning.

🛑 A client who is actively hallucinating may perceive touch as threatening and may respond in an aggressive manner, causing harm to others.

  3. Accept the client and encourage to share the content of hallucinations.
  4. Do not reinforce the hallucination. Use "the voices" instead of words like "they" that imply validation.
  5. Let client know that you do not share the perception. Say, "Even though I realize the voices are real to you, I do not hear any voices speaking."

MAKING THE CONNECTION

Denying the client's belief or arguing with a hallucinating or delusional client serves no useful purpose because delusional ideas and/or hallucinations are not eliminated by this approach. This may also impede the development of a trusting relationship. Discussions that focus on the false ideas are purposeless and useless and may even aggravate the psychosis.

  6. Help the client understand the connection between increased anxiety and the presence of hallucinations.
  7. Distract the client from the hallucination.
  8. For persistent hallucinations, encourage client to listen to the radio, watch television, or hum a tune to distract him or her from the voices.

DID YOU KNOW?

An intervention called "voice dismissal" can be used to counteract persistent auditory hallucinations. With this technique, the client is taught to say loudly, "Go away!" or "Leave me alone!" in a conscious effort to dismiss the auditory perception.

B. Interventions for clients experiencing paranoid delusions
  1. Convey acceptance of client's need for the false belief but indicate that you do not share the belief.
  2. Do not argue or deny the belief. Use "reasonable doubt" as a therapeutic technique: "I understand that you believe this is true, but I personally find it hard to accept."
  3. Reinforce and focus on reality. Discourage long ruminations about the irrational thinking. Talk about real events and real people.
  4. If client is highly suspicious, the following interventions may be helpful:
    a. Use same staff; be honest and keep all promises.
    b. Avoid physical contact; warn client before touching to perform a procedure, such as taking a blood pressure.
    c. Avoid laughing, whispering, or talking quietly in client's presence.
    d. Provide canned food with can opener or serve food family style.
    e. Conduct mouth checks to verify that client is swallowing pills.
    f. Provide activities that encourage a one-to-one relationship with the nurse or therapist.
    g. Maintain an assertive, matter-of-fact, yet genuine approach.

DID YOU KNOW?

Suspicious clients often feel threatened by a friendly or overly cheerful attitude. They do not have the capacity to relate to this approach.

C. Interventions for socially isolated clients
  1. Convey an accepting attitude by making brief, frequent contacts.
  2. Show unconditional positive regard.
  3. Accompany client to groups and activities.
  4. Give recognition and positively reinforce client's voluntary interactions with others.

5. Encourage verbalization of fears.
6. Teach and role-play effective communication techniques.
D. Interventions for clients at risk for self-directed or other-directed violence
   1. Maintain low level of stimuli in client's environment (low lighting, few people, simple decor, low noise level).

🛈 A stimulating environment may increase anxiety levels. An anxious, suspicious, agitated client may perceive individuals as threatening and strike out defensively. Increased anxiety may also precipitate impulsive acts of self-harm.

   2. Observe client's behavior frequently while carrying out routine activities.
   3. Remove all dangerous objects from client's environment.
   4. Intervene at the first sign of increased anxiety, agitation or verbal or behavioral aggression. Offer empathetic responses: "You seem anxious (frustrated, angry) about this situation. How can I help?"
   5. Maintain a calm attitude. As the client's anxiety increases, offer some alternatives: participating in a physical activity (e.g., punching bag, physical exercise), talking about the situation, taking some antianxiety medication.

DID YOU KNOW?

The avenue of the "least restrictive alternative" must be selected when planning interventions for a potentially violent client. Restraints should be used only as a last resort after all other interventions have failed and the client is clearly at risk of harm to self or others.

   6. Have sufficient staff available to indicate a show of strength if necessary.
   7. If client does not respond to verbal interventions or medication, use of mechanical restraints may be necessary.
E. Interventions for clients with impaired communication
   1. Attempt to decode incomprehensible communication patterns. Seek validation and clarification. Example: "I don't understand what you mean by that. Would you please explain it to me?"
   2. Maintain staff assignments as consistently as possible.
   3. Anticipate and fulfill client's needs until functional communication pattern returns.
   4. Orient client to reality. Call the client by name. Validate those aspects of communication that help differentiate between what is real and not real.
   5. Provide explanations based on the client's level of comprehension. Example: "Pick up the spoon,

---

MAKING THE CONNECTION

If restraint is deemed necessary, ensure that sufficient staff members are available to assist. Follow institution protocols. The Joint Commission requires that an in-person evaluation by a physician or other licensed independent practitioner (LIP) be conducted within 1 hour of the initiation of the restraint or seclusion. The physician or LIP must reissue a new order for restraints every 4 hours for adults 18 years of age or older, every 2 hours for children and adolescents 9 to 17 years of age, and every 1 hour for children under 9 years of age. The Joint Commission requires that the client in restraints be continually observed and assessed at least every 15 minutes to ensure that circulation to extremities is not compromised (check temperature, color, pulses); to assist the client with needs related to nutrition, hydration, and elimination; and to position the client so that comfort is facilitated and aspiration is prevented. Some institutions may require continuous one-to-one monitoring of restrained clients, particularly those who are highly agitated and for whom there is a high risk of self- or accidental injury. As agitation decreases, assess the client's readiness for restraint removal or reduction. Remove one restraint at a time while assessing the client's response.

MAKING THE CONNECTION

When a client is mute (unable or unwilling to speak), the technique of *verbalizing the implied* is useful. Example: "That must have been a very difficult time for you when your mother left. You must have felt very alone."

---

scoop some mashed potatoes into it, and put it in your mouth."

DID YOU KNOW?

Because concrete thinking is a symptom of schizophrenia, abstract phrases and clichés must be avoided because they are likely to be misinterpreted.

F. Interventions for clients with self-care deficits
   1. Provide assistance with self-care needs as required.
   2. Encourage client to perform independently. Provide positive reinforcement for independent accomplishments.
   3. Use concrete communication to show client what is expected. Provide step-by-step instructions for assistance in performing activities of daily living. Example: "Take your pajamas off and put them in the drawer. Take your shirt and pants from the closet and put them on. Comb your hair and brush your teeth."

4. If the client is not eating, allow client to open his or her own canned or packaged foods, or serve food family style.
5. Establish a structured schedule for meeting toileting needs.

VIII. Nursing Process: Evaluation

Evaluation of the nursing actions for the client diagnosed with schizophrenia may be facilitated by gathering information using the following types of questions:

A. Has the client established trust with at least one staff member?
B. Is the anxiety level maintained at a manageable level?
C. Is delusional thinking still prevalent?
D. Is hallucinogenic activity evident? Does the client share content of hallucinations, particularly if commands are heard?
E. Is the client able to interrupt escalating anxiety with adaptive coping mechanisms?
F. Is the client easily agitated?
G. Is the client able to interact with others appropriately?
H. Does the client voluntarily attend therapy activities?
I. Is verbal communication comprehensible?
J. Is the client compliant with medication? Does the client verbalize the importance of taking medication regularly and on a long-term basis? Does he or she verbalize understanding of possible side effects and when to seek assistance from the physician?
K. Does the client spend time with others rather than isolating self?
L. Is the client able to carry out all activities of daily living independently?
M. Is the client able to verbalize resources from which he or she may seek assistance outside the hospital?
N. Does the client's family have information regarding support groups in which they may participate and from which they may seek assistance in dealing with their family member who is ill?
O. If the client lives alone, does he or she have a source for assistance with home maintenance and health management?

IX. Treatment Modalities

A. Psychological treatments
  1. Individual psychotherapy.
     a. Intensive psychodynamic- and insight-oriented psychotherapy is generally not recommended.
     b. Reality-oriented individual therapy is the most suitable approach.
     c. Primary focus is to decrease anxiety and increase trust.
     d. Establishing a relationship is difficult because the client with schizophrenia is desperately lonely yet defends against closeness and trust.
     e. Client is likely to respond to attempts at closeness with suspicion, anxiety, aggression, or regression.
     f. Successful intervention may be achieved with honesty, simple directness, and a manner that respects the client's privacy and human dignity.
     g. Exaggerated warmth and professions of friendship are likely to be met with confusion and suspicion.
     h. Individual psychotherapy paired with pharmacological treatment involves:
        i. Problem-solving
        ii. Reality testing
        iii. Psychoeducation
        iv. Supportive and cognitive-behavioral techniques
     i. Goal is to improve medication compliance, enhance social and occupational functioning, and prevent relapse.
     j. Individual psychotherapy is a long-term endeavor that requires patience, with the recognition that a great deal of change may not occur.
  2. Group therapy.
     a. Better success in outpatient setting when symptoms are in control.
     b. Can be intensive and highly stimulating so may be counterproductive early in treatment.
     c. Focuses on real-life plans, problems, and relationships.
     d. Supportive environment more helpful than a confrontational approach.
     e. Effective in:
        i. Reducing social isolation
        ii. Increasing the sense of cohesiveness
        iii. Improving reality testing
  3. Behavior therapy.
     a. Behavior modification has been successful in reducing bizarre, disturbing, and deviant behaviors and increasing appropriate behaviors.
     b. Features that have led to the most positive results include:
        i. Clearly defining goals and how they will be measured
        ii. Attaching positive, negative, and aversive reinforcements to adaptive and maladaptive behavior
        iii. Using simple, concrete instructions to elicit the desired behavior
     c. Limitation is the inability of some individuals with schizophrenia to generalize what they have

learned from the treatment setting to the community setting.

4. Social skills training.
   a. Social dysfunction is a hallmark of schizophrenia.
   b. Complex interpersonal skills involve the smooth integration of a combination of simpler behaviors, including:
      i. Nonverbal behaviors (facial expression, eye contact)
      ii. Paralinguistic features (voice loudness and affect)
      iii. Verbal content (the appropriateness of what is said)
      iv. Interactive balance (response latency, amount of time talking)
   c. These skills can be taught, and through the process of shaping (rewarding successful steps toward the target behavior), complex behavior can be acquired.
   d. Educational procedure focuses on role-play.
   e. Progress is geared toward the client's needs and limitations.
   f. Focus is on small units of behavior.
   g. Training proceeds gradually.
   h. Highly threatening issues are avoided.
   i. Emphasis is placed on functional skills that relate to activities of daily living.

B. Social treatments
   1. Milieu therapy.
      a. Emphasizes group and social interaction.
      b. Rules and expectations are mediated by peer pressure for normalization of adaptation.
      c. Needs to be combined with psychotropic medication.
      d. Necessary to have high staff-to-client ratio.
      e. Usually requires longer hospitalizations.
   2. Family therapy.
      a. Expanded role of family in the aftercare of relatives with schizophrenia.
      b. Family intervention programs are designed to:
         i. Support the family system
         ii. Prevent or delay relapse
         iii. Help to maintain the client in the community
      c. Programs treat the family as a resource rather than a stressor.
      d. Focus is on concrete problem-solving and specific helping behaviors for coping with stress.
      e. Programs are long term (usually 9 months to 2 years or more).
      f. Provide client and family with information about the illness and its management.
      g. Focus on improving adherence to prescribed medications.
      h. Strive to decrease stress in the family, and improve family functioning.

3. Program of Assertive Community Treatment (PACT).
   a. Program of case management that takes a team approach in providing comprehensive, community-based psychiatric treatment, rehabilitation, and support to persons with serious and persistent mental illness such as schizophrenia.

DID YOU KNOW?

The National Alliance on Mental Illness (NAMI) uses the terms "PACT" and "Assertive Community Treatment" ("ACT") interchangeably. Some states use other terms for this type of treatment, such as Mobile Treatment Teams (MTTs) and Community Support Programs (CSPs).

   b. Responsibilities shared by multiple team members: psychiatrists, nurses, social workers, vocational rehabilitation therapists, and substance abuse counselors.
   c. Services are provided in the person's home, within the neighborhood, in local restaurants, parks, stores, or wherever assistance is required.
   d. Services available 24 hours a day, 365 days a year.
   e. Aggressive programs of treatment individually tailored for each client.
   f. Teach basic living skills.
   g. Help clients work with community agencies.
   h. Assist clients in developing a social support network.
   i. Emphasis on vocational expectations and supported work settings (sheltered workshops).
   j. Substance abuse treatment.
   k. Psychoeducational programs.
   l. Family support and education.
   m. Mobile crisis intervention.
   n. Attention to health care needs.
   o. Goals.
      i. To meet basic needs and enhance quality of life
      ii. To improve functioning in adult social and employment roles
      iii. To enhance ability to live independently in the community
      iv. To lessen the family's burden of providing care
      v. To lessen or eliminate debilitating symptoms
      vi. To minimize or prevent recurrent acute episodes

C. Psychopharmacology
   1. Antipsychotic medications are effective in the treatment of acute and chronic manifestations of schizophrenia and in maintenance therapy to prevent exacerbation of schizophrenic symptoms.

DID YOU KNOW?

Antipsychotic medications are also called neuroleptics or major tranquilizers. Without drug treatment, an estimated 72% of individuals who have experienced a psychotic episode relapse within a year. This relapse rate can be reduced to about 23% with continuous medication administration.

2. Prognosis.
   a. One-third achieves significant and lasting improvement (may never experience another episode of psychosis).
   b. One-third may achieve some improvement with intermittent relapses and residual disability (occupational level may have decreased because of their illness, or they may be socially isolated).
   c. One-third experiences severe and permanent incapacity (do not respond to medication and remain severely ill for much of their lives).
   d. Men have poorer outcomes than women.
   e. Women respond better to treatment with antipsychotic medications.
   f. Efficacy of antipsychotic medications is enhanced by adjunct psychosocial therapy.
3. More cooperative with the psychosocial therapies when symptoms are controlled by neuroleptics.
4. Lag time for effectiveness (several weeks) can lead to nonadherence.
5. Classified as either "typical" (first generation, conventional antipsychotics) or "atypical" (newer, novel antipsychotics). See Table 10.3 for a list of antipsychotic agents.
6. Contraindications/precautions.
   a. Typical antipsychotics.
      i. Contraindicated with known hypersensitivity (cross-sensitivity with phenothiazines)

MAKING THE CONNECTION

Clients and families need to be taught that it takes several weeks for antipsychotics to effectively treat positive symptoms. Appreciating the importance of waiting is critical to medication adherence.

Table 10.3 Antipsychotic Agents

Category	Generic (Trade Name)	Pregnancy Categories/ Half-Life (hr)	Daily Dosage Range (mg)
Typical Antipsychotic Agents (first generation, conventional)	Chlorpromazine	C/24	40–400
	Fluphenazine	C/HCl: 18 hr; decanoate: 6.8–9.6 days	2.5–10
	Haloperidol (Haldol)	C/~18 (oral); ~3 wk (intramuscular decanoate)	1–100
	Loxapine	C/8	20–250
	Perphenazine	C/9–12	12–64
	Pimozide (Orap)	C/~55	1–10
	Prochlorperazine	C/3–5 (oral), 6.9 (intravenous)	15–150
	Thioridazine	C/24	150–800
	Thiothixene (Navane)	C/34	6–30
	Trifluoperazine	C/18	4–40
Atypical Antipsychotic Agents (second generation; novel)	Aripiprazole (Abilify)	C/75–146	10–30
	Asenapine (Saphris)	C/24	10–20
	Clozapine (Clozaril)	B/8 (single dose); 12 (at steady state)	300–900
	Iloperidone (Fanapt)	C/18–33	12–24
	Lurasidone (Latuda)	B/18	40–80
	Olanzapine (Zyprexa)	C/21–54	5–20
	Paliperidone (Invega)	C/23	6–12
	Quetiapine (Seroquel)	C/~6	300–400
	Risperidone (Risperdal)	C/3–20	4–8
	Ziprasidone (Geodon)	C/~7 (oral); 2–5 (intramuscular)	40–160

   ii. Should not be used:
1) In comatose states
2) When central nervous system (CNS) depression is evident
3) When blood dyscrasias exist
4) In clients with Parkinson's disease or narrow-angle glaucoma
5) In clients with liver, renal, or cardiac insufficiency
6) In clients with poorly controlled seizure disorders
7) In elderly clients with dementia-related psychosis

   iii. Thioridazine, pimozide, and haloperidol have been shown to prolong the QT interval and are contraindicated if the client is taking other drugs that also produce this side effect

   iv. Caution with the elderly, severely ill, or debilitated clients

   v. Caution with diabetic clients or clients with respiratory insufficiency, prostatic hypertrophy, or intestinal obstruction

   vi. Antipsychotics may lower seizure threshold

   vii. Clients should avoid exposure to extreme temperatures

   viii. Safety in pregnancy and lactation has not been established

b. Atypical antipsychotics.
   i. Contraindicated in hypersensitivity, comatose, or severely depressed clients

   ii. Contraindicated with elderly clients with dementia-related psychosis

   iii. Contraindicated with lactation

   iv. Ziprasidone, risperidone, paliperidone, asenapine, and iloperidone are contraindicated in clients with a history of QT prolongation or cardiac arrhythmias, recent myocardial infarction (MI), uncompensated heart failure, and concurrent use with other drugs that prolong the QT interval

   v. Clozapine is contraindicated in clients with myeloproliferative disorders, with a history of clozapine-induced agranulocytosis or severe granulocytopenia, and with uncontrolled epilepsy

   vi. Lurasidone is contraindicated in concomitant use with strong inhibitors of cytochrome P450 isozyme 3A4 (CYP3A4) (e.g., ketoconazole) and strong CYP3A4 inducers (e.g., rifampin)

   vii. Caution in administering these drugs to elderly or debilitated clients

   viii. Caution with clients with cardiac, hepatic, or renal insufficiency

   ix. Caution with clients with a history of seizures, diabetes, or risk factors for diabetes

   x. Clients should avoid exposure to extreme temperatures

   xi. Caution with conditions that cause hypotension (dehydration, hypovolemia, treatment with antihypertensive medication)

   xii. Not recommended for pregnant clients or children (safety not established)

7. Interactions.
a. Typical antipsychotics.
   i. Additive hypotensive effects with antihypertensive agents

   ii. Additive CNS effects with CNS depressants

   iii. Additive anticholinergic effects when taken with drugs that have anticholinergic properties

   iv. Phenothiazines may reduce the effectiveness of oral anticoagulants

   v. Concurrent use of phenothiazines or haloperidol with epinephrine or dopamine may result in severe hypotension

   vi. Additive effects of QT prolongation occur when haloperidol, thioridazine, or pimozide are taken concurrently with other drugs that prolong the QT interval

   vii. Pimozide is contraindicated with CYP3A inhibitors, and thioridazine is contraindicated with cytochrome P450 isozyme 2D6 (CYP2D6) inhibitors

   viii. Concurrent use of haloperidol and carbamazepine results in decreased therapeutic effects of haloperidol and increased effects of carbamazepine

b. Atypical antipsychotics.
   i. Additive hypotensive effects when taken with antihypertensive agents

   ii. Additive CNS effects with CNS depressants

   iii. Additive anticholinergic effects when risperidone or paliperidone are taken with other drugs that have anticholinergic properties

   iv. Additive effects of QT prolongation occur when ziprasidone, risperidone, paliperidone, asenapine, and iloperidone are taken with other drugs that prolong the QT interval

   v. Decreased effects of levodopa and dopamine agonists occur with concurrent use of ziprasidone, olanzapine, quetiapine, risperidone, or paliperidone

vi. Increased effects of ziprasidone, clozapine, quetiapine, aripiprazole, lurasidone, and iloperidone occur with CYP3A4 inhibitors

vii. Decreased effects of lurasidone occur with CYP3A4 inducers

viii. Increased effects of iloperidone with CYP2D6 inhibitors

ix. Decreased effects of ziprasidone, clozapine, olanzapine, risperidone, paliperidone, asenapine, and aripiprazole occur with cytochrome P450 isozyme 1A2 (CYP1A2) inducers, and increased effects occur with CYP1A2 inhibitors

x. Concurrent use of asenapine and paroxetine results in decreased therapeutic effects of asenapine and increased effects of paroxetine

xi. Additive orthostatic hypotension occurs with risperidone, paliperidone, or iloperidone and other drugs

8. Side effects.
   a. Related to blockage of a number of receptors.
      i. Blockage of the dopamine receptors controls positive symptoms
      ii. Dopamine blockage also results in **extrapyramidal symptoms** (EPS) and prolactin elevation (galactorrhea; gynecomastia)
      iii. Cholinergic blockade causes anticholinergic side effects (dry mouth, blurred vision, constipation, urinary retention, tachycardia)
      iv. Blockage of the alpha$_1$-adrenergic receptors produces dizziness, orthostatic hypotension, tremors, and reflex tachycardia
      v. Histamine blockade is associated with weight gain and sedation
   b. A profile of side effects comparing various antipsychotic medications is presented in Table 10.4.
   c. Stopping an antipsychotic drug abruptly after long-term use might produce withdrawal symptoms, such as nausea, vomiting, dizziness, gastritis, headache, tachycardia, insomnia, tremulousness.

Table 10.4 Comparison of Side Effects Among Antipsychotic Agents

Class	Generic (Trade) Name	EPS†	Sedation	Anti-cholinergic	Orthostatic Hypotension	Weight Gain
Typical Antipsychotic Agents	Chlorpromazine	3	4	3	4	*
	Fluphenazine	5	2	2	2	
	Haloperidol (Haldol)	5	2	2	2	
	Loxapine	3	2	2	2	*
	Perphenazine	4	2	2	2	*
	Pimozide (Orap)	4	2	3	2	*
	Prochlorperazine	3	2	2	2	*
	Thioridazine	2	4	4	4	*
	Thiothixene (Navane)	4	2	2	2	*
	Trifluoperazine	4	2	2	2	*
Atypical Antipsychotic Agents	Aripiprazole (Abilify)	1	2	1	3	2
	Asenapine (Saphris)	1	3	1	3	4
	Clozapine (Clozaril)	1	5	5	4	5
	Iloperidone (Fanapt)	1	3	2	3	3
	Lurasidone (Latuda)	1	3	1	3	3
	Olanzapine (Zyprexa)	1	3	2	2	5
	Paliperidone (Invega)	1	2	1	3	2
	Quetiapine (Seroquel)	1	3	1	3	4
	Risperidone (Risperdal)	1	2	1	3	4
	Ziprasidone (Geodon)	1	3	1	2	2

Key: 1 = Very low; 2 = Low; 3 = Moderate; 4 = High; 5 = Very high. EPS = extrapyramidal symptoms
* Weight gain occurs, but incidence is unknown.
Source: Adapted from Black & Andreasen (2011); *Drug Facts and Comparisons* (2012); Schatzberg, Cole, & DeBattista (2010).

d. Smoking increases the metabolism of antipsychotics, requiring an adjustment in dosage to achieve a therapeutic effect.

e. Body temperature is harder to maintain. Exposure to very high or low temperatures should be avoided.

f. Alcohol potentiates the effects of antipsychotics.

g. Many medications (including over-the-counter products) contain substances that interact in a harmful way with antipsychotics.

h. Safe use of antipsychotics during pregnancy has not been established. Antipsychotics cross the placental barrier potentially affecting the fetus.

i. Anticholinergic effects and nursing interventions.
  i. Dry mouth
    1) Provide sugarless candy or gum, ice, and frequent sips of water
    2) Ensure client practices strict oral hygiene
  ii. Blurred vision
    1) Explain that this symptom is transient lasting only a few weeks
    2) Advise client not to drive a car until vision clears
    3) Clear small items from pathway to prevent falls
  iii. Constipation
    1) Encourage foods high in fiber
    2) Promote increased physical activity
    3) Increase fluid intake if not contraindicated
  iv. Urinary retention
    1) Instruct client to report any difficulty urinating
    2) Monitor intake and output

j. Nausea; gastrointestinal (GI) upset (may occur with all classifications) and Nursing Interventions.
  i. Administer medications with food to minimize GI upset
  ii. Dilute concentrates and administer with fruit juice or other liquid; mix immediately before administration

k. Skin rash (may occur with all classifications) and Nursing Interventions.
  i. Report any rash on skin to physician
  ii. Avoid spilling liquid concentrate on skin; may cause contact dermatitis

l. Sedation and Nursing Interventions.
  i. Advocate for administering the drug at bedtime
  ii. Advocate for a possible dosage decrease or a change to a less sedating drug
  iii. Instruct client not to drive or operate dangerous equipment while experiencing sedation

m. Orthostatic hypotension and Nursing Interventions.
  i. Instruct client to rise slowly from a lying or sitting position

  ii. Monitor blood pressure (lying and standing) each shift; document and report significant changes

n. Photosensitivity (may occur with all classifications) and Nursing Interventions.
  i. Ensure the use of sunblock
  ii. Encourage the use of protective clothing and sunglasses

o. Hormonal effects (may occur with all classifications, but more common with typical antipsychotics) and Nursing Interventions.
  i. Decreased libido, retrograde ejaculation, gynecomastia (men)
    1) Explain the effects and reassure of reversibility
    2) If necessary, advocate for alternate medication
  ii. Amenorrhea (women) and Nursing Interventions
    1) Reassure of reversibility
    2) Instruct client to continue use of contraception, because amenorrhea does not indicate cessation of ovulation
  iii. Weight gain (may occur with all classifications; has been problematic with the atypical antipsychotics) and Nursing Interventions
    1) Weigh client every other day
    2) Order calorie-controlled diet
    3) Provide opportunity for physical exercise
    4) Provide diet and exercise instruction

p. Electrocardiogram (ECG) changes and Nursing Interventions.
  i. Monitor vital signs every shift
  ii. Observe for symptoms of dizziness, palpitations, syncope, weakness, dyspnea, and peripheral edema

q. Reduction of seizure threshold (more common with the typical than the atypical

MAKING THE CONNECTION

ECG changes, including prolongation of the QT interval, are possible with most antipsychotic medications. This is particularly true with ziprasidone, thioridazine, pimozide, haloperidol, paliperidone, iloperidone, asenapine, and clozapine. Caution is advised in prescribing these medications to individuals with history of arrhythmias. Conditions that produce hypokalemia and/or hypomagnesemia, such as diuretic therapy or diarrhea, should be taken into consideration when prescribing. Routine ECG should be administered before initiation of therapy and periodically during therapy. Clozapine has also been associated with other cardiac events, such as ischemic changes, arrhythmias, congestive heart failure, myocarditis, and cardiomyopathy.

antipsychotics, with the exception of clozapine) and Nursing Interventions.
   i. Closely observe clients with history of seizures
   ii. Particularly important with clients taking clozapine (Clozaril)

🛑 Seizures have been frequently associated with the administration of clozapine. Dose appears to be an important predictor, with a greater likelihood of seizures occurring at higher doses. Extreme caution is advised in prescribing clozapine for clients with a history of seizures.

   r. Agranulocytosis (more common with the typical than the atypical antipsychotics, with the exception of clozapine).
      i. Usually occurs within the first 3 months of treatment
         a) Observe for symptoms of sore throat, fever, malaise
         b) Monitor complete blood count if these symptoms appear

🛑 There is a significant risk of agranulocytosis with clozapine (Clozaril). Agranulocytosis is a potentially fatal blood disorder in which the client's white blood cell (WBC) count can drop to extremely low levels. A baseline WBC count and absolute neutrophil count (ANC) must be taken before initiation of treatment with clozapine and weekly for the first 6 months of treatment. Only a 1-week supply of medication is dispensed at a time. If the counts remain within the acceptable levels (i.e., WBC at least 3500/mm^3 and the ANC at least 2000/mm^3) during the 6-month period, blood counts may be monitored biweekly, and a 2-week supply of medication may then be dispensed. If the counts remain within the acceptable level for the biweekly period, counts may then be monitored every 4 weeks thereafter. When the medication is discontinued, weekly WBC counts are continued for an additional 4 weeks.

   s. Hypersalivation (most common with clozapine).

DID YOU KNOW?

A significant number of clients receiving clozapine (Clozaril) therapy experience extreme salivation. Not only is this an embarrassing situation, it is an extremely visible sign that the client is being treated with antipsychotic drugs. It may also be a safety issue (risk of aspiration) if the problem is severe. Management has included the use of sugar-free gum to increase the swallowing rate and medications such as an anticholinergic (scopolamine patch) or alpha$_2$-adrenoceptor agonist (clonidine) to directly decrease salivation.

   t. Extrapyramidal symptoms and Nursing Interventions.
      i. Observe for symptoms and report
      ii. Administer antiparkinsonian drugs, as ordered (see Table 10.5)

   iii. EPS symptoms
      a) Pseudoparkinsonism (tremor, shuffling gait, drooling, rigidity)
         • Symptoms may appear 1 to 5 days after initiation of antipsychotic medication
         • Occurs most often in women, the elderly, and dehydrated clients
      b) Akinesia (muscular weakness)
         • Symptoms may appear 1 to 5 days after initiation of antipsychotic medication
         • Occurs most often in women, the elderly, and dehydrated clients
      c) Akathisia (continuous restlessness and fidgeting)
         • Occurs most frequently in women
         • Symptoms may occur 50 to 60 days after initiation of therapy
      d) Dystonia (involuntary muscular movements [spasms] of face, arms, legs, and neck)
         • Occurs most often in men
         • Occurs in people younger than 25 years of age
      e) Oculogyric crisis (uncontrolled rolling back of the eyes)
         • May appear as part of the syndrome called dystonia
         • May be mistaken for seizure activity

🛑 Dystonia and/or oculogyric crisis are emergency situations. Notify the physician immediately upon assessment of these symptoms. Expect the physician to order intravenous benztropine mesylate (Cogentin) and stay with client and offer reassurance and support.

      f) Tardive dyskinesia (TD) (bizarre facial and tongue movements, stiff neck, and difficulty swallowing; may occur with all classifications, but more common with typical antipsychotics).
         • All clients receiving long-term (months or years) antipsychotic therapy are at risk
         • Symptoms are potentially irreversible
         • Withdraw drug at first sign of TD (usually vermiform movements of the tongue)
         • Prompt action may prevent irreversibility

MAKING THE CONNECTION

The terms "akinesia" and "akathisia" are similar sounding but have very different meanings. Akinesia is the descriptive term for "muscular weakness," and akathisia is the descriptive term for "continuous restlessness and fidgeting." To differentiate these terms, you can associate "weak knees" with akinesia (aki-*knees*-ia).

Table 10.5 Antiparkinsonian Agents Used to Treat Extrapyramidal Side Effects of Antipsychotic Drugs

Indication	Used to treat parkinsonism of various causes and drug-induced extrapyramidal reactions.
Action	Restores the natural balance of acetylcholine and dopamine in the central nervous system. The imbalance is a deficiency in dopamine that results in excessive cholinergic activity.
Contraindications/Precautions	Antiparkinsonian agents are contraindicated in individuals with hypersensitivity. Anticholinergics should be avoided by individuals with angle-closure glaucoma; pyloric, duodenal, or bladder neck obstructions; prostatic hypertrophy; or myasthenia gravis.
	Caution should be used in administering these drugs to clients with hepatic, renal, or cardiac insufficiency; elderly and debilitated clients; those with a tendency toward urinary retention; or those exposed to high environmental temperatures.
Common side effects	Anticholinergic effects (dry mouth, blurred vision, constipation, paralytic ileus, urinary retention, tachycardia, elevated temperature, decreased sweating), nausea/gastrointestinal upset, sedation, dizziness, orthostatic hypotension, exacerbation of psychoses.

Chemical Class	Generic (Trade Name)	Pregnancy Categories/ Half-Life (hr)	Daily Dosage Range (mg)
Anticholinergics	Benztropine (Cogentin)	C/UKN	1–8
	Biperiden (Akineton)	C/18.4–24.3	2–6
	Trihexyphenidyl	C/5.6–10.2	1–15
Antihistamines	Diphenhydramine (Benadryl)	C/4–15	25–200
Dopaminergic Agonists	Amantadine	C/10–25	200–300

MAKING THE CONNECTION

The Abnormal Involuntary Movement Scale (AIMS) is a rating scale that was developed to measure involuntary movements associated with tardive dyskinesia. The AIMS aids in early detection of movement disorders and provides a means for ongoing surveillance. The AIMS assessment tool, examination procedure, and interpretation of scoring are presented in Box 10.2.

  u. Neuroleptic malignant syndrome (NMS) (more common with the typical than the atypical antipsychotics) and Nursing Interventions.
   i. Relatively rare
   ii. Potentially fatal
   iii. Assessments should include temperature and observation for parkinsonian symptoms
   iv. Onset can occur within hours or up to years after drug initiation
   v. Progression can be rapid over 24 to 72 hours
   vi. Symptoms include:
    1) Severe parkinsonian muscle rigidity
    2) Very high fever
    3) Tachycardia

    4) Tachypnea
    5) Fluctuations in blood pressure
    6) Diaphoresis
    7) Rapid deterioration of mental status to stupor and coma

🛑 The rapid deterioration of mental status that accompanies NMS can be misinterpreted as worsening symptoms of schizophrenia. This can lead to physicians increasing dosages of antipsychotic medications. If NMS is the cause of this deterioration, higher dosages of antipsychotics can be life threatening. Look for other symptoms such as high fever and muscle rigidity to determine whether the problem is NMS.

   vii. Discontinue antipsychotic medications and notify physician immediately
   viii. Monitor vital signs, degree of muscle rigidity, intake and output, level of consciousness
   ix. Bromocriptine (Parlodel) or dantrolene (Dantrium) may be ordered to counteract the effects of NMS
  v. Hyperglycemia and diabetes (more common with atypical antipsychotics) and Nursing Interventions.
   i. Monitor clients diagnosed with diabetes regularly for worsening glucose control

Box 10.2 Abnormal Involuntary Movement Scale (AIMS)

Name _____ **Rater Name** _____

Date _____

Instructions: Complete the examination procedure before making ratings. For movement ratings, circle the highest severity observed. Rate movements that occur on activation one *less* than those observed spontaneously. Circle movement as well as code number that applies.

Code: 0 = None

1 = Minimal, may be normal

2 = Mild

3 = Moderate

4 = Severe

Facial and Oral Movements	**1. Muscles of Facial Expression** (e.g., movements of forehead, eyebrows, periorbital area, cheeks, including frowning, blinking, smiling, grimacing)	0 1 2 3 4
	2. Lips and Perioral Area (e.g., puckering, pouting, smacking)	0 1 2 3 4
	3. Jaw (e.g., biting, clenching, chewing, mouth opening, lateral movement)	0 1 2 3 4
	4. Tongue (Rate only increases in movement both in and out of mouth. NOT inability to sustain movement. Darting in and out of mouth.)	0 1 2 3 4
Extremity Movements	**5. Upper (arms, wrists, hands, fingers)** (Include choreic movements (i.e., rapid, objectively purposeless, irregular, spontaneous) and athetoid movements (i.e., slow, irregular, complex serpentine). *Do not include tremor* (i.e., repetitive, regular, rhythmic)	0 1 2 3 4
	6. Lower (legs, knees, ankles, toes) (e.g., lateral knee movement, foot tapping, heel-dropping, foot squirming, inversion and eversion of foot)	0 1 2 3 4
Trunk Movements	**7. Neck, shoulders, hips** (e.g., rocking, twisting, squirming, pelvic gyrations)	0 1 2 3 4
Global Judgments	**8. Severity of abnormal movements overall**	0 1 2 3 4
	9. Incapacitation due to abnormal movements	0 1 2 3 4
	10. Patient's awareness of abnormal movements (Rate only the client's report) No awareness Aware, no distress Aware, mild distress Aware, moderate distress Aware, severe distress	0 1 2 3 4
Dental Status	**11. Current problems with teeth and/or dentures?**	No Yes
	12. Are dentures usually worn?	No Yes
	13. Edentia?	No Yes
	14. Do movements disappear in sleep?	No Yes

Continued

| Box 10.2 | AIMS Examination Procedure—cont'd |

Either before or after completing the Examination Procedure, observe the client unobtrusively, at rest (e.g., in waiting room). The chair to be used in this examination should be a hard, firm one without arms.

1. *Ask client to remove shoes and socks.*
2. *Ask client whether there is anything in his or her mouth (e.g., gum, candy, etc.), and if there is, to remove it.*
3. *Ask client about the current condition of his or her teeth. Ask client if he or she wears dentures. Do teeth or dentures bother client now?*
4. *Ask client whether he or she notices any movements in mouth, face, hands, or feet. If yes, ask to describe and to what extent they currently bother client or interfere with his or her activities.*
5. *Have client sit in chair with both hands on knees, legs slightly apart, and feet flat on floor. (Look at entire body for movements while in this position.)*
6. *Ask client to sit with hands hanging unsupported. If male, between legs, if female and wearing a dress, hanging over knees. (Observe hands and other body areas.)*
7. *Ask client to open mouth. (Observe tongue at rest within mouth.) Do this twice.*
8. *Ask client to protrude tongue. (Observe abnormalities of tongue movement.) Do this twice.*
9. *Ask client to tap thumb with each finger as rapidly as possible for 10 to 15 seconds, separately with right hand then with left hand. (Observe facial and leg movements.)*
10. *Flex and extend client's left and right arms (one at a time). (Note any rigidity.)*
11. *Ask client to stand up. (Observe in profile. Observe all body areas again, hips included.)*
12. *Ask client to extend both arms outstretched in front with palms down. (Observe trunk, legs, and mouth.)*
13. *Have client walk a few paces, turn, and walk back to chair. (Observe hands and gait.) Do this twice.*

Interpretation of AIMS Score

Add client scores and note areas of difficulty.
Score of:
- *0 to 1 = Low risk*
- *2 in only ONE of the areas assessed = borderline/observe closely*
- *2 in TWO or more of the areas assessed **or** 3 to 4 in ONLY ONE area = indicative of TD*

Source: U.S. Department of Health and Human Services. Available for use in the public domain.

ii. Clients with risk factors for diabetes should undergo fasting blood glucose testing at the beginning of treatment and periodically thereafter

iii. All clients taking these medications should be monitored for symptoms of hyperglycemia (polydipsia, polyuria, polyphagia, and weakness) and should undergo fasting blood glucose testing if necessary

w. Increased risk of mortality in elderly clients with dementia-related psychosis.

🛑 Causes of death in the elderly who are taking antipsychotic medications are commonly related to infections or cardiovascular problems. All antipsychotic drugs now carry black-box warnings to this effect. They are not approved for treatment of elderly clients with dementia-related psychosis.

REVIEW QUESTIONS

1. A nurse is assessing a client diagnosed with paranoid schizophrenia for the presence of hallucinations. Which therapeutic communication technique used by the nurse is an example of "making observations"?
   1. "I notice that you are talking to someone who I do not see."
   2. "Please tell me what they are telling you."
   3. "Why do you continually look up at the ceiling?"
   4. "I understand that you see someone in the hall, but I do not see anyone."

2. A nurse would recognize which medication as most effective in providing a client immediate relief from neuroleptic-induced extrapyramidal side effects (EPS)?
   1. Lorazepam (Ativan) 1 mg by mouth (PO)
   2. Diazepam (Valium) 5 mg PO
   3. Haloperidol (Haldol) 2 mg intramuscular (IM)
   4. Benztropine (Cogentin) 2 mg PO

3. To deal with a client's hallucinations therapeutically, which nursing intervention should be implemented?
   1. Reinforce the perceptual distortions until the client develops new defenses
   2. Provide an unstructured environment
   3. Avoid making connections between anxious situations and hallucinations
   4. Distract the client's attention

4. A client is experiencing paranoid delusions. What behaviors could the nurse expect to assess?
   1. Altered speech and extreme suspiciousness
   2. Psychomotor retardation
   3. Regressive and primitive behaviors
   4. Anger and aggressive acts

5. A client diagnosed with schizophrenia experiences identity confusion and communicates with the nurse using echolalia. What is the client attempting to do by using this form of speech?
   1. Identify with the person speaking
   2. Imitate the nurse's movements
   3. Alleviate alogia
   4. Alleviate avolition

6. _____ are false personal beliefs that are inconsistent with the person's intelligence or cultural background.

7. Family members ask the nurse about their relative's chance of a positive outcome after being diagnosed with schizophrenia. Which of the following information should the nurse provide the family? **Select all that apply.**
   1. Good premorbid functioning can predict a positive outcome.
   2. Early age of onset can predict a positive outcome.
   3. Being male can predict a positive outcome.
   4. An abrupt onset of symptoms can predict a positive outcome.
   5. An associated mood disturbance can predict a positive outcome.

8. A client diagnosed with schizophrenia states, "Look, color, hate me, get away, yes, yes." Which is an appropriate charting entry to describe this client's statement?
   1. "The client is experiencing command hallucinations."
   2. "The client is verbalizing a neologism."
   3. "The client is experiencing a delusion of control."
   4. "The client is verbalizing a word salad."

9. Which of the following nursing interventions would correctly follow the Joint Commission's requirements for monitoring a hallucinating client while in restraints? **Select all that apply.**
   1. Ensure that an in-person evaluation has occurred within 1 hour of restraint initiation.
   2. Ensure that a new restraint order has been reissued for a child every one to 2 hours.
   3. Ensure that a new restraint order has been reissued for an adult every 6 hours.
   4. Observe the client at least every 30 minutes.
   5. Observe the adolescent client at least every 15 minutes.

10. _____ symptoms of schizophrenias tend to reflect an alteration or distortion of normal mental functions.

11. Place the following symptoms in the order they would occur in the schizophrenia spectrum phases of development.
    1. _____ The client experiences sleep disturbance, anxiety, and depressed mood.
    2. _____ The client's acute symptoms are either absent or no longer prominent.
    3. _____ The client experiences social maladjustment and social withdrawal.
    4. _____ The client's psychotic symptoms are prominent.

12. Which of the following personality disorders are most commonly susceptible to the diagnosis of *brief psychotic disorder*? **Select all that apply.**
    1. Antisocial personality disorder
    2. Paranoid personality disorder
    3. Borderline personality disorder
    4. Schizoid personality disorder
    5. Histrionic personality disorder

13. During an admission assessment, a nurse asks a client diagnosed with schizophrenia, "Have you ever felt that certain objects or persons have control over your behavior?" The nurse is assessing for which type of thought disruption?
    1. Delusions of persecution
    2. Delusions of influence
    3. Delusions of reference
    4. Delusions of grandeur

14. A nurse admits a client who is exhibiting delusional thinking, auditory hallucinations, incoherent speech, suicidal ideations, and a mood rating of 2 out of 10. Given this clinical picture, the client is manifesting symptoms in which diagnostic category?
    1. Paranoid schizophrenia
    2. Brief psychotic disorder
    3. Schizoaffective disorder
    4. Schizophreniform disorder

15. A client states, "I can't go into my bathroom because I saw a demon in the tub." Which nursing diagnosis reflects this client's problem?
    1. Self-care deficit
    2. Ineffective health maintenance
    3. Disturbed sensory perception
    4. Disturbed thought processes

16. The nurse is interacting with a client diagnosed with schizophrenia. Number the nurse's interventions in the correct sequence.
    _____3_____ Present and refocus on reality
    _____5_____ Educate the client about the disease process
    _____1_____ Establish a trusting nurse-client relationship
    _____2_____ Empathize with the client about feelings generated by disease symptoms
    _____4_____ Encourage compliance with antipsychotic medications

17. A client has been adherent with olanzapine (Zyprexa) 4 mg QHS for the past year. On assessment, the nurse notes that the client has bizarre facial and tongue movements. Which is a priority nursing intervention?
    1. With the next dose of olanzapine (Zyprexa), give the ordered prn dose of benztropine (Cogentin).
    2. Notify the physician of the observed side effects, place a hold on the Zyprexa, and request discontinuation of the medication.
    3. Ask the physician to increase the dose of Zyprexa to assist with the bizarre behaviors.
    4. Explain to the client that these side effects are temporary and should subside in 2 to 3 weeks.

18. A client diagnosed with schizophrenia exhibits a flat affect, apathy, and avolition. Which medication should a nurse expect a physician to order to address these symptoms?
    1. Olanzapine (Zyprexa) to address these negative symptoms
    2. Haloperidol (Haldol) to address these positive symptoms
    3. Risperidone (Risperdal) to address these positive symptoms
    4. Chlorpromazine (Thorazine) to address these negative symptoms

19. A nurse has received a client's white blood cell count (WBC) result. Which client was most likely to have had this blood work ordered?
    1. A client diagnosed with schizophrenia prescribed aripiprazole (Abilify)
    2. A client diagnosed with schizophrenia prescribed clozapine (Clozaril).
    3. A client diagnosed with schizophrenia prescribed haloperidol (Haldol)
    4. A client diagnosed with schizophrenia prescribed risperidone (Risperdal)

20. Which of the following are negative symptoms of schizophrenia that are categorized as psychomotor behavior? **Select all that apply.**
    1. Anergia
    2. Apathy
    3. Waxy flexibility
    4. Emotional ambivalence
    5. Posturing

REVIEW ANSWERS

1. ANSWER: 1

Rationale:

1. The nurse is using the communication technique of *making an observation* when stating, "I notice that you are talking to someone that I do not see." Making observations involves verbalizing what is observed or perceived. This encourages the client to recognize specific behaviors and make comparisons with the nurse's perceptions.

2. The nurse is using the communication technique of *exploring*, not *making observations* when stating, "Please tell me what they are telling you." *Exploring* helps the nurse to gather information related to a subject, idea, experience or relationship. Also by using the term "they," the nurse has inadvertently validated the client's hallucination. Better to ask, "What are the voices telling you?"

3. The nurse is using the communication block of *requesting an explanation,* not *making an observation,* when asking, "Why do you continually look up at the ceiling?" *Requesting an explanation* asks the client to provide the reasons for thoughts, feelings, behavior, and events. Asking "why" a client did something or feels a certain way can be intimidating and implies that the client must defend his or her behavior or feelings.

4. The nurse is using the communication technique of *presenting reality,* not *making an observation* when stating, "I understand that you see someone in the hall, but I do not see anyone." *Presenting reality* indicates the nurse's perception of the situation when a client is out of touch with objective reality.

TEST-TAKING TIP: Review the communication techniques presented in Chapter 5 of this text.
Content Area: Safe and Effective Care Environment: Management of Care;
Integrated Process: Nursing Process: Implementation;
Client Need: Safe and Effective Care Environment: Management of Care;
Cognitive Level: Application
Concept: Cognition

2. ANSWER: 4

Rationale:

1. Ativan is an anxiolytic medication used for the management of anxiety and/or insomnia, not for relief of EPS.

2. Valium is an anxiolytic medication used for the management of anxiety, preoperative sedation, and conscious sedation, not for relief of EPS.

3. Haldol is an antipsychotic medication used for acute and chronic psychotic disorders. One of this drug's side effects is EPS. To give more Haldol would only increase the intensity of EPS.

4. The symptoms of neuroleptic induced EPS include, but are not limited to, tremors, chorea, dystonia, akinesia, and akathisia. Cogentin 1 to 4 mg given once or twice daily is the drug of choice to treat these symptoms.

TEST-TAKING TIP: Understand that EPS is a side effect of antipsychotic or neuroleptic medications. This knowledge would immediately eliminate Option 3.

Content Area: Safe and Effective Care Environment: Management of Care;
Integrated Process: Nursing Process: Implementation;
Client Need: Safe and Effective Care Environment: Management of Care;
Cognitive Level: Application;
Concept: Medication

3. ANSWER: 4

Rationale:

1. Hallucinations should never be reinforced.

2. A client experiencing hallucinations needs a structured, not unstructured, environment. A structured environment can decrease confusion and may decrease disorganized thinking.

3. The nurse should help the client to see relationships between anxiety-producing situations and the onset of hallucinations. Exploring this relationship should not be avoided.

4. The nurse should first empathize with the client by focusing on feelings generated by the hallucination, present objective reality, and then distract or redirect the client to reality-based activities.

TEST-TAKING TIP: Review the appropriate nursing interventions for clients experiencing hallucinations.
Content Area: Safe and Effective Care Environment: Management of Care;
Integrated Process: Nursing Process: Implementation;
Client Need: Safe and Effective Care Environment: Management of Care;
Cognitive Level: Application
Concept: Cognition

4. ANSWER: 4

Rationale:

1. Clients experiencing paranoia do exhibit suspicious behaviors. But although thoughts may be disorganized during delusional thinking, speech is rarely altered.

2. Clients experiencing catatonic schizophrenia exhibit motor behavior abnormalities. Clients experiencing paranoid delusions do not usually exhibit these behaviors.

3. Clients experiencing disorganized thinking may exhibit regressive and primitive behaviors. Clients experiencing paranoid delusions do not usually exhibit these behaviors.

4. Clients experiencing paranoid delusions are often angry, aggressive, and guarded due to their belief that others are threatening harm. Angry and aggressive behaviors are the client's attempt to protect self from this fictitious threat.

TEST-TAKING TIP: Remember that if two parts of an answer are presented in a multiple-choice option, both parts must be correct for the answer to be acceptable.
Content Area: Safe and Effective Care Environment: Management of Care;
Integrated Process: Nursing Process: Assessment;
Client Need: Safe and Effective Care Environment: Management of Care;
Cognitive Level: Application
Concept: Assessment

5. ANSWER: 1

Rationale:

1. **Echolalia is a parrot-like repetition of overheard words or fragments of speech. It is an attempt by the client to identify with the person who is speaking.**

2. The term used for imitating a person's movements is echopraxia, not echolalia. The client in the question is not demonstrating this imitating motor behavior.

3. The term "alogia," when used in the context of describing the symptoms of schizophrenia, refers to a severe limitation of speech. The client in the question is not demonstrating this limitation and therefore does not need to alleviate the problem.

4. Avolition is a lack of initiative and goal-directed activities. The client in the question is not demonstrating a lack of motivation and therefore does not need to alleviate the problem.

TEST-TAKING TIP: Review the various types of schizophrenia symptoms under the *Nursing Process: Assessment* section of this chapter.

Content Area: Safe and Effective Care Environment: Management of Care;

Integrated Process: Nursing Process: Assessment;

Client Need: Safe and Effective Care Environment: Management of Care;

Cognitive Level: Application

Concept: Cognition

6. ANSWER: Delusions

Rationale: Delusions are false personal beliefs that are inconsistent with the person's intelligence or cultural background. The individual continues to have the belief despite obvious proof that it is false or irrational.

TEST-TAKING TIP: To understand this definition, review the key words at the beginning of this chapter.

Content Area: Psychosocial Integrity;

Integrated Process: Nursing Process: Assessment;

Client Need: Psychosocial Integrity;

Cognitive Level: Knowledge;

Concept: Cognition

7. ANSWERS: 1, 4, 5

Rationale:

1. **Good premorbid functioning is a factor associated with positive outcomes for clients diagnosed with schizophrenia.**

2. A later age of onset, not an early age of onset, is a factor associated with positive outcomes for clients diagnosed with schizophrenia.

3. Being female, not male, is a factor associated with positive outcomes for clients diagnosed with schizophrenia.

4. **An abrupt onset of symptoms is a factor associated with positive outcomes for clients diagnosed with schizophrenia.**

5. **Having an associated mood disturbance is a factor associated with positive outcomes for clients diagnosed with schizophrenia.**

TEST-TAKING TIP: Review the factors associated with positive outcomes for clients diagnosed with schizophrenia.

Content Area: Psychosocial Integrity;

Integrated Process: Nursing Process: Evaluation;

Client Need: Psychosocial Integrity;

Cognitive Level: Application;

Concept: Cognition

8. ANSWER: 4

Rationale:

1. The situation presented in the question does not indicate that the client is experiencing command hallucinations. Command hallucinations are "voices" that issue commands that may include violent acts.

2. The situation presented in the question does not indicate that the client is verbalizing a neologism. A neologism is when a client invents a new word that is meaningless to others but may have symbolic meaning to the client.

3. The situation presented in the question does not indicate that the client is experiencing a delusion of control. A delusion of control or influence refers to the individual's belief that certain objects or persons have control over his or her behavior.

4. **The nurse should chart that the client is verbalizing a word salad. A word salad refers to a group of words that are put together randomly without any logical connection.**

TEST-TAKING TIP: Review the positive symptoms of schizophrenia and be able to distinguish the various forms of thought that are affected by this disease.

Content Area: Safe and Effective Care Environment: Management of Care;

Integrated Process: Nursing Process: Assessment;

Client Need: Safe and Effective Care Environment: Management of Care;

Cognitive Level: Application

Concept: Cognition

9. ANSWERS: 1, 2, 5

Rationale:

1. **The Joint Commission requires that an in-person evaluation by a physician or other licensed independent practitioner (LIP) be conducted within 1 hour of the initiation of the restraint or seclusion. This nursing intervention would correctly follow The Joint Commission's requirements for monitoring a hallucinating client while in restraints.**

2. **The physician or LIP must reissue a new order for restraints every 4 hours for adults and every 1 to 2 hours for children and adolescents. This nursing intervention would correctly follow The Joint Commission's requirements for monitoring a hallucinating client while in restraints.**

3. The physician or LIP must reissue a new order for restraints every 4, not 6, hours for adults and every 1 to 2 hours for children and adolescents. This nursing intervention does *not* correctly follow The Joint Commission's requirements for monitoring a hallucinating client while in restraints.

4. The Joint Commission requires that the client in restraints be observed at least every 15, not 30, minutes to ensure that circulation to extremities is not compromised (check temperature, color, pulses); to assist the client with needs related to nutrition, hydration, and elimination; and to position the client so that comfort is facilitated and aspiration is prevented.

5. **The Joint Commission requires that all clients in restraints be observed at least every 15 minutes to ensure that circulation to extremities is not compromised (check temperature, color, pulses); to assist the client with needs**

related to nutrition, hydration, and elimination; and to position the client so that comfort is facilitated and aspiration is prevented. This nursing intervention would correctly follow the Joint Commission's requirements for monitoring a hallucinating client while in restraints.
TEST-TAKING TIP: Review the Joint Commission's requirements for caring for a client in restraints.
Content Area: Safe and Effective Care Environment: Management of Care;
Integrated Process: Nursing Process: Implementation;
Client Need: Safe and Effective Care Environment: Management of Care;
Cognitive Level: Application
Concept: Nursing

10. **ANSWER: Positive**
Rationale: Positive symptoms of schizophrenia tend to reflect an alteration or distortion of normal mental functions. Positive symptoms are associated with normal brain structures on computed tomography (CT) scan and relatively good responses to treatment. Some examples of positive symptoms are delusions and hallucinations.
TEST-TAKING TIP: To understand this definition, review the key words at the beginning of this chapter.
Content Area: Psychosocial Integrity;
Integrated Process: Nursing Process: Assessment;
Client Need: Psychosocial Integrity;
Cognitive Level: Knowledge;
Concept: Cognition

11. **ANSWER: The correct order is 2, 4, 1, 3**
Rationale: The pattern of development of schizophrenia may be viewed in four phases: the premorbid phase, the prodromal phase, the active psychotic phase (schizophrenia), and the residual phase.
1. Premorbid phase (the premorbid personality often indicates social maladjustment, social withdrawal, irritability, and antagonistic thoughts and behavior).
2. Prodromal phase (the prodrome of an illness refers to certain signs and symptoms that precede the characteristic manifestations of the acute, fully developed illness like sleep disturbance, anxiety, and depressed mood).
3. Active psychotic phase (in the active phase of the disorder, psychotic symptoms are prominent).
4. Residual phase (a residual phase usually follows an active phase of the illness. During the residual phase, symptoms of the acute stage are either absent or no longer prominent).
TEST-TAKING TIP: Review the phases through which schizophrenia spectrum develops.
Content Area: Safe and Effective Care Environment: Management of Care;
Integrated Process: Nursing Process: Assessment;
Client Need: Safe and Effective Care Environment: Management of Care;
Cognitive Level: Analysis;
Concept: Cognition

12. **ANSWERS: 2, 3, 5**
Rationale:
1. Individuals with preexisting personality disorders (most commonly, histrionic, narcissistic, paranoid,

schizotypal, and borderline personality disorders), *not* antisocial personality disorder, appear to be susceptible to *brief psychotic disorder.*
2. **Individuals with preexisting personality disorders such as paranoid personality disorder appear to be susceptible to *brief psychotic disorder.***
3. **Individuals with preexisting personality disorders such as borderline personality disorder appear to be susceptible to *brief psychotic disorder.***
4. Individuals with preexisting personality disorders (most commonly, histrionic, narcissistic, paranoid, schizotypal, and borderline personality disorders), *not* schizoid personality disorder, appear to be susceptible to *brief psychotic disorder.*
5. **Individuals with preexisting personality disorders such as histrionic personality disorder appear to be susceptible to *brief psychotic disorder.***
TEST-TAKING TIP: Review the assessment data presented about brief psychotic disorder presented in this chapter.
Content Area: Safe and Effective Care Environment: Management of Care;
Integrated Process: Nursing Process: Assessment;
Client Need: Safe and Effective Care Environment: Management of Care;
Cognitive Level: Application;
Concept: Self

13. **ANSWER: 2**
Rationale:
1. An individual experiencing a delusion of persecution, irrationally and without cause, believes that he or she is being persecuted or malevolently treated in some way. The nurse's question does not assess for the presence of a persecutory delusion.
2. **The nurse in the question is assessing the client for delusions of influence when asking whether the client has ever felt that objects or persons have control of his or her behavior. Delusions of control or influence occur when the client believes that behavior is being externally controlled. An example would be if a client believes that a hearing aid receives transmissions that control thoughts and behaviors.**
3. An individual experiencing a delusion of reference believes that all events within the environment are referring to him or her. The nurse's question does not assess for the presence of delusions of reference.
4. An individual experiencing a grandiose delusion has irrational ideas regarding his or her own worth, talent, knowledge, or power. The nurse's question does not assess for the presence of grandiose delusions.
TEST-TAKING TIP: Review the positive symptoms of schizophrenia and be able to distinguish the various thought content that is affected by this disease.
Content Area: Safe and Effective Care Environment: Management of Care;
Integrated Process: Nursing Process: Assessment;
Client Need: Safe and Effective Care Environment: Management of Care;
Cognitive Level: Application;
Concept: Cognition

14. ANSWER: 3

1. A client diagnosed with paranoid schizophrenia exhibits delusions of persecution or grandeur. Auditory hallucinations related to a persecutory theme may be present. The client is tense, suspicious, and guarded and may be argumentative, hostile, and aggressive. These symptoms are not described in the question. The auditory hallucinations experienced by the client in the question are not described as persecutory in nature.

2. The essential feature of brief psychotic disorder is the sudden onset of psychotic symptoms that may or may not be preceded by a severe psychosocial stressor. These symptoms last at least 1 day but less than 1 month, and there is eventual full return to the premorbid level of functioning. There is no mood component to the symptoms experienced during a brief psychotic disorder.

3. Schizoaffective disorder is manifested by schizo-phrenic behaviors with a strong element of symptoms associated with the mood disorders (mania or depression). The client may appear depressed with suicidal ideations. When the mood disorder has been assessed, the decisive factor in the diagnosis is the presence of characteristic schizophrenia symptoms, such as delusional thinking, prominent hallucinations, or incoherent speech.

4. The essential features of schizophreniform disorder are identical to schizophrenia, with the exception that the duration is at least 1 month but less than 6 months. There is no mood component to the symptoms experienced in schizophreniform disorder.

TEST-TAKING TIP: The clinical picture of schizoaffective disorder must include *both* psychotic and mood symptoms. All the other diagnostic categories presented in the answer choices do not include mood symptoms and can be eliminated.

Content Area: Safe and Effective Care Environment: Management of Care;
Integrated Process: Nursing Process: Evaluation;
Client Need: Safe and Effective Care Environment: Management of Care;
Cognitive Level: Application;
Concept: Cognition

15. ANSWER: 3

Rationale:

1. *Self-care deficit* is defined as the impaired ability to perform or complete activities of daily living. The hallucination that the client is experiencing may affect the client's self-care, but the presenting symptom, a visual hallucination, is not directly related to a self-care deficit problem.

2. *Ineffective health maintenance* is defined as the inability to identify, manage, or seek out help to maintain health. Noncompliance with antipsychotic medications is one form of ineffective health maintenance that is common in clients diagnosed with thought disorders, but there is no indication that the client described in the question has this problem.

3. *Disturbed sensory perception* is defined as a change in the amount or patterning of incoming stimuli (either internally or externally initiated), accompanied by a diminished, exaggerated, distorted, or impaired response to such stimuli. The client's statement in the question indicates that the client is experiencing a visual hallucination, which is an example of a disturbed sensory perception.

4. *Disturbed thought processes* is defined as the disruption in cognitive operations and activities. An example of a disturbed thought process is a delusion. The client's statement in the question is an example of a visual hallucination, a disturbed sensory perception, not a disturbed thought process.

TEST-TAKING TIP: Differentiate disturbed thought processes from disturbed sensory perceptions to answer this question correctly. Disturbed sensory perceptions predominantly refer to hallucinations, which are false sensory perceptions not associated with real external stimuli. Disturbed thought processes refer predominantly to delusions, which are false beliefs.

Content Area: Safe and Effective Care Environment: Management of Care;
Integrated Process: Nursing Process: Evaluation;
Client Need: Safe and Effective Care Environment: Management of Care;
Cognitive Level: Analysis;
Concept: Cognition

16. ANSWER: The correct sequence of nursing interventions is 3, 5, 1, 2, 4.

Rationale:

(1) The establishment of a trusting nurse-client relationship should be the first nursing intervention because all further interventions will be affected by the trust the client has for the nurse. (2) Empathizing with the client helps the nurse to connect with the client and further enhances trust. (3) Presenting reality in a matter-of-fact way helps the client to distinguish what is real from what is not. (4) Encouraging compliance with antipsychotic medications helps to decrease symptoms of the disorder and increases the client's cooperation with psychosocial therapies. (5) Educating the client about the disease process comes later in the therapeutic plan of care. A trusting nurse-client relationship has to be established and the client needs to be stabilized before initiating any effective teaching.

TEST-TAKING TIP: Understand that the establishment of trust is the basis for any other effective nursing intervention. Educating the client would be later in the therapeutic process because trust must be established and the client's symptoms must be stabilized for learning to occur.

Content Area: Safe and Effective Care Environment: Management of Care;
Integrated Process: Nursing Process: Evaluation;
Client Need: Safe and Effective Care Environment: Management of Care;
Cognitive Level: Analysis;
Concept: Nursing

17. ANSWER: 2

Rationale:

1. Bizarre facial and tongue movements, stiff neck, and difficulty swallowing all are signs of tardive dyskinesia (TD). All clients receiving long-term antipsychotic medications, from months to years, are at risk. The symptoms are potentially permanent, and the medication should be discontinued as soon as symptoms are noted. Benztropine (Cogentin), an anticholinergic medication, works for extrapyramidal symptoms, such as pseudoparkinsonism (tremor, shuffling gait, drooling, and rigidity), akinesia (muscular weakness), akathisia (restlessness and fidgeting),

dystonia (involuntary muscular movements or spasms of the face, arms, legs, and neck), and oculogyric crisis (uncontrolled rolling back of the eyes). If the nurse continues to administer olanzapine, the TD will continue to worsen and have the potential to be irreversible.

2. When the nurse notes signs of TD, the nurse should notify the physician of the observed side effects and the hold placed on the Zyprexa and request discontinuation of the medication. It is important for nurses to assess for the beginning signs of TD throughout antipsychotic therapy to avoid permanent damage.

3. These bizarre behaviors are not signs of psychosis, and if more olanzapine is given, the symptoms may worsen and potentially become irreversible.

4. TD can be a permanent side effect of long-term antipsychotic medications; however, if the medication is discontinued immediately when symptoms arise, the chance decreases that TD will become permanent. Because this answer does not mention discontinuing the medication, it is incorrect.

TEST-TAKING TIP: Recognize that in Option 1, giving benztropine may be appropriate; however, if the nurse continues to give the olanzapine, TD could become irreversible. Recognize that if one part of the answer is incorrect, the entire answer is incorrect.

Content Area: Safe and Effective Care Environment: Management of Care;
Integrated Process: Nursing Process: Evaluation;
Client Need: Safe and Effective Care Environment: Management of Care;
Cognitive Level: Analysis;
Concept: Medication

18. **ANSWER: 1**
Rationale:
1. The nurse should expect the physician to order olanzapine to address the negative symptoms of schizophrenia. Olanzapine is an atypical antipsychotic used to reduce negative symptoms, including flat affect (lack of emotional reactivity), apathy (indifference to or disinterest in the environment), and avolition (general lack of drive or motivation to pursue meaningful goals). Negative symptoms do not respond well to any medication, but the atypical drugs (like olanzapine) do better than the older typical antipsychotics, such as chlorpromazine.

2. The symptoms presented in the question are negative, not positive symptoms.

3. The symptoms presented in the question are negative, not positive symptoms.

4. Negative symptoms do not respond well to any medication, but the atypical drugs (like olanzapine) do better than the older typical antipsychotics, such as chlorpromazine.

TEST-TAKING TIP: Negative symptoms of schizophrenia do not respond well to antipsychotic drugs. The newer, second-generation, atypical antipsychotic medications are more effective than the older, typical, first-generation medications. Also recognize that if one part of the answer is incorrect, the entire answer is incorrect.

Content Area: Safe and Effective Care Environment: Management of Care;
Integrated Process: Nursing Process: Evaluation;
Client Need: Safe and Effective Care Environment: Management of Care;

Cognitive Level: Application;
Concept: Medication

19. **ANSWER: 2**
Rationale:
1. There is no indication to perform a white blood cell count on a client diagnosed with schizophrenia taking Abilify.

2. Clozapine can have a serious side effect of agranulocytosis, in which a potentially fatal drop in white blood cells can occur. It is appropriate to monitor white blood cell count on clients receiving this medication.

3. There is no indication to perform a white blood cell count on a client diagnosed with schizophrenia taking Haldol.

4. There is no indication to perform a white blood cell count on a client diagnosed with schizophrenia taking Risperdal.

TEST-TAKING TIP: Review the side effects of antipsychotic medications.

Content Area: Safe and Effective Care Environment: Management of Care;
Integrated Process: Nursing Process: Evaluation;
Client Need: Safe and Effective Care Environment: Management of Care;
Cognitive Level: Application;
Concept: Medication

20. **ANSWERS: 1, 3, 5**
Rationale:
1. Anergia is a deficiency of energy. The client lacks sufficient energy to carry out activities of daily living or to interact with others. Anergia is a negative symptom of schizophrenia categorized as psychomotor behavior.

2. Apathy is defined as indifference to or disinterest in the environment. Apathy is a negative symptom of schizophrenia, but it is categorized under affect, not psychomotor behavior.

3. Waxy flexibility is when a client allows body parts to be placed in bizarre or uncomfortable positions. Once placed in position, the body part remains in that position for long periods, regardless of discomfort. Waxy flexibility is a negative symptom of schizophrenia categorized as psychomotor behavior.

4. Emotional ambivalence is the coexistence of opposite emotions toward the same object, person, or situation. Emotional ambivalence interferes with the client's ability to make even a very simple decision. It is a negative symptom of schizophrenia, but it is categorized under impaired volition, not psychomotor behavior.

5. Posturing is the voluntary assumption of inappropriate or bizarre postures. Posturing is a negative symptom of schizophrenia categorized as psychomotor behavior.

TEST-TAKING TIP: Review the positive and negative symptoms of schizophrenia.

Content Area: Psychosocial Integrity;
Integrated Process: Nursing Process: Assessment;
Client Need: Psychosocial Integrity;
Cognitive Level: Application;
Concept: Cognition

CASE STUDY: Putting it All Together

Monique is a 30-year-old woman who received gastric lavage and was stabilized in the emergency department after she was found by her sister, unconscious with an empty pill bottle by her side. On the psychiatric unit, Monique's sister tells the psychiatric nurse practitioner (PNP), Ms. Williams, that Monique had stopped taking her medications and had been threatening suicide ever since losing custody of her three young children to her ex-husband. The sister also tells Ms. Williams that when Monique was a teenager, she began acting paranoid and often heard voices that told her to do bad things. She also said that when Monique was 17 years old, she was hospitalized, given medication, and told never to stop taking the pills. The sister claims that after that, Monique was able to finish high school, graduate from college, get married, and have three children. However, she relates that over the past 2 years things seemed to have fallen apart. The sister also tells Ms. Williams that their father was, in the past, institutionalized for "bizarre" behavior.

During the initial assessment, Ms. Williams notes that Monique's affect is hostile, her eyes dart around the room, and her lips silently move as if interacting with someone. As Ms. Williams approaches, Monique screams out, "Are you the one having an affair with my husband, or are you the one who kidnapped my kids?" Once reassurance and prn medication take effect, Monique is reoriented, begins to understand what happened, and agrees to talk about her problems. She tells Ms. Williams that she knows that she should never have stopped taking her meds but states, "I hate taking them. They increase my food appetite and decrease my sex appetite. I think that's what ended my marriage. Now the voices are telling me that my ex has paid off someone to kill me. First I lost my husband and then my kids. I just don't care anymore." In a very soft monotone, Monique whispers, "Please help me. I love my kids and want them back."

1. On the basis of these symptoms and client actions, what medical diagnosis would Ms. Williams assign to Monique?
2. What predisposing factors may have led to Monique's disorder?
3. What are Monique's subjective symptoms that would lead to the determination of this diagnosis?
4. What are Monique's objective symptoms that would lead to the determination of this diagnosis?
5. What NANDA nursing diagnosis would address Monique's current problem?
6. On the basis of this nursing diagnosis, what short-term outcome would be appropriate for Monique?
7. On the basis of this nursing diagnosis, what long-term outcome would be appropriate for Monique?
8. List the psychological treatments the PNP might employ to treat Monique.
9. What classification of medications might be prescribed for the long-term treatment of Monique's symptoms?
10. List the nursing interventions (actions) that will assist Monique in successfully meeting these outcomes.
11. List the questions that should be asked to determine the success of the nursing interventions.

Chapter 11

Depression

KEY TERMS

Affect—A behavioral expression of emotion; may be appropriate (congruent to the situation); constricted or blunted (diminished range of intensity); or flat (absence of emotional expression)

Apathy—An affective alteration exhibited by a lack of emotion and interest; listless condition; unconcern; indifference; observed in clients diagnosed with severe depression

Automatic thoughts—Thoughts that occur rapidly in response to a situation and without rational analysis; they are often negative and based on erroneous logic

Bereavement overload—An accumulation of grief that occurs when an individual experiences many losses over a short period of time and is unable to resolve one before another is experienced; this phenomenon is common among the elderly

"Black box" label warning for antidepressants—An advisory issued by the Federal Drug Administration (FDA) warning the public about the increased risk of suicidal thoughts and behavior in children and adolescents being treated with antidepressant medications

Cognitive therapy—A form of therapy in which the individual is taught to control thought distortions that are considered to be a factor in the development and maintenance of emotional disorders

Depression—An alteration in mood that is expressed by feelings of sadness, despair, and pessimism

Disruptive mood dysregulation disorder (DMDD)—DMMD in children is a chronic, severe, and persistent irritability; this irritability is often displayed by the child as a temper tantrum or temper outburst that occurs frequently (three or more times per week)

Dysthymia—A chronically depressed or dysphoric mood

Failure to thrive—A condition in which infants and children not only fail to gain weight but also may lose it; a contributing factor may be emotional deprivation as a result of parental withdrawal, rejection, or hostility

Melancholia—A profoundly painful dejection, cessation of interest in the outside world, loss of the capacity to love, inhibition of all activity, and a lowering of self-regarding feelings to a degree that self-reproach and self-reviling culminate in a delusional expectation of punishment

Mood—An individual's sustained emotional tone, which significantly influences behavior, personality, and perception

Persistent Depressive Disorder (dysthymia)—Formerly known as dysthymic disorder, the essential feature of this disorder is a depressed mood that occurs for most of the day, for more days than not, for at least 2 years (at least 1 year for children and adolescents)

Postpartum depression—A period of heightened maternal emotions that follow the birth of a baby, typically beginning in the first three to 5 days after childbirth but occurring any time within the first year postpartum

Premenstrual dysphoric disorder—Characterized by symptoms such as a markedly depressed mood, anxiety, affective lability, and decreased interest in activities

Psychomotor retardation—A generalized slowing of physical and mental reactions; seen frequently in depression, intoxications, and other conditions

Tyramine—An intermediate product in the conversion of tyrosine to epinephrine; tyramine is found in cheeses and in beer, broad bean pods, yeast, wine, and chicken liver

Depression is likely the oldest and still one of the most frequently diagnosed psychiatric illnesses. Symptoms of depression have been described almost as far back as there is evidence of written documentation. An occasional bout with the "blues," a feeling of sadness or downheartedness, is common among healthy people and considered to be a normal response to everyday disappointments in life. These episodes are short-lived as the individual adapts to the loss, change, or failure (real or perceived) that has been experienced. Pathological depression occurs when adaptation is ineffective.

I. Epidemiology

A. Major depressive disorder (MDD) is one of the leading causes of disability in the United States
B. More than 1 in 25 adults reported a major depressive episode with severe impairment
C. Twenty-one percent of women and 13% of men will become clinically depressed at some point during their lifetime

DID YOU KNOW?
The widespread occurrence of depression has led researchers to consider the disorder "the common cold of psychiatric disorders" and this generation the "age of **melancholia**."

D. Age and gender
  1. MDD more prevalent in women than men by almost 2 to 1.
  2. Women experience more depression than men beginning at about age 10 and continuing through midlife.
  3. The gender difference is less pronounced between ages 44 and 65.
  4. After age 65, women are again more likely to be depressed than men.
  5. May be related to gender stereotypes and gender socialization.
     a. "Feminine" characteristics (helplessness, passivity, and emotionality) are associated with depression.
     b. Research suggests that "masculine" characteristics are associated with higher self-esteem and less depression.
E. Social class

DID YOU KNOW?
Research shows that both depression and personality disorders are associated with low socioeconomic status. However, it has not yet been determined whether poor socioeconomic conditions predispose people to mental disability or if mental disabilities predispose people to poor socioeconomic conditions.

F. Race and culture
  1. No *consistent* relationship between race and depression has been established, but depression is more prevalent in whites than in blacks.
  2. Research is ongoing.
  3. Clinicians underdiagnose mood disorders in clients who have racial or cultural backgrounds different from their own.

Misdiagnosis of depression may result from language barriers between clients and physicians who are unfamiliar with the cultural aspects of nonwhite clients' behavior and language.

G. Marital status
  1. Studies suggest that marriage has a positive effect on psychological well-being.
  2. Studies suggest that the effect of marital status on depression may be contingent on age, with a protective effect against major depression only in the oldest age category (65+).
H. Seasonality
  1. Two prevalent periods of seasonal involvement:
     a. Spring (March, April, and May).
     b. Fall (September, October, and November).
  2. Congruent with suicide patterns, which peak in spring and decrease in the fall
  3. Theories include:
     a. Drastic temperature and barometric pressure changes affect mental instability.
     b. Biochemical variables related to seasonal variations in serotonergic function.

II. Types of Depressive Disorders

A. Major depressive disorder (MDD)
  1. Characterized by:
     a. Depressed **mood** or loss of interest or pleasure in usual activities.
     b. An **affect** that expresses sadness.

DID YOU KNOW?
Mood describes an individual's emotional feeling tone. It is a subjective symptom that can only be described by the individual. *Affect* is the expression of emotion. It is an objective symptom that can be observed. Mood and affect are not always congruent. People can present a happy face while experiencing extreme sadness.

     c. **Apathy:** a state of indifference, unconcern, and listlessness.
     d. Impaired social and occupational functioning for at least 2 weeks.
     e. No history of manic behavior.
     f. Symptoms that cannot be attributed to substances or medical condition.

g. Whether depression is a single episode or recurrent.
2. Diagnosis may also note:
   a. Degree of severity (mild, moderate, or severe).
   b. Evidence of psychotic, catatonic, or melancholic features.
   c. Presence of anxiety.
   d. Severity of suicide risk.
B. Persistent depressive disorder
1. Persists for most of the day, more days than not, for at least 2 years (1 year for children or adolescents).
2. Similar to, but milder form of, MDD.
3. Early onset, occurring before age 21 years.
4. Chronic, irritable mood observed in children or adolescents.
5. Late onset, occurring at age 21 years or later.
6. Mood described as chronically feeling sad or "down in the dumps."
C. Premenstrual dysphoric disorder
1. Essential features include markedly depressed mood, excessive anxiety, mood swings, and decreased interest in activities.
2. Occurs the week before menses and subsides shortly after the onset of menstruation.
D. Substance-induced depressive disorder
1. Depressive symptoms are the direct result of a substance.
2. Depressive symptoms may cause impairment in social, occupational, or other areas of functioning.
3. Substances from which intoxication or withdrawal evokes mood symptoms:
   a. Alcohol.
   b. Amphetamines.
   c. Cocaine.
   d. Hallucinogens.
   e. Opioids.
   f. Phencyclidine-like substances.
   g. Sedatives, hypnotics, or anxiolytics.
E. Medications that may evoke mood symptoms include:
1. Anesthetics.
2. Analgesics.
3. Anticholinergics.
4. Anticonvulsants.
5. Antihypertensives.
6. Antiparkinsonian agents.
7. Antiulcer agents.
8. Cardiac medications.
9. Oral contraceptives.
10. Psychotropic medications.
11. Muscle relaxants.
12. Steroids.
13. Sulfonamides.

F. Depressive disorder due to another medical disorder
1. Characterized by depressive symptoms associated with direct physiological effects of another medical condition.
2. Depressive symptoms may cause impairment in social, occupational, or other areas of functioning.

III. Predisposing Factors

A. Biological theories (genetics)
1. Research suggests a genetic link.
2. The heritability of recurrent major depression is approximately 37% in monozygotic twins.
3. MDD is more common among first-degree biological relatives than among the general population.

DID YOU KNOW?
Studies show that biological children of parents with mood disorders are at higher risk of developing the disorder, even if adoptive parents who do not have the disorder raise them.

B. Biochemical influences (neurotransmitters)
1. Precise role of neurotransmitters is unknown.
2. Neurotransmitter deficiencies that may contribute to the disorder include (see Fig. 11-1):
   a. Norepinephrine: key component in ability to deal with stressful situations.
   b. Serotonin: regulates mood, anxiety, arousal, vigilance, irritability, thinking, cognition, appetite, aggression, and circadian rhythm.
   c. Dopamine: thought to exert strong influence over mood and behavior.
   d. Acetylcholine: contributes to arousal, attention span, and REM sleep.
C. Neuroendocrine disturbances
1. Persistent depressive illness noted with endocrine disease.
2. Disturbance of mood noted with the administration of certain hormones.
3. Hypothalamic-pituitary-adrenocortical axis disturbance.
   a. Normal system of hormonal inhibition fails.
   b. This failure results in hypersecretion of cortisol.
   c. Cortisol level is basis for dexamethasone suppression test to determine whether client has somatically treatable depression.
4. Hypothalamic-pituitary-thyroid axis disturbance.
   a. Thyrotropin-releasing factor (TRF) stimulates the release of thyroid-stimulating hormone (TSH).
   b. TSH stimulates the thyroid gland.
   c. Diminished TSH response to administered TRF is observed in approximately 25% of depressed persons.
   d. Test has potential for identifying clients at high risk for affective disorders.

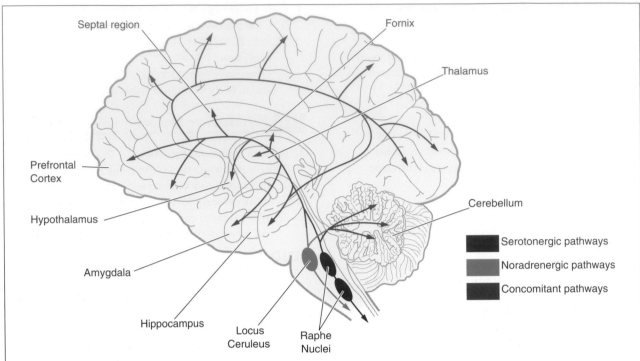

Fig 11.1 Neurobiology of depression.

NEUROTRANSMITTERS

Although other neurotransmitters have also been implicated in the pathophysiology of depression, distur-bances in serotonin and norepinephrine have been the most extensively scrutinized.

Cell bodies of origin for the serotonin pathways lie within the raphe nuclei located in the brainstem. Those for norepinephrine originate in the locus ceruleus. Projections for both neurotransmitters extend throughout the forebrain, prefrontal cortex, cerebellum, and limbic system.

AREAS OF THE BRAIN AFFECTED

Areas of the brain affected by depression and the symptoms that they mediate include the following:

- Hippocampus: memory impairments, feelings of worthlessness, hopelessness, and guilt
- Amygdala: anhedonia, anxiety, reduced motivation
- Hypothalamus: increased or decreased sleep and appetite; decreased energy and libido
- Other limbic structures: emotional alterations
- Frontal cortex: depressed mood; problems concentrating
- Cerebellum: psychomotor retardation/agitation

MEDICATIONS AND THEIR EFFECTS ON THE BRAIN

All medications that increase serotonin, norepinephrine, or both can improve the emotional and vegetative symptoms of depression. Medications that produce these effects include those that block the presynaptic reuptake of the neurotransmitters or block receptors at nerve endings (tricyclics, SSRIs, SNRIs) and those that inhibit monoamine oxidase, an enzyme that is involved in the metabolism of the monoamines serotonin, norepinephrine, and dopamine (MAOIs).

Side effects of these medications relate to their specific neurotransmitter receptor-blocking action. Tricyclic and tetracyclic drugs (e.g., imipramine, amitriptyline, mirtazapine) block reuptake and/or receptors for sero-tonin, norepinephrine, acetylcholine, and histamine. SSRIs are selective serotonin reuptake inhibitors. Others, such as bupropion, venlafaxine, and duloxetine, block serotonin and norepinephrine reuptake, and also are weak inhibitors of dopamine.

Blockade of norepinephrine reuptake results in side effects of tremors, cardiac arrhythmias, sexual dysfunc-tion, and hypertension. Blockade of serotonin reuptake results in side effects of gastrointestinal disturbances, in-creased agitation, and sexual dysfunction. Blockade of dopamine reuptake results in side effects of psychomotor activation. Blockade of acetylcholine reuptake results in dry mouth, blurred vision, constipation, and urinary retention. Blockade of histamine reuptake results in sedation, weight gain, and hypotension.

5. Physiological influences (secondary depression) may include:
  a. Medication side effects.
    i. Alone or in combination, drugs can produce a depressive syndrome
    ii. Common drugs having a direct effect on the central nervous system include:
      a) Anxiolytics
      b) Antipsychotics and sedative-hypnotics
      c) Antihypertensive medications, such as propranolol (Inderal) and reserpine
      d) The acne medication isotretinoin (Accutane)
      e) Steroids: prednisone and cortisone
      f) Hormones: estrogen and progesterone
      g) Sedatives: barbiturates and benzodiazepines
      h) Antibacterial drugs: ampicillin, cycloserine, tetracycline
      i) Antifungal drugs: sulfonamides
      j) Antineoplastics: vincristine and zidovudine
      k) Analgesics and anti-inflammatory drugs: opiates, ibuprofen, and phenylbutazone
      l) Antiulcer: cimetidine (Tagamet)
  b. Neurological disorders that might contribute to affective disorders:
    i. Cerebrovascular accident (CVA)
    ii. Brain tumors, particularly in the area of the temporal lobe
    iii. Alzheimer's disease
    iv. Parkinson's disease
    v. Huntington's disease
    vi. Multiple sclerosis
  c. Electrolyte disturbances that might contribute to affective disorders:
    i. Excessive levels of sodium bicarbonate or calcium
    ii. Deficits in magnesium and sodium
    iii. Excessive levels or deficits in potassium
  d. Hormonal disturbances that might contribute to affective disorders:
    i. Dysfunctional adrenal cortex observed in both Addison's disease and Cushing's syndrome
    ii. Hypoparathyroidism, hyperparathyroidism, hypothyroidism, and hyperthyroidism
    iii. Estrogen and progesterone imbalance leading to **premenstrual dysphoric disorder**
  e. Nutritional deficiencies that might contribute to affective disorders:
    i. Vitamin B_1 (thiamine)
    ii. Vitamin B_6 (pyridoxine)
    iii. Vitamin B_{12} (niacin)
    iv. Vitamin C
    v. Iron, folic acid, zinc, calcium, and potassium
  f. Physiological conditions associated with secondary depression that might contribute to affective disorders:
    i. Systemic lupus erythematosus and polyarteritis nodosa
    ii. Cardiomyopathy, congestive heart failure, and myocardial infarction
    iii. Infections, such as encephalitis, hepatitis, mononucleosis, pneumonia, and syphilis
    iv. Metabolic disorders, such as diabetes mellitus and porphyria

C. Psychosocial theories
  1. Psychoanalytical theory (Freud) "mourning and melancholia."
    a. Occurs after the loss of a loved object by death or rejection.
    b. Rage is internalized because of identification with the lost object.
    c. Individuals predisposed to melancholia experience ambivalence in love relationships.
  2. Learning theory (Seligman) "learned helplessness."
    a. Occurs in individuals who have experienced numerous real or perceived failures.
    b. Individuals then abandon further attempts to succeed.
    c. Individuals feel lack of control over life situation.
    d. Depression and helplessness develop because they have learned that whatever they do is futile.
    e. Especially damaging very early in life.
    f. Failure in mastery over one's environment undermines the foundation for future emotional development.
  3. Object loss theory
    a. Mother is child's main source of security (the "object").
    b. Depression occurs with "loss" of mother during first 6 months of life.
    c. Absence of attachment leads to feelings of helplessness and despair and may result in the following behaviors:
      i. Excessive crying
      ii. Anorexia
      iii. Withdrawal
      iv. **Psychomotor retardation**
      v. Stupor
      vi. Generalized impairment in growth and development

MAKING THE CONNECTION

Freud postulated that once the loss had been incorporated into the self (ego), the anger part of the ambivalence that had been felt for the lost object is then turned inward against the ego leading to depression.

vii. Depression from loss in adult life more severe if the subjects suffered loss in early childhood

4. **Cognitive theory.**
   a. Suggests the primary disturbance in depression is cognitive versus affective.
   b. Three cognitive distortions resulting in negative, defeated attitudes include:
      i. Negative expectations of the environment
      ii. Negative expectations of the self
      iii. Negative expectations of the future
   c. Distortions arise out of a defect in cognitive development.
   d. Individual feels inadequate, worthless, and rejected by others.

IV. Developmental Implications

A. Childhood
1. Symptoms of depression present differently in childhood, and symptoms change with age.
   a. Up to age 3:
      i. Feeding problems
      ii. Tantrums
      iii. Lack of playfulness
      iv. Lack of emotional expressiveness
      v. **Failure to thrive**
      vi. Delays in speech and gross motor development
   b. Ages 3 to 5:
      i. Accident proneness
      ii. Phobias
      iii. Aggressiveness
      iv. Excessive self-reproach for minor infractions
   c. Ages 6 to 8:
      i. Vague physical complaints
      ii. Aggression
      iii. Clinging behavior
      iv. Avoidance of new people and challenges
      v. Lagging behind classmates in social skills and academic competence
   d. Ages 9 to 12:
      i. Morbid thoughts and excessive worry
      ii. Lack of interest in play and friendships
      iii. Depression may be caused by their perception of parental disappointment

MAKING THE CONNECTION

Cognitive therapy focuses on helping the individual to alter mood by changing the way he or she thinks. The individual is taught to control negative thought distortions that lead to pessimism, lethargy, procrastination, and low self-esteem.

2. **Disruptive mood dysregulation disorder (DMDD)**
   a. A chronic, severe and persistent irritability with severe, recurrent temper outbursts. Symptoms include:
      i. Onset of symptoms before the age of 10
      ii. Temper outbursts grossly out of proportion in intensity or duration to the situation
      iii. Temper outbursts inconsistent with developmental level
      iv. Temper outbursts occur, on average, three or more times per week
      v. Irritable or angry mood is observable by others (e.g., parents, teachers, peers)
3. Other symptoms of childhood depression may include:
   a. Hyperactivity.
   b. Delinquency.
   c. School problems.
   d. Psychosomatic complaints.
   e. Sleeping and eating disturbances.
   f. Social isolation.
   g. Delusional thinking.
   h. Suicidal thoughts or actions.
4. Common precipitating factors include:
   a. Genetic predisposition.
   b. Physical or emotional detachment by the primary caregiver.
   c. Parental separation or divorce.
   d. Death of a loved one (person or pet).
   e. A move, academic failure, or physical illness.
   f. The common denominator is loss.
5. Therapies for depressed children include:
   a. Strengthening coping and adaptive skills.
   b. Prevention of future psychological problems.
   c. Treatment usually on an outpatient basis.
   d. Parental and family therapy used with the younger depressed child.
   e. Emotional support and guidance to family members.
   f. Children older than age 8 years can participate in family therapy.
   g. Individual treatment may be appropriate for older children.
   h. Untreated childhood depression may lead to adolescent and adult life problems.
   i. Hospitalization occurs:
      i. Only if child is actively suicidal
      ii. When home environment precludes adherence to a treatment regimen
      iii. If child needs to be separated from home because of psychosocial deprivation

j. Medications
  i. Antidepressants (more serious and recurrent forms of depression)
  ii. Selective serotonin reuptake inhibitors (SSRIs) in combination with psychosocial therapies
  iii. Antidepressant medications may cause suicidal behavior in young people
  iv. The U.S. Food and Drug Administration (FDA) has applied a "black box" label warning to all antidepressant medications.

🛑 The **black-box warning label** on all antidepressant medications describes the risk of suicidal thoughts and behavior in children and adolescents and emphasizes the need for ongoing medical monitoring. The advisory language does not prohibit the use of antidepressants in children and adolescents. Rather, it warns of the risk of suicidality and encourages prescribers to balance this risk with clinical need. Children already taking an antidepressant should remain on the medication if it has been helpful but should be carefully monitored by a doctor for side effects. Parents should promptly seek medical advice and evaluation if their child or adolescent experiences suicidal thinking or behavior, nervousness, agitation, irritability, mood instability, or sleeplessness that either emerges or worsens during treatment with antidepressant medications.

B. Adolescents
1. Depression is often mistaken for the normal stress of growing up.
2. Often do not get the help they need.
3. Depression is a major cause of suicide among teens.
4. Suicide is the second leading cause of death in the 15- to 24-year-old age group.
5. Common symptoms of depression (often inappropriately expressed):
   a. Anger.
   b. Aggressiveness.
   c. Running away.
   d. Delinquency.
   e. Social withdrawal.
   f. Sexual acting out.
   g. Substance abuse.
   h. Restlessness and apathy.
   i. Loss of self-esteem.
   j. Sleeping and eating disturbances.
   k. Psychosomatic complaints.
6. Indicators that differentiate mood disorder from the typical stormy behavior.
   a. Visible manifestation of behavioral change that lasts for several weeks.
   b. Normally outgoing adolescent who becomes withdrawn and antisocial.

c. Classroom performance goes from high marks to failing grades and truancy.
d. Self-confidence changes to inappropriate irritability and defensiveness.

🛑 Depression is a common manifestation of the stress and independence conflicts associated with the normal maturation process. Depression may be the response to death of a parent, relative, or friend, or to a breakup with a boyfriend or girlfriend. The perception of abandonment by parents or closest peer relationship is thought to be the most frequent immediate precipitant to adolescent suicide.

7. Therapies for depressed adolescents include:
   a. Outpatient treatment.
   b. Hospitalization:
     i. In cases of severe depression or threat of imminent suicide
     ii. When a family situation is such that treatment cannot be carried out in the home
     iii. When the physical condition precludes self-care of biological needs
     iv. When the adolescent has indicated possible harm to self or others in the family
   c. Medications (see Black Box Warning Alert).
     i. Fluoxetine (Prozac) has been approved by the FDA to treat depression in children and adolescents
     ii. Escitalopram (Lexapro) was approved in 2009 for treatment of MDD in adolescents aged 12 to 17 years
     iii. Other SSRI medications that have not yet been approved for use in adolescents include:
       1) Sertraline
       2) Citalopram
       3) Paroxetine
     iv. SNRI medications, that have not yet been approved for use in adolescents include:
       1) Duloxetine
       2) Venlafaxine
       3) Desvenlafaxine

C. Senescence (old age)
1. The elderly make up 13.1% of the population of the United States.
2. Depression is the most common psychiatric disorder of the elderly.
3. This population accounts for approximately 16% of the suicides in the United States.
4. The highest number of suicides in the United States is among white men 85 years of age and older.
5. Elderly suicide is almost four times the national rate.
6. Our society places value on youth, vigor, and uninterrupted productivity.

7. Problems that accompany advanced age include:
   a. Low self-esteem.
   b. Helplessness and hopelessness.
   c. Maladaptive coping strategies.
   d. Financial problems.
   e. Physical illness.
   f. Changes in bodily functioning.
   g. Increasing awareness of approaching death.
   h. Losses of significant others, home, and independence.
   i. Cumulative effect results in a phenomenon called **bereavement overload.**
      i. Unable to resolve one grief response before another one begins
      ii. Predisposes elderly individuals to depressive illness
8. Symptoms of depression are often confused with other illnesses associated with the aging process.
9. Depression accompanies many illnesses that affect the elderly such as:
   a. Parkinson's disease.
   b. Cancer.
   c. Arthritis.
   d. Early stages of Alzheimer's disease.
10. Therapies for the depressed elderly.
    a. Goal to reduce suffering and increase adaptive cope skills.
    b. Therapeutic approaches include:
       i. Interpersonal
       ii. Behavioral
       iii. Cognitive
       iv. Group and family psychotherapies
       v. Antidepressant medications
          1) Administered with consideration for age-related physiological changes in absorption, distribution, elimination, and brain receptor sensitivity
          2) Because of these changes, plasma concentrations of medications can reach very high levels despite moderate oral doses
       vi. Electroconvulsive therapy (ECT) considered safe and effective especially for suicidal

MAKING THE CONNECTION

The elderly are at high risk for a diagnosis of depression because of many variables. Symptoms of both depression and dementia include memory loss, confused thinking, and apathy. Medical conditions, such as endocrine, neurological, nutritional, and metabolic disorders, often present with classic symptoms of depression. Many medications commonly used by the elderly, such as antihypertensives, corticosteroids, and analgesics, can also produce a depressant effect.

elderly and those who are unable to tolerate antidepressant medications

D. Postpartum depression
1. Etiology of postpartum depression remains unclear.
2. A combination of hormonal, metabolic, and psychosocial influences.
3. "Maternity blues" associated with hormonal changes including.
   a. Alterations in tryptophan metabolism.
   b. Alterations in membrane transport during the early postpartum period.
4. Women experiencing moderate to severe symptoms are probably vulnerable to depression related to:
   a. Heredity.
   b. Upbringing.
   c. Early life experiences.
   d. Personality.
   e. Social circumstances.
5. Types of postpartum depression.
   a. "Maternity blues," "baby blues."
      i. Affects 50% to 85% of postpartum women
      ii. Symptoms begin within 48 hours of delivery, peak at about 3 to 5 days, and last approximately 2 weeks
      iii. Symptoms include:
         a) Mood swings
         b) Anxiety
         c) Sadness
         d) Irritability
         e) Tearfulness
         f) Impaired concentration
   b. Moderate depression.
      i. Affects 10% to 20% of postpartum women
      ii. Symptoms begin later than those in the "maternity blues" and take from a few weeks to several months to abate
      iii. Symptoms include:
         a) Depressed mood varying from day to day, with more bad days than good
         b) Tends to be worse toward evening
         c) Fatigue
         d) Irritability
         e) Loss of appetite
         f) Sleep disturbances
         g) Loss of libido
         h) Excessive concern about inability to care for infant
   c. Postpartum melancholia or depressive psychosis.
      i. Affects 1 or 2 out of 1000 women postpartum
      ii. Symptoms usually develop during the first few days after birth, but may occur later

iii. Symptoms include:
  a) Depressed mood
  b) Agitation
  c) Indecision
  d) Lack of concentration
  e) Guilt
  f) Abnormal attitude toward bodily functions
  g) Lack of interest in, or rejection of, infant
  h) Morbid fear that the baby may be harmed
  i) Suicide and infanticide may be contemplated

6. Treatment options determined by severity of illness:
  a. "Maternity blues": no treatment beyond reassurance from the physician or nurse and extra support and comfort from significant others.
  b. Moderate depression relieved with supportive psychotherapy and continuing assistance with home management.
  c. Psychotic depression treated with antidepressants, supportive psychotherapy, group therapy, and possibly family therapy.

V. Nursing Process for Depression: Assessment

DID YOU KNOW?
All individuals become depressed from time to time. Symptomatology can be viewed on a continuum according to the severity of the illness. The continuum of depression is presented in Figure 11.2.

A. Symptoms of depression can be described as alterations in four spheres of human functioning (affective, behavioral, cognitive, and physiological)

B. Types of depression
  1. Transient depression.
    a. Symptoms that accompany the everyday disappointments of life.
    b. Symptoms subside relatively quickly.

  c. Symptoms not necessarily dysfunctional. Alterations include:
    i. Affective:
      a) Sadness
      b) Dejection
      c) Feeling downhearted, having the "blues"
    ii. Behavioral: some crying possible
    iii. Cognitive: some difficulty getting mind off one's disappointment
    iv. Physiological: feeling tired and listless

  2. Mild depression.
    a. Loss of a valued object, such as a loved one, pet, friend, home, job, significant other.
    b. Individual able to work through stages of grief.
    c. Loss is accepted, and symptoms subside.
    d. Activities of daily living are resumed within a few weeks.
    e. Symptoms at this level similar to uncomplicated grieving. Alterations include:
      i. Affective:
        a) Denial of feelings
        b) Anger
        c) Anxiety
        d) Guilt
        e) Helplessness, hopelessness
        f) Sadness
        g) Despondency
      ii. Behavioral:
        a) Tearfulness
        b) Regression
        c) Restlessness
        d) Agitation
        e) Withdrawal
      iii. Cognitive:
        a) Preoccupation with the loss
        b) Self-blame
        c) Ambivalence
        d) Blaming others
      iv. Physiological:
        a) Anorexia or overeating
        b) Insomnia or hypersomnia
        c) Headache, backache, chest pain

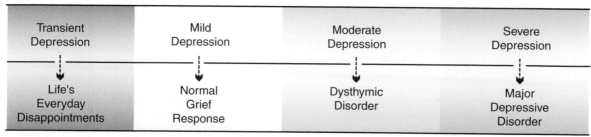

Fig 11.2 A continuum of depression.

3. Moderate depression.
    a. Persistent depressive disorder (dysthymia) is an example of moderate depression.
    b. Occurs when grief is prolonged or exaggerated.
    c. Individual becomes fixed in the anger stage of the grief response.
    d. Anger is turned inward on the self.
    e. All feelings of normal grieving are exaggerated out of proportion.
    f. Individual is unable to function without assistance.
    g. Poor appetite or overeating.
    h. Insomnia or hypersomnia.
    i. Low energy or fatigue.
    j. Low self-esteem.
    k. Poor concentration or difficulty making decisions.
    l. Feelings of hopelessness.

DID YOU KNOW?
Because symptoms of persistent depressive disorder have become a part of the individual's day-to-day experience, particularly in the case of early onset (e.g., "I've always been this way"), they may not be reported unless the individual is directly prompted. During the 2-year period (1 year for children or adolescents), any symptom-free intervals last no longer than 2 months.

    m. In children and adolescents, the mood can be irritable.
    n. In children and adolescents, symptoms must last for at least 1 year.
    o. Alterations include:
        i. Affective:
            a) Feelings of sadness ("feeling down in the dumps")
            b) Dejection
            c) Helplessness
            d) Powerlessness
            e) Hopelessness; gloomy and pessimistic outlook
            f) Low self-esteem
            g) Difficulty experiencing pleasure in activities
        ii. Behavioral:
            a) Slowed physical movements (i.e., psychomotor retardation)
            b) Slumped posture
            c) Slowed speech
            d) Limited verbalizations, with ruminations about life's failures or regrets
            e) Social isolation with a focus on the self
            f) Potential increased use of substances
            g) Potential self-destructive behavior
            h) Decreased interest in personal hygiene and grooming

        iii. Cognitive:
            a) Retarded thinking processes
            b) Difficulty concentrating and directing attention
            c) Obsessive and repetitive thoughts
            d) Generally portraying pessimism and negativism
            e) Verbalizations and behavior reflecting suicidal ideation
        iv. Physiological:
            a) Anorexia or overeating
            b) Insomnia or hypersomnia and sleep disturbances
            c) Amenorrhea
            d) Decreased libido
            e) Headaches, backaches, chest pain, abdominal pain
            f) Low energy level; fatigue and listlessness
            g) Feeling best early in the morning and worse as the day progresses (may be related to the diurnal variation in the level of neurotransmitters that affect mood and level of activity)
4. Severe depression.
    a. Intensified symptoms associated with the moderate level.
    b. May demonstrate a loss of contact with reality.
    c. May demonstrate complete lack of pleasure (anhedonia) in all activities.
    d. Ruminations about suicide are common.
    e. Major depressive disorder and bipolar depression are examples of severe depression.
    f. Alterations include:
        i. Affective:
            a) Feelings of total despair, hopelessness, and worthlessness
            b) Flat (unchanging) affect, appearing devoid of emotional tone
            c) Prevalent feelings of nothingness and emptiness
            d) Apathy; loneliness; sadness; inability to feel pleasure
        ii. Behavioral:
            a) Psychomotor retardation-physical movement may come to a standstill
            b) Psychomotor agitation—rapid purposeless movements
            c) Slumped posture; sitting in a curled-up position; walking slowly and rigidly
            d) Virtually no communication; may reflect delusional thinking when it occurs
            e) No personal hygiene and grooming
            f) Social isolation is common, with virtually no interaction with others

iii. Cognitive:
   a) Prevalent delusional thinking, with delusions of persecution and somatic delusions being most common
   b) Confusion, indecisiveness, and an inability to concentrate
   c) Hallucinations reflecting misinterpretations of the environment
   d) Excessive self-deprecation, self-blame, and thoughts of suicide
iv. Physiological:
   a) A general slowdown of the entire body
   b) Sluggish digestion, constipation, and urinary retention; amenorrhea; impotence; diminished libido; anorexia; weight loss
   c) Difficulty falling asleep; awakening very early in the morning
   d) Feeling worse early in the morning and somewhat better as the day progresses (may be related to the diurnal variation in the level of neurotransmitters that affect mood and level of activity)

DID YOU KNOW?

A number of assessment rating scales are available for measuring the severity of depressive symptoms. Some are meant to be clinician administered, whereas others may be self-administered. Examples of self-rating scales include the Zung Self-Rating Depression Scale and the Beck Depression Inventory. One of the most widely used clinician-administered scales is the Hamilton Depression Rating Scale (HDRS). It has been reviewed and revised over the years and exists today in several versions. The original version contains 17 items and is designed to measure mood, guilty feelings, suicidal ideation, sleep disturbances, anxiety levels, and weight loss. The Hamilton Depression Rating Scale is presented in Box 11.1.

🛑 Because of the low energy level and retarded thought processes, the individual with severe depression may not be able to follow through on suicidal ideations. However, the desire is strong at this level. The nurse must be vigilant to watch for any indication of self-harm behaviors, especially when antidepressant medications begin to relieve symptoms.

Box 11.1 Hamilton Depression Rating Scale (HDRS)

Instructions: For each item, circle the number to select the one "cue" that best characterizes the patient.

1. **Depressed Mood** *(sadness, hopeless, helpless, worthless)*
   0 = Absent
   1 = These feeling states indicated only on questioning.
   2 = These feeling states spontaneously reported verbally.
   3 = Communicates feeling states nonverbally, i.e., through facial expression, posture, voice, tendency to weep.
   4 = Patient reports virtually only these feeling states in spontaneous verbal and nonverbal communication.
2. **Feelings of Guilt**
   0 = Absent.
   1 = Self reproach; feels he/she has let people down.
   2 = Ideas of guilt or rumination over past errors or sinful deeds.
   3 = Present illness is a punishment. Delusions of guilt.
   4 = Hears accusatory or denunciatory voices and/or experiences threatening visual hallucinations.
3. **Suicide**
   0 = Absent.
   1 = Feels life is not worth living.
   2 = Wishes he/she were dead or any thoughts of possible death to self.
   3 = Suicidal ideas or gesture.
   4 = Attempts at suicide (any serious attempt rates 4)
4. **Insomnia: Early in the Night**
   0 = No difficulty falling asleep
   1 = Complains of occasional difficulty falling asleep, i.e., more than a half hour.
   2 = Complains of nightly difficulty falling asleep.
5. **Insomnia: Middle of the Night**
   0 = No difficulty
   1 = Complains of being restless and disturbed during the night.
   2 = Waking during the night—any getting out of bed rates 2 (except for purposes of voiding)

6. **Insomnia: Early Hours of the Morning**
   0 = No difficulty.
   1 = Waking in early hours of the morning, but goes back to sleep.
   2 = Unable to fall asleep again if he/she gets out of bed.
7. **Work and Activities**
   0 = No difficulty
   1 = Thoughts and feelings of incapacity, fatigue, or weakness related to activities, work, or hobbies.
   2 = Loss of interest in activity, hobbies, or work—either directly reported by patient, or indirectly in listlessness, indecision, and vacillation (feels he/she has to push self to work or activities).
   3 = Decrease in actual time spent in activities or decrease in productivity. Rate 3 if patient does not spend at least 3 hours a day in activities (job or hobbies), excluding routine chores.
   4 = Stopped working because of present illness. Rate 4 if patient engages in no activities except routine chores, or if does not perform routine chores unassisted.
8. **Psychomotor Retardation** *(slowness of thought and speech, impaired ability to concentrate, decreased motor activity)*
   0 = Normal speech and thought.
   1 = Slight retardation during the interview.
   2 = Obvious retardation during the interview.
   3 = Interview difficult.
   4 = Complete stupor.
9. **Agitation**
   0 = None.
   1 = Fidgetiness.
   2 = Playing with hands, hair, etc.
   3 = Moving about, can't sit still.
   4 = Hand wringing, nail biting, hair pulling, biting of lips

Continued

Box 11.1 Hamilton Depression Rating Scale (HDRS)—cont'd

10. *Anxiety (Psychic)*
    0 = No difficulty.
    1 = Subjective tension and irritability.
    2 = Worrying about minor matters.
    3 = Apprehensive attitude apparent in face or speech.
    4 = Fears expressed without questioning.
11. *Anxiety (Somatic):* Physiological concomitants of anxiety (e.g., dry mouth, indigestion, diarrhea, cramps, belching, palpitations, headache, tremor, hyperventilation, sighing, urinary frequency, sweating, flushing)
    0 = Absent
    1 = Mild
    2 = Moderate
    3 = Severe
    4 = Incapacitating
12. *Somatic Symptoms (Gastrointestinal)*
    0 = None
    1 = Loss of appetite, but eating without encouragement. Heavy feelings in abdomen.
    2 = Difficulty eating without urging from others. Requests or requires medication for constipation or gastrointestinal symptoms.
13. *Somatic Symptoms (General)*
    0 = None
    1 = Heaviness in limbs, back or head. Backaches, headache, muscle aches. Loss of energy and fatigability.
    2 = Any clear-cut symptom rates 2

14. *Genital Symptoms* (e.g., loss of libido, impaired sexual performance, menstrual disturbances)
    0 = Absent
    1 = Mild
    2 = Severe
15. *Hypochondriasis*
    0 = Not present.
    1 = Self-absorption (bodily)
    2 = Preoccupation with health
    3 = Frequent complaints, requests for help, etc.
    4 = Hypochondriacal delusions
16. *Loss of Weight (Rate either A or B)*
    A. *According to subjective patient history:*
       0 = No weight loss
       1 = Probable weight loss associated with present illness
       2 = Definite weight loss associated with present illness
    B. *According to objective weekly measurements:*
       0 = Less than 1 pound weight loss in week.
       1 = Greater than 1 pound weight loss in week.
       2 = Greater than 2 pound weight loss in week.
17. *Insight*
    0 = Acknowledges being depressed and ill
    1 = Acknowledges illness but attributes cause to bad food, climate, overwork, virus, need for rest, etc.
    2 = Denies being ill at all.

TOTAL SCORE _____

SCORING:
0–6 = No evidence of depressive illness
7–17 = Mild depression
18–24 = Moderate depression
>24 = Severe depression

Source: Hamilton, M. (1960). A rating scale for depression. *Journal of Neurology, Neurosurgery, & Psychiatry, 23,* 56–62. The HDRS is in the public domain.

VI. Nursing Process for Depression: Diagnosis (Analysis)

Table 11.1 presents a list of client behaviors and the NANDA nursing diagnoses that correspond to those behaviors, which may be used in planning care for the client with a depressive disorder.

VII. Nursing Process for Depression: Planning

The following outcomes may be developed to guide the care of a client with a depressive disorder. **The client will:**

A. Do no physical harm to self
B. Discuss the loss with staff and family members
C. No longer idealize or obsess about the lost entity/concept
D. Set realistic goals for self
E. No longer be afraid to attempt new activities

F. Identify aspects of self-control over life situations
G. Verbalize personal satisfaction and support from spiritual practices
H. Be able to interact willingly and appropriately with others
I. Be able to maintain reality orientation
J. Be able to concentrate, reason, and solve problems
K. Eat a well-balanced diet with snacks, to prevent weight loss and maintain nutritional status
L. Be able to sleep 6 to 8 hours per night and report feeling well rested
M. Bathe, wash, comb hair, and dress in clean clothing without assistance

VIII. Nursing Process for Depression: Implementation

A. Interventions for clients who are experiencing complicated grieving:
   1. Determine the stage of grief in which the client is fixed.

Table 11.1 Assigning Nursing Diagnoses to Behaviors Commonly Associated with Depression

Behaviors	Nursing Diagnosis
Depressed mood; feelings of hopelessness and worthlessness; anger turned inward in the self; misinterpretations of reality; suicidal ideation, plan, and available means	Risk for suicide
Depression, preoccupation with thoughts of loss, self-blame, grief avoidance, inappropriate expression of anger, decreased functioning in life roles	Complicated grieving
Expressions of helplessness, uselessness, guilt, and shame; hypersensitivity to slight or criticism; negative, pessimistic outlook; lack of eye contact; self-negating verbalizations	Low self-esteem
Apathy, verbal expressions of having no control, dependence on others to fulfill needs	Powerlessness
Expresses anger toward God, expresses lack of meaning in life, sudden changes in spiritual practices, refuses interactions with significant others or with spiritual leaders	Spiritual distress
Withdrawn, uncommunicative, seeks to be alone, dysfunctional interaction with others, discomfort in social situations	Social isolation/impaired social interaction
Inappropriate thinking, confusion, difficulty concentrating, impaired problem-solving ability, inaccurate interpretation of environment, memory deficit	Disturbed thought processes*
Weight loss, poor muscle tone, pale conjunctiva and mucous membranes, poor skin turgor, weakness	Imbalanced nutrition: less than body requirements
Difficulty falling asleep, difficulty staying asleep, lack of energy, difficulty concentrating, verbal reports of not feeling well rested	Insomnia
Uncombed hair, disheveled clothing, offensive body odor	Self-care deficit (hygiene, grooming)

*This diagnosis has been resigned from the NANDA-I list of approved diagnoses. It is used in this instance because it is most compatible with the identified behaviors.

2. Identify behaviors associated with this stage.
3. Develop a trusting relationship.
4. Show empathy, concern, and unconditional positive regard.
5. Be honest and keep all promises.
6. Convey an accepting attitude and enable the client to express feelings openly.
7. Encourage the client to express anger.
8. Do not become defensive if the initial expression of anger is displaced on the nurse or therapist.
9. Help the client explore angry feelings so that they may be directed toward the actual intended person or situation.
10. Help the client to discharge pent-up anger through participation in large motor activities (e.g., brisk walks, jogging, physical exercises, volleyball, punching bag, exercise bike).
11. Teach the normal stages of grief and behaviors associated with each stage.
12. Help the client to understand that feelings such as guilt and anger toward the lost concept are appropriate and acceptable during the grief process and should be expressed rather than held inside.
13. Encourage the client to review the relationship with the lost concept.

MAKING THE CONNECTION

The client must give up an idealized perception and be able to accept both positive and negative aspects about the lost concept before the grief process is complete. For example, a wife whose recently deceased husband was narcissistic and demanding now thinks of him as perfect in every way. This idealized perception may negatively influence the wife's ability to effectively move through the grieving process.

14. With support and sensitivity, point out the reality of the situation in areas where misrepresentations are expressed.
15. Communicate that crying is acceptable. (Use of touch may also be therapeutic but must be used discretely to avoid misinterpretation.)
B. Interventions for clients who exhibit low self-esteem
1. Be accepting and spend time with client even though pessimism and negativism may seem objectionable.
2. Focus on strengths and accomplishments and minimize limitations and failures.
3. Promote attendance in therapy groups that offer simple methods of accomplishment.

4. Encourage client to be as independent as possible.
5. Encourage client to recognize positive change and provide assistance toward this effort.
6. Teach assertiveness techniques:
   a. Ability to recognize the differences among passive, assertive, and aggressive behaviors.
   b. Importance of respecting the human rights of others while protecting one's own basic human rights.
   c. Teach effective communication techniques, such as the use of "I" messages.

DID YOU KNOW?

"I" statements like "I feel hurt when you say those things" help an individual to avoid making judgmental statements such as, "You hurt my feelings when you say those things."

C. Interventions for clients who experience powerlessness
   1. Encourage client to take responsibility for own self-care practices.
      a. Include client in setting the goals of care he or she wishes to achieve.
      b. Allow client to establish own schedule for self-care activities.
      c. Provide client with privacy as need is determined.
      d. Provide positive feedback for decisions made.
      e. Respect client's right to make those decisions independently.
      f. Refrain from influencing client toward decisions that seem more logical.
   2. Help client set realistic goals.
   3. Help client identify areas of life that he or she can control.
   4. Help identify areas of life that he or she can't control.
   5. Encourage verbalization of feelings related to this inability.
D. Interventions for clients who experience spiritual distress
   1. Be accepting and nonjudgmental when client expresses anger and bitterness toward God. Stay with client.
   2. Encourage client to ventilate feelings related to meaning of own existence in the face of current loss.
   3. Encourage client as part of grief work to reach out to previous religious or spiritual practices for support.
   4. Encourage client to discuss these practices and how they provided support in the past.
   5. Reassure client that he or she is not alone when feeling inadequate in the search for life's answers.
   6. After request, contact spiritual leader of client's choice.

E. Interventions for clients who experience hopelessness
   1. Identify stressors in client's life that precipitated current crisis.
   2. Determine coping behaviors previously used and client's perception of effectiveness then and now.
   3. Encourage client to explore and verbalize feelings and perceptions.
   4. Provide expressions of hope to client in positive, low-key manner:
      a. "I know you feel you cannot go on, but I believe that things can get better for you."
      b. "What you are feeling is temporary."
      c. "It is okay if you don't see it just now."
      d. "You are very important to the people who care about you."
   5. Help client identify areas of life situations that are under his or her own control.

DID YOU KNOW?

The client's emotional condition may interfere with ability to problem solve. Assistance may be required to perceive the benefits and consequences of available alternatives accurately.

   6. Identify resources or services that can be used after discharge when crises occur or hopelessness or suicidal ideations prevail.

IX. Nursing Process for Depression: Evaluation

A. Evaluation of the nursing actions for the client diagnosed with depression may be facilitated by gathering information using the following types of questions:
   1. Has the client discussed the recent loss with staff and family members?
   2. Is he or she able to verbalize feelings and behaviors associated with each stage of the grieving process and recognize own position in the process?
   3. Have obsession with and idealization of the lost object subsided?
   4. Is anger toward the lost object expressed appropriately?
   5. Does the client set realistic goals for self?
   6. Is he or she able to verbalize positive aspects about self, past accomplishments, and future prospects?

MAKING THE CONNECTION

The nursing role of client teacher is important in the psychiatric area, as it is in all areas of nursing. A list of topics for client/family education relevant to depression is presented in Box 11.2.

Box 11.2 Topics for Client/Family Education Related to Depression

Nature of the Illness

1. *Stages of grief and symptoms associated with each stage.*
2. *What is depression?*
3. *Why do people get depressed?*
4. *What are the symptoms of depression?*

Management of the Illness

1. *Medication Management*
   a. *Nuisance side effects*
   b. *Side effects to report to physician*
   c. *Importance of taking regularly*
   d. *Length of time to take effect*
   e. *Diet (related to monoamine oxidase inhibitors)*
2. *Assertiveness techniques*
3. *Stress-management techniques*
4. *Ways to increase self-esteem*
5. *Electroconvulsive therapy*

Support Services

1. *Suicide hotline*
2. *Support groups*
3. *Legal/financial assistance*

7. Can the client identify areas of life situation over which he or she has control?
8. Is the client able to participate in usual religious or spiritual practices and feel satisfaction and support from them?
9. Is the client seeking out interaction with others in an appropriate manner?
10. Does the client maintain reality orientation with no evidence of delusional thinking?
11. Is he or she able to concentrate and make decisions concerning own self-care?
12. Is the client selecting and consuming foods sufficiently high in nutrients and calories to maintain weight and nutritional status?
13. Does the client sleep without difficulty and wake feeling rested?
14. Does the client show pride in appearance by attending to personal hygiene and grooming?
15. Have somatic complaints subsided?

X. Treatment Modalities for Depression

A. Individual psychotherapy
   1. Research has documented the importance of close and satisfactory interpersonal attachments/relationships in the prevention of depression.
   2. Research has documented the role of disrupted attachments in the development of depression.
   3. Interpersonal psychotherapy focuses on the client's current interpersonal relations.

4. Phases of interpersonal psychotherapy.
   a. Phase I.
      i. Client is assessed to determine the extent of the illness
      ii. Information given to the individual regarding:
         a) The nature of depression
         b) Symptom pattern
         c) Frequency of experiencing symptoms
         d) Clinical course
         e) Treatment options
      iii. For severe depression, interpersonal psychotherapy is combined with antidepressant medication
      iv. Client is encouraged to continue working and participating in regular activities during therapy
      v. A mutually agreeable therapeutic contract is negotiated
   b. Phase II.
      i. Client is helped to resolve complicated grief reactions
         a) Addresses ambivalence with a lost relationship
         b) Therapeutic relationship serves as a temporary substitute for the lost relationship
         c) Assists with establishing new relationships
      ii. Client is helped to resolve interpersonal disputes between himself or herself and a significant other
      iii. Client is helped with difficult role transitions at various developmental life cycles
      iv. Client is helped to correct interpersonal deficits that may interfere with his or her ability to initiate or sustain interpersonal relationships
   c. Phase III: The therapeutic alliance is terminated with emphasis on:
      i. Reassurance
      ii. Clarification of emotional states
      iii. Improvement of interpersonal communication
      iv. Testing of perceptions
      v. Performance in interpersonal settings
B. Group therapy (once the acute phase of the illness is passed)
   1. Important dimension of multimodal treatment.
   2. Discussion of issues that cause, maintain, or arise out of having a serious affective disorder.
   3. Peer support provides a feeling of security, as troublesome or embarrassing issues are discussed and resolved.
   4. Other specific purposes of groups.
      a. Serves to monitor medication or related issues.
      b. Promotes education related to the affective disorder and its treatment.

c. Helps members gain a sense of perspective on their condition.

d. Encourages members to link up with others who have common problems.

e. Conveys that members are not alone or unique in experiencing affective illness.

5. Self-help groups offer support.
    a. Peer led.
    b. Not meant to substitute for, or compete with, professional therapy.
    c. Offer supplementary support and enhance compliance with the medical regimen.
    d. Examples of self-help groups:
        i. Depression and Bipolar Support Alliance (DBSA)
        ii. Depressives Anonymous
        iii. Recovery International
        iv. GriefShare (grief recovery support groups)

DID YOU KNOW?

Although self-help groups are not psychotherapy groups, they do provide important adjunctive support experiences, which often have therapeutic benefit for participants.

C. Family therapy
    1. Objective is to resolve the symptoms and initiate or restore adaptive family functioning.
    2. Examines the role of the mood-disordered member in the overall psychological well-being of the whole family.
    3. Examines the role of the entire family in the maintenance of the client's symptoms.
    4. A combination of psychotherapeutic and pharmacotherapeutic treatments are most effective.
    5. Family therapy is indicated when:
        a. Disorder jeopardizes the client's marriage or family functioning.
        b. The mood disorder is promoted or maintained by the family situation.

D. **Cognitive therapy**
    1. The individual is taught to control thought distortions that are considered to be a factor in the development and maintenance of mood disorders.

DID YOU KNOW?

In the cognitive model, depression is characterized by a triad of negative distortions related to expectations of the environment, self, and future. The environment and activities within it are viewed as unsatisfying, the self is unrealistically devalued, and the future is perceived as hopeless.

2. Goals include:
    a. Obtaining symptom relief as quickly as possible.
    b. Assisting the client in identifying dysfunctional patterns of thinking and behaving.

c. Guiding the client to evidence and logic that tests the validity of the dysfunctional thinking.

3. Focuses on changing "**automatic thoughts**" that occur spontaneously and contribute to the distorted affect.

4. Examples of automatic thoughts in depression:
    a. Personalizing: "I'm the only one who failed."
    b. All or nothing: "I'm a complete failure."
    c. Mind reading: "He thinks I'm foolish."
    d. Discounting positives: "The other questions were so easy. Any dummy could have gotten them right."

E. Electroconvulsive therapy (ECT)
    1. The induction of a grand mal (generalized) seizure through the application of electrical current to the brain.
    2. Considered for treatment only after a trial of therapy with antidepressant medication has proved ineffective.
    3. Used for clients experiencing:
        a. Severe depression.
        b. Acute suicidal ideations.
        c. Psychotic symptoms.
        d. Psychomotor retardation.
        e. Neurovegetative changes (disturbances in sleep, appetite, and energy).
    4. Mechanism of action.
        a. Exact mechanism is unknown.
        b. Biochemical theory postulates that electrical stimulation increases the same biogenic amines that are affected by antidepressant drugs.
        c. Evidence suggests that ECT may also result in increases in glutamate and gamma-aminobutyric acid.
        d. Electrical stimulation increases the circulating levels of the following neurotransmitters:
            i. Serotonin
            ii. Norepinephrine
            iii. Dopamine
    5. Side effects.
        a. Temporary memory loss.

MAKING THE CONNECTION

During cognitive therapy, the client is asked to describe evidence that both supports and disputes the automatic thought. The logic underlying the inferences is then reviewed with the client. Another technique involves evaluating what would most likely happen if the client's automatic thoughts were true. Implications of the consequences are then discussed. The results of several studies with depressed clients show that cognitive therapy may be equally or even more effective than antidepressant medication.

b. Aside from time immediately surrounding ECT, most individual report no problems with memory loss.

c. Rarely reported retrograde amnesia extending back months before treatment.

d. Confusion.

e. Critics argue that these changes represent irreversible brain damage.

f. Proponents insist they are temporary and reversible.

g. It is unclear whether the memory loss is due to the ECT or to ongoing depressive symptoms.

DID YOU KNOW?

The controversy continues regarding the choice of unilateral versus bilateral ECT. While unilateral placement of the electrodes decreases the amount of memory disturbance, unilateral ECT often requires a greater number of treatments to match the efficacy of bilateral ECT in the relief of depression.

6. Risks
   a. Mortality rate about 2 per 100,000 treatments
   b. Major cause of death is cardiovascular complication

🛑 Assessment and management of cardiovascular disease before treatment is vital in the reduction of morbidity and mortality rates associated with ECT.

   c. Critics remain adamant in their belief that ECT always results in some degree of immediate brain damage.
   d. Although brain damage remains a concern, proponents view ECT as a useful treatment for depression.

7. Medications used with ECT include:
   a. Atropine sulfate or glycopyrrolate (Robinal).
      i. Decreases secretions
      ii. Prevents aspiration
      iii. Counteracts vagal stimulation and bradycardia
   b. Propofol (Diprivan) or etomidate (Amidate).
      i. Short-acting anesthetic
      ii. Given intravenously
   c. Intravenous succinylcholine chloride (Anectine).
      i. Prevents severe muscle contractions, fractures, and dislocations during induced seizure
      ii. Induces respiratory paralysis making client oxygenation necessary

F. Transcranial magnetic stimulation (TMS)
   1. Uses very short pulses of magnetic energy to stimulate nerve cells in the brain.
   2. Unlike ECT, the electrical waves generated by TMS do not result in generalized seizure activity.
   3. Waves are passed through a coil placed on the scalp to areas of the brain involved in mood regulation.

4. Proponents believe that TMS holds a great deal of promise, whereas critics remain skeptical.

G. Light therapy
   1. Between 15% and 25% of people with recurrent depressive disorder exhibit a seasonal pattern.
   2. Symptoms exacerbated during winter and subside during spring and summer.
   3. Could be related to the increase of the hormone melatonin during dark hours.
   4. Commonly identified as seasonal affective disorder (SAD) or "winter blues."
   5. Treated by a 10,000-lux light box, which contains white fluorescent light tubes covered with a plastic screen that blocks ultraviolet rays.
   6. Therapy usually begins with 10 to 15 minute sessions and gradually progresses to 30 to 45 minutes.
   7. Some show rapid improvement, whereas for others it may take several weeks.
   8. Side effects appear to be dosage related and include:
      a. Headache, eyestrain, nausea, irritability, photophobia (eye sensitivity to light).
      b. Insomnia (when light therapy is used late in the day) and (rarely) hypomania.
   9. Studies show no significant outcome difference between light therapy and antidepressant medication.

H. Psychopharmacology
   1. Antidepressant medications are used in the treatment of:
      a. Persistent depressive disorder.
      b. Major depression with melancholia or psychotic symptoms.
      c. Depression associated with organic disease, alcoholism, schizophrenia, or mental retardation.
      d. Depressive phase of bipolar disorder; and depression accompanied by anxiety.
   2. Selected medications are also used to treat anxiety disorders, bulimia nervosa, and premenstrual dysphoric disorder.
   3. Antidepressant medications work to increase the concentration of norepinephrine, serotonin, and/or dopamine by:
      a. Blocking the reuptake of neurotransmitters by the neurons.
         i. Tricyclic antidepressants (TCAs)
         ii. Heterocyclics
         iii. Selected serotonin reuptake inhibitors (SSRIs)
         iv. Selected norepinephrine reuptake inhibitors (SNRIs)
      b. Blocking monoamine oxidase.
         i. Monoamine oxidase inactivates norepinephrine, serotonin, and dopamine
         ii. Class of drugs referred to as monoamine oxidase inhibitor (MAOIs)
   4. Examples of commonly used antidepressant medications are presented in Table 11.2

Table 11.2 Medications Used in the Treatment of Depression

Chemical Class	Generic (Trade) Name*	Pregnancy Category/ Half-Life (hr)	Range (mg)	Plasma Ranges†
Tricyclics	Amitriptyline	D/31–46	50–300	110–250 (including metabolite)
	Amoxapine	C/8	50–300	200–500
	Clomipramine (Anafranil)	C/19–37	25–250	80–100
	Desipramine (Norpramin)	C/12–24	25–300	125–300
	Doxepin	C/8–24	25–300	100–200 (including metabolite)
	Imipramine (Tofranil)	D/11–25	30–300	200–350 (including metabolite)
	Nortriptyline (Aventyl; Pamelor)	D/18–44	30–100	50–150
	Protriptyline (Vivactil)	C/67–89	15–60	100–200
	Trimipramine (Surmontil)	C/7–30	50–300	180 (including metabolite)
Selective Serotonin Reuptake Inhibitors (SSRIs)	Citalopram (Celexa)	C/~35	20–40	Not well established
	Escitalopram (Lexapro)	C/27–32	10–20	Not well established
	Fluoxetine (Prozac; Sarafem)	C/1–16 days (including metabolite)	20–80	Not well established
	Fluvoxamine (Luvox)	C/13.6–15.6	50–300	Not well established
	Paroxetine (Paxil)	D/21 (controlled release: 15–20)	10–50 (CR: 12.5–75)	Not well established
	Sertraline (Zoloft)	C/26–104 (including metabolite)	25–200	Not well established
	Vilazodone (Viibryd) (also acts as a partial serotonergic agonist)	C/25	40	Not well established
Monoamine Oxidase Inhibitors	Isocarboxazid (Marplan)	C/Not established	20–60	Not well established
	Phenelzine (Nardil)	C/2–3	45–90	Not well established
	Tranylcypromine (Parnate)	C/2.4–2.8	30–60	Not well established
	Selegiline Transdermal System (Emsam)	C/18–25 including metabolites	6/24 hr – 12/24 hr patch	Not well established
Heterocyclics	Bupropion (Wellbutrin)	C/8–24	200–450	Not well established
	Maprotiline	B/21–25	25–225	200–300 (incl. metabolite)
	Mirtazapine (Remeron)	C/20–40	15–45	Not well established
	Nefazodone‡	C/2–4	200–600	Not well established
	Trazodone	C/4–9	150–600	800–1600
Serotonin-Norepinephrine Reuptake Inhibitors (SNRIs)	Desvenlafaxine (Pristiq)	C/11	50–400	Not well established
	Duloxetine (Cymbalta)	C/8–17	40–60	Not well established
	Venlafaxine (Effexor)	C/5–11 (including metabolite)	75–375	Not well established
Psychotherapeutic Combinations	Olanzapine and fluoxetine (Symbyax)	C/see individual drugs	6/25–12/50	Not well established
	Chlordiazepoxide and fluoxetine (Limbitrol)	D/see individual drugs	20/50–40/100	Not well established
	Perphenazine and amitriptyline (Etrafon)	C-D/see individual drugs	6/30–16/200	Not well established

*Drugs without trade names are available in generic form only.
†Dosage requires slow titration; onset of therapeutic response may be 1 to 4 weeks.
‡Bristol Myers Squibb voluntarily removed their brand of nefazodone (Serzone) from the market in 2004. The generic equivalent is currently available through various other manufacturers.

5. Antidepressant medications may take 7 to 28 days to elevate mood and 6 to 8 weeks for major depression symptoms to subside.

🛑 Antidepressant medications are contraindicated in individuals with hypersensitivity. TCAs are contraindicated in the acute recovery phase after myocardial infarction and in individuals with angle-closure glaucoma. TCAs, heterocyclics, SSRIs, and SNRIs are contraindicated with concomitant use of MAOIs. Caution should be used in administering these medications to elderly or debilitated clients and those with hepatic, renal, or cardiac insufficiency. (The dosage usually must be decreased.) Caution is also required with psychotic clients, with clients who have benign prostatic hypertrophy, and with individuals who have a history of seizures (may decrease seizure threshold). All antidepressants carry an FDA black box warning for increased risk of suicidality in children and adolescents. As these drugs take effect and mood begins to lift, the individual may have increased energy with which to implement a suicide plan. Suicide potential often *increases* as level of depression *decreases*. The nurse should be particularly alert to sudden lifts in mood.

6. Interactions.
   a. Tricyclic antidepressants (TCAs):
      i. Increased effects may occur with bupropion, cimetidine, haloperidol, SSRIs, and valproic acid
      ii. Decreased effects may occur with carbamazepine, barbiturates, and rifamycins
      iii. Hyperpyretic crisis, convulsions, and death may occur with MAOIs
      iv. Coadministration with clonidine may produce hypertensive crisis
      v. Decreased effects of levodopa and guanethidine may occur
      vi. Potentiation of pressor response may occur with direct-acting sympathomimetics
      vii. Increased anticoagulation effects may occur with dicumarol
      viii. Increased serum levels of carbamazepine occur with concomitant use of tricyclics
      ix. Increased risk of seizures with concomitant use of maprotiline and phenothiazines
   b. MAOIs.
      i. Serious, potentially fatal adverse reactions may occur with concurrent use of all other antidepressants, carbamazepine, cyclobenzaprine, buspirone, sympathomimetics, tryptophan, dextromethorphan, anesthetic agents, central nervous system (CNS) depressants, and amphetamines
      ii. Avoid using within 2 weeks of each other (5 weeks after therapy with fluoxetine)
      iii. Hypertensive crisis may occur with amphetamines, methyldopa, levodopa, dopamine, epinephrine, norepinephrine, guanethidine, guanadrel, reserpine, or vasoconstrictors
      iv. Hypertension or hypotension, coma, convulsions, and death may occur with opioids (avoid use of meperidine within 14–21 days of MAOI therapy)
      v. Excess CNS stimulation and hypertension may occur with methylphenidate
      vi. Additive hypotension may occur with antihypertensives, thiazide diuretics, or spinal anesthesia
      vii. Additive hypoglycemia may occur with insulins or oral hypoglycemic agents
      viii. Doxapram may increase pressor response
      ix. Serotonin syndrome may occur with concomitant use of St. John's wort

🛑 When MAOIs are used, hypertensive crisis may occur with ingestion of foods or other products containing high concentrations of **tyramine**. Consumption of foods or beverages with high caffeine content increases the risk of hypertension and arrhythmias. Bradycardia may occur with concurrent use of MAOIs and beta blockers. There is a risk of toxicity from the 5-hydroxytryptamine (5-HT) receptor agonists with concurrent use of MAOIs (see Table 11.3).

   c. Selective Serotonin Reuptake Inhibitors (SSRIs).
      i. Toxic, sometimes fatal, reactions have occurred with concomitant use of MAOIs
      ii. Increased effects of SSRIs may occur with cimetidine, L-tryptophan, lithium, linezolid, and St. John's wort
      iii. Serotonin syndrome may occur with concomitant use of SSRIs and metoclopramide, sibutramine, tramadol, or 5-HT-receptor agonists (triptans)
      iv. Concomitant use of SSRIs may increase effects of hydantoins, tricyclic antidepressants, cyclosporine, benzodiazepines, beta blockers, methadone, carbamazepine, clozapine, olanzapine, pimozide, haloperidol, phenothiazines, St. John's wort, sumatriptan, sympathomimetics, tacrine, theophylline, and warfarin
      v. Concomitant use of SSRIs may decrease effects of buspirone and digoxin
      vi. Lithium levels may be increased or decreased by concomitant use of SSRIs
      vii. There may be decreased effects of SSRIs with concomitant use of carbamazepine and cyproheptadine

Table 11.3 Diet and Drug Restrictions for Clients on MAOI Therapy: Foods Containing Tyramine

High Tyramine Content *(Avoid while on MAOI Therapy)*	Moderate Tyramine Content *(May eat occasionally while on MAOI Therapy)*	Low Tyramine Content *(Limited quantities permissible on MAOI Therapy)*
Aged cheeses (cheddar, Swiss, Camembert, blue cheese, Parmesan, provolone, Romano, brie)	Gouda cheese, processed American cheese, mozzarella, yogurt, sour cream, avocados, bananas	Pasteurized cheeses (cream cheese, cottage cheese, ricotta), figs, distilled spirits (in moderation)
Raisins, fava beans, flat Italian beans, Chinese pea pods	Beer, white wine, coffee, colas, tea, hot chocolate	
Red wines (e.g., Chianti, burgundy, cabernet sauvignon)	Meat extracts, such as bouillon, chocolate	
Smoked and processed meats (salami, bologna, pepperoni, summer sausage)		
Caviar, pickled herring, corned beef, chicken or beef liver		
Soy sauce, brewer's yeast, meat tenderizer (MSG)		

Drug Restrictions

Ingestion of the following substances while on MAOI therapy could result in life-threatening hypertensive crisis. A 14-day interval is recommended between use of these drugs and an MAOI.

- *All other antidepressant medications (e.g., SSRIs, TCAs, SNRIs, heterocyclics)*
- *Sympathomimetics: (epinephrine, dopamine, norepinephrine, ephedrine, pseudoephedrine, phenylephrine, phenylpropanolamine, over-the-counter cough and cold preparations)*
- *Stimulants (amphetamines, cocaine, diet drugs)*
- *Antihypertensives (methyldopa, guanethidine, reserpine)*
- *Meperidine and (possibly) other opioid narcotics (morphine, codeine)*
- *Antiparkinsonian agents (levodopa)*

Sources: Black & Andreasen (2010); Sadock & Sadock (2007); Martinez, Marangell, & Martinez (2008).

d. Others (heterocyclics and SNRIs).
   i. Concomitant use with MAOIs results in serious, sometimes fatal, effects resembling neuroleptic malignant syndrome
   ii. Serotonin syndrome may occur when any of the following are used together: St. John's wort, sibutramine, trazodone, nefazodone, venlafaxine, desvenlafaxine, duloxetine, SSRIs, 5-HT-receptor agonists (triptans)
   iii. Increased effects of haloperidol, clozapine, and desipramine may occur when used concomitantly with venlafaxine
   iv. Increased effects of venlafaxine may occur with cimetidine
   v. Increased effects of duloxetine may occur with cytochrome P450 (CYP) 1A2 inhibitors (e.g., fluvoxamine, quinolone antibiotics) and CYP2D6 inhibitors (e.g., fluvoxamine, quinolone antibiotics) and CYP2D6 inhibitors (e.g., fluoxetine, quinidine, paroxetine)
   vi. Increased risk of liver injury occurs with concomitant use of alcohol and duloxetine

   vii. Increased risk of toxicity or adverse effects from drugs extensively metabolized by CYP2D6 (e.g., flecainide, phenothiazines, propafenone, tricyclic antidepressants, thioridazine) when used concomitantly with duloxetine, desvenlafaxine, or bupropion
   viii. Decreased effects of bupropion and trazodone may occur with carbamazepine
   ix. Altered anticoagulant effect of warfarin may occur with bupropion, venlafaxine, desvenlafaxine, duloxetine, or trazodone
7. Side effects that may occur with all chemical classes and their nursing interventions:
   a. Dry mouth.
      i. Offer the client sugarless candy, ice, frequent sips of water
      ii. Provide strict oral hygiene
   b. Sedation.
      i. Advocate for medication to be given at bedtime
      ii. Advocate for decreased dosage or use of less sedating drug
      iii. Instruct the client not to drive or use dangerous equipment

c. Nausea.
  i. Administer with food to minimize gastrointestinal distress
  ii. Advocate for decreased dosage, medication change, or antiemetic
d. Discontinuation syndrome.

🛑 All classes of antidepressants have varying potentials to cause discontinuation syndromes. Following long-term therapy with SSRIs, such as venlafaxine, desvenlafaxine, or duloxetine, abrupt withdrawal may result in dizziness, lethargy, headache, and nausea. Because of its long half-life, fluoxetine is less likely to result in withdrawal symptoms. Abrupt withdrawal from tricyclics may produce hypomania, akathisia, cardiac arrhythmias, gastrointestinal upset, and panic attacks. The discontinuation syndrome associated with MAOIs includes flulike symptoms, confusion, hypomania, and worsening of depressive symptoms. **All antidepressant medication should be tapered gradually to prevent withdrawal symptoms.**

8. Side effects that most commonly occur with tricyclics and heterocyclics and their nursing interventions:
  a. Blurred vision.
    i. Offer reassurance that this symptom should subside after a few weeks
    ii. Instruct the client not to drive until vision is clear
    iii. Clear small items from routine pathway to prevent falls
  b. Constipation.
    i. Order foods high in fiber
    ii. Increase fluid intake if not contraindicated
    iii. Encourage client to increase physical exercise, if possible
  c. Urinary retention.
    i. Instruct client to report hesitancy or inability to urinate
    ii. Monitor intake and output
    iii. Stimulate urination by running water in the bathroom or pouring water over the perineal area
  d. Orthostatic hypotension.
    i. Instruct the client to rise slowly from a lying or sitting position
    ii. Monitor blood pressure (lying and standing) frequently, document, and report significant changes
    iii. Instruct client to avoid long hot showers or tub baths
  e. Reduction of seizure threshold.
    i. Observe clients with history of seizures closely
    ii. Institute seizure precautions as specified in hospital procedure manual

iii. Bupropion (Wellbutrin) should be administered in doses of no more than 150 mg and should be given at least 4 hours apart

🛑 Bupropion has been associated with a relatively high incidence of seizure activity in anorexic and cachectic clients.

  f. Tachycardia, arrhythmias.
    i. Carefully monitor blood pressure, pulse rate, and rhythm
    ii. Report any significant change to physician
  g. Photosensitivity.
    i. Ensure that client wears sunblock lotion
    ii. Advise using protective clothing and sunglasses outdoors
  h. Weight gain.
    i. Provide instructions for reduced-calorie diet
    ii. Encourage increased level of activity, if appropriate
9. Side effects that most commonly occur with SSRIs and SNRIs and their nursing interventions:
  a. Insomnia; agitation.
    i. Administer or instruct client to take dose early in the day
    ii. Instruct client to avoid caffeinated food and drinks
    iii. Teach relaxation techniques to use before bedtime
  b. Headache.
    i. Administer analgesics, as prescribed
    ii. Without relief, advocate for antidepressant medication change
  c. Weight loss (may occur early in therapy).
    i. Provide caloric intake sufficient to maintain desired weight
    ii. Weigh client daily or every other day, at the same time, and on the same scale if possible
    iii. Alert physician if client is anorectic
    iv. After prolonged use, some clients may gain weight
  d. Sexual dysfunction.
    i. Advise men to report any abnormal ejaculation or impotence
    ii. Advise women to report any delay or loss of orgasm
    iii. Advocate for medication change if side effect becomes intolerable
  e. Serotonin syndrome (may occur when two drugs that potentiate serotonergic neurotransmission are used concurrently).
    i. Most frequent symptoms include changes in mental status, restlessness, myoclonus, hyperreflexia, tachycardia, labile blood

pressure, diaphoresis, shivering, and
tremors

ii. Advocate for immediate discontinuation
of the medication

🛑 If a client experiences serotonin syndrome, the physician
may prescribe medications to block serotonin receptors,
relieve hyperthermia and muscle rigidity, and prevent seizures.
In severe cases, artificial ventilation may be required. The
histamine-1 receptor antagonist, cyproheptadine, is commonly used to treat the symptoms of serotonin syndrome.
Monitoring vital signs, providing safety measures to prevent
injury when muscle rigidity and changes in mental status are
present, providing cooling blankets and tepid baths to assist
with temperature regulation, and monitoring intake and
output are supporting nursing measures that are vital to
the comfort and safety of the client. Once the offending
medication has been discontinued, the condition will usually
resolve on its own. However, if left untreated, the condition
may progress to life-threatening complications, which
include seizures, coma, hypotension, ventricular arrhythmias,
disseminated intravascular coagulation, rhabdomyolysis,
metabolic acidosis, and renal failure.

10. Side effects that most commonly occur with
MAOIs and their nursing interventions:
a. Hypertensive crisis.
i. Occurs if individual consumes foods
containing tyramine while receiving
MAOI therapy
ii. Has not been shown to be a problem
with selegiline transdermal system at the
6 mg/24 hr dosage, and dietary restrictions at this dose are not recommended
iii. Dietary modifications are recommended,
however, at the 9 mg/24 hr and 12 mg/
24 hr dosages
iv. Symptoms of hypertensive crisis include
severe occipital headache, palpitations,
nausea/vomiting, nuchal rigidity, fever,
sweating, marked increase in blood
pressure, chest pain, and coma
v. Advocate for immediate discontinuation
of the medication
vi. Monitor vital signs
vii. Administer prescribed short-acting
antihypertensive medication
viii. Use external cooling measures to control
hyperpyrexia
b. Application site reactions (with selegiline
transdermal system [Emsam])
i. Most common reactions include rash,
itching, erythema, irritation, swelling,
or urticarial lesions
ii. Assure client that most reactions resolve
spontaneously, requiring no treatment

iii. Advise to report reactions that do not
resolve
iv. Advocate for the use of topical
corticosteroids
11. Miscellaneous side effects and their nursing
interventions:
a. Priapism is a rare side effect, but it has
occurred in some men taking trazodone.
i. If prolonged or inappropriate penile erection occurs, withhold medication and
immediately notify physician
ii. If severe, may require surgical intervention;
if not treated successfully, it can result in
impotence
b. Life-threatening hepatic failure has been
reported in clients treated with nefazodone.
i. Advise clients to immediately report signs
or symptoms suggestive of liver dysfunction
ii. Symptoms may include jaundice, anorexia,
gastrointestinal complaints, or malaise
12. Possible risks can occur when taking antidepressants during pregnancy
13. Anyone taking antidepressants should carry a
card or other identification at all times describing
the medications

🛑 More than 36,000 persons in the United States end their
lives each year by suicide. Suicide is the third leading cause of
death among young Americans ages 15 to 24 years, the fourth
leading cause of death for ages 25 to 44, and the eighth leading cause of death for individuals 45 to 64. Many more people
attempt suicide than succeed, and countless others seriously
contemplate the act without carrying it out. Almost 95% of
all people who commit or attempt suicide have a diagnosed
mental disorder. Depressive disorders account for 80% of
this figure. Over the years, some mistaken beliefs have been
accepted as truth regarding suicide. Some facts and fables
related to suicide are presented in Table 11.4.

MAKING THE CONNECTION

It is important to teach the client to follow the correct
procedure for applying the selegiline transdermal patch.
The patch must be applied to dry, intact skin on the
upper torso, upper thigh, or outer surface of upper arm.
Teach the client to apply the patch at approximately
the same time each day to a new spot on the skin, after
removing and discarding the old patch. Instruct the client
to wash his or her hands thoroughly after applying the
patch. Teach the client to avoid exposing the application
site to direct heat (e.g., heating pads, electric blankets,
heat lamps, hot tub, or prolonged direct sunlight). Tell
the client if the patch falls off to apply a new patch to a
new site and resume the previous schedule.

Table 11.4 Facts and Fables About Suicide

Fables	Facts
People who talk about suicide do not commit suicide. Suicide happens without warning.	Eight out of ten people who kill themselves have given definite clues and warnings about their suicidal intentions. Very subtle clues may be ignored or disregarded by others.
You cannot stop a suicidal person. He or she is fully intent on dying.	Most suicidal people are very ambivalent about their feelings regarding living or dying. Most are "gambling with death" and see it as a cry for someone to save them.
Once a person is suicidal, he or she is suicidal forever.	People who want to kill themselves are only suicidal for a limited time. If they are saved from feelings of self-destruction, they can go on to lead normal lives.
Improvement after severe depression means that the suicidal risk is over.	Most suicides occur within about 3 months after the beginning of "improvement," when the individual has the energy to carry out suicidal intentions.
Suicide is inherited, or "runs in families."	Suicide is not inherited. It is an individual matter and can be prevented. However, suicide by a close family member increases an individual's risk factor for suicide.
All suicidal individuals are mentally ill, and suicide is the act of a psychotic person.	Although suicidal persons are extremely unhappy, they are not necessarily psychotic or otherwise mentally ill. They are merely unable at that point in time to see an alternative solution to what they consider an unbearable problem.
Suicidal threats and gestures should be considered manipulative or attention-seeking behavior and should not be taken seriously.	All suicidal behavior must be approached with the gravity of the potential act in mind. Attention should be given to the possibility that the individual is issuing a cry for help.
People usually commit suicide by taking an overdose of drugs.	Gunshot wounds are the leading cause of death among suicide victims.
If an individual has attempted suicide, he or she will not do it again.	Between 50% and 80% of all people who ultimately kill themselves have a history of a previous attempt.

Sources: Friends for Survival, Inc. (2012); NAMI (2011); The Samaritans (2012).

XI. Nursing Process for Suicide: Assessment

A. Suicide assessment demographics include:
1. Age: highest in persons older than 50. Adolescents are also at high risk.
2. Gender: males are at higher risk than females.
3. Ethnicity: Caucasians are at higher risk than Native Americans, who are at higher risk than African Americans.
4. Marital status: single, divorced, and widowed are at higher risk than married.

MAKING THE CONNECTION

The following items should be considered when conducting a suicidal assessment: demographics, presenting symptoms/medical-psychiatric diagnosis, suicidal ideas or acts, interpersonal support system, analysis of the suicidal crisis, psychiatric/medical/family history, and coping strategies. Risk factors are associated with a greater potential for suicide and suicidal behavior, whereas protective factors are associated with reduced potential for suicide. These risk and protective factors are outlined in Table 11.5.

5. Socioeconomic status: individuals in the highest and lowest socioeconomic classes are at higher risk than those in the middle classes.
6. Occupation: professional health-care personnel and business executives are at highest risk.
7. Method: use of firearms presents a significantly higher risk than overdose of substances.
8. Religion: individuals who are not affiliated with any religious group are at higher risk than those who have this type of affiliation.
9. Family history: higher risk exists if individual has a family history of suicide.

B. Assess presenting symptoms/medical-psychiatric diagnosis
1. Major depression and bipolar disorders are the most common disorders that precede suicide.
2. Individuals with substance use disorders are also at high risk.
3. Other psychiatric disorders in which suicide may be a risk include:
   a. Anxiety disorders.
   b. Schizophrenia.
   c. Borderline and antisocial personality disorders.
   d. Other chronic and terminal physical illnesses.

Table 11.5 **Suicide Risk Factors and Protective Factors**

Risk Factors	Protective Factors
• *Previous suicide attempt* • *Mental disorders—particularly mood disorders such as depression and bipolar disorder* • *Co-occurring mental and alcohol and substance abuse disorders* • *Family history of suicide* • *Hopelessness* • *Impulsive and/or aggressive tendencies* • *Barriers to accessing mental health treatment* • *Relational, social, work, or financial loss* • *Physical illness* • *Easy access to lethal methods, especially guns* • *Unwillingness to seek help because of stigma attached to mental and substance abuse disorders and/or suicidal thoughts* • *Influence of significant people—family members, celebrities, peers who have died by suicide—both through direct personal contact or inappropriate media representations* • *Cultural and religious beliefs—for instance, the belief that suicide is a noble resolution of a personal dilemma* • *Local epidemics of suicide that have a contagious influence* • *Isolation, a feeling of being cut off from other people*	• *Effective and appropriate clinical care for mental, physical, and substance abuse disorders* • *Easy access to a variety of clinical interventions and support for help seeking* • *Restricted access to highly lethal methods of suicide* • *Family and community support* • *Support from ongoing medical and mental health care relationships* • *Learned skills in problem-solving, conflict resolution, and nonviolent handling of disputes* • *Cultural and religious beliefs that discourage suicide and support self-preservation instincts*

Source: U.S. Public Health Service (1999). *The Surgeon General's Call to Action to Prevent Suicide.* Washington, DC: Author.

C. Assess suicidal ideas or acts
1. How serious is the intent?
2. Does the person have a plan?
3. Does the person have the means?
4. How lethal are the means?
5. Are there any previous attempts?
6. Does the person have any meaningful network of relationships?
7. Does the person have any support system to access?

D. Assess behavioral and verbal clues to suicidal intent
1. Giving away prized possessions.
2. Getting financial affairs in order.
3. Writing suicide notes.
4. Sudden lifts in mood (may indicate a decision to carry out the intent).
5. Direct and indirect verbal clues:
    a. Direct: "I want to die."
    b. Direct: "I'm going to kill myself."
    c. Indirect: "This is the last time you'll see me."
    d. Indirect: "I won't be around much longer for the doctor to have to worry about."
    e. Indirect: "I don't have anything worth living for anymore."

E. Assess precipitating stressors:
1. Depression.
2. Loss of a loved person either by death or divorce.
3. Problems in major relationships.
4. Changes in role or serious physical illness.
5. Relevant history:
    a. Experiences numerous failures or rejections.
    b. Dysfunctional response to current situation.

6. Life-stage issues:
    a. During various stages of life, inability to tolerate losses and disappointment.
    b. Struggles with developmental issues (e.g., adolescence, midlife).

F. Assess psychiatric/medical/family history
1. Assess for previous depression, alcoholism, suicide attempts.
2. Assess for presence of chronic, debilitating, or terminal illness.
3. Assess for family history involving depression and suicide.

G. Assess coping strategies
1. How has the individual handled previous crisis?
2. How does this situation differ from previous ones?

XII. Nursing Process for Suicide: Diagnoses (Analysis)

A. Risk for suicide R/T feelings of hopelessness and desperation

MAKING THE CONNECTION

By discussing fear related to end of life issues, including pain control, the nurse can therapeutically offer the terminal client an opportunity to ask questions and vent feelings about impending death.

B. Hopelessness R/T absence of support systems and perception of worthlessness AEB statement "Life isn't worth living anymore."

XIII. Nursing Process for Suicide: Planning

The following outcomes may be developed to guide the care of a suicidal client. **The client will:**

A. Experience no physical harm to self
B. Set realistic goals for self
C. Express some optimism and hope for the future

XIV. Nursing Process for Suicide: Implementation

A. Ask client directly: "Have you thought about killing yourself?"
B. If so, "what do you plan to do? Do you have the means to carry out this plan?"

🛑 The risk of suicide is greatly increased if the client has developed a plan and particularly if means exist for the client to execute the plan. Client safety is always a nursing priority.

C. Create a safe environment for the client
D. Remove all potentially harmful objects from client's access (sharp objects, straps, belts, ties, glass items, alcohol)
E. Supervise closely during meals and medication administration
F. Perform room searches as deemed necessary
G. Depending on level of suicide precaution, provide one-to-one contact, constant visual observation, or every-15-minute checks
H. Place in room close to nurse's station; do not assign to private room
I. Monitor during off-unit activities
J. Monitor bathroom use
K. Maintain special care in administration of medications
　1. To prevent saving up medications to overdose.
　2. To prevent nonadherence.
L. Make rounds at frequent, *irregular* intervals (especially at night, toward early morning, at change of shift, or other predictably busy times for staff)
M. Encourage client to express honest feelings, including anger
N. Provide hostility release if needed

MAKING THE CONNECTION

Depression and suicidal behaviors may be viewed as anger turned inward on the self. If this anger can be verbalized in a nonthreatening environment, the client may be able to eventually resolve these feelings.

O. Help client to identify the true source of anger
P. Encourage client to work on adaptive coping skills

XV. Intervention With the Suicidal Client Following Discharge (or Outpatient Suicidal Client)

A. The person should not be left alone
　1. Arrange for the client to stay with family or friends.
　2. If not possible, hospitalization should be reconsidered.
B. Establish a written no-suicide plan with the client
C. Enlist family or friends to ensure a safe home environment
D. Provide telephone numbers of counselor or emergency contact
E. Schedule appointments daily or every other day until crisis has subsided
F. Establish rapport and promote a trusting relationship
G. Be direct; talk openly and matter-of-factly about suicide
H. Listen actively and encourage expression of feelings, including anger
I. Nonjudgmentally accept the client's feelings
J. Discuss the client's current crisis
K. Offer alternatives to suicide:
　1. "It is my belief that you are incorrect in your idea that suicide is the only and best solution to your problem."
　2. "There are alternatives, and they are good. What is more, you will be alive to test them."
L. Help the client identify areas of life that can and cannot be controlled
M. Discuss feelings associated with these control issues
N. Some control over life situations may increase self-worth
O. No more than a 3-day supply of antidepressant medications should be dispensed; no refills should be prescribed

🛑 As depression lifts, clients can become energized and are thus able to put their suicide plans into action. Sometimes, depressed clients with or without treatment suddenly appear to be at peace with themselves because they have reached a secret decision to commit suicide. Clinicians should be especially suspicious of such a dramatic clinical change, which may portend a suicidal attempt.

P. Information for family and friends of the suicidal client
　1. Take any hint of suicide seriously.
　2. Anyone expressing suicidal feelings needs immediate attention.

3. Do not keep secrets. If a suicidal person says, "Promise you won't tell anyone," do not make that promise.

🛑 Suicidal individuals are ambivalent about dying, and suicidal behavior may be a cry for help. It is that ambivalence that leads the person to confide suicidal thoughts. The decision to commit suicide can be impulsive. Immediate interventions can serve to prevent the act thereby giving the opportunity to present to the client the idea that suicide is a permanent solution to a temporary problem. It is critical to seek help. A national suicide hotline is available 24 hours a day at 1-800-SUICIDE.

4. Avoid showing anger or attempting to provoke guilt in individuals who are suicidal.
5. Don't discount feelings or tell them to "snap out of it." This is a very real and serious situation to them, and they are in real pain.
6. Be a good listener. If people express suicidal thoughts or feel depressed, hopeless, or worthless, be supportive.

Q. Interventions for families and friends of suicide victims

DID YOU KNOW?
Suicide has a profound effect on the family, friends, and associates of the victim that transcends the immediate loss. As those close to the victim suffer through bereavement, a variety of reactions and coping mechanisms are engaged as each individual sorts through individual reactions to the difficult loss. Bereavement after suicide is complicated by the complex psychological impact of the act on those close to the victim. It is further complicated by the societal perception that the act of suicide is a failure by the victim and the family to deal with some emotional issue and ultimately society affixes blame for the loss on the survivors. This individual or societal stigma introduces a unique stress on the bereavement process that in some cases requires clinical intervention.

1. Encourage the clients to talk about the suicide, each responding to the others' viewpoints and reconstructing of events. Share memories.
2. Be aware of any blaming or scapegoating of specific family members. Discuss how each

person fits into the family situation, both before and after the suicide.
3. Listen to feelings of guilt and self-persecution. Gently move the individuals toward the reality of the situation.
4. Encourage the family members to discuss individual relationships with the lost loved one.
5. Focus on both positive and negative aspects of the relationships.
6. Gradually point out the irrationality of any idealized concepts of the deceased person.
7. The family must be able to recognize both positive and negative aspects about the person before grief can be resolved.

DID YOU KNOW?
No two people grieve in the same way. It may appear that some family members are getting over the grief faster than others. All family members must be made to understand that if this occurs, it is not because they care less, just that they grieve differently. Variables that enter into this phenomenon include individual past experiences, personal relationship with the deceased person, and individual temperament and coping abilities.

XXI. Nursing Process for Suicide: Evaluation

A. Has self-harm to the individual been avoided?
B. Have suicidal ideations subsided?
C. Does the individual know where to seek assistance outside the hospital when suicidal thoughts occur?
D. Can the client identify areas of life situations over which he or she has control?

MAKING THE CONNECTION
Evaluation of the suicidal client is an ongoing process accomplished through continuous reassessment of the client, as well as determination of goal achievement. Once the immediate crisis has been resolved, extended psychotherapy may be indicated. A suicidal person feels worthless and hopeless.

REVIEW QUESTIONS

1. Which symptom is an example of an affective alteration exhibited by clients diagnosed with severe depression?
   1. Apathy
   2. Somatic delusion
   3. Difficulty falling asleep
   4. Social isolation

2. When asked about interactions with friends and family, the client states, "I'm a loner. I don't like small talk. I keep to myself." A nursing diagnosis of impaired social isolation is recorded. Which of the following client outcomes are appropriate? **Select all that apply.**
   1. By day 4, the client verbalizes a plan to maintain control over life situations.
   2. By day 5, the client demonstrates willingness and desire to socialize with others.
   3. By discharge, the client appropriately approaches others for a one-to-one interaction.
   4. By day 3, the client voluntarily attends group therapy.
   5. By end of day 1, the client will no longer seek to be alone.

3. A client notifies a staff member of current suicidal ideations. Which nursing intervention would take priority?
   1. Place the client on a one-to-one observation.
   2. Determine whether the client has a specific plan to commit suicide.
   3. Assess for past history of suicide attempts.
   4. Notify all staff members and place the client on suicide precautions.

4. A client on an inpatient psychiatric unit has been prescribed tranylcypromine (Parnate) 30 mg daily. Which client statement indicates that discharge teaching has been successful?
   1. "I can't wait to order liver and fava beans with a nice Chianti!"
   2. "Chicken teriyaki with soy sauce, apple sauce, and tea sounds great!"
   3. "I'm craving a hamburger with lettuce and onion, potato chips, and milk."
   4. "For lunch tomorrow, I'm having bologna and cheese, a banana, and a cola."

5. A client with a history of a suicide attempt has been discharged and is being followed in an outpatient clinic. At this time, which is the most appropriate nursing intervention?
   1. Provide the client with a safe and structured environment.
   2. Isolate the client from all stressful situations that may precipitate a suicide attempt.
   3. Observe the client continuously to prevent self-harm.
   4. Assist the client to develop more effective coping mechanisms.

6. A nurse should recognize which of the following statements as being a misconception about suicide? **Select all that apply.**
   1. Eight out of 10 people who commit suicide give warnings about their intentions.
   2. Most suicidal people are very ambivalent about their feelings about suicide.
   3. Most individuals commit suicide by taking an overdose of drugs.
   4. Initial mood improvement can precipitate suicide.
   5. All suicidal individuals are mentally ill and psychotic.

7. A client is being treated with sertraline (Zoloft) for a major depressive episode. The client tells the nurse, "I've only been taking this drug for 2 weeks, but I'm sleeping better, and my appetite has improved." Which is the correct response by the nurse?
   1. "It will take a minimum of 8 weeks for any mood elevation to occur."
   2. "Sleep disturbances and appetite problems are not affected by Zoloft."
   3. "A change in your environment and activity is the reason for this improvement."
   4. "Zoloft therapy can improve insomnias and appetite by the second week."

8. All antidepressants carry an FDA _____ _____ warning for increased risk of suicide in children and adolescents.

9. A nurse practitioner is counseling a depressed client. The nurse determines that the client is using the cognitive distortion of "automatic thoughts." Which client statement is evidence of the "automatic thought" of *personalizing*?
   1. "I'm the only one responsible for my divorce."
   2. "There is nothing good about me."
   3. "I know they all hate me."
   4. "You must need glasses if you think I'm slim."

10. A nursing instructor is teaching about disruptive mood dysregulation disorder (DMDD). Which of the following statements should the instructor include? **Select all that apply.**
    1. The onset of symptoms is after age 10 years.
    2. Temper outbursts are out of proportion in intensity or duration to the situation.
    3. Temper outbursts are inconsistent with developmental level.
    4. Temper outbursts occur, on average, two times per week.
    5. The irritable or angry mood is observable by others (e.g., parents, teachers, peers).

11. A client diagnosed with persistent depressive disorder (dysthymia) is describing ongoing mood disturbances. Which would the nurse expect the client to state?
    1. "My anxiety seems to be getting worse by the day."
    2. "One minute I'm feeling sad, and the next I feel upbeat and happy."
    3. "I'm scared because the voices keep telling me to kill myself."
    4. "I'm feeling low, and the whole world looks pretty dismal all the time."

12. _____ is a pervasive and sustained emotional tone, which significantly influences behavior, personality, and perception.

13. A nursing student is preparing an epidemiological research paper on the prevalence of major depressive disorders (MDD) in the United States. Which of the following statements should the student include? **Select all that apply.**
    1. More than 1 in 25 adults report having a major depressive episode during their life span.
    2. Approximately 21% of men and 13% of women will become clinically depressed during their life span.
    3. Men experience more depression than women beginning at about age 10 and continuing through midlife.
    4. Researchers consider depression the "common cold" of psychiatric disorders.
    5. It has not yet been determined that poor socioeconomic conditions predispose people to mental disability.

14. A nursing student is writing a paper about the various types of depressive disorders. Which symptoms would the student include that characterize major depressive disorder (MDD)? **Select all that apply.**
    1. Depressed mood or loss of interest or pleasure in usual activities
    2. Impaired social and occupational functioning for at least a 1 week duration
    3. History of no more than two manic episodes during the past year
    4. Symptoms cannot be attributed to substances or medical condition
    5. Fatigue or loss of energy nearly every day

15. The normal level of norepinephrine is to the ability to deal with stressful situations as the normal level of serotonin is to the ability to
    1. Exert strong influence over mood and behavior
    2. Regulate mood, anxiety, aggression, irritability, cognition
    3. Contribute to arousal and attention span
    4. Control REM sleep

16. Symptoms of depression present differently in childhood and change with age. List in chronological order the symptoms of childhood depression.
    _____ a. Vague physical complaints and aggressive behavior. They may cling to parents and avoid new people and challenges.
    _____ b. Feeding problems, tantrums, lack of playfulness and emotional expressiveness, failure to thrive, or delays in speech and gross motor development.
    _____ c. Morbid thoughts and excessive worrying. There may be lack of interest in playing with friends.
    _____ d. Accident proneness, phobias, aggressiveness, and excessive self-reproach for minor infractions.

17. A malnourished elderly widow of 2 years is angry, obsesses about her loss, and refuses to eat. Which priority nursing diagnosis would be appropriate for this client?
    1. Risk for suicide
    2. Disturbed sensory perception
    3. Social isolation
    4. Complicated grieving

18. After a spouse dies, a client is diagnosed with complicated grieving with depressed mood. Symptoms include self-care deficit, denial and obsession with loss, social isolation, and anger. Which of the following client outcomes are correct? **Select all that apply.**
    1. By discharge, the client will discuss loss of spouse with staff and family members.
    2. By discharge, the client will interact willingly and appropriately with others.
    3. By discharge, the client will bathe, comb hair, and dress without assistance.
    4. By discharge, the client will eat appropriate meals and gain weight.
    5. By discharge, the client will verbalize feelings about life situations that he or she has no control over.

19. A client diagnosed with major depressive disorder recently fled from a physically abusive spouse. She states, "I probably deserve everything I got." Which is the priority nursing diagnosis for this client?
    1. Suicide R/T depressed mood AEB anger turned inward on the self.
    2. Low self-esteem R/T underdeveloped ego and punitive superego AEB negative self-evaluation.
    3. Powerlessness R/T lifestyle of helplessness AEB client's statement, "I probably deserve everything I got."
    4. Ineffective role performance R/T dysfunctional family system AEB needing to flee from a physically abusive spouse.

20. A severely depressed, sullen adolescent has been taking fluoxetine (Prozac) for 10 days. During a follow-up visit, the client smiles euphorically and states, "I feel so much better now." How might the nurse interpret this behavioral change?
    1. The Prozac has potentiated serotonin syndrome.
    2. The medication dosage should be decreased.
    3. The client's behavioral change is normal and expected.
    4. The client may have decided to carry out suicide plan.

21. A client scheduled for electroconvulsive therapy (ECT) asks the nurse to explain procedures and medications that will be administered. Which of the following would the nurse include? **Select all that apply.**
    1. Atropine sulfate or glycopyrrolate (Robinul) is administered intramuscularly before the treatment to decrease secretions.
    2. Glycopyrrolate (Robinul) paralyzes respiratory muscles making the administration of oxygen necessary before treatment.
    3. Succinylcholine chloride (Anectine) is given intravenously to prevent muscle contractions and bone fractures during the seizure.
    4. Ventilation with pure oxygen will be initiated before, during, and after the treatment.
    5. The anesthesiologist will administer an intravenous, short-acting anesthetic, such as propofol (Diprivan) or etomidate (Amidate).

REVIEW ANSWERS

1. ANSWER: 1

Rationale: Severe depression is characterized by an intensification of the symptoms described for moderate depression.

1. **Apathy is defined as indifference, insensibility, and lack of emotion. Apathy is an affective alteration exhibited by clients diagnosed with severe depression.**
2. Somatic delusion is a cognitive, not an affective, alteration exhibited by clients diagnosed with severe depression.
3. Difficulty falling asleep is a physiological, not an affective, alteration exhibited by clients diagnosed with severe depression.
4. Social isolation is a behavioral, not an affective, alteration exhibited by clients diagnosed with severe depression.

TEST-TAKING TIP: Review the symptoms of severe depression to recognize affective symptoms associated with this disorder.

Content Area: Psychosocial Integrity;
Integrated Process: Nursing Process: Assessment;
Client Need: Psychosocial Integrity;
Cognitive Level: Application;
Concept: Mood

2. ANSWERS: 2, 3, 4

Rationale: Correctly written outcomes must be client centered, specific, realistic, and measurable and must also include a time frame.

1. This outcome is correctly written; however, nothing in the question indicates that this client is powerless and is unable to control his or her life situations.
2. **The client demonstrating willingness and desire to socialize with others by day 5 is an appropriate and correctly written statement.**
3. **The client approaching others for a one-to-one interaction by discharge is an appropriate and correctly written statement.**
4. **The client voluntarily attending group therapy by day 3 is an appropriate and correctly written statement.**
5. It is an unrealistic expectation for the client to no longer seek to be alone by the end of day 1.

TEST-TAKING TIP: Follow the criteria for correctly written outcomes in Chapter 4, and then match the appropriate outcome to the client's nursing diagnosis presented in the question.

Content Area: Safe and Effective Care Environment;
Management of Care;
Integrated Process: Nursing Process: Planning;
Client Need: Safe and Effective Care Environment;
Management of Care;
Cognitive Level: Application;
Concept: Critical Thinking

3. ANSWER: 2

Rationale:

1. To intervene by placing a client on a one-on-one observation before completing a full suicide risk assessment is premature. One-on-one observation may be too extreme an intervention to impose in this situation.

2. **Assessment is the first step in the nursing process. Assessing a client's plan for suicide would give the nurse the information needed to intervene appropriately and therefore should be prioritized.**

3. Although it is important to assess for a past history of suicide attempts, and this does place the client at an increased risk for suicide, a current plan indicates an immediate risk and would therefore be the priority.

4. If the nurse notifies all staff members of a client's suicidal intentions and places the client on suicide precautions before a full suicide assessment, the nurse may be basing this intervention on inaccurate information. Suicide precautions may be necessary for clients experiencing suicidal ideations; however, suicide precaution levels would be based on assessed client risk.

TEST-TAKING TIP: Recognize that the action of assessing a client is considered a nursing intervention. Gathering assessment data should take priority so that later interventions are appropriate. When a client has a viable plan, the suicide risk is increased and requires immediate intervention.

Content Area: Safe and Effective Care Environment;
Management of Care;
Integrated Process: Nursing Process: Implementation;
Client Need: Safe and Effective Care Environment;
Management of Care;
Cognitive Level: Application;
Concept: Nursing

4. ANSWER: 3

Rationale: Tranylcypromine (Parnate) is a monoamine oxidase inhibitor (MAOI) used in the treatment of major depressive disorder. When MAOIs are prescribed, teaching about drug and food interactions is of critical importance in order to avoid the potential for a hypertensive crisis.

1. Liver, fava beans, and Chianti ingested when taking an MAOI would put the client at risk for a hypertensive crisis.
2. Soy sauce ingested when taking an MAOI would put the client at risk for a hypertensive crisis.
3. **All of the foods chosen in this meal are safe to ingest when taking an MAOI. This indicates that discharge teaching has been successful.**
4. Bologna, aged cheese, bananas, and cola ingested when taking an MAOI would put the client at risk for a hypertensive crisis.

TEST-TAKING TIP: Review and memorize all MAOI antidepressants, and then know which foods would be contraindicated while taking this medication.

Content Area: Safe and Effective Care Environment;
Management of Care;
Integrated Process: Nursing Process: Evaluation;
Client Need: Safe and Effective Care Environment;
Management of Care;
Cognitive Level: Application;
Concept: Medication

5. ANSWER: 4

Rationale:

1. Manipulating the environment is impossible in an outpatient setting. Only in an inpatient setting can a safe and structured environment be provided.

2. Isolating the client from all stressful situations is an unrealistic intervention in both inpatient and outpatient settings. In the real world, not all stressful situations can be avoided.

3. Observing the client continuously is impossible in an outpatient setting. Only in an inpatient setting can continual observation be implemented.

4. Assisting the client to develop more effective coping mechanisms is a nursing intervention that can and should be implemented in outpatient settings as ongoing follow-up.

TEST-TAKING TIP: Know the difference between realistic and unrealistic interventions. Always keep the client's safety a priority.

Content Area: Safe and Effective Care Environment; Management of Care;
Integrated Process: Nursing Process: Evaluation;
Client Need: Safe and Effective Care Environment; Management of Care;
Cognitive Level: Application;
Concept: Nursing

6. ANSWERS: 3, 5
Rationale:
1. It is a valid statement that 8 out of 10 individuals who commit suicide give clues and warnings about their intentions. Very subtle clues may be ignored or disregarded by others.

2. It is a valid statement that most suicidal individuals are very ambivalent about their feelings regarding living or dying. Most of these individuals are "gambling with death" and see it as a cry for someone to save them.

3. It is a misconception that individuals usually commit suicide by taking an overdose of drugs. Gunshot wounds are the leading cause of death among suicide victims.

4. It is a valid statement that initial mood improvement can precipitate suicide. Clients experiencing a deep depression are at lower risk for suicide because they may not have the energy to formulate and carry out a suicide plan. When mood begins to elevate and energy levels improve, these clients are at higher risk for suicide.

5. It is a misconception that all suicidal individuals are mentally ill and psychotic. Although these individuals are extremely unhappy, they are not necessarily psychotic or otherwise mentally ill.

TEST-TAKING TIP: Review Table 11.4, "Facts and Fables About Suicide."

Content Area: Safe and Effective Care Environment; Management of Care;
Integrated Process: Nursing Process: Evaluation;
Client Need: Safe and Effective Care Environment; Management of Care;
Cognitive Level: Analysis;
Concept: Assessment

7. ANSWER: 4
Rationale:
1. After initially taking Zoloft, some mood elevation can occur in a minimum of 1 to 4 weeks, not 8 weeks. This nursing response is incorrect.

2. Sleep disturbances and appetite problems are two of the symptoms targeted within the first week of administration of Zoloft. This nursing response is incorrect.

3. Change in environment can have a positive effect on the client but will not likely be sufficient to improve sleep patterns or appetite. It is also unlikely that the client's activity level has changed such that it would improve the condition of the mood. There is nothing presented in the question to imply that the client has had a change in environment or activity.

4. Zoloft is known to elevate mood and improve insomnia, appetite disturbances, and anxiety as early as 2 weeks after drug initiation.

TEST-TAKING TIP: Remember that for SSRIs, mood elevation may take 7 to 28 days, but may take 6 to 8 weeks for major depression symptoms to subside.

Content Area: Safe and Effective Care Environment; Management of Care;
Integrated Process: Nursing Process: Implementation;
Client Need: Safe and Effective Care Environment; Management of Care;
Cognitive Level: Application;
Concept: Medication

8. ANSWER: black box
Rationale: All antidepressants carry an FDA black box warning for increased risk of suicide in children and adolescents. The black box warning label on all antidepressant medications describes the risk for suicide and emphasizes the need for close monitoring of children and adolescents started on these medications.

TEST-TAKING TIP: Review the key terms at the beginning of the chapter.

Content Area: Psychosocial Integrity;
Integrated Process: Nursing Process: Assessment;
Client Need: Psychosocial Integrity;
Cognitive Level: Knowledge
Concept: Medication

9. ANSWER: 1
Rationale:
1. "I'm the only one responsible for my divorce" is an example of the cognitive distortion of the "automatic thought" *personalizing*.

2. "There is nothing good about me" is an example of the cognitive distortion of the "automatic thought" *all or nothing*.

3. "I know they all hate me" is an example of the cognitive distortion of the "automatic thought" *mind reading*.

4. "You must need glasses if you think I'm slim" is an example of the cognitive distortion of the "automatic thought" *discounting positives*.

TEST-TAKING TIP: Review and be able to distinguish the difference between the various cognitive distortions of "automatic thoughts."

Content Area: Psychosocial Integrity;
Integrated Process: Nursing Process: Implementation;
Client Need: Psychosocial Integrity;
Cognitive Level: Application;
Concept: Assessment

10. ANSWERS: 2, 3, 5
Rationale:
1. The age of onset of symptoms is before, not after, 10 years.
2. **Temper outbursts are grossly out of proportion in intensity or duration to the situation.**
3. **Temper outbursts are inconsistent with developmental level.**
4. Temper outbursts occur, on average, three or more, times per week. Having temper outbursts only 2 times per week would not meet the conditions for this diagnosis.
5. **The irritable or angry mood is observable by others (e.g., parents, teachers, peers).**
TEST-TAKING TIP: Review the symptoms of the childhood disorder *disruptive mood dysregulation disorder.*
Content Area: Safe and Effective Care Environment;
Management of Care;
Integrated Process: Nursing Process: Implementation;
Client Need: Safe and Effective Care Environment;
Management of Care;
Cognitive Level: Application;
Concept: Nursing Roles

11. ANSWER: 4
Rationale:
1. The statement "My anxiety seems to be getting worse by the day" describes an anxiety, not a persistent depressive disorder.
2. The statement, "One minute I'm feeling sad, and the next, I feel upbeat and happy," describes a cyclothymic, not a persistent depressive disorder.
3. The statement, "I'm scared because the voices keep telling me to kill myself," describes a paranoid psychosis, not a persistent depressive disorder.
4. **"I'm feeling low, and the whole world looks pretty dismal all the time" is a statement that the nurse would expect a client diagnosed with persistent depressive disorder to make. Characteristics of this disorder are similar to, if somewhat milder than, those ascribed to major depressive disorder. Individuals with this mood disturbance describe their mood as sad or "down in the dumps." To be diagnosed with this disorder, a client must experience symptoms for at least 2 years (1 year for children and adolescents).**
TEST-TAKING TIP: Review the symptoms of persistent depressive disorder (dysthymia) and recognize how these symptoms differ from both major depressive disorder and bipolar disorder.
Content Area: Psychosocial Integrity;
Integrated Process: Nursing Process: Assessment;
Client Need: Psychosocial Integrity;
Cognitive Level: Application
Concept: Mood

12. ANSWER: Mood
Rationale: Mood is an individual's sustained emotional tone, which significantly influences behavior, personality, and perception. Mood may have a major influence on a person's perception of the world.
TEST-TAKING TIP: Review the key terms at the beginning of the chapter.
Content Area: Psychosocial Integrity;
Integrated Process: Nursing Process: Assessment;

Client Need: Psychosocial Integrity;
Cognitive Level: Knowledge;
Concept: Mood

13. ANSWERS: 1, 4, 5
Rationale:
1. **Researchers have concluded that more than 1 in 25 adults report having a major depressive episode during their life span.**
2. Approximately 21% of *women* and 13% of *men* will become clinically depressed during their life span.
3. Women, not men, experience more depression beginning at about age 10 and continuing through midlife. The incidence of major depressive disorder is higher in women than men by almost two to one.
4. **Researchers consider depression the "common cold" of psychiatric disorders. Researchers also consider the current generation the "age of melancholia."**
5. **Research shows that both depression and personality disorders are associated with low socioeconomic status. However, it has not yet been determined whether poor socioeconomic conditions predispose people to mental disability or if mental disabilities predispose people to poor socioeconomic conditions.**
TEST-TAKING TIP: Review the epidemiological information related to depression.
Content Area: Psychosocial Integrity;
Integrated Process: Nursing Process: Evaluation;
Client Need: Psychosocial Integrity;
Cognitive Level: Analysis;
Concept: Assessment

14. ANSWERS: 1, 4, 5
Rationale:
1. **Major depressive disorder (MDD) is characterized by depressed mood or loss of interest or pleasure in usual activities.**
2. Impaired social and occupational functioning has existed for a duration of at least 2 weeks, not 1 week.
3. To be diagnosed with MDD, there can be no history of manic behavior.
4. **To be diagnosed with MDD, symptoms cannot be attributed to the use of substances or a general medical condition.**
5. **MDD is characterized by fatigue or loss of energy nearly every day.**
TEST-TAKING TIP: Review the different types of depressive disorders, specifically characteristics associated with major depressive disorder.
Content Area: Safe and Effective Care Environment;
Management of Care;
Integrated Process: Nursing Process: Implementation;
Client Need: Safe and Effective Care Environment;
Management of Care;
Cognitive Level: Application;
Concept: Mood

15. ANSWER: 2
Rationale:
1. Dopamine, not serotonin, is the neurotransmitter that exerts a strong influence over mood and behavior.
2. **Serotonin is the neurotransmitter that regulates mood, anxiety, arousal, vigilance, irritability,**

thinking, cognition, appetite, aggression, and
circadian rhythm.
3. Acetylcholine, not serotonin, is the neurotransmitter
that contributes to arousal and attention span.
4. Acetylcholine, not serotonin, is the neurotransmitter
that contributes to the control of REM sleep.
TEST-TAKING TIP: Review the biochemical influences of
neurotransmitters.
*Content Area: Safe and Effective Care Environment;
Management of Care;*
Integrated Process: Nursing Process: Assessment;
*Client Need: Safe and Effective Care Environment;
Management of Care;*
Cognitive Level: Analysis;
Concept: Assessment

16. **ANSWER: The correct order is 3, 1, 4, 2**
Rationale:
1. Up to age 3 years, the symptoms of depression may include feeding problems, tantrums, lack of playfulness and
emotional expressiveness, failure to thrive, or delays in
speech and gross motor development.
2. From ages 3 to 5 years, common symptoms may include
accident proneness, phobias, aggressiveness, and excessive
self-reproach for minor infractions.
3. From ages 6 to 8 years, there may be vague physical
complaints and aggressive behavior. They may cling to
parents and avoid new people and challenges. They may
lag behind their classmates in social skills and academic
competence.
4. From ages 9 to 12 years, common symptoms include
morbid thoughts and excessive worrying. They may reason
that they are depressed because they have disappointed
their parents in some way. There may be lack of interest in
playing with friends.
TEST-TAKING TIP: Review the developmental implications
of childhood depression and understand that symptoms of
depression present differently in childhood and change
with age.
*Content Area: Safe and Effective Care Environment;
Management of Care;*
Integrated Process: Nursing Process: Assessment;
*Client Need: Safe and Effective Care Environment;
Management of Care;*
Cognitive Level: Analysis;
Concept: Mood

17. **ANSWER: 4**
Rationale:
1. There is nothing presented in the question indicating
that this client is at risk for suicide.
2. There is nothing presented in the question indicating
that this client is delirious, demented, or psychotic,
as seen in clients diagnosed with disturbed sensory
perception.
3. There is nothing presented in the question indicating
that this client is socially isolated.
4. **Complicated grieving is the priority nursing diagnosis for this client in that after being widowed for
2 years, she remains angry, obsesses about her loss,
and refuses to eat. Complicated grieving occurs after
the death of a significant other in which the experience**

of distress accompanying bereavement fails to follow
normative expectations and manifests in functional
impairment.
TEST-TAKING TIP: Review Table 11.1, "Assigning Nursing
Diagnoses to Behaviors Commonly Associated With
Depression"; then match the appropriate nursing diagnosis
to the client's symptoms presented in the question.
*Content Area: Safe and Effective Care Environment;
Management of Care;*
Integrated Process: Nursing Process: Diagnosis (Analysis);
*Client Need: Safe and Effective Care Environment;
Management of Care;*
Cognitive Level: Analysis;
Concept: Critical Thinking

18. **ANSWERS: 1, 2, 3, 5**
Rationale: Correctly written outcomes must be client
centered, specific, realistic, measurable, and must also
include a time frame.
1. **The client's ability to discuss loss of spouse with staff
and family members by discharge meets all the criteria
for a correctly written outcome and addresses the
client's denial issues.**
2. **The client's ability to interact willingly and appropriately with others by discharge meets all the criteria for
a correctly written outcome and addresses the client's
social isolation issues.**
3. **The client's ability to bathe, comb hair, and dress
without assistance by discharge meets all the criteria for
a correctly written outcome and addresses the client's
self-care deficit issues.**
4. There is nothing presented in the question indicating
that the client is suffering from a nutritional deficit. Also,
the outcome is incorrectly written. Although the phrase
"by discharge" meets time frame criteria, "weight gain" is
a vague term and cannot be measured.
5. **The client's ability to verbalize feelings about life
situations that he or she has no control over by discharge
meets all the criteria for a correctly written outcome and
addresses the client's anger issues.**
TEST-TAKING TIP: Follow the criteria for correctly written
outcomes in Chapter 2 and then match the appropriate
outcome to the client's symptoms presented in the
question.
Content Area: Psychosocial Integrity;
Integrated Process: Nursing Process: Planning;
Client Need: Psychosocial Integrity;
Cognitive Level: Application;
Concept: Critical Thinking

19. **ANSWER: 2**
Rationale:
1. Suicide indicates that the act has already occurred and
assigning a nursing diagnosis would become a moot point.
Correctly written, this nursing diagnosis would be "Risk
for suicide R/T lifestyle of helplessness." "Risk for" nursing
diagnoses do not have an AEB statement because the problem has not yet occurred.
2. **"Low self-esteem R/T underdeveloped ego and punitive superego AEB negative self-evaluation" is the priority NANDA nursing diagnosis. It is correctly written and
corresponds to this client's behavior.**

3. "Powerlessness R/T lifestyle of helplessness AEB client's statement, 'I probably deserve everything I got'" is a NANDA nursing diagnosis that may eventually correspond to this client's behavior; however, low self-esteem takes priority because good self-esteem must be established in order for the client to feel empowered.

4. "Ineffective role performance R/T dysfunctional family system AEB needing to flee from a physically abusive spouse" is a NANDA nursing diagnosis; however, ineffective role performance implies that the client, by being ineffective in her family role, is responsible for the abuse. There is nothing in the question that indicates client responsibility.

TEST-TAKING TIP: Review the concept and follow the criteria for correctly written NANDA nursing diagnoses in Chapter 4 and then match the appropriate nursing diagnosis to the client's symptoms presented in the question.

Content Area: Safe and Effective Care Environment; Management of Care;
Integrated Process: Nursing Process: Diagnosis (Analysis);
Client Need: Safe and Effective Care Environment; Management of Care;
Cognitive Level: Analysis;
Concept: Critical Thinking

20. **ANSWER: 4**
Rationale:

1. Serotonin syndrome occurs when two drugs that potentiate serotonergic neurotransmission are used concurrently causing symptoms that include changes in mental status, restlessness, myoclonus, hyperreflexia, tachycardia, labile blood pressure, diaphoresis, shivering, and tremors. There is no indication that the client is experiencing serotonin syndrome.

2. The client's symptoms do not indicate a change in dosage.

3. Mood elevation can be evidenced in 2 to 4 weeks; however, it will take 6 to 8 weeks for major depressive symptoms to subside. This client's behavioral changes would not be normal or expected.

4. **This client has not been taking Prozac long enough to warrant the positive response exhibited. Therefore, the client's euphoria may indicate a decision to carry out a suicide plan. The black box warning label on all antidepressant medications describes this risk and emphasizes the need for close monitoring of clients started on these mediations. The advisory language does not prohibit the use of antidepressants in children and adolescents;**

rather, it warns of the risk of suicide and encourages prescribers to balance this risk with clinical need.

TEST-TAKING TIP: Review Table 11.2, "Medications Used in the Treatment of Depression.: Read and review the "black box" warning, especially as it pertains to adolescence.

Content Area: Safe and Effective Care Environment; Management of Care;
Integrated Process: Nursing Process: Assessment;
Client Need: Safe and Effective Care Environment; Management of Care;
Cognitive Level: Application;
Concept: Medication

21. **ANSWERS: 1, 3, 5**
Rationale:

1. **A pretreatment medication, such as atropine sulfate or glycopyrrolate (Robinul) is administered intramuscularly approximately 30 minutes before the treatment. Either of these medications may be ordered to decrease secretions (to prevent aspiration) and counteract the effects of vagal stimulation (bradycardia) induced by the ECT.**

2. Glycopyrrolate (Robinul) decreases secretions. Succinylcholine chloride (Anectine) paralyzes respiratory muscles.

3. **Succinylcholine chloride (Anectine) is administered intravenously during treatment to prevent severe muscle contractions during the seizure, thereby reducing the possibility of fractured or dislocated bones. Because succinylcholine paralyzes respiratory muscles as well, the client is ventilated with pure oxygen during and after the treatment.**

4. Succinylcholine is given during and not before treatment; therefore, no oxygenation is needed before treatment.

5. **In the treatment room, the anesthesiologist will intravenously administer a short-acting anesthetic, such as propofol (Diprivan) or etomidate (Amidate).**

TEST-TAKING TIP: Review all ECT medications and their actions.

Content Area: Safe and Effective Care Environment; Management of Care;
Integrated Process: Nursing Process: Implementation;
Client Need: Safe and Effective Care Environment; Management of Care;
Cognitive Level: Analysis;
Concept: Nursing Roles

CASE STUDY: Putting it All Together

Melanie, a disheveled 41-year-old woman, has been admitted to an inpatient psychiatric unit. Since her 16-year-old son's suicide 4 months ago, Melanie has been despondent, has difficulty sleeping, claims a 20-pound weight loss, and says she has no right to live. She has bouts of crying that no amount of comfort consoles, and when approached by Jim, the psychiatric nurse practitioner (PNP), she once again dissolves into tears. Melanie accepts the prn Xanax Jim offers and seems to collect herself as Jim sits quietly by her side. Looking at Jim with a doleful expression, she says in a shaky voice, "Let me tell you about my wonderful boy." Jim listens carefully as Melanie's story unfolds.

"He was smart, athletic, handsome, and talented. His future was so bright, and his father and I couldn't have been prouder of him. Then about a year ago, he began looking miserable saying he couldn't live up to everyone's expectations, and sometimes it just wasn't worth going on. I remember feeling the same way when I was a teenager, and my mother said that all teenagers, including her, had felt the same way. When my concerns only grew, I took him to our family doctor who listened and told me that the feelings my son was experiencing were just the normal emotional stresses of growing up. He prescribed Zoloft and said that my

son should be right as rain in 2 to 3 weeks. Two weeks after starting the medication, my son seemed just like his old self. Two days later, I found him hanging in the closet. I never read the "black box" label warning, and now he's dead because of me. It's all my fault. I will never be okay." Melanie's eyes fill with tears as she whispers, "I just want to end it all and be with him."

1. The PNP would document which tentative medical diagnosis for Melanie?
2. What are Melanie's subjective symptoms that would lead to the determination of this diagnosis?
3. What are Melanie's objective symptoms that would lead to the determination of this diagnosis?
4. What treatment modality may Melanie's PNP use to address the symptoms of her disorder?
5. What NANDA nursing diagnosis would be appropriate for Melanie?
6. On the basis of this nursing diagnosis, what short-term outcome would be appropriate for Melanie?
7. On the basis of this nursing diagnosis, what long-term outcome would be appropriate for Melanie?
8. List the nursing interventions (actions) that will assist Melanie in successfully meeting these outcomes.
9. List the questions that should be answered in determining the success of the nursing actions.

Chapter 12

Bipolar and Related Disorders

KEY TERMS

Bipolar disorder—A chronic mood disturbance characterized by mood swings from profound depression to extreme euphoria (mania), with intervening periods of normalcy; psychotic symptoms may or may not be present

Clouding of consciousness—A mental state in which a client is not fully aware of the immediate surroundings

Cyclothymic disorder—A chronic mood disturbance involving numerous episodes of hypomania and depressed mood, of insufficient severity or duration to meet the criteria for bipolar disorder

Depression—An alteration in mood that is expressed by feelings of sadness, despair, and pessimism; there is a loss of interest in usual activities, and somatic symptoms may be evident; changes in appetite and sleep patterns are common

Distractibility—Inability to focus one's attention; the loss of the ability to concentrate

Euphoria—An exaggerated feeling of well-being or elation

Grandiosity—An unrealistic and exaggerated concept of self-worth, importance, wealth, and ability

Hypomania—A mild form of mania; symptoms are excessive hyperactivity, but not severe enough to cause marked impairment in social or occupational functioning or to require hospitalization

Mania—An alteration in mood that is expressed by feelings of elation, inflated self-esteem, grandiosity, hyperactivity, agitation, and accelerated thinking and speaking

Monotherapy—Treatment with a single drug

Mood swings—Periods of variation of how one feels, changing from a sense of well-being to one of depression; this occurs normally but may become abnormally intense in persons with bipolar disorder

Pressured speech—Loud and emphatic speech that is increased in amount, accelerated, and usually difficult or impossible to interrupt; the speech is not in response to a stimulus and may continue even though no one is listening

Bipolar disorder is a mood disorder manifested by cycles of mania and depression. Mania is an alteration in mood that is expressed by feelings of elation, inflated self-esteem, grandiosity, hyperactivity, agitation, and accelerated thinking and speaking.

DID YOU KNOW?

Mania can occur as a biological (organic) or psychological disorder or as a response to substance use or a general medical condition.

I. Epidemiology of **Bipolar Disorder**

A. The incidence of bipolar disorder is roughly equal in both genders, with a ratio of women to men of about 1.2 to 1

B. The average age of onset is the early 20s

C. After the first manic episode, the disorder tends to be recurrent

D. As with depression, bipolar disorder appears to be more common in unmarried than in married persons

E. Unlike depressive disorders, bipolar disorder appears to occur more frequently among the higher socioeconomic classes
F. Bipolar disorder is the sixth leading cause of disability in the middle-age population

II. Predisposing Factors

A. The exact etiology of bipolar disorder is unknown
B. Scientific evidence supports a chemical imbalance in the brain although the cause of the imbalance remains unclear
C. Theories that consider a combination of hereditary factors and environmental triggers (stressful life events) appear to hold the most credibility
D. Biological theories
   1. Genetics.
      a. Research suggests that bipolar disorder strongly reflects an underlying genetic vulnerability.
      b. Evidence from family, twin, and adoption studies exists to support this observation.

DID YOU KNOW?
Twin studies have indicated a concordance rate for bipolar disorder among monozygotic twins at 60% to 80% compared with 10% to 20% in dizygotic twins. Family studies have shown that if one parent has bipolar disorder, the risk that a child will have the disorder is around 28%. If both parents have the disorder, the risk is two to three times as great.

   c. Children born to parents with bipolar disorder and adopted at birth and reared by adoptive parents without evidence of the disorder have a higher risk of developing the disorder. These results strongly indicate that genes play a role separate from that of the environment.
   d. Genetic studies have shown that an alteration in particular genes contributes to the risk of developing bipolar disorder.
   2. Biochemical influences.
      a. Early studies have associated symptoms of depression with a functional deficiency of norepinephrine and dopamine and symptoms of mania with a functional excess of these amines.
      b. The neurotransmitter serotonin appears to remain low in both states.
      c. Some support of this neurotransmitter hypothesis has been demonstrated by the effects of neuroleptic drugs that influence the levels of these biogenic amines to produce the desired effect.
      d. Because cholinergic agents do have profound effects on mood, electroencephalogram (EEG), sleep, and neuroendocrine function, it has been suggested that the problem in depression and mania may be an imbalance between the biogenic amines and acetylcholine.
      e. Cholinergic transmission is thought to be excessive in depression and inadequate in mania.
   3. Physiological influences that have been shown to induce secondary mania:
      a. Right-sided lesions in the limbic system, temporobasal areas, basal ganglia, and thalamus.
      b. Magnetic resonance imaging (MRI) studies have revealed enlarged third ventricles and subcortical white matter and periventricular hyperintensities in clients with bipolar disorder.
   4. Medication side effects.

DID YOU KNOW?
Certain medications used to treat somatic illnesses have been known to trigger a manic response. These medications include steroids, amphetamines, antidepressants, and high doses of anticonvulsants and narcotics.

E. Psychosocial theories
   1. The credibility of psychosocial theories has declined in recent years.
   2. Bipolar disorder is viewed as a disease of the brain with biological etiologies.

III. Types of Bipolar Disorders:

A. Bipolar I disorder
   1. Characterized by mood swings from profound depression to extreme euphoria (mania), with intervening periods of normalcy.
   2. Psychotic features, including delusions or hallucinations, may be present.
   3. Onset of symptoms may reflect a seasonal pattern.
   4. During a manic episode, the mood is elevated, expansive, or irritable.
   5. The disturbance is sufficiently severe to cause marked impairment in occupational functioning or in usual social activities or relationships with others or to require hospitalization to prevent harm to self or others.
   6. Motor activity is excessive and frenzied.
B. Bipolar II disorder
   1. Characterized by recurrent bouts of depression with episodic occurrence of **hypomania.**
   2. May present with symptoms (or history) of depression or hypomania.

🛑 A client diagnosed with bipolar II disorder must never have experienced a full manic episode. If a full manic episode has ever been part of the client's clinical history, then a diagnosis of bipolar I is assigned.

3. The current or most recent episode can be:
   a. Hypomanic.
   b. Depressed.
   c. Mixed features.
4. Psychotic or catatonic features may be noted in the severe depression phase of bipolar II disorder.
5. The hypomania phase of bipolar II disorder does not include psychotic features.

C. Cyclothymic disorder
   1. A chronic mood disturbance of at least 2 years' duration.
   2. Numerous periods of elevated mood that do not meet the criteria for a hypomanic episode.
   3. Numerous periods of depressed mood of insufficient severity or duration to meet the criteria for major depressive episode.
   4. Individual is never without the symptoms for more than 2 months.

D. Substance-induced bipolar disorder
   1. Disturbance of mood considered to be the direct result of physiological effects of a substance (e.g., a drug of abuse, a medication, or other treatment).
   2. The mood disturbance may involve elevated, expansive, or irritable mood, with inflated self-esteem, decreased need for sleep, and distractibility.
   3. Clinically significant distress or impairment in social, occupational, or other important areas of functioning.
   4. Mood disturbances are associated with *intoxication* from substances such as alcohol, amphetamines, cocaine, hallucinogens, inhalants, opioids, phencyclidine, sedatives, hypnotics, and anxiolytics.
   5. Symptoms can occur with *withdrawal* from substances such as alcohol, amphetamines, cocaine, sedatives, hypnotics, and anxiolytics.
   6. A number of medications have been known to evoke mood symptoms.
      a. Anesthetics.
      b. Analgesics.
      c. Anticholinergics.
      d. Anticonvulsants.
      e. Antihypertensives.
      f. Antiparkinsonian agents.
      g. Antiulcer agents.
      h. Cardiac medications.
      i. Oral contraceptives.
      j. Psychotropic medications.
      k. Muscle relaxants.
      l. Steroids.
      m. Sulfonamides.

E. Bipolar disorder associated with another medical condition
   1. Characterized by an abnormally and persistently elevated, expansive, or irritable mood and excessive activity or energy that is judged to be the result of direct physiological effects of another medical condition.
   2. Causes clinically significant distress or impairment in social, occupational, or other important areas of functioning.

IV. Nursing Process: Assessment: Bipolar Mania

A. Three stages of the symptoms of manic states
   1. Hypomania.
   2. Acute mania.
   3. Delirious mania.

B. Hypomania
   1. Symptoms not sufficiently severe to cause marked impairment in social or occupational functioning or to require hospitalization.
   2. Mood.
      a. Cheerful and expansive.
      b. Underlying irritability surfaces rapidly with unfulfilled wishes or desires.
      c. Client's nature is volatile and fluctuating.
   3. Cognition and perception.
      a. Perceptions of the self are grandiose with ideas of great worth and ability.
      b. Flight of ideas.
      c. Perception of the environment is heightened.
      d. Individual is easily distracted by irrelevant stimuli.
      e. Increase in goal-directed activities.
   4. Activity and behavior.
      a. Increased motor activity.
      b. Very extroverted and sociable; attract numerous acquaintances.
      c. Lack the depth of personality and warmth to formulate close friendships.
      d. Talk and laugh very loudly and often inappropriately.
      e. Increased libido.
      f. May experience anorexia, decreased need for sleep, insomnia, and weight loss.
      g. Exalted self-perception leads to inappropriate behaviors, such as buying huge amounts on a credit card without having the resources to pay.

C. Stage II: acute mania
   1. Symptoms of acute mania may be a progression in intensification of those experienced in hypomania, or they may manifest directly.
   2. Most individuals experience marked impairment in functioning and require hospitalization.
   3. Mood.
      a. Characterized by **euphoria** and elation.
      b. Appears to be on a continuous "high."
      c. Mood is subject to frequent variation, easily changing to irritability and anger, or even to sadness and crying.

4. Cognition and perception.
   a. An inflated self-esteem or grandiosity.
   b. Cognition and perception become fragmented.
   c. Cognition and perception often psychotic in acute mania.
   d. Rapid thinking proceeds to racing and disjointed thinking (flight of ideas).
   e. May be manifested by a continuous flow of accelerated, **pressured speech** (loquaciousness), with abrupt changes from topic to topic.
   f. When flight of ideas is severe, speech may be disorganized and incoherent.
   g. **Distractibility** becomes all pervasive.
   h. Attention can be diverted by even the smallest of stimuli.
   i. Hallucinations and delusions (usually paranoid and grandiose) are common.
5. Activity and behavior.
   a. Psychomotor activity is excessive.
   b. Sexual interest is increased.
   c. Poor impulse control; socially and sexually uninhibited, intrudes on others' space.
   d. Excessive spending is common.
   e. Clients may manipulate others to carry out their wishes, and if things go wrong, they can skillfully project responsibility for the failure onto others.
   f. Energy seems inexhaustible.

DID YOU KNOW?

During a full manic state, a client's metabolic rate is increased leading to increased caloric and oxygen requirements.

   g. Need for sleep is diminished.
   h. Hygiene and grooming is neglected.
   i. Dress may be disorganized, flamboyant, or bizarre.

   j. Wearing excessive make-up or jewelry is common.
D. Stage III: Delirious Mania
   1. Grave form of the disorder.
   2. Intensification of the symptoms associated with acute mania.
   3. Relatively rare since the availability of antipsychotic medications.
   4. Mood.
      a. Mood very labile.
      b. Exhibits feelings of despair, quickly converting to unrestrained merriment and ecstasy.
      c. Can become irritable or totally indifferent to the environment.
      d. Panic anxiety may be evident.
   5. Cognition and perception.
      a. Severe **clouding of consciousness.**
      b. Confusion, disorientation, and sometimes stupor.
      c. Delusions of grandeur or persecution.
      d. Auditory or visual hallucinations.
      e. Extremely distractible and incoherent.
   6. Activity and behavior.
      a. Psychomotor activity is frenzied and characterized by agitated, purposeless movements.

🛑 Agitated, frenzied movement puts the client at risk for injury. A nurse's first priority is always client safety.

      b. Exhaustion, injury to self or others, and eventually death could occur without intervention.

V. Nursing Process: Diagnosis (Analysis)

See Table 12-1 for a list of client behaviors and the NANDA nursing diagnoses that correspond to those behaviors, which may be used in planning care for the client experiencing a manic episode.

Table 12.1 Assigning Nursing Diagnoses to Behaviors Commonly Associated with Bipolar Mania

Behaviors	Nursing Diagnoses
Extreme hyperactivity; increased agitation and lack of control over purposeless and potentially injurious movements	**Risk for injury**
Manic excitement, delusional thinking, hallucinations, impulsivity	**Risk for violence: self-directed or other-directed**
Loss of weight, amenorrhea, refusal or inability to sit still long enough to eat	**Imbalanced nutrition: less than body requirements**
Delusions of grandeur and persecution; inaccurate interpretation of the environment	**Disturbed thought processes***
Auditory and visual hallucinations; disorientation	**Disturbed sensory-perception***
Inability to develop satisfying relationships, manipulation of other for own desires, use of unsuccessful social interaction behaviors	**Impaired social interaction**
Difficulty falling asleep, sleeping only short periods	**Insomnia**

*These diagnoses have been resigned from the NANDA-I list of approved diagnoses. They are used in this instance because they are most compatible with the identified behaviors.

VI. Nursing Process: Planning

The following outcomes may be assigned when planning care for the client experiencing a manic episode.
By discharge, the client will:
A. Exhibit no evidence of physical injury
B. Have not harmed self or others
C. No longer exhibit signs of physical agitation
D. Eat a well-balanced diet with snacks to prevent weight loss and maintain nutritional status
E. Verbalize an accurate interpretation of the environment
F. Verbalize that hallucinatory activity has ceased and demonstrate no outward behavior indicating hallucinations
G. Accept responsibility for own behaviors
H. Not manipulate others for gratification of own needs
I. Interact appropriately with others
J. Be able to fall asleep within 30 minutes of retiring
K. Be able to sleep 6 to 8 hours per night without medication

VII. Nursing Process: Implementation

A. Reduce stimuli and maintain a calm attitude

DID YOU KNOW?
Anxiety is contagious and can be transmitted from a staff member to client.

B. Provide structured schedule with limited group activities (e.g., 1:1 basketball with staff) and established rest periods
C. Assign private room

A client experiencing mania is extremely distractible, and responses to even the slightest stimuli are exaggerated. A milieu unit may be too stimulating. Decreasing stimuli will minimize anxiety, agitation, and suspiciousness.

D. Observe client every 15 min
E. Stay with agitated client
F. Remove sharps, belts, and other dangerous objects from environment

A client who is experiencing active mania can be irrational and may harm self inadvertently. Dangerous objects must be removed so that the client (in an agitated, hyperactive state) cannot use them to harm self or others.

G. Provide sufficient staff for show of strength if necessary
H. Administer ordered tranquilizers as needed

DID YOU KNOW?
Antipsychotics are commonly used when a client is extremely manic and are effective for providing rapid relief from symptoms of hyperactivity.

I. After attempts to verbally deescalate client, mechanical restraints may be necessary
J. Provide favorite foods that are high-protein, high-calorie fingers foods
K. Provide juice and snacks on unit
L. Monitor intake and output, calorie count, daily weights
M. Provide vitamin and mineral supplements
N. Sit with client during meals
O. Provide physical activities

DID YOU KNOW?
Physical activities help relieve pent-up tension.

P. Set limits on manipulative behaviors
Q. Explain what is expected and the consequences if limits are violated
R. Do not argue, bargain, or try to reason with client; simply state limits
S. Confront manipulative or exploitative behaviors immediately

MAKING THE CONNECTION
Clients should be offered an avenue of the "least restrictive alternative." Restraints should be used only as a last resort, after all other interventions (e.g., verbal interactions, physical exercise, offering antianxiety medications) have been unsuccessful, and the client is clearly at risk of harm to self or others. Follow The Joint Commission guidelines for the use of restraints and seclusion presented in Chapter 6.

MAKING THE CONNECTION
Clients experiencing mania have difficulty sitting still long enough to eat a meal. Providing high calorie finger foods will increase the likelihood that the client will consume food and drinks. Sandwiches and hot dogs, for example, are good choices. Nutritious intake is required on a regular basis to compensate for increased caloric requirements due to hyperactivity.

MAKING THE CONNECTION

Because of a strong id influence, the client experiencing mania is unable to establish limits so this must be done for him or her. Unless consequences for violation of limits are consistent, manipulative behavior will not be eliminated. Inconsistency creates confusion and encourages testing of limits.

T. Follow through with consequences
U. Provide positive reinforcement for nonmanipulative behaviors

VIII. Nursing Process: Evaluation

Evaluation of the nursing actions for the client with bipolar mania may be facilitated by gathering information using the following types of questions.
A. Has the individual avoided personal injury?
B. Has violence to client or others been prevented?
C. Has agitation subsided?
D. Have nutritional status and weight been stabilized? Is the client able to select foods to maintain adequate nutrition?
E. Have delusions and hallucinations ceased? Is the client able to interpret the environment correctly?
F. Is the client able to make decisions about own self-care? Have hygiene and grooming improved?
G. Is behavior socially acceptable? Is client able to interact with others in a satisfactory manner? Has the client stopped manipulating others to fulfill own desires?
H. Is the client able to sleep 6 to 8 hours per night and awaken feeling rested?
I. Does the client understand the importance of maintenance medication therapy? Does he or she understand that symptoms may return if medication is discontinued?

DID YOU KNOW?
Clients diagnosed with bipolar disorder often purposefully are nonadherent with their medications. They take pleasure from the expansive mood and creativity characteristic of a manic state and stop their medications to reexperience this "high."

J. Can the client taking lithium verbalize early signs of lithium toxicity? Does he or she understand the necessity for blood level checks?

IX. Treatment Modalities for Bipolar Disorder (Mania)

A. Individual psychotherapy
   1. Assists with relationships that tend to be shallow and rigid.
   2. Focuses on grief, role conflicts, role transitions, and interpersonal deficiencies.
   3. Provides psychoeducation about bipolar disorder.
   4. Encourages treatment adherence.
B. Group therapy (Should not be implemented until acute phase of the illness is stabilized)
   1. Provides an atmosphere in which individuals may discuss issues in their lives that cause, maintain, or arise out of having a serious affective disorder.
   2. Peer support may provide a feeling of security, as troublesome or embarrassing issues are discussed and resolved.
   3. Support groups help members gain a sense of perspective on their condition.
   4. Hope is conveyed when the individual is able to see that he or she is not alone or unique in experiencing affective illness.
   5. Peer led, self-help groups are not meant to substitute for, or compete with, professional therapy.
C. Family therapy
   1. Objective is to resolve the symptoms and initiate or restore adaptive family functioning.
   2. Combination of psychotherapeutic and pharmacotherapeutic treatments is the most effective approach.
D. Cognitive therapy
   1. Individual is taught to control thought distortions that are considered to be a factor in the development and maintenance of mood disorders.
   2. Mania is characterized by exaggeratedly positive cognitions and perceptions.
   3. Goals in cognitive therapy:
      a. Obtain symptom relief as quickly as possible.
      b. Assist the client in identifying dysfunctional patterns of thinking and behaving.
      c. Guide the client to evidence and logic that effectively tests the validity of the dysfunctional thinking.
      d. Therapy focuses on changing "automatic thoughts" that occur spontaneously and contribute to the distorted affect.
         i. Personalizing: "She's this happy only when she's with me."
         ii. All or nothing: "Everything I do is great."
         iii. Mind reading: "She thinks I'm wonderful."
         iv. Discounting negatives: "None of those mistakes are really important."
      e. Cognitive therapy should be considered a secondary treatment to pharmacological treatment.
E. The recovery model
   1. Recovery is a continuous process.
   2. The clinician and client work together to develop a treatment plan that is in alignment with the goals set forth by the client.

3. Client and clinician work on strategies to help the individual with bipolar disorder take control of and manage his or her illness.
   a. Become an expert on the disorder.
   b. Take medications regularly.
   c. Become aware of earliest symptoms.
   d. Develop a plan for emergencies.
   e. Identify and reduce sources of stress: know when to seek help.
   f. Develop a personal support system.
4. Recovery is possible in the sense of learning to prevent and minimize symptoms and to successfully cope with the effects of the illness on mood, career, and social life.
F. Electroconvulsive therapy
   1. Used when the client does not tolerate or fails to respond to drug treatment.
   2. Used when life is threatened by dangerous behavior or exhaustion.
G. Psychopharmacology with mood-stabilizing agents
   1. In past, drug of choice for treatment and management of bipolar mania was lithium carbonate.
   2. Practitioners have achieved satisfactory results with several other medications, either alone or in combination with lithium.

3. Table 12.2 provides information about the indication, action, and contraindications and precautions of various medications being used as mood stabilizers.
4. Side effects.
   a. Side effects and nursing implications for mood-stabilizing agents are presented in Table 12.3.
   b. Lithium Toxicity.

(!) The margin between the therapeutic and toxic levels of lithium carbonate is narrow. Clients should be screened for adequate liver and kidney functioning before initiating lithium therapy. Serum lithium levels should be monitored once or twice a week after initial treatment until dosage and serum levels are stable. Then levels should be monitored monthly during maintenance therapy.

   i. The usual ranges of therapeutic serum concentrations are:
      1) For acute mania: 1.0 to 1.5 mEq/L
      2) For maintenance: 0.6 to 1.2 mEq/L
   ii. Blood samples should be drawn 12 hours *after* the last dose
   iii. Symptoms of lithium toxicity begin to appear at blood levels greater than 1.5 mEq/L and are dosage determinate.

Table 12.2 Mood-Stabilizing Agents

Classification: Generic (Trade)	Pregnancy Category/ Half-life Indications	Mechanism of Action	Contraindications/ Therapeutic	Daily Adult Dosage Range/Therapeutic Plasma Range
ANTIMANIC Lithium carbonate (Eskalith, Lithobid)	D/24 hr/ • *Prevention and treatment of manic episodes of bipolar disorder.* *Unlabeled uses:* • *Neutropenia* • *Cluster headaches (prophylaxis)* • *Alcohol dependence* • *Bulimia* • *Postpartum affective psychosis* • *Corticosteroid-induced psychosis*	Not fully understood, but may modulate the effects of various neurotransmitters such as norepinephrine, serotonin, dopamine, glutamate, and GABA, that are thought to play a role in the symptomatology of bipolar disorder (may take 1–3 weeks for symptoms to subside).	Hypersensitivity. Cardiac or renal disease, dehydration; sodium depletion; brain damage; pregnancy and lactation. Caution with thyroid disorders, diabetes, urinary retention, history of seizures, and with the elderly.	Acute mania: 1800–2400 mg Maintenance: 900–1200 mg Acute mania: 1.0–1.5 mEq/L Maintenance: 0.6–1.2 mEq/L
Anticonvulsants Carbamazepine (Tegretol)	D/25–65 hr (initial); 12–17 hr (repeated doses)/ • *Epilepsy* • *Trigeminal neuralgia* *Unlabeled uses:* • *Bipolar disorder* • *Resistant schizophrenia* • *Management of alcohol withdrawal* • *Restless legs syndrome* • *Postherpetic neuralgia*	Action in the treatment of bipolar disorder is unclear.	Hypersensitivity. With MAOIs, lactation. Caution with elderly, liver/renal/cardiac disease, pregnancy.	200–1600 mg/ 4–12 mcg/mL

Continued

Table 12.2 Mood-Stabilizing Agents—cont'd

Classification: Generic (Trade)	Pregnancy Category/ Half-life Indications	Mechanism of Action	Contraindications/ Therapeutic	Daily Adult Dosage Range/Therapeutic Plasma Range
Clonazepam (Klonopin)	C/18–60 hr/ • *Petit mal, akinetic, and myoclonic seizures* • *Panic disorder* *Unlabeled uses:* • *Acute manic episodes* • *Uncontrolled leg movements during sleep* • *Neuralgias*	Action in the treatment of bipolar disorder is unclear.	Hypersensitivity, glaucoma, liver disease, lactation. Caution in elderly, liver/renal disease, pregnancy.	0.5–20 mg/ 20–80 ng/mL
Valproic acid (Depakene, Depakote)	D/5–20 hr/ • *Epilepsy* • *Manic episodes* • *Migraine prophylaxis* • *Adjunct therapy in schizophrenia*	Action in the treatment of bipolar disorder is unclear.	Hypersensitivity; liver disease. Caution in elderly, renal/cardiac diseases, pregnancy and lactation.	5 mg/kg to 60 mg/kg/ 50–150 µg/mL
Lamotrigine (Lamictal)	C/~33 hr/ • *Epilepsy* *Unlabeled use:* • *Bipolar disorder*	Action in the treatment of bipolar disorder is unclear.	Hypersensitivity. Caution in renal and hepatic insufficiency, pregnancy, lactation, and children <16 years old.	100–200 mg/not established
Gabapentin (Neurontin)	C/5–7 hr/ • *Epilepsy* • *Postherpetic neuralgia* *Unlabeled uses:* • *Bipolar disorder* • *Migraine prophylaxis* • *Neuropathic pain* • *Tremors associated with multiple sclerosis*	Action in the treatment of bipolar disorder is unclear.	Hypersensitivity and children <3 years. Caution in renal insufficiency, pregnancy, lactation, children, and the elderly.	900–1800 mg/not established
Topiramate (Topamax)	C/21 hr/ • *Epilepsy* • *Migraine prophylaxis* *Unlabeled uses:* • *Bipolar disorder* • *Cluster headaches* • *Bulimia* • *Binge eating disorder* • *Weight loss in obesity*	Action in the treatment of bipolar disorder is unclear.	Hypersensitivity. Caution in renal and hepatic impairment, pregnancy, lactation, children, and the elderly.	50–400 mg/not established
Oxcarbazepine (Trileptal)	C/2–9/ • *Epilepsy* *Unlabeled uses:* • *Bipolar disorder* • *Diabetic neuropathy* • *Neuralgia*	Action in the treatment of bipolar disorder is unclear.	Hypersensitivity. Caution in renal and hepatic impairment, pregnancy, lactation, children, and the elderly.	600–2400 mg/not established
Calcium Channel Blocker Verapamil (Calan; Isoptin)	C/ 3–7 hr (initially); 4.5–12 hr (repeated dosing) • *Angina* • *Arrhythmias* • *Hypertension* *Unlabeled uses:* • *Bipolar mania* • *Migraine headache prophylaxis*	Action in the treatment of bipolar disorder is unclear.	Hypersensitivity; severe left ventricular dysfunction, heart block, hypotension, cardiogenic shock, congestive heart failure. Caution in liver or renal disease, cardiomyopathy, intracranial pressure, elderly patients, pregnancy and lactation.	80–320 mg/not established

Table 12.2 Mood-Stabilizing Agent—cont'd

Classification: Generic (Trade)	Pregnancy Category/ Half-life Indications	Mechanism of Action	Contraindications/ Therapeutic	Daily Adult Dosage Range/Therapeutic Plasma Range
Antipsychotics Olanzapine (Zyprexa)	C/21–54 hr/ • Schizophrenia • Acute manic episodes • Management of bipolar disorder • Agitation associated with schizophrenia or mania Unlabeled uses: • Obsessive-compulsive disorder	All antipsychotics: Efficacy in schizophrenia is achieved through a combination of dopamine and serotonin type 2 (5HT$_2$) antagonism. Mechanism of action in the treatment of mania is unknown.	All antipsychotics: Hypersensitivity, children, lactation. Caution with hepatic or cardiovascular disease, history of seizures, comatose or other CNS- depression, prostatic hypertrophy, narrow-angle glaucoma, diabetes or risk factors for diabetes, pregnancy, elderly and debilitated patients.	10–20 mg/not established
Olanzapine and fluoxetine (Symbyax)	C/(see individual drugs)/ • For the treatment of depressive episodes associated with bipolar disorder			6/25–12/50 mg/not established
Aripiprazole (Abilify)	C/50–80 hr/ • Bipolar mania • Schizophrenia			10–30 mg/not established
Chlorpromazine (Thorazine)	C/24 hr/ • Bipolar mania • Schizophrenia • Emesis/ hiccoughs • Acute intermittent porphyria • Preoperative apprehension Unlabeled uses: • Migraine headaches			75–400 mg/not established
Quetiapine (Seroquel)	C/6 hr/ • Schizophrenia • Acute manic episodes			100–800 mg/not established
Risperidone (Risperdal)	C/3–20 hr/ • Bipolar mania • Schizophrenia Unlabeled uses: • Severe behavioral problems in children • Behavioral problems associated with autism • Obsessive-compulsive disorder			1–6 mg/not established
Ziprasidone (Geodon)	C/7 hr (oral)/ • Bipolar mania • Schizophrenia • Acute agitation in schizophrenia			40–160 mg/not established
Asenapine (Saphris)	C/24 hr/ • Schizophrenia • Bipolar mania			10–20 mg/not established

Table 12.3 Side Effects and Nursing Implications of Mood-Stabilizing Agents

Medication	Side Effects	Nursing Implications
Antimanic: Lithium carbonate (Eskalith, Lithane, Lithobid)	1. Drowsiness, dizziness, headache 2. Dry mouth, thirst 3. Gastrointestinal (GI) upset; nausea/vomiting 4. Fine hand tremors 5. Hypotension, arrhythmias, pulse irregularities 6. Polyuria, dehydration 7. Weight gain	1. Ensure that client does not participate in activities that require alertness, or operate dangerous machinery. 2. Provide sugarless candy, ice, frequent sips of water. Ensure that strict oral hygiene is maintained. 3. Administer medications with meals to minimize GI upset. 4. Report to physician, who may decrease dosage. Some physicians prescribe a small dose of the beta blocker propranolol to counteract this effect. 5. Monitor vital signs two or three times a day. Physician may decrease dose of medication. 6. May subside after initial week or two. Monitor daily intake and output and weight. Monitor skin turgor daily. 7. Provide instructions for reduced calorie diet. Emphasize importance of maintaining adequate intake of sodium.
Anticonvulsants: Clonazepam (Klonopin) Carbamazepine (Tegretol) Valproic acid (Depakote, Depakene) Gabapentin (Neurontin) Lamotrigine (Lamictal) Topiramate (Topamax) Oxcarbazepine (Trileptal)	1. Nausea/vomiting 2. Drowsiness; dizziness 3. Blood dyscrasias 4. Prolonged bleeding time (with valproic acid) 5. Risk of severe rash (with lamotrigine) 6. Decreased efficacy with oral contraceptives (with topiramate) 7. Risk of suicide with all antiepileptic drugs (warning by U.S. Food and Drug Administration, December 2008).	1. May give with food or milk to minimize GI upset. 2. Ensure that client does not operate dangerous machinery or participate in activities that require alertness. 3. Ensure that client understands importance of regular blood tests while receiving anticonvulsant therapy. 4. Ensure that platelet counts and bleeding time are determined before initiation of therapy with valproic acid. Monitor for spontaneous bleeding or bruising. 5. Ensure that client is informed that he or she must report evidence of skin rash to physician immediately. 6. Ensure that client is aware of decreased efficacy of oral contraceptives with concomitant use. 7. Monitor for worsening of depression, suicidal thoughts or behavior, or any unusual changes in mood or behavior.
Calcium Channel Blocker: Verapamil (Calan, Isoptin)	1. Drowsiness, dizziness 2. Hypotension; bradycardia 3. Nausea 4. Constipation	1. Ensure that client does not operate dangerous machinery or participate in activities that require alertness. 2. Take vital signs just before initiation of therapy and before daily administration of the medication. Physician will provide acceptable parameters for administration. Report marked changes immediately. 3. May give with food to minimize GI upset. 4. Encourage increased fluid (if not contraindicated) and fiber in the diet.
Antipsychotics: Aripiprazole (Abilify) Asenapine (Saphris) Chlorpromazine Olanzapine (Zyprexa) Quetiapine (Seroquel) Risperidone (Risperdal)) Ziprasidone (Geodon)	1. Drowsiness, dizziness 2. Dry mouth, constipation 3. Increased appetite, weight gain 4. Electrocardiogram changes 5. Extrapyramidal symptoms 6. Hyperglycemia and diabetes	1. Ensure that client does not operate dangerous machinery or participate in activities that require alertness. 2. Provide sugarless candy or gum, ice, and frequent sips of water. Provide foods high in fiber. Encourage physical activity and fluid if not contraindicated. 3. Provide calorie-controlled diet; provide opportunity for physical exercise; provide diet and exercise instruction. 4. Monitor vital signs. Observe for symptoms of dizziness, palpitations, syncope, or weakness. 5. Monitor for symptoms. Administer prn medications at first sign. 6. Monitor blood glucose regularly. Observe for the appearance of symptoms of polydipsia, polyuria, polyphagia, and weakness at any time during therapy.

iv. Symptoms include the following:
    1) At serum levels of 1.5 to 2.0 mEq/L: blurred vision, ataxia, tinnitus, persistent nausea and vomiting, severe diarrhea.
    2) At serum levels of 2.0 to 3.5 mEq/L: excessive output of dilute urine, increasing tremors, muscular irritability, psychomotor retardation, mental confusion, giddiness
    3) At serum levels greater than 3.5 mEq/L: impaired consciousness, nystagmus, seizures, coma, oliguria/anuria, arrhythmias, myocardial infarction, cardiovascular collapse
  viii. If left untreated, lithium toxicity can be life threatening

X. Client/Family Education Related to Pharmacotherapy for Bipolar Disorder

A. Lithium
1. Take medication on a regular basis, even when feeling well. Discontinuation can result in return of symptoms.
2. Do not drive or operate dangerous machinery until lithium levels are stabilized. Drowsiness and dizziness can occur.
3. Do not skimp on dietary sodium intake. Client should eat a variety of healthy foods and avoid "junk" foods. The client should drink 6 to 8 large glasses of water (2500–3000 mL) each day and avoid excessive use of beverages containing caffeine (coffee, tea, colas), which promote increased urine output.
4. Notify the physician if vomiting or diarrhea occurs. These symptoms can result in sodium loss and an increased risk of lithium toxicity.
5. Carry card or other identification noting that client is taking lithium.
6. Be aware of appropriate diet should weight gain become a problem. Include adequate sodium and other nutrients while decreasing number of calories.

🛑 It is important to make a client aware of risks of becoming pregnant while receiving lithium therapy. Provide information regarding methods of contraception. Instruct the client to notify the physician as soon as possible if pregnancy is suspected or planned.

7. Be aware of side effects and symptoms associated with toxicity. Notify the physician if any of the following symptoms occur:
  a. Persistent nausea and vomiting.
  b. Severe diarrhea.
  c. Ataxia.
  d. Blurred vision.
  e. Tinnitus.

MAKING THE CONNECTION

Mild lithium toxicity can be treated with minimal intervention; often only cessation or reduction of lithium doses is sufficient. Moderate and severe toxicity both require more aggressive approaches such as antipoisoning measures, gastric lavage, and, in extreme cases, hemodialysis or peritoneal dialysis.

  f. Excessive urine output.
  g. Increasing tremors.
  h. Mental confusion.
8. Refer to written materials furnished by health-care providers while receiving self-administered maintenance therapy.
9. Keep appointments for outpatient follow-up.
10. Have serum lithium level checked every 1 to 2 months, or as advised by physician.

B. Anticonvulsants
1. Refrain from discontinuing the drug abruptly. Physician will taper the drug when therapy is to be discontinued.
2. Report the following symptoms to the physician immediately:
  a. Skin rash.
  b. Unusual bleeding.
  c. Spontaneous bruising.
  d. Sore throat.
  e. Fever.
  f. Malaise.
  g. Dark urine.
  h. Yellow skin or eyes.
3. Do not drive or operate dangerous machinery until reaction to the medication has been established.
4. Avoid consuming alcoholic beverages and nonprescription medications without approval from physician.
5. Encourage alternate methods of birth control because of decreased efficacy of oral contraceptives.
6. Carry card at all times identifying the name of medications being taken.

C. Calcium channel blockers
1. Take medication with meals if gastrointestinal (GI) upset occurs.
2. Use caution when driving or when operating dangerous machinery. Dizziness, drowsiness, and blurred vision can occur.

🛑 Make sure the client who is taking a calcium channel blocker refrains from discontinuing the drug abruptly. To do so may precipitate cardiovascular problems. The physician will taper the drug when therapy is to be discontinued.

3. Report occurrence of any of the following symptoms to physician immediately:
   a. Irregular heartbeat.
   b. Shortness of breath.
   c. Swelling of the hands and feet.
   d. Pronounced dizziness.
   e. Chest pain.
   f. Profound mood swings.
   g. Severe and persistent headache.
4. Rise slowly from a sitting or lying position to prevent a sudden drop in blood pressure.
5. Avoid taking other medications (including over-the-counter medications) without physician's approval.
6. Carry card at all times describing medications being taken.

D. Antipsychotics
1. Use caution when driving or operating dangerous machinery. Drowsiness and dizziness can occur.

🛈 Make sure the client who is taking an antipsychotic refrains from discontinuing the drug abruptly after long-term use. To do so might produce withdrawal symptoms, such as nausea, vomiting, dizziness, gastritis, headache, tachycardia, insomnia, and tremulousness. The physician will taper the drug when therapy is to be discontinued.

2. Use sunblock lotion and wear protective clothing when spending time outdoors. Skin is more susceptible to sunburn, which can occur in as little as 30 minutes.
3. Report the occurrence of any of the following symptoms to the physician immediately:
   a. Sore throat.
   b. Fever.
   c. Malaise.
   d. Unusual bleeding.
   e. Easy bruising.
   f. Persistent nausea and vomiting.
   g. Severe headache.
   h. Rapid heart rate.
   i. Difficulty urinating.
   j. Muscle twitching.
   k. Tremors.
   l. Darkly colored urine.
   m. Excessive urination.
   n. Excessive thirst.
   o. Excessive hunger.
   p. Weakness.
   q. Pale stools.
   r. Yellow skin or eyes.
   s. Muscular incoordination.
   t. Skin rash.
   u. Extrapyramidal symptoms.
4. Rise slowly from a sitting or lying position to prevent a sudden drop in blood pressure.

5. Take frequent sips of water, chew sugarless gum, or suck on hard candy, if dry mouth is a problem. Good oral care (frequent brushing, flossing) is important.
6. Consult the physician regarding smoking while on antipsychotic therapy. Smoking increases the metabolism of these drugs, requiring an adjustment in dosage to achieve a therapeutic effect.
7. Dress warmly in cold weather, and avoid extended exposure to very high or low temperatures. Body temperature is harder to maintain with this medication.
8. Avoid drinking alcohol while on antipsychotic therapy. These drugs potentiate each other's effects.
9. Avoid taking other medications (including over-the-counter products) without the physician's approval. Many medications contain substances that interact with antipsychotic medications in a way that may be harmful.
10. Be aware of possible risks of taking antipsychotics during pregnancy. Safe use during pregnancy has not been established. Antipsychotics are thought to readily cross the placental barrier; if so, a fetus could experience adverse effects of the drug. Inform the physician immediately if pregnancy occurs, is suspected, or is planned.
11. Be aware of side effects of antipsychotic medications. Refer to written materials furnished by health-care providers for safe self-administration.
12. Continue to take the medication, even if feeling well. Symptoms may return if medication is discontinued.
13. Carry a card or other identification at all times describing medications being taken.

XI. Developmental Implications: Childhood and Adolescence

A. The lifetime prevalence of pediatric and adolescent bipolar disorders is estimated to be about 1%
B. Tends to be a chronic condition with high rate of relapse
C. Often difficult to diagnose

DID YOU KNOW?
Symptoms of bipolar disorder are often difficult to assess in children, and they may also present with comorbid conduct disorders or attention deficit-hyperactivity disorder (ADHD). Because of the genetic predisposition to bipolar disorder, family history is particularly important when assigning a bipolar diagnosis.

D. Guidelines for the diagnosis and treatment of children with bipolar disorder

1. To differentiate between occasional spontaneous behaviors of childhood and behaviors associated with bipolar disorder, the Consensus Group recommends that clinicians use the FIND (frequency, intensity, number, and duration) strategy (Kowatch et al., 2005):

   a. Frequency: symptoms occur most days in a week.

   b. Intensity: symptoms are severe enough to cause extreme disturbance in one domain or moderate disturbance in two or more domains.

   c. Number: symptoms occur three or four times a day.

   d. Duration: symptoms occur 4 or more hours a day.

2. For any symptoms to be counted as a manic symptom, they must:

   a. Exceed the FIND threshold.

   b. Occur in concert with other manic symptoms because no one symptom is diagnostic of mania.

   c. Symptoms associated with mania in children and adolescents are as follows:

      i. Euphoric/expansive mood: extremely happy, silly, or giddy

      ii. Irritable mood: hostility and rage, often over trivial matters; the irritability may be accompanied by aggressive and/or self-injurious behavior

      iii. Grandiosity: believing that his or her abilities are better than everyone else's

      iv. Decreased need for sleep: may sleep only 4 or 5 hours per night and wake up fresh and full of energy the next day, or client may get up in the middle of the night and wander around the house looking for things to do

      v. Pressured speech: rapid speech that is loud, intrusive, and difficult to interrupt

      vi. Racing thoughts: topics of conversation change rapidly, in a manner confusing to anyone listening

      vii. Distractibility: to consider distractibility a manic symptom, it needs to:

      • Reflect a change from baseline functioning

      • Occurs in conjunction with a "manic" mood shift

      • Cannot be accounted for exclusively by another disorder, particularly ADHD

      • May be reflected in school performance

      viii. Increase in goal-directed activity/psychomotor agitation: A child who is not usually highly productive becomes very project oriented during a manic episode, increasing goal-directed activity to an obsessive level; psychomotor agitation represents a distinct change from baseline behavior

      ix. Excessive involvement in pleasurable or risky activities: Children with bipolar disorder are often hypersexual, exhibiting behavior that has an erotic, pleasure-seeking quality about it. Adolescents may seek out sexual activity multiple times in a day

      x. Psychosis: in addition to core symptoms of mania, psychotic symptoms, including hallucinations and delusions, are frequently present in children with bipolar disorder

      xi. Suicidality: although not a core symptom of mania, children with bipolar disorder are at risk of suicidal ideation, intent, plans, and attempts during a depressed episode or when psychotic (Geller et al., 2002)

E. Treatment Strategies for Children and Adolescents

1. Psychopharmacology: primary method of stabilizing an acutely ill bipolar child and/or adolescent client.

   a. **Monotherapy** with traditional mood stabilizers (e.g., lithium, divalproex, carbamazepine) or atypical antipsychotics (e.g., olanzapine, quetiapine, risperidone, aripiprazole) has been determined to be the first-line treatment.

   b. Augmentation with a second medication is indicated if monotherapy fails.

   c. ADHD has been identified as the most common comorbid condition in children and adolescents with bipolar disorder.

   d. Because stimulants can exacerbate mania, it is suggested that medication for ADHD be initiated only after bipolar symptoms have been controlled with a mood stabilizer.

   e. Nonstimulant medications indicated for ADHD (e.g., atomoxetine, bupropion, the tricyclic antidepressants) may also induce switches to mania or hypomania.

   f. Because of the high risk of relapse, maintenance therapy is indicated with the same medications used to treat acute symptoms.

   g. Few research studies exist that deal with long-term maintenance of bipolar disorder in children.

   h. Medication tapering or discontinuation should be considered after remission has been achieved for a minimum of 12 to 24 consecutive months.

   i. Some clients may require long-term or even lifelong pharmacotherapy.

2. Family interventions.
   a. Family-focused therapy (FFT) plays an important role in preventing relapses and improving adjustment.
   b. Psychoeducation occurs in FFT therapy, which familiarizes both the client and the family with the etiology, symptoms, early recognition, course, and effect of the disorder and the available treatment options. Also self-management, communication training, and problem-solving skills training can be addressed.
   c. Clients and family need counseling because of the disruption in both social and family functioning.
   d. Emphasis is on relapse prevention and treatment adherence.
   e. Educate family to promote understanding that behaviors are attributable to an illness that must be managed, as opposed to the client being willful and deliberate.
   f. Research suggests that the addition of psychosocial therapy enhances the effectiveness of psychopharmacological therapy in the maintenance of bipolar disorder in children and adolescents.

REVIEW QUESTIONS

1. A client prescribed lithium carbonate (Lithobid) 300 mg twice daily 3 months ago comes to the emergency department with mental confusion, excessive diluted urine output, and consistent tremors. Which lithium level would the nurse expect?
   1. 1.2 mEq/L
   2. 1.5 mEq/L
   3. 1.7 mEq/L
   4. 2.2 mEq/L

2. A nursing instructor is teaching about cyclothymic disorder. Which of the following should be included in the lesson plan? **Select all that apply.**
   1. For adults, symptoms must last at least 2 years.
   2. Symptoms are attributable to the physiological effects of a substance.
   3. During a 2-year period, clients can't be symptom free for more than 2 months at a time.
   4. Symptoms cause significant distress in social or occupational functioning.
   5. The client has never experienced a major depressive, manic, or hypomanic episode.

3. A nursing instructor is teaching about the prevalence of bipolar disorder. Which student statement indicates that learning has occurred?
   1. "This disorder is more prevalent in the lower socioeconomic groups."
   2. "This disorder is equally prevalent in females and males."
   3. "This disorder is more prevalent in married than unmarried persons."
   4. "This disorder's prevalence can't be evaluated based on demographic data."

4. A physician orders clonazepam (Klonopin) 50 mg/day for a client diagnosed with bipolar disorder. How would a nurse evaluate this medication order?
   1. This dosage is within the recommended dosage range.
   2. This dosage is lower than the recommended dosage range.
   3. This dosage is more than twice the recommended dosage range.
   4. This dosage is four times higher than the recommended dosage range.

5. A nurse practitioner is counseling a client exhibiting manic behaviors. The nurse determines that the client is using the cognitive distortion of "automatic thoughts." Which client statement is evidence of the "automatic thought" of *personalizing*?
   1. "I'm the only one who can make this family run smoothly."
   2. "I expect to pass my tests with A's."
   3. "I know they all want to be like me."
   4. "My tardiness doesn't make a real difference."

6. A family describes a client diagnosed with bipolar disorder as being "on the move." The client sleeps 3 to 4 hours nightly, spends excessively, and has recently lost 10 pounds. During the initial client assessment, which client response would the nurse expect?
   1. Short, polite responses to interview questions
   2. Introspection related to present situation
   3. Disorganized thinking and the inability to remain seated
   4. Feelings of helplessness and hopelessness

7. A client who is prescribed lithium carbonate is being discharged from inpatient care. Which medication information should the nurse teach this client?
   1. Do not skimp on dietary sodium intake.
   2. Have serum lithium levels checked every 6 months.
   3. Limit fluid intake to 1000 mL of fluid per day.
   4. Adjust the medication dose if you feel out of control.

8. A nursing instructor is teaching about bipolar disorders. Which statement differentiates the symptoms of a manic episode from a hypomanic episode?
   1. During a manic episode, clients are more talkative than usual and experience pressure to keep talking; these symptoms are absent in hypomania.
   2. During a manic episode, there may be an increase in goal-directed activity or psychomotor agitation; these symptoms are absent in hypomania.
   3. During a manic episode, clients may have excessive involvement in pleasurable but risky activities; this symptom is absent in hypomania.
   4. During a manic episode, there is a marked impairment in social or occupational functioning; this symptom is absent in hypomania.

9. An instructor is listing the symptoms that a client could experience during a hypomanic episode. Which of the following should be included in this list? **Select all that apply.**
   1. Perceptions of the self are grandiose
   2. Decrease in goal directed activities
   3. Decreased need for sleep
   4. Flight of ideas
   5. Distractibility

10. A parent tells the nurse, "The doctor said that my son who has attention deficit-hyperactivity disorder (ADHD) may also have bipolar disorder, but this diagnosis is still uncertain." Which is the nurse's most appropriate response?
    1. "Children diagnosed with bipolar disorder are rarely diagnosed with ADHD."
    2. "Having ADHD rules out the diagnosis of bipolar disorder."
    3. "Symptoms of ADHD and bipolar disorder can be so similar that a diagnosis is hard to assign."
    4. "Symptoms of bipolar disorder must be present for 6 months to assign this diagnosis."

11. How would the nurse determine whether a child or adolescent is experiencing manic symptoms? **Select all that apply.**
    1. Symptoms must exceed the FIND (frequency, intensity, number, and duration) threshold.
    2. Symptoms must occur in concert with other manic symptoms because no one symptom is diagnostic of mania.
    3. Symptoms must include an increased need for sleep.
    4. Symptoms must include suicidality.
    5. Symptoms must occur on a monthly basis.

12. A nurse is caring for an adolescent who has a diagnosis of both attention deficit-hyperactivity disorder (ADHD) and bipolar disorder. When administering medication for ADHD, which should the nurse consider?
    1. Medication for bipolar disorder should be initiated only after ADHD symptoms have been controlled.
    2. Medications for ADHD should be initiated only after bipolar symptoms have been controlled with a mood stabilizer.
    3. Stimulants work to calm the adolescent experiencing mania.
    4. Nonstimulant medications indicated for ADHD rarely precipitate mania.

13. A nurse documents a client's problem with the following nursing diagnosis: impaired social interaction. Which client symptom led to this conclusion?
    1. Manipulation of others
    2. Inaccurate interpretations of the environment
    3. Disorientation
    4. Increased agitation and lack of control

14. Which medication used in the treatment of bipolar disorder is correctly classified?
    1. The antimanic medication valproic acid (Depakote)
    2. The anticonvulsant medication lamotrigine (Lamictal)
    3. The calcium channel blocker medication aripiprazole (Abilify)
    4. The antipsychotic medication verapamil (Isoptin)

15. Which medication is correctly matched with its significant side effect? **Select all that apply.**
    1. Valproic acid (Depakote): prolonged bleeding time
    2. Lamotrigine (Lamictal): severe rash
    3. Topiramate (Topamax): decreased efficacy of oral contraceptives
    4. Lithium carbonate (Lithobid): weight loss
    5. Clonazepam (Klonopin): extrapyramidal symptoms

16. Bipolar I disorder is the diagnosis given to an individual who has experienced a(n) _____ episode.

17. Family-focused treatment is used for children and adolescents diagnosed with bipolar disorder. What are the goals of this psychoeducational intervention? **Select all that apply.**
    1. To assist the client and family to control thought distortions
    2. To assist the client and family to determine goals based on personal values
    3. To reduce the incidence of relapse
    4. To increase medication adherence
    5. To promote the understanding that behavior can be attributable to the illness

18. _____ theory suggests that bipolar disorder strongly reflects an underlying genetic vulnerability.

19. A client diagnosed with bipolar disorder is experiencing a severe depressive episode. Which client symptom would require a priority nursing intervention?
    1. The client is not responding to other clients on the unit.
    2. The client is refusing to take his or her prescribed mood stabilizer.
    3. The client states, "There is no future when you feel so depressed."
    4. The client angrily argues with another client stating, "God is dead."

20. Conditions such as schizophrenia and bipolar disorder are viewed as diseases of the _____.

REVIEW ANSWERS

1. ANSWER: 4

Rationale:

1. A lithium level of 1.2 mEq/L is within the normal range for lithium maintenance, and therefore the client would not exhibit the symptoms listed in the question.

2. The lithium level necessary for managing acute mania is 1.0 to 1.5 mEq/L, and 1.5 mEq/L is within this range. Therefore, the client would not exhibit the symptoms listed in the question.

3. When the serum lithium level is 1.5 to 2.0 mEq/L, the client exhibits signs such as blurred vision, ataxia, tinnitus, persistent nausea, vomiting, and diarrhea, but not the symptoms listed in the question.

4. When the serum lithium level is 2.0 to 3.5 mEq/L, the client may exhibit signs such as excessive output of diluted urine, increased tremors, muscular irritability, psychomotor retardation, mental confusion, and giddiness. The client's symptoms described in the question support a lithium serum level of 2.2 mEq/L.

TEST-TAKING TIP: Pair the lithium level with the client's symptoms presented in the question. Lithium has a narrow therapeutic range, and levels outside this range place the client at high risk for injury.

Content Area: Safe and Effective Care Environment: Management of Care;

Integrated Process: Nursing Process: Evaluation;

Client Need: Safe and Effective Care Environment: Management of Care;

Cognitive Level: Application;

Concept: Medication

2. ANSWERS. 1, 3, 4, 5

Rationale:

1. Adults who are diagnosed with cyclothymic disorder must have symptoms that last at least 2 years.

2. The symptoms experienced by clients who are diagnosed with cyclothymic disorder must **not** be attributable to the physiological effects of a substance.

3. Clients diagnosed with cyclothymic disorder can't be symptom free for more than 2 months at a time during a 2-year period.

4. Clients diagnosed with substance-induced bipolar disorder, not cyclothymia, experience symptoms that cause significant distress or impairment in social, occupational, or other important areas of functioning.

5. To be diagnosed with cyclothymic disorder, a client must never have experienced a major depressive, manic, or hypomanic episode.

TEST-TAKING TIP: Review the symptoms of cyclothymic disorder.

Content Area: Safe and Effective Care Environment: Management of Care;

Integrated Process: Nursing Process: Implementation;

Client Need: Safe and Effective Care Management of Care;

Cognitive Level: Application;

Concept: Nursing Roles

3. ANSWER: 2

Rationale:

1. The nursing student is inaccurate when stating that bipolar disorder is more prevalent in lower socioeconomic groups. Unlike depressive disorder, bipolar disorder is more prevalent in the higher socioeconomic groups.

2. The nursing student is accurate when stating that bipolar disorder is equally prevalent in females and males.

3. The nursing student is inaccurate when stating that bipolar disorder is more prevalent in married than unmarried persons. As with depression, bipolar disorder appears to be more prevalent in unmarried than married persons.

4. The nursing student is inaccurate when stating that bipolar disorder's prevalence cannot be evaluated based on demographic data. Prevalence is based on the consideration of age, gender, marital, and socioeconomic status.

TEST-TAKING TIP: Review the demographics and prevalence rates for bipolar disorder.

Content Area: Psychosocial Integrity: Management of Care;

Integrated Process: Nursing Process: Evaluation;

Client Need: Psychosocial Integrity: Management of Care;

Cognitive Level: Application;

Concept: Nursing Roles

4. ANSWER: 3

Rationale:

1. The recommended dosage range for clonazepam is 0.5 to 20 mg/day. The nurse should determine that the ordered medication is more than twice the recommended dosage range.

2. The recommended dosage range for clonazepam is 0.5 to 20 mg/day. The nurse should determine that the ordered medication is higher, not lower, than the recommended dosage range.

3. The recommended dosage range for clonazepam is 0.5 to 20 mg/day. The nurse should determine that the ordered medication is more than twice the recommended dosage range.

4. The recommended dosage range for clonazepam is 0.5 to 20 mg/day. The nurse should determine that the ordered medication is more than twice, not more than four times, the recommended dosage range.

TEST-TAKING TIP: Review the therapeutic daily adult dosage range for mood-stabilizing agents in clients diagnosed with bipolar disorder. A review of Table 12.2 will provide the test-taker with this information.

Content Area: Safe and Effective Care Environment: Management of Care;

Integrated Process: Nursing Process: Evaluation;

Client Need: Safe and Effective Care Environment: Management of Care;

Cognitive Level: Application;

Concept: Medication

5. ANSWER: 1

Rationale:

1. The statement "I'm the only one who can make this family run smoothly" is a good example of the automatic thought of *personalizing*.

2. The statement "I expect to pass my tests with A's" is an example of the automatic thought of *all or nothing,* not the automatic thought of *personalizing.*

3. The statement "I know they all want to be like me" is an example of the automatic thought of *mind reading,* not the automatic thought of *personalizing.*

4. The statement "My tardiness doesn't make a real difference" is an example of the automatic thought of *discounting negatives,* not the automatic thought of *personalizing.*

TEST-TAKING TIP: Review the four automatic thoughts that may occur spontaneously and contribute to the distorted affect in an individual diagnosed with bipolar disorder.

Content Area: Psychosocial Integrity;
Integrated Process: Nursing Process: Implementation;
Client Need: Psychosocial Integrity;
Cognitive Level: Application;
Concept: Assessment

6. **ANSWER: 3**

Rationale:

1. During the manic phase of bipolar disorder, clients have short attention spans and may be impatient and hostile toward authority figures. These clients would not provide short, polite answers.

2. Introspection requires focusing and concentration. Clients in the manic phase of bipolar disorder experience flight of ideas and have short attention spans, making them unable to focus and concentrate.

3. In the manic phase of bipolar disorder, the client experiences hyperactivity, restlessness, and flight of ideas. This would cause the client to have difficulty remaining seated and have problems organizing his or her thoughts.

4. Feelings of helplessness and hopelessness are symptoms of the depressive phase of bipolar disorder. The symptoms presented in the question describe the manic, not depressive, phase of bipolar disorder.

TEST-TAKING TIP: When treating clients diagnosed with bipolar disorder, know and recognize what a manic episode might look like.

Content Area: Safe and Effective Care Environment: Management of Care;
Integrated Process: Nursing Process: Assessment;
Client Need: Safe and Effective Care Environment: Management of Care;
Cognitive Level: Application;
Concept: Assessment

7. **ANSWER: 1**

Rationale:

1. Clients taking lithium should consume a diet adequate in sodium and drink 2500 to 3000 mL of fluid per day. The recommended daily allowance of dietary sodium is 2.3 grams, or approximately one teaspoon of table salt per day. Lithium is a salt and competes in the body with sodium. If sodium is lost, the body will retain lithium resulting in possible toxicity. Maintaining normal sodium and fluid levels is critical to maintaining therapeutic levels of lithium.

2. The margin between therapeutic and toxic levels of lithium is very narrow. Serum lithium levels should be monitored once or twice a week after initial treatment until dosage and serum levels are stable, then monthly during maintenance therapy to check for toxic levels.

3. Clients taking lithium should consume a diet adequate in sodium and drink 2500 to 3000 mL, not 1000 mL of fluid per day. Lithium is a salt and competes in the body with sodium. If sodium is lost, the body will retain lithium, resulting in possible toxicity. Maintaining normal sodium and fluid levels is critical to maintaining therapeutic levels of lithium.

4. The margin between therapeutic and toxic levels of lithium is very narrow. It is critical that clients maintain the prescribed dosage of lithium and comply with regularly scheduled blood work to monitor lithium levels.

TEST-TAKING TIP: Review the information that must be taught to a client who is being treated with lithium.

Content Area: Safe and Effective Care Environment: Management of Care;
Integrated Process: Nursing Process: Implementation;
Client Need: Safe and Effective Care Environment: Management of Care;
Cognitive Level: Application;
Concept: Medication

8. **ANSWER: 4**

Rationale:

1. During both manic and hypomanic episodes, clients are more talkative than usual and experience pressure to keep talking.

2. During both manic and hypomanic episodes, there may be an increase in goal-directed activity or psychomotor agitation.

3. During both manic and hypomanic episodes, clients may have excessive involvement in pleasurable but risky activities.

4. During a manic episode there is a marked impairment in social or occupational functioning; however, these symptoms are absent in hypomania.

TEST-TAKING TIP: Review the differences between the symptoms of a hypomanic episode and a manic episode.

Content Area: Safe and Effective Care Environment: Management of Care;
Integrated Process: Nursing Process: Evaluation;
Client Need: Safe and Effective Care Environment: Management of Care;
Cognitive Level: Analysis;
Concept: Assessment

9. **ANSWERS: 1, 3, 4, 5**

Rationale:

1. An inflated self-esteem or grandiosity is one of the symptoms that a client could experience during a hypomanic episode.

2. An increase (either socially, at work or school, or sexually), not a decrease in goal directed activities, is one of the symptoms a client could experience during a hypomanic episode.

3. A decreased need for sleep (e.g., feels rested after only 3 hours of sleep) is one of the symptoms a client could experience during a hypomanic episode.

4. A flight of ideas or subjective experience that thoughts are racing is one of the symptoms a client could experience during a hypomanic episode.

5. Distractibility (i.e., attention is easily drawn to unimportant or irrelevant stimuli) is one of the symptoms a client could experience during a hypomanic episode.

TEST-TAKING TIP: Review the variety of symptoms a client could experience during a hypomanic episode.
Content Area: Safe and Effective Care Environment: Management of Care;
Integrated Process: Nursing Process: Assessment;
Client Need: Safe and Effective Care Management of Care;
Cognitive Level: Application;
Concept: Mood

10. **ANSWER: 3**
Rationale:
1. ADHD has been identified as the most common comorbid condition in children and adolescents diagnosed with bipolar disorder.
2. Having ADHD does not rule out the diagnosis of bipolar disorder. Bipolar disorder in a child or adolescent often presents with comorbid conduct disorders or ADHD.
3. A child or adolescent diagnosed with bipolar disorder may also present with comorbid conduct disorders or ADHD, making a diagnosis of bipolar disorder difficult to determine. Because of the genetic predisposition to bipolar disorder, knowledge of family history is particularly important when assigning a bipolar diagnosis.
4. Symptoms of mania in bipolar disorder must last at least 1 week, not 6 months, and be present most of the day, nearly every day.
TEST-TAKING TIP: Review the symptoms of ADHD, conduct disorder, and bipolar disorder with the understanding that it is difficult to differentiate these diagnoses.
Content Area: Safe and Effective Care Environment: Management of Care;
Integrated Process: Nursing Process: Implementation;
Client Need: Safe and Effective Care Environment: Management of Care;
Cognitive Level: Analysis;
Concept: Assessment

11. **ANSWER: 1, 2**
Rationale:
1. For a symptom experienced by a child or adolescent to be counted as a manic symptom, the symptom must exceed the FIND threshold.
2. For a symptom experienced by a child or adolescent to be counted as a manic symptom, the symptom must have occurred in concert with other manic symptoms. No one symptom is diagnostic of mania.
3. One of the manic symptoms that can be experienced by a child or adolescent is a decreased, not increased, need for sleep.

4. Although suicidality is not a core symptom of mania, children with bipolar disorder are at risk of suicidal ideation, intent, plans, and attempts during a depressed or mixed episode or when psychotic.
5. The FIND threshold for frequency is that symptoms occur most days in a week, not monthly.
TEST-TAKING TIP: Review the FIND strategy used to evaluate symptoms in order to diagnose bipolar disorder in children and adolescents.
Content Area: Safe and Effective Care Environment: Management of Care;
Integrated Process: Nursing Process: Assessment;
Client Need: Safe and Effective Care Environment: Management of Care;
Cognitive Level: Application;
Concept: Assessment

12. **ANSWER: 2**
Rationale:
1. Because stimulants can exacerbate mania, bipolar symptoms must be addressed before administering stimulant medications for the symptoms of ADHD.
2. Because stimulants can exacerbate mania, bipolar symptoms must be controlled with a mood stabilizer before administering stimulant medications for ADHD.
3. Stimulants can exacerbate mania. They do not work to calm the adolescent experiencing mania.
4. Nonstimulant medications indicated for ADHD (e.g., atomoxetine, bupropion, the tricyclic antidepressants) may precipitate a manic or hypomanic episode.
TEST-TAKING TIP: Understand that stimulants and nonstimulant medications used to treat ADHD can exacerbate mania in a child or adolescent diagnosed with bipolar disorder.
Content Area: Safe and Effective Care Environment: Management of Care;
Integrated Process: Nursing Process: Implementation;
Client Need: Safe and Effective Care Environment: Management of Care;
Cognitive Level: Application;
Concept: Nursing

13. **ANSWER: 1**
Rationale:
1. The nursing diagnosis of *impaired social interaction* would document the client's manipulation of others.
2. The nursing diagnosis of *disturbed thought processes,* not *impaired social interaction,* would document the client's inaccurate interpretations of the environment.
3. The nursing diagnosis of *disturbed sensory-perception,* not *impaired social interaction,* would document the client's disorientation.
4. The nursing diagnosis of *risk for injury,* not *impaired social interaction,* would document the client's increased agitation and lack of control.
TEST-TAKING TIP: Review Table 12.1 to familiarize yourself with behaviors that are associated with nursing diagnoses for bipolar mania.

Content Area: Safe and Effective Care Environment: Management of Care;
Integrated Process: Nursing Process: Diagnosis (Analysis);
Client Need: Safe and Effective Care Environment: Management of Care;
Cognitive Level: Analysis;
Concept: Critical Thinking

14. **ANSWER: 2**
Rationale:
1. Valproic acid is classified as an anticonvulsant, not as an antimanic medication.
2. Lamotrigine is correctly classified as an anticonvulsant medication.
3. Aripiprazole is classified as an antipsychotic, not as a calcium channel blocker medication.
4. Verapamil is classified as a calcium channel blocker medication, not as an antipsychotic.
TEST-TAKING TIP: See Table 12.2 to review the various classifications of medications used in the treatment of bipolar disorder.
Content Area: Safe and Effective Care Environment: Management of Care;
Integrated Process: Nursing Process: Evaluation;
Client Need: Safe and Effective Care Environment: Management of Care;
Cognitive Level: Application;
Concept: Medication

15. **ANSWERS: 1, 2, 3**
Rationale:
1. Prolonged bleeding time is a serious side effect of valproic acid.
2. Stevens-Johnson syndrome, which causes a severe rash, is a side effect of lamotrigine.
3. Decreased efficacy of oral contraceptives is a side effect of topiramate.
4. Weight gain, not loss, is a side effect of lithium carbonate.
5. Extrapyramidal symptoms are side effects of antipsychotics, not the anticonvulsant clonazepam.
TEST-TAKING TIP: See Table 12.3 to review the various side effects of medications used in the treatment of bipolar disorder.
Content Area: Safe and Effective Care Environment: Management of Care;
Integrated Process: Nursing Process: Evaluation;
Client Need: Safe and Effective Care Environment: Management of Care;
Cognitive Level: Application;
Concept: Medication

16. **ANSWER: manic**
Rationale: Bipolar I disorder is the diagnosis given to an individual who has experienced a **manic** episode or has a history of one or more manic episodes. Episodes of depression are also part of the clinical picture of bipolar I disorder.
TEST-TAKING TIP: Review the symptoms of bipolar I disorder and remember that experiencing a manic episode rules out a diagnosis of major depressive episode.

Content Area: Psychosocial Integrity;
Integrated Process: Nursing Process: Assessment;
Client Need: Psychosocial Integrity;
Cognitive Level: Comprehension;
Concept: Mood

17. **ANSWER: 3, 4, 5**
Rationale:
1. Cognitive therapy, not FFT, assists the client and family to control thought distortions.
2. The recovery model, not FFT, assists the client and family in determining goals based on personal values or what they define as giving meaning and purpose to life
3. Studies show that FFT is an effective method of reducing relapses in clients diagnosed with bipolar disorder.
4. Studies show that FFT is an effective method of increasing medication adherence in clients diagnosed with bipolar disorder.
5. FFT promotes the understanding that at least part of the client's negative behaviors are attributable to an illness that must be managed, as opposed to being willful and deliberate.
TEST-TAKING TIP: Review the treatment strategies for children and adolescents diagnosed with bipolar disorder including family-focused therapy.
Content Area: Safe and Effective Care Environment: Management of Care;
Integrated Process: Nursing Process: Planning;
Client Need: Safe and Effective Care Environment: Management of Care;
Cognitive Level: Application
Concept: Nursing

18. **ANSWER: Biological**
Rationale: Research suggests that bipolar disorder strongly reflects an underlying genetic vulnerability. Evidence from family, twin, and adoption studies exists to support this observation. Theories that are associated with genetics are included in the category of **biological** theory.
TEST-TAKING TIP: Review the theories of origin for bipolar disorder
Content Area: Psychosocial Integrity;
Integrated Process: Nursing Process: Assessment;
Client Need: Psychosocial Integrity;
Cognitive Level: Comprehension;
Concept: Evidenced-based Practice

19. **ANSWER: 3**
Rationale:
1. The nurse should address the issue of the client not responding to other clients on the unit, but compared with the other client behaviors presented, this symptom does not take priority.
2. The nurse should address the issue of the client not taking his or her prescribed mood-stabilizing medication, but compared with the other client behaviors presented, this symptom does not take priority.
3. When a severely depressed client states, "There is no future when you feel so depressed," the nurse should

recognize the possibility that the client may have intentions of self-harm. With safety and security being a priority, the nurse should implement immediate suicide precautions.

4. A nurse observing two clients arguing may decide to closely monitor and deescalate the situation, if needed, but, compared with the other client behaviors presented, this symptom does not take priority.

TEST-TAKING TIP: Recognize signs of both overt and covert intentions of self-harm and remember that safety and security issues are always prioritized. Review Maslow's hierarchy of needs. Note that safety and security is the second highest level of need after physiological needs have been met.

Content Area: Safe and Effective Care Environment: Management of Care;
Integrated Process: Nursing Process: Implementation;

Client Need: Safe and Effective Care Environment: Management of Care;
Cognitive Level: Analysis;
Concept: Critical Thinking

20. **ANSWER: brain**

Rationale: The credibility of psychosocial theories to explain the origins of schizophrenia and bipolar disorder have declined in recent years. Schizophrenia and bipolar disorder are viewed as diseases of the **brain.**

TEST-TAKING TIP: Review the theories of origin for bipolar disorder

Content Area: Psychosocial Integrity;
Integrated Process: Nursing Process: Assessment;
Client Need: Psychosocial Integrity;
Cognitive Level: Comprehension;
Concept: Assessment

CASE STUDY: Putting it All Together

Rick is an emaciated 30-year-old attorney who was brought to the emergency department (ED) by his distraught wife. She tells the emergency department (ED) physician that her husband hasn't eaten or slept in days, and that he is talking and acting bizarrely. After the ED assessment, Rick is admitted to the hospital's psychiatric unit. He is dressed in a flamboyant shirt and mismatched socks. He is loud, restless and sexually suggestive calling his assigned nurse practitioner (NP), Melanie, "honey" and "darlin'," until admonished and corrected. As the antianxiety medication, administered in the ED begins to take effect, Melanie is able to direct Rick into a quiet area for an assessment interview. Rick admits to being moody and easy to anger when frustrated. He claims to be able to multitask with great success, but then bangs his fist on the table and angrily states, "I always 'crash' into despair. It happened again last week. I took out a second mortgage on our house and opened three law offices in the tri-city area. It was a brilliant move, but my wife found out and threatened to divorce me. She's a real pain! Keeps fixing me food. I tell her I don't need to eat, and sleeping is such a waste of time. Her parents never liked me, and I'll bet they're telling her things about me that aren't true." As Rick delves further into his story, Melanie has difficulty keeping up with his racing, disjointed thoughts. She also notes that his speech is becoming louder and more pressured. He begins rapidly pacing. After an exaggerated breath, Rick rolls his eyes and continues, "Then the bills were coming in faster than I could pay them, and my secretary informed me that I'm the father of her unborn child. It's so frustrating! I don't seem to be able to complete plans that I set in motion before my world turns upside down. Believe me, my ideas are really great! So great, I stay awake at night just basking in my own brilliance."

1. On the basis of the symptoms described here and the client's actions, what medical diagnosis would Melanie assign to Rick?
2. What are Rick's subjective symptoms?
3. What are Rick's objective symptoms?
4. What treatment modalities might Melanie use to address the symptoms of Rick's disorder?
5. What NANDA nursing diagnosis would address Rick's main problem?
6. Based on this nursing diagnosis, what short-term outcome would be appropriate for Rick?
7. On the basis of this nursing diagnosis, what long-term outcome would be appropriate for Rick?
8. List the nursing interventions (actions) that will assist Rick in successfully meeting these outcomes.
9. List the questions that should be asked to determine the success of the nursing interventions.

Chapter 13

Personality Disorders

KEY TERMS

Antisocial personality disorder—A pervasive pattern of socially irresponsible, exploitive, and guiltless behavior that reflects a disregard for the rights of others

Borderline personality disorder—A pattern of intense and chaotic relationships with affective instability and fluctuating attitudes

Depersonalization—An alteration in the perception or experience of the self so that the feeling of one's own reality is temporarily lost

Derealization—An alteration in the perception or experience of the external world so that it seems strange or unreal

Helicopter parenting—A style of child rearing in which an overprotective mother or father discourages a child's independence by being too involved in the child's life

Impulsivity—The urge or inclination to act without consideration of the possible consequences of one's behavior

Limit setting—A reasonable setting of parameters for client behavior that provides control and safety

Manipulation—Purposeful behavior directed at getting one's needs met

Object constancy—The phase in the separation/ individuation process when the child learns to

relate to objects in an effective, constant manner

Personality—The habitual patterns and qualities of behavior of any individual as expressed by physical and mental activities and attitudes

Personality disorders—A class of mental disorders characterized by enduring maladaptive patterns of behavior, cognition, and inner experience, exhibited across many contexts and deviating markedly from those accepted by the individual's culture; these patterns develop early, are inflexible, and are associated with significant distress or disability

Personality traits—An enduring and consistent pattern of values, desires, attitudes, beliefs, and behaviors; when personality traits become inflexible or maladaptive and cause significant impairment, a personality disorder may be diagnosed

Self-mutilative behaviors—Self-injurious behavior common in, but not limited to, borderline personality disorder

Splitting—The failure to integrate and accept the positive and negative qualities of self or others; the individual tends to think in extremes (e.g., actions and motivations are *all* good or *all* bad with no middle ground); splitting creates instability in relationships

---

Personality is defined as a deeply ingrained pattern of behavior, which includes the way one relates to, perceives, and thinks about the environment and oneself. **Personality traits** may be defined as characteristics with which an individual is born or that develop early in life, such as values, desires, attitudes, beliefs, and behaviors. **Personality disorders** occur when these traits become rigid and inflexible and contribute to maladaptive patterns of behavior or impairment in functioning. Nurses working in psychiatric settings are likely to encounter clients diagnosed with borderline and antisocial personality disorders, whereas

individuals diagnosed with other personality disorders are not often treated in acute care settings. Therefore, in this chapter, the nursing process will be applied only to borderline and antisocial personality disorders.

DID YOU KNOW?

Personality disorders are not diagnosed until early adulthood. An individual must complete all stages of personality development before his or her maladaptive patterns of behavior can be attributed to a personality disorder.

I. Personality Development

A. Biological and psychological influences
   1. Heredity.
   2. Temperament.
   3. Experiential learning.
   4. Social interaction.
B. Personality maturation occurs:
   1. At different rates in different individuals.
   2. In an orderly, stepwise fashion.
   3. With some degree of stage overlap.

DID YOU KNOW?
The nurse should understand "normal" personality development before learning about what is considered maladaptive.

C. Table 13.1 compares three theories of normal personality development

II. Classification of Personality Disorders

A. Cluster A: behaviors described as odd or eccentric
   1. Paranoid personality disorder.
   2. Schizoid personality disorder.
   3. Schizotypal personality disorder.

MAKING THE CONNECTION
The *Diagnostic and Statistical Manual of Mental Disorders,* Fifth Edition (DSM-5) has established a diagnostic system that classifies the 10 personality disorders into three clusters according to the description of personality traits.

B. Cluster B: behaviors described as dramatic, emotional, or erratic
   1. Antisocial personality disorder.
   2. Borderline personality disorder.
   3. Histrionic personality disorder.
   4. Narcissistic personality disorder.
C. Cluster C: behaviors described as anxious or fearful
   1. Avoidant personality disorder.
   2. Dependent personality disorder.
   3. Obsessive-compulsive personality disorder.

III. Types of Personality Disorders

A. Paranoid personality disorder
   1. Definition and epidemiological statistics:
      a. Paranoid personality disorder is characterized by a pervasive pattern of detachment from

Table 13.1 Comparison of Personality Development—Sullivan, Erikson, and Mahler: Major Developmental Tasks and Designated Ages

Sullivan	Erikson	Mahler
Birth to 18 months: Relief from anxiety through oral gratification of needs.	Birth to 18 months: To develop a basic trust in the mothering figure and be able to generalize it to others.	Birth to 1 month: Fulfillment of basic needs for survival and comfort
18 months to 6 years: Learning to experience a delay in personal gratification without undue anxiety.	18 months to 3 years: To gain some self-control and independence within the environment.	1–5 months: Developing awareness of external source of need fulfillment.
6–9 years: Learning to form satisfactory peer relationships.	3–6 years: To develop a sense of purpose and the ability to initiate and direct own activities.	5–10 months: Commencement of a primary recognition of separateness from the mothering figure.
9–12 years: Learning to form satisfactory relationships with persons of the same gender; the initiation of feelings of affection for another person.	6–12 years: To achieve a sense of self-confidence by learning, competing, performing successfully, and receiving recognition from significant others, peers, and acquaintances.	10–16 months: Increased independence through locomotor functioning; increased sense of separateness of self.
12–14 years: Learning to form satisfactory relationships with persons of the opposite gender; developing a sense of identity.	12–20 years: To integrate the tasks mastered in the previous stages into a secure sense of self.	16–24 months: Acute awareness of separateness of self; learning to seek "emotional refueling" from mothering figure to maintain feeling of security.
14–21 years: Establishing self-identity; experiences satisfying relationships; working to develop a lasting, intimate opposite-gender relationship.	20–30 years: To form an intense, lasting relationship or a commitment to another person, a cause, an institution, or a creative effort.	24–36 months: Sense of separateness established; on the way to object constancy: able to internalize a sustained image of loved object/person when it is out of sight; resolution of separation anxiety.
	30–65 years: To achieve the life goals established for oneself, while also considering the welfare of future generations.	
	65 years to death: To review one's life and derive meaning from both positive and negative events, while achieving a positive sense of self-worth.	

social relationships and a restricted range of expression of emotions in interpersonal settings.
    b. Experiences an inappropriate mistrust of others' motives.
    c. Present in 1% to 4% of general population.
    d. More commonly diagnosed in men.
  2. Clinical picture:
    a. Constantly on guard and hypervigilant.
    b. Insensitive to feelings of others.
    c. Feels others are there to take advantage of him or her.
    d. Attempts to intimidate others.
    e. Takes no responsibility for own behavior.
    f. Reprisal and vindication can lead to aggression and violence.
  3. Predisposing factors:
    a. Possible hereditary link (relatives diagnosed with schizophrenia).
    b. Subjected to parental antagonism, harassment, and aggression.
    c. Subjected to scapegoating.
    d. Perceives world as harsh, unkind; a place for vigilance and mistrust.
    e. Has "chip-on-the-shoulder" attitude.

B. Schizoid personality disorder
  1. Definition and epidemiological statistics.
    a. Characterized by a pervasive pattern of detachment from social relationships and a restricted range of expression of emotions in interpersonal settings.
    b. Lifelong pattern of social withdrawal.
    c. Discomfort with human interaction.
    d. Affects 3% to 7.5% of general population.
    e. Diagnosed more frequently in men.
  2. Clinical picture.
    a. Cold, aloof, and indifferent to others.
    b. Isolative, unsociable, introverted with no desire for emotional ties.
    c. Spends enormous energy in intellectual pursuits.
    d. Shy, anxious, and exhibits little or no spontaneity.
    e. Unable to experience pleasure.
    f. Affect is bland and constricted.
  3. Predisposing factors.
    a. Introversion is highly inheritable.
    b. Childhood: bleak, cold, and lacking empathy and nurturing.
    c. Poor parenting results in devaluing relationships.

C. Schizotypal personality disorder
  1. Definition and epidemiological statistics.
    a. Characterized by a pervasive pattern of social and interpersonal deficits marked by acute discomfort with, and reduced capacity for, close relationships as well as a cognitive or perceptual distortions and eccentric behavior.
    b. Odd and eccentric but not to the level of schizophrenia.
    c. Less severe than schizoid personality pattern.
    d. Effects 1% to 2% of the general population.
    e. Slightly more common in males.
  2. Clinical picture.
    a. Cognitive or perceptual distortions commonly include:
      i. Magical thinking
      ii. Ideas of reference
      iii. Illusions
      iv. Depersonalization
      v. Belief in superstitions
      vi. Belief in clairvoyance, telepathy, or "sixth sense"
      vii. Belief that "others can feel my feelings"
    b. Bizarre speech patterns.
    c. Illogical thinking.
      i. Thoughts lost in personal irrelevancies
      ii. Thoughts tangential, vague, digressive, and not pertinent
      iii. Illogical thinking alienates individual from others
    d. Under stress may demonstrate brief psychotic symptoms:
      i. Delusional thoughts
      ii. Hallucinations
      iii. Bizarre behavior
    e. Affect is bland and inappropriate.
    f. Low self-esteem.
    g. Distrust in personal relationships.
    h. Inability to cope.
    i. Lives in inner world versus reality.
    j. Likely to be shunned, overlooked, rejected, and humiliated by others.
  3. Predisposing factors.
    a. Possible hereditary link (first-degree biological relatives diagnosed with schizophrenia).

DID YOU KNOW?
Schizotypal personality disorder is now considered part of the schizophrenia spectrum of disorders.

    b. Biogenic factors:
      i. Anatomical deficits
      ii. Neurochemical dysfunctions
      iii. Minimal pleasure-pain sensibilities
      iv. Impaired cognitive functions
    d. Family dynamics:
      i. Indifference
      ii. Impassivity or formality
      iii. Discomfort with personal affection and closeness

D. Antisocial personality disorder
 1. Definition.
  a. Antisocial personality disorder is characterized by a pervasive pattern of disregard for the rights of others.
  b. This behavior has occurred since the age of 15 years.
 2. Epidemiological statistics.
  a. Prevalent in 2% to 4% of men and 1% of women.
  b. More common in lower socioeconomic classes.
 Note: The clinical picture, predisposing factors, and the steps of the nursing process used for care of clients diagnosed with antisocial personality disorder are presented later in this chapter.

E. Borderline personality disorder
 1. Definition.
  a. Characterized by intense chaotic relationships with affective instability and fluctuating attitudes toward others.
  b. Individuals are impulsive, directly and indirectly self-destructive, and lack a clear sense of identity.
 2. Epidemiological statistics.
  a. Diagnosed in 1% to 2% of the population.
  b. More common in women (4 to 1).
 Note: The clinical picture, predisposing factors, and the steps of the nursing process used for care of clients diagnosed with borderline personality disorder are presented later in this chapter.

F. Histrionic personality disorder
 1. Definition and epidemiological statistics.
  a. Characterized by a pervasive pattern of excessive emotionality and attention-seeking behaviors.
  b. Difficulty maintaining long-lasting relationships.
  c. Requires constant approval and acceptance.
  d. Effects 2% to 3% of general population.
  e. More common in women.
 2. Clinical picture:
  a. Self-dramatizing, attention seeking, overly gregarious, and seductive.
  b. Gains attention by manipulative and exhibitionistic behaviors.
  c. Has need to be well liked, successful, popular.
  d. Extroverted, attractive, and sociable.
  e. Failure to evoke attention and approval results in feelings of dejection and anxiety.
  f. Highly distractible and flighty.
  g. Difficulty paying attention to detail.
  h. Sophisticated persona on one hand; inhibited and naive persona on the other.
  i. Highly suggestible, impressionable, and easily influenced.
  j. Demonstrates dependent behavior.
  k. Unable to sustain genuine affection.
  l. Somatic complaints common.
  m. Psychosis may occur during periods of extreme stress.
 3. Predisposing factors:
  a. Enhanced sensitivity and reactivity to environmental stimuli (heightened noradrenergic activity).
  b. Impulsivity associated with decreased serotonergic activity.
  c. More common among first-degree biological relatives of people with the disorder.
  d. Disorder associated with biogenetically determined temperament.

DID YOU KNOW?
Learning experiences in childhood may contribute to the later diagnosis of histrionic personality disorder. When parents withhold positive or negative feedback and are inconsistent with acceptance and approval or ignore their children, the children learn to become dependent on parental expectations. Such children enter adolescence with a nearly insatiable thirst for attention and love.

G. Narcissistic personality disorder
 1. Definition and epidemiological statistics:
  a. Characterized by a pervasive pattern of grandiosity, a need for admiration, and a lack of empathy.
  b. Hypersensitive to evaluation of others.
  c. Feel entitled to get what they what when they want it.
  d. Diagnosed more often in men.
 2. Clinical picture:
  a. Lacks humility.
  b. Overly self-centered.
  c. Exploits others to fulfill own desires.
  d. Little insight into inappropriate or objectionable behaviors.
  e. Feels superior and entitled to special rights and privileges.
  f. Experiences grandiose distortions of reality.
  g. Mood is optimistic, relaxed, cheerful, and carefree.
  h. Moody if self-expectations are not met or if criticized by others.
  i. May respond with rage, shame, humiliation, or dejection.
  j. Fragile self-esteem.
  k. Fantasizes continued stature and perfection.
  l. Exploitation and self-gratification impair interpersonal relationships.
  m. Will choose self-sacrificing mate.

3. Predisposing factors:
   a. Children had their fears, failures, or dependency needs criticized, disdained, or neglected.
   b. Parents demanding, perfectionistic, and critical, with unrealistic expectations.
   c. Unable to view others as sources of comfort and support.
   d. Projected invulnerability and self-sufficiency conceal their true sense of emptiness, contributing to shallowness.
   e. Parents often model narcissistic behaviors.
   f. Possible parental physical or emotional abuse.
   g. Child believes he or she is above that which is required for everyone else.

H. Avoidant personality disorder
1. Definition and epidemiological statistics.
   a. Characterized by a pervasive pattern of social inhibition, feelings of inadequacy, and hypersensitivity to negative evaluation.
   b. Individuals may have a strong desire for companionship.
   c. Extreme shyness, fears rejection, needs unconditional acceptance.
   d. Affects about 1% of general population.
   e. Equally common in men and women.
2. Clinical picture.
   a. Awkward and uncomfortable in social situations.
   b. Generally perceived as timid, withdrawn, or cold and strange.
   c. In closer relationships, perceived as sensitive, touchy, evasive, and mistrustful.
   d. Speech is slow, constrained, with frequent hesitations.
   e. Thoughts are fragmentary with occasional confused and irrelevant digressions.
   f. Expresses feelings of loneliness and being unwanted.

MAKING THE CONNECTION

Some parents pamper and indulge their children in ways that teach them that their every wish is their command, that they can receive without giving in return, and that they deserve prominence without effort. Therefore, these children learn to associate the self with positive affect and develop favorable representations of self. However, because the world will not be as accepting, personal failures, humiliations, and weaknesses undermine the individual's self-esteem. Overblown parental expectations lead to a sense of entitlement, and perceptions of falling short of these expectations undermine the child's self-esteem.

   g. Views others as critical, betraying, and humiliating.
   h. Desires close relationships but avoids them for fear of rejection.
   i. Depressed, anxious, and angry at self for failing to develop social relations.
3. Predisposing factors.
   a. No clear cause.
   b. A combination of biological, genetic, and psychosocial influences.
   c. Infantile temperament:
     i. Hyperirritability
     ii. Crankiness
     iii. Tension
     iv. Withdrawal behaviors
   d. Parental and/or peer rejection and censure.
   e. Family belittlement, abandonment, and criticism.
   f. Low self-worth and social alienation replace natural optimism.
   g. Suspiciousness is learned, and the world is viewed as hostile and dangerous.

IV. Dependent Personality Disorder

1. Definition and epidemiological statistics.
   a. Characterized by a pervasive and excessive need to be taken care of that leads to submissive and clinging behavior and fears of separation.
   b. Allows others to make decisions.
   c. Feels helpless when alone.
   d. Submissive.
   e. Tolerates mistreatment by others.
   f. Demeans self to gain acceptance.
   g. Inadequate assertive or dominant behavior.
   h. Is more common in women and in the youngest children of a family.
2. Clinical picture.
   a. Lacks self-confidence; often apparent in posture, voice, and mannerisms.
   b. Passive and acquiescent to the desires of others.
   c. Overly generous and thoughtful, underplaying own attractiveness and achievements.
   d. Sees the world through "rose-colored glasses."
   e. When alone, may feel pessimistic, discouraged, and dejected.
   f. Suffers in silence.
   g. Assumes passive and submissive role in relationships.
   h. Allows others to make important decisions.
   i. Feels fearful and vulnerable.
   j. Lacks confidence in ability to care for self.
   k. Establishes relationships with dominant others to meet dependent needs.

l. Avoids positions of responsibility.

m. Pervasive feelings of low self-worth.

n. Easily hurt by criticism and disapproval.

o. Tolerates unpleasant or demeaning situations to earn acceptance of others.

3. Predisposing factors.

   a. May be genetically predisposed.

   b. Twin studies measuring submissiveness show a higher correlation between identical twins than fraternal twins.

   c. Dependency is fostered in infancy when stimulation and nurturance are experienced exclusively from one source.

   d. **Helicopter parenting:**

      i. Overprotection

      ii. Discouraging independent behaviors and autonomy

      iii. Making new experiences unnecessarily easy

      iv. Refusing to allow child to learn by experience

      v. Subtly rewarding dependent behaviors

      vi. Threatened rejection if autonomy is attempted

DID YOU KNOW?

A helicopter parent is a parent who pays extremely close attention to a child's or to children's experiences and problems, particularly at educational institutions. Helicopter parents are so named because, like helicopters, they hover overhead.

J. Obsessive-compulsive personality disorder

   1. Definition and epidemiological statistics.

      a. Characterized by a pervasive pattern of preoccupation with orderliness, perfectionism, and interpersonal control at the expense of flexibility, openness, and efficiency.

      b. Very serious and formal; have difficulty expressing emotions.

      c. Overly disciplined, perfectionistic, and preoccupied with rules.

      d. Inflexible about the way in which things must be done.

      e. Devoted to productivity to the exclusion of personal pleasure.

      f. Extreme fear of making mistakes leading to difficulty with decision-making.

      g. Relatively common.

      h. Occurs more often in men.

      i. Most common in oldest children.

   2. Clinical picture.

      a. Inflexible and lack spontaneity.

      b. Meticulously work at tasks that require accuracy and discipline.

      c. Overly concerned with matters of organization and efficiency.

      d. Rigid and unbending about rules and procedures.

      e. Polite and formal.

      f. Solicitous to and ingratiating with authority figures.

      g. Autocratic and condemnatory, pompous and self-righteous with subordinates.

      h. See themselves as conscientious, loyal, dependable, and responsible.

      i. Contemptuous of people whose behavior they consider frivolous and impulsive.

      j. Emotional behavior is considered immature and irresponsible.

      k. Appear calm and controlled.

      l. Under the surface are ambivalent, conflicted, and hostile.

      m. Commonly use the defense mechanisms of reaction formation, intellectualization, rationalization, and undoing.

   3. Predisposing factors.

      a. Overcontrolling parenting.

      b. Parents imposed standards of conduct; condemnation if standards were not met.

      c. Parental praise is less frequent than punishment.

      d. Child learns to heed rigid restrictions and rules.

      e. Positive achievements are expected, taken for granted.

      f. Parental comments and judgments are limited to pointing out transgressions and infractions of rules.

   4. Differences between obsessive-compulsive disorder (OCD) and obsessive-compulsive personality disorder (OCPD)

      a. OCD symptoms change in severity over time, whereas OCPD reflects an overly rigid personality style that remains unchanged over a lifetime.

      b. The obsessions and compulsions associated with OCD, an anxiety disorder, are attempts to control extreme anxiety.

      c. OCPD is not associated with the obsessions and compulsions that are prominent in OCD.

         i. Both carry out repetitive behaviors

         ii. Underlying motive is very different

            1) Clients with OCD might be compelled to repeatedly write out lists with the motivation being prevention of a catastrophe, thereby avoiding excessive anxiety

            2) Clients with OCPD would likely write out lists, but the motivation would be to increase efficiency and productivity

      d. Clients with OCD want to alleviate their symptoms.

e. Clients with OCPD see nothing wrong with their behavior and feel that "other people" are the problem.

V. Antisocial Personality Disorder: Further Information and Nursing Process

A. Predisposing factors
1. Biological influences.
   a. More common among first-degree biological relatives of those with the disorder than among the general population.
   b. Twin and adoptive studies implicate the role of genetics.
   c. Higher number with relatives diagnosed with antisocial personality or alcoholism, even with separation at birth.
   d. Temperament in newborn may be significant (e.g., temper tantrums).
   e. May develop bullying attitudes.
   f. Undaunted by punishment, generally unmanageable.
   g. Display risky behaviors and seem unaffected by pain.
   h. Often diagnosed with attention deficit-hyperactivity disorder (ADHD) and conduct disorder.
   i. May be mediated by serotonergic dysregulation in the septohippocampal system.
   j. May find abnormalities in the prefrontal brain system and reduced autonomic activity, which may account for low arousal, poor fear conditioning, and decision-making deficits.
2. Family dynamics.
   a. Chaotic home environment.
   b. Parental deprivation during the first 5 years of life.
   c. Separation due to delinquency.
   d. Inconsistent and impulsive parenting.
   e. Physical abuse during childhood might damage child's central nervous system and may provide a model for behavior.
   f. Abuse engenders rage, which is then displaced onto others.
   g. Absence of parental discipline.
   h. Extreme poverty.
   i. Removal from home.
   j. Not having parental figures of both sexes.
   k. Erratic and inconsistent methods of discipline.
   l. Being rescued and not suffering consequences of own behavior.
   m. Maternal deprivation.

B. Nursing process: assessment
1. Displays socially irresponsible, exploitative, and guiltless behavior.
2. Manipulates for personal gain.
3. Disregards laws and authority figures.
4. Poor employment history.
5. Unstable relationships.
6. Avoids legal consequences through voluntary hospitalization.
7. Can become furious and vindictive when desires are not met.
8. Shows low tolerance for frustration, acts impetuously.
9. Unable to delay gratification.
10. Restless and easily bored, often taking chances and seeking thrills.
11. Can act cheerful, even gracious and charming, when desires are met.
12. Easily provoked to attack, first inclination is to demean and dominate.
13. Believes that "good guys come in last."
14. Shows contempt for the weak and underprivileged.
15. See themselves as victims.
16. Uses projection as the primary ego defense mechanism.
17. Does not take responsibility for the consequences of behavior.

Nursing process: diagnosis (analysis): Table 13.2 presents a list of client behaviors and the NANDA nursing diagnoses that correspond to those behaviors, which may be used in planning care.

C. Nursing process: planning
1. Short-term goal: within 24 hours after admission, client will verbalize understanding of facility rules and regulations and the consequences for violating them.
2. Long-term goal: by discharge from treatment, client will be able to delay gratification of own desires when interacting with others.

D. Nursing process: implementation
1. Convey an accepting attitude toward the client.
2. Explore with client alternative ways to handle frustration.
3. Explain acceptable behaviors and consequences of violation of rules.
4. Enforce **limit-setting** on unacceptable behaviors.

MAKING THE CONNECTION

The client must come to understand that certain behaviors will not be tolerated within society and that severe consequences will be imposed on those individuals who refuse to comply. The client must be motivated to become a productive member of society before he or she can be helped.

Table 13.2 Assigning Nursing Diagnoses to Behaviors Commonly Associated With Antisocial Personality Disorder

Behaviors	Nursing Diagnoses
Body language (e.g., rigid posture, clenching of fists and jaw, hyperactivity, pacing, breathlessness, threatening stances); cruelty to animals; rage reactions; history of childhood abuse; history of violence against others; impulsivity; substance abuse; negative role-modeling; inability to tolerate frustration	Risk for other-directed violence
Disregard for societal norms and laws; absence of guilty feelings; inability to delay gratification; denial of obvious problems; grandiosity; hostile laughter; projection of blame and responsibility; ridicule of others; superior attitude toward others	Defensive coping
Manipulation of others to fulfill own desires; inability to form close, personal relationships; frequent lack of success in life events; passive-aggressiveness; overt aggressiveness (hiding feelings of low self-esteem)	Chronic low self-esteem
Inability to form a satisfactory, enduring, intimate relationship with another; dysfunctional interaction with others; use of unsuccessful social interaction behaviors	Impaired social interaction
Demonstration of inability to take responsibility for meeting basic health practices; history of lack of health-seeking behavior; demonstrated lack of knowledge regarding basic health practices; lack of expressed interest in improving health behaviors	Ineffective health maintenance

5. Clearly explain client expectations.
6. Give positive feedback and rewards for acceptable behavior.
7. Provide appropriate milieu environment.
8. Help client gain insight into his or her own behavior.
9. Talk about past client behaviors.
10. Help identify ways client has exploited others.
11. Explore how client would feel if circumstances were reversed.
12. Assure client that while behaviors may be unacceptable, the client is valued.

F. Nursing process: evaluation: reassessment is conducted to determine whether the nursing actions have been successful. The following questions may be used to evaluate the objectives of care.
1. Does the client recognize when anger is getting out of control?
2. Can the client seek out staff instead of expressing anger in an inappropriate manner?
3. Can the client use other sources for rechanneling anger (e.g., physical activities)?
4. Has harm to others been avoided?
5. Can the client follow rules and regulations of the therapeutic milieu with little or no reminding?
6. Can the client verbalize which behaviors are appropriate and which are not?
7. Does the client express a desire to change?
8. Can the client delay gratifying own desires in deference to those of others when appropriate?
9. Does the client refrain from manipulating others to fulfill own desires?

VI. Borderline Personality Disorder: Further Information and Nursing Process

A. Predisposing factors
1. Biological influences.
   a. Possible serotonergic defect.
   b. Mood disorders are common in the family background.
2. Psychosocial influences.
   a. Reared in families with chaotic environments.
   b. Family environments characterized by trauma, neglect, and/or separation.
   c. Exposed to sexual and physical abuse and serious parental psychopathology, such as substance abuse and antisocial personality disorder.
   d. Has been linked to post-traumatic stress disorder (PTSD) in response to childhood trauma and abuse.
3. Mahler's theory of object relations: six phases from birth to 36 months when a sense of separateness from the parenting figure is finally established. These phases include the following:
   a. **Phase 1 (Birth–1 Month), Autistic Phase:** baby spends most of his or her time in a half-waking, half-sleeping state. The main goal is fulfillment of needs for survival and comfort.
   b. **Phase 2 (1–5 Months), Symbiotic Phase:** there is a type of psychic fusion of mother and child. Sees self as an extension of the parenting figure, although baby is developing awareness of external sources of need fulfillment.

   c. **Phase 3 (5–10 Months), Differentiation Phase:** recognizes that there is a separateness between the self and the parenting figure.

   d. **Phase 4 (10–16 Months), Practicing Phase:** increased locomotor functioning and the ability to explore the environment independently. A sense of separateness of the self is increased.

   e. **Phase 5 (16–24 Months), Rapprochement Phase:** separateness of the self becomes acute. Frightening to child, who wants to regain some lost closeness but not return to symbiosis. Child wants mother there as needed for "emotional refueling" and security.

   f. **Phase 6 (24–36 Months), On the Way to Object Constancy Phase:** Child completes the individuation process and learns to relate to objects in an effective, constant manner. Separateness is established, and child is able to internalize a sustained image of the loved object or person when out of sight. Separation anxiety is resolved.

DID YOU KNOW?

The individual with borderline personality disorder becomes fixed in the rapprochement phase of development. This occurs when the child shows increasing separation and autonomy. The mother, who feels secure in the relationship as long as the child is dependent, begins to feel threatened by the child's increasing independence. The mother may indeed be experiencing her own fears of abandonment. In response to separation behaviors, the mother withdraws the emotional support or "refueling" that is so vitally needed during this phase for the child to feel secure. Instead, the mother rewards clinging, dependent behaviors, and punishes (withholding emotional support) independent behaviors. With his or her sense of emotional survival at stake, the child learns to behave in a manner that satisfies the parental wishes. An internal conflict develops within the child, based on fear of abandonment. He or she wants to achieve independence common to this stage of development but fears that the mother will withdraw emotional support as a result. This unresolved fear of abandonment remains with the child into adulthood. Unresolved grief for the nurturing they failed to receive results in internalized rage that manifests itself in the depression so common in people with borderline personality disorder.

B. Nursing process: assessment

DID YOU KNOW?

Individuals with borderline personality always seem to be in a state of crisis. Their affect is one of extreme intensity, and their behavior reflects frequent changeability. These changes can occur within days, hours, or even minutes. Often these individuals exhibit a single, dominant affective tone, such as depression, which may give way periodically to anxious agitation or inappropriate outbursts of anger.

1. Chronic depression.
   a. Many diagnosed with major depressive disorder.
   b. Depression occurs in response to feelings of abandonment by mother.
   c. Rage turns both inward and externally on the environment.
   d. Client unaware of these feelings until well into long-term therapy.
2. Inability to be alone.
   a. Occurs in response to abandonment by mother.
   b. Frantic search for companionship regardless of quality.
   c. Prefers unsatisfactory relationship to feelings of loneliness, emptiness, and boredom.
3. Clinging and distancing (patterns of interaction).
   a. When clinging to another individual, may exhibit helpless, dependent, or even childlike behaviors.
   b. Overidealizes an individual with whom they want to spend all their time.
   c. Expresses a frequent need to talk; seeks constant reassurance.
   d. Acting-out behaviors, even self-mutilation, result when unable to be with chosen individual.
   e. Behavior characterized by hostility, anger, and devaluation of others.
   f. Arises from feelings of discomfort with closeness.
   g. Occurs in response to separations, confrontations, or attempts to limit certain behaviors.
   h. Devaluation of others is manifested by discrediting or undermining strengths and personal significance of others.
4. **Splitting.**
   a. A primitive ego defense mechanism common in people with borderline personality disorder.
   b. Arises from lack of achievement of **object constancy** (see Mahler's theory of object relations).
   c. Manifested by an inability to integrate and accept both positive and negative feelings.
   d. See people and situations in black-and-white terms, all bad or all good, with no shades of gray.
   e. Intention to disrupt staff cohesiveness.

MAKING THE CONNECTION

In the view of individuals diagnosed with borderline personality disorder, people—including themselves—and life situations are either all good or all bad. For example, if a caregiver is nurturing and supportive, he or she is lovingly idealized. Should the nurturing relationship be threatened in any way (e.g., the caregiver must move because of his or her job), suddenly the individual is devalued, and the idealized image changes from beneficent caregiver to one of hateful and cruel persecutor.

5. **Manipulation.**
   a. To prevent feared separation.
   b. Any behavior is acceptable in achieving relief from separation anxiety.
   c. Playing one individual against another is a common ploy to allay fears of abandonment.
6. Self-destructive behaviors.

Repetitive, **self-mutilative behaviors** are classic manifestations of borderline personality disorder. Although these acts can be fatal, most commonly they are manipulative gestures designed to elicit a rescue response from significant others. Suicide attempts are quite common and result from feelings of abandonment after separation from a significant other. The endeavor is often attempted, however, incorporating a measure of "safety" into the plan (e.g., swallowing pills in an area where the person will surely be discovered by others or swallowing pills and making a phone call to report the act to someone).

   a. Other types of destructive behaviors include cutting, scratching, and burning.
   b. May have higher levels of endorphins, thereby increasing pain threshold.

   c. May be in a state of **depersonalization** and **derealization** and unable initially to feel pain.
   d. Mutilation continues until pain is felt in an attempt to counteract the feelings of unreality.
   e. Some clients report that "to feel pain is better than to feel nothing," and the pain validates their existence.
7. **Impulsivity:** These acting-out behaviors occur in response to real or perceived feelings of abandonment.
   a. Substance abuse.
   b. Gambling.
   c. Promiscuity.
   d. Reckless driving.
   e. Binging and purging.
C. Nursing process: diagnosis (analysis): Table 13.3 presents a list of client behaviors and the NANDA nursing diagnoses that correspond to those behaviors, which may be used in planning care
D. Nursing process: planning
   1. Short-term goal: client will seek out staff member if feelings of harming self emerge.
   2. Long-term goal: by discharge, client will exhibit no evidence of splitting during social and therapeutic activities.
E. Nursing process: implementation
   1. Create a trusting relationship.
   2. Observe client's behavior frequently.
   3. Establish safety contract with client.
   4. Care for wounds matter-of-factly.
   5. Encourage verbalization of feelings.
   6. Provide safe environment.
   7. Act as role model.
   8. Encourage appropriate expressions of anger.
   9. Enforce **limit-setting** on acting-out behavior.

Table 13.3 Assigning Nursing Diagnoses to Behaviors Commonly Associated With Borderline Personality Disorder

Behaviors	Nursing Diagnoses
History of self-injurious behavior; history of inability to plan solutions; impulsivity; irresistible urge to damage self; feels threatened with loss of significant relationship	Risk for self-mutilation
History of suicide attempts; suicidal ideation; suicidal plan; impulsiveness; childhood abuse; fears of abandonment; internalized rage	Risk for self-directed violence; risk for suicide
Body language (e.g., rigid posture, clenching of fists and jaw, hyperactivity, pacing, breathlessness, threatening stances); history of childhood abuse; impulsivity; transient psychotic symptomatology	Risk for other-directed violence
Depression; persistent emotional distress; rumination; separation distress; traumatic distress; verbalizes feeling empty; inappropriate expression of anger	Complicated grieving
Alternating clinging and distancing behaviors; staff splitting; manipulation	Impaired social interaction
Feelings of depersonalization and derealization	Disturbed personal identity
Transient psychotic symptoms (disorganized thinking; misinterpretation of the environment); increased tension; decreased perceptual field	Anxiety (severe to panic)
Dependent on others; excessively seeks reassurance; manipulation of others; inability to tolerate being alone	Chronic low self-esteem

10. Encourage independence and give positive reinforcement.
11. Rotate staff.
    a. Prevents inappropriate attachments.
    b. Prevents feelings of abandonment.
    c. Prevents splitting behaviors by client.
    d. Prevents staff burnout.
F. Nursing process: evaluation—evaluation of the nursing actions for the client with borderline personality disorder may be facilitated by gathering information using the following types of questions:
    1. Has the client been able to seek out staff when feeling the desire for self-harm?
    2. Has the client avoided self-harm?
    3. Can the client correlate times of desire for self-harm to times of elevation in level of anxiety?
    4. Can the client discuss feelings with staff (particularly feelings of depression and anger)?
    5. Can the client identify the true target toward which anger is directed?
    6. Can the client verbalize understanding of the basis for his or her anger?
    7. Can the client express anger appropriately?
    8. Can the client function independently?
    9. Can the client relate to more than one staff member?
    10. Can the client verbalize the knowledge that the staff members will return and are not abandoning the client when leaving for the day?
    11. Can the client separate from the staff in an appropriate manner?
    12. Can the client delay gratification and refrain from manipulating others to fulfill own desires?

VII. Treatment Modalities

A. Interpersonal psychotherapy
   1. Brief and time-limited: addresses problems with interpersonal style.
   2. Long-term: addresses maladjusted behaviors, cognition, and affect that dominate personal lives and relationships.

MAKING THE CONNECTION

Clients diagnosed with a personality disorder do not recognize their maladaptive personality traits as undesirable or in need of change; therefore, treatment is difficult and, in some instances, may even seem impossible. The selection of intervention is generally based on the area of greatest dysfunction, such as cognition, affect, behavior, or interpersonal relations.

3. Establishment of empathetic therapist-client relationship (therapist as role model).
4. Therapy suggested for clients diagnosed with paranoid, schizoid, schizotypal, borderline, dependent, narcissistic, and obsessive-compulsive personality disorders.
5. From a psychoanalytic perspective, treatment focuses on the unconscious motivation for seeking total satisfaction from others and the inability to commit oneself to a stable, meaningful relationship.
B. Milieu or group therapy
   1. Feedback from peers more effective than one-on-one with therapist.
   2. Homogenous supportive groups increase social skills.
   3. Helpful in overcoming anxiety and developing trust and rapport.
   4. Suggested for clients diagnosed with histrionic, antisocial, dependent, and avoidant personality disorders.
C. Cognitive behavioral therapy
   1. Behavioral strategies offer reinforcement for positive change.
   2. Social skills and assertiveness training teach alternative ways to deal with frustration.
   3. Strategies help to correct inaccurate internal mental schemata.
   4. Suggested for clients diagnosed with antisocial, dependent, obsessive-compulsive, and avoidant personality disorders.
D. Dialectical behavioral therapy (DBT)
   1. Combination of cognitive, behavioral, and interpersonal therapies with Eastern mindfulness practices.
   2. Suggested for clients diagnosed with borderline personality disorder.
   3. Five functions of DBT:
      a. Enhances behavioral capabilities.
      b. Improves motivation to change.
      c. Ensures that new capabilities generalize to the natural environment.
      d. Structures the treatment environment such that client and therapist capabilities are supported and effective behaviors are reinforced.
      e. Enhances therapist capabilities and motivation to treat clients effectively.
   4. Four primary modes of DBT:
      a. Group skills training.
      b. Individual psychotherapy.
      c. Telephone contact.
      d. Therapist consultation/team meetings.
E. Psychopharmacology
   1. Medication has no effect in the direct treatment of personality disorders.

2. Symptomatic treatment includes:
   a. Antipsychotic medication.
      i. Prescribed for clients diagnosed with paranoid, schizotypal, and borderline personality disorders
      ii. May decrease psychotic decompensation, ideas of reference, paranoid thinking, anxiety, and hostility
   b. Antidepressants: selective serotonin reuptake inhibitors (SSRIs).
      i. Prescribed for clients diagnosed with borderline personality disorders to decrease impulsivity and self-destructive acts
      ii. A combination of SSRIs and an atypical antipsychotic medication may treat dysphoria, mood instability, and impulsivity
   c. Lithium carbonate and propranolol prescribed for clients diagnosed with antisocial personality disorder.
      i. May decrease violent episodes
      ii. Used with caution because of high risk for substance abuse
   d. Anxiolytics and antidepressants such as sertraline and paroxetine may be prescribed for clients diagnosed with avoidant personality disorders.
      i. Help during stressful periods
      ii. Help when episodes of panic are experienced

REVIEW QUESTIONS

1. Which predisposing factor would be implicated in the etiology of an avoidant personality disorder?
   1. Parents were demanding and perfectionist with unrealistic expectations
   2. Parental rejection and censure
   3. Parental bleakness and pervasive, unfeeling coldness
   4. Parental approval only when behaviors met parental expectations

2. A client is being assessed for schizotypal personality disorder. Which of the following behaviors would the nurse expect to note? **Select all that apply.**
   1. The client experiences magical thinking and ideas of reference.
   2. The client has an intense fear of making mistakes, leading to difficulty with decision-making.
   3. Under stress, the client may decompensate and demonstrate various psychotic behaviors.
   4. The client is extremely vulnerable and constantly on the defensive.
   5. The client is aloof and may have an affect that is bland or inappropriate.

3. The nurse expects to establish a supportive therapeutic relationship with a client diagnosed with schizotypal personality disorder. Which nursing intervention is most appropriate?
   1. Set limits on acting-out behaviors and explain consequences.
   2. Present reality when client is experiencing magical thinking.
   3. Encourage client to gradually verbalize hostile feelings.
   4. Remove all dangerous objects from the environment.

4. Which nursing intervention takes priority when caring for a client with a nursing diagnosis: risk for other-directed violence R/T rage reactions, negative role-modeling, and the inability to tolerate frustration?
   1. Assess for self-injurious intent and available means.
   2. Observe the client's behavior frequently.
   3. Place the client in strict seclusion.
   4. Help the client identify situations that provoke defensiveness.

5. _____ personality disorder is characterized by a pattern of intense and chaotic relationships with affective instability and fluctuating attitudes toward other people.

6. A client is diagnosed with narcissistic personality disorder. Which of the following symptoms must be present to be assigned this diagnosis? **Select all that apply.**
   1. The client's exaggerated self-appraisal may be inflated, deflated, or vacillate between extremes.
   2. The client's goal setting is based on gaining approval from others.
   3. The client's personal standards are unreasonably high based on a sense of entitlement.
   4. The client is reluctant to get involved with people unless certain of being liked.
   5. The client's relationships are largely superficial and exist to serve self-esteem.

7. An instructor is teaching students about clients diagnosed with borderline personality disorder. Which of the following student statements indicate(s) that further instruction is needed? **Select all that apply.**
   1. "Individuals consider relationships to be more intimate then they actually are."
   2. "Individuals always seem to be in a state of crisis."
   3. "Individuals read hidden threatening meanings into benign remarks."
   4. "Individuals have little tolerance for being alone and have chronic fear of abandonment."
   5. "Individuals manifest an inability to integrate and accept both positive and negative feelings."

8. A client is being assessed for dependent personality disorder. Which of the following behaviors would the nurse expect to note? **Select all that apply.**
   1. The client has an ability to work diligently and patiently at tasks that require accuracy and discipline.
   2. The client is unable to tolerate being alone.
   3. The client may appear to others to "see the world through rose-colored glasses."
   4. The client is overly generous and thoughtful and underplays his or her own attractiveness and achievements.
   5. The client lacks confidence in his or her ability to care for self.

9. During group therapy, which client action should a nurse identify as the dramatic and extroverted behavior commonly associated with histrionic personality disorder?
   1. The client suddenly lifts her blouse and exposes her breasts to her peers.
   2. The client suddenly cuts her wrist with a broken light-bulb shard.
   3. The client lights up a cigarette and demands the right to receive special consideration for her habit.
   4. The client laughingly declares that her cat is actually her grandmother reincarnated.

10. When employing dialectal behavior therapy (DBT) for a client diagnosed with borderline personality disorder, which of the following would be included in this therapy? **Select all that apply.**
    1. Group skills training
    2. Symptom relief psychopharmacology
    3. Individual psychotherapy
    4. Telephone contact
    5. Therapist consultation/team meeting

11. A client is being assessed for antisocial personality disorder. Which of the following behaviors would the nurse expect to note? **Select all that apply.**
    1. The client is socially irresponsible, exploitive, and exhibits guiltless behavior.
    2. The client has difficulty sustaining consistent employment and stable relationships.
    3. The client lacks warmth and compassion and displays a brusque and belligerent manner.
    4. The client attempts suicide and self-injurious behaviors.
    5. The client exhibits a low tolerance for frustration and is unable to delay gratification.

12. Obsessive-compulsive personality disorder is characterized by being perfectionistic, overly disciplined, and preoccupied with rules, whereas schizotypal personality disorder is characterized by being:
    1. Aloof, isolative, while behaving in a bland and apathetic manner
    2. Overly generous and thoughtful while underplaying own worth
    3. Overly self-centered, while exploiting others to fulfill own desires
    4. Extremely sensitive to rejection, which leads to a socially withdrawn life

13. A 27-year-old man has been diagnosed with antisocial personality disorder. Which of the following nursing interventions might be identified for this client? **Select all that apply.**
    1. Explain which behaviors are acceptable on the unit and which are not
    2. Ensure that all sharp objects have been removed from the environment
    3. Determine appropriate consequences for violations of unit rules
    4. Don't be taken in by charming, manipulative behavior
    5. Encourage client to talk about his past misdeeds

14. An instructor is teaching students the difference between obsessive-compulsive disorder (OCD) and obsessive-compulsive personality disorder (OCPD). Which student statement indicates that further instruction is needed?
    1. "OCD symptoms change in severity over time, whereas OCPD symptoms remain unchanged over a lifetime."
    2. "OCPD is not associated with the obsessions and compulsions that are prominent in OCD."
    3. "Clients with OCD want to alleviate their symptoms , whereas clients with OCPD see nothing wrong with their behavior."
    4. "OCD becomes OCPD when symptoms of anxiety reach the level of uncontrolled panic."

15. The mother of a teenage client asks what the term "helicopter parent" means. Which explanation by the nurse would be most accurate?
    1. A parent who hires a drone to hover overhead and protect his or her child from harm.
    2. A parent who is basically depressed and fears his or her child will succumb to the same affliction if not protected and controlled.
    3. A parent who pays extremely close attention to his or her child's experiences and problems.
    4. A parent who, as a child, once experienced the same parental overprotection and overcontrol.

16. Using _____ as a primary ego defense mechanism, individuals diagnosed with antisocial personality disorder see themselves as victims and do not accept responsibility for the consequences of their behavior.

17. When faced with a confrontational situation, to which of the following clients would the nurse most likely employ interventions that minimize manipulative behavior? **Select all that apply.**
    1. A client diagnosed with borderline personality disorder
    2. A client diagnosed with avoidant personality disorder
    3. A client diagnosed with schizoid personality disorder
    4. A client diagnosed with antisocial personality disorder
    5. A client diagnosed with obsessive-compulsive personality disorder

18. Which of the following behavioral patterns is characteristic of individuals diagnosed with narcissistic personality disorder? **Select all that apply.**
    1. Suspicious and mistrustful of others
    2. Appears to lack humility
    3. Entitled to special rights and privileges
    4. Justified in possessing whatever they seek
    5. Indirectly and directly self-destructive

19. Understanding the typical problems faced by clients diagnosed with dependent personality disorder, which nursing diagnosis would the nurse most likely assign?
    1. Risk for injury R/T seeking attention by self-harm
    2. Altered self-image R/T exaggerated sense of self AEB pressured speech
    3. Risk for altered communication process R/T inability to establish meaningful relationships
    4. Impaired social interaction R/T lack of confidence AEB friends who take advantage

20. Order the following nursing interventions used in the care of clients diagnosed with antisocial personality disorder.
    _____ Immediately set limits on maladaptive behaviors that defy rules
    _____ Review unit rules and regulations
    _____ Consistently implement consequences of rule infractions
    _____ Clearly explain the consequences of rule infractions

21. A nurse is planning care for a client diagnosed with obsessive-compulsive personality disorder. Which one of the following behavioral characteristics is the nurse most likely to observe? **Select all that apply.**
    1. Colorful, dramatic, and extroverted behavior
    2. Efficient, organized, and rigid behavior
    3. Contemptuous of frivolous and impulsive behavior in others
    4. Extremely sensitive to rejection
    5. Unbending about rules and procedures

REVIEW ANSWERS

1. **ANSWER: 2**
   Rationale:
   1. Having parents who were demanding and perfectionistic and who had unrealistic expectations is a predisposing factor for an individual diagnosed with narcissistic, not avoidant, personality disorder.
   2. The primary psychological predisposing influence to avoidant personality disorder is parental rejection and censure, which is often reinforced by peers. These children are often reared in families in which they are belittled, abandoned, and criticized.
   3. Having parents who were bleak and unfeelingly cold is a predisposing factor for an individual diagnosed with schizoid, not avoidant, personality disorder.
   4. Having parents who showed approval only when the child's behaviors met parental expectations is a predisposing factor for an individual diagnosed with histrionic, not avoidant, personality disorder.
   TEST-TAKING TIP: Review the predisposing factors for and recognize the parenting styles that contribute to each of the 10 personality disorders.
   Content Area: Safe and Effective Care Environment: Management of Care;
   Integrated Process: Nursing Process: Assessment;
   Client Need: Safe and Effective Care Environment: Management of Care;
   Cognitive Level: Application;
   Concept: Assessment

2. **ANSWERS: 1, 3, 5**
   Rationale:
   1. Experiencing magical thinking and having ideas of reference are characteristic behaviors of schizotypal personality disorder. Some individuals assume the passive and submissive role in relationships.
   2. Intense fear of making mistakes leading to difficulty with decision-making is a characteristic behavior of an obsessive-compulsive, not schizotypal, personality disorder.
   3. Decompensating and demonstrating various psychotic behaviors when under stress are characteristic of schizotypal personality disorder. However, delusional thoughts, hallucinations, or bizarre behaviors are usually of brief duration.
   4. Being extremely vulnerable and constantly on the defensive is a characteristic behavior of a paranoid, not schizotypal, personality disorder.
   5. Being aloof and having an affect that is bland or inappropriate is a characteristic behavior of schizotypal personality disorder. These individuals also have a bland and apathetic manner.
   TEST-TAKING TIP: Review the clinical picture for schizoid personality disorder to recognize characteristic behaviors of this disorder.
   Content Area: Safe and Effective Care Environment: Management of Care;
   Integrated Process: Nursing Process: Assessment;
   Client Need: Safe and Effective Care Environment: Management of Care;

Cognitive Level: Application;
Concept: Self

3. **ANSWER: 2**
   Rationale:
   1. Clients diagnosed with schizotypal personality disorder are aloof and isolative, and they behave in a bland and apathetic manner. Rarely, if ever, would there be a need to set limits on acting-out behaviors.
   2. Magical thinking, ideas of reference, illusions, and depersonalization are part of the world for a client diagnosed with schizotypal personality disorder. The most appropriate nursing intervention when a client is experiencing magical thinking is for the nurse to present reality.
   3. Under stress, individuals diagnosed with schizotypal personality disorder will decompensate and demonstrate psychotic symptoms. Their affect is bland or inappropriate, such as laughing at their own problems. Anger and hostility are not characteristic of this disorder.
   4. There would be no need to remove all dangerous objects from the environment. Individuals diagnosed with schizotypal personality disorder do not typically have thoughts of self-harm or suicide.
   TEST-TAKING TIP: Review the clinical picture for schizotypal personality in order to recognize and match problems with appropriate nursing interventions.
   Content Area: Safe and Effective Care Environment: Management of Care;
   Integrated Process: Nursing Process: Implementation;
   Client Need: Safe and Effective Care Environment: Management of Care;
   Cognitive Level: Application;
   Concept: Critical Thinking

4. **ANSWER: 2**
   Rationale:
   1. The client in the question is at risk for other-directed, not self-directed, violence.
   2. Clients who are at risk for other-directed violence need to be observed frequently. Close observation is prioritized so that interventions can be implemented to ensure unit safety. The nurse should avoid appearing watchful and suspicious while observing the client's activities and interactions.
   3. Client seclusion would only be implemented if the client exhibited behaviors that indicate imminent harm or injury to others.
   4. The nurse could help the client identify situations that provoke defensiveness by role-playing more appropriate responses. Role-playing provides confidence to deal with difficult situations when they actually occur. Although this is an important intervention, it does not take priority over safety.
   TEST-TAKING TIP: Remember when choosing a nursing intervention, safety is always prioritized.
   Content Area: Safe and Effective Care Environment: Management of Care;
   Integrated Process: Nursing Process: Implementation;
   Client Need: Safe and Effective Care Environment: Management of Care;

Cognitive Level: Application;
Concept: Critical Thinking

5. **ANSWER: Borderline**
Rationale: Borderline personality disorder is characterized by a pattern of intense and chaotic relationships, with affective instability and fluctuating attitudes toward other people. These individuals are impulsive, directly and indirectly self-destructive, and lack a clear sense of identity.
TEST-TAKING TIP: Review and become familiar with the characteristics of borderline personality disorder.
Content Area: Psychosocial Integrity;
Integrated Process: Nursing Process: Assessment;
Client Need: Psychosocial Integrity;
Cognitive Level: Knowledge;
Concept: Self

6. **ANSWERS: 1, 2, 3, 5**
Rationale:
1. To assign the diagnosis of narcissistic personality disorder, the client must experience an exaggerated self-appraisal that may be inflated, deflated, or vacillate between extremes.
2. To assign the diagnosis of narcissistic personality disorder, the client's goal setting must be based on gaining approval from others.
3. To assign the diagnosis of narcissistic personality disorder, the client must have personal standards that are unreasonably high based on a sense of entitlement.
4. Reluctance to get involved with people unless there is a certainty of being liked is not a symptom that is required for a diagnosis of narcissistic personality disorder.
5. To assign the diagnosis of narcissistic personality disorder, clients must experience relationships that are largely superficial and exist to serve their self-esteem.
TEST-TAKING TIP: Review the clinical picture for narcissistic personality to recognize and match behaviors with the appropriate assigned medical diagnosis.
Content Area: Safe and Effective Care Environment: Management of Care;
Integrated Process: Nursing Process: Assessment;
Client Need: Safe and Effective Care Environment: Management of Care;
Cognitive Level: Application;
Concept: Assessment

7. **ANSWERS: 1, 3**
Rationale:
1. An individual diagnosed with histrionic, not borderline, personality disorder might consider relationships to be more intimate than they actually are. This student statement indicates that further instruction is needed.
2. The student's statement that individuals diagnosed with borderline personality disorder always seem to be in a state of crisis is accurate and indicates that learning has occurred.
3. An individual diagnosed with paranoid, not borderline, personality disorder might read hidden threatening meanings into benign remarks. This student statement indicates that further instruction is needed.

4. The student's statement that individuals diagnosed with borderline personality disorder have little tolerance for being alone and have chronic fear of abandonment is accurate and indicates that learning has occurred.
5. The student's statement that individuals diagnosed with borderline personality are unable to integrate and accept both positive and negative feelings is accurate and indicates that learning has occurred.
TEST-TAKING TIP: Review the clinical picture for borderline personality to recognize characteristic behaviors of this disorder.
Content Area: Safe and Effective Care Environment: Management of Care;
Integrated Process: Nursing Process: Evaluation;
Client Need: Safe and Effective Care Environment: Management of Care;
Cognitive Level: Analysis;
Concept: Nursing Roles

8. **ANSWERS: 3, 4, 5**
Rationale:
1. Working diligently and patiently at tasks that require accuracy and discipline is a characteristic behavior of a client diagnosed with obsessive-compulsive, not dependent, personality disorder.
2. Having an inability to tolerate being alone is a characteristic behavior of a client diagnosed with borderline, not dependent, personality disorder.
3. Appearing to others to "see the world through rose-colored glasses" is a characteristic behavior of a dependent personality disorder. Although when alone, they may feel pessimistic, discouraged, and dejected.
4. Being overly generous and thoughtful and underplaying one's own attractiveness and achievements are characteristic behaviors of a dependent personality disorder. Some individuals assume the passive and submissive role in relationships.
5. Lacking confidence in the ability to care for themselves is a characteristic behavior of persons with a dependent personality disorder. They are willing to let others make their decisions.
TEST-TAKING TIP: Review the clinical picture for dependent personality disorder to recognize characteristic behaviors of this disorder.
Content Area: Safe and Effective Care Environment: Management of Care;
Integrated Process: Nursing Process: Assessment;
Client Need: Safe and Effective Care Environment: Management of Care;
Cognitive Level: Application;
Concept: Self

9. **ANSWER: 1**
Rationale:
1. A nurse would identify a client who suddenly lifts her blouse and exposes her breasts to her peers as dramatic and extroverted. This behavior is associated with histrionic personality disorder. Individuals with this disorder tend to be self-dramatizing, attention seeking, overly gregarious, and seductive.

2. A nurse would identify a client who suddenly cuts her wrist as impulsive and self-destructive. This behavior is associated with borderline personality disorder. Individuals with this disorder seem to be in a constant state of crisis, and their behavior reflects frequent changeability. These changes can occur within days, hours, or even minutes.

3. A nurse would identify a client who lights up a cigarette and demands the right to receive special consideration as dramatic, emotional, and entitled. This behavior is associated with narcissistic personality disorder. Individuals with this disorder have an exaggerated sense of self-worth. They lack empathy and believe they have the inalienable right to receive special consideration.

4. A nurse would identify a client who declares that her cat is actually her grandmother reincarnated as odd or eccentric. This behavior is associated with schizoid personality disorder. Under stress, these individuals may decompensate and demonstrate psychotic symptoms such as delusional thoughts, but these thoughts are usually of brief duration.

TEST-TAKING TIP: Review the definition and clinical picture for histrionic personality disorder to recognize characteristic behaviors of this disorder.

Content Area: Safe and Effective Care Environment: Management of Care;
Integrated Process: Nursing Process: Evaluation;
Client Need: Safe and Effective Care Environment: Management of Care;
Cognitive Level: Application;
Concept: Assessment

10. **ANSWERS: 1, 3, 4, 5**
Rationale:
1. **Group skills training is one of the four primary modes of DBT. In these groups, clients are taught skills considered relevant to their particular problems.**
2. Symptom relief psychopharmacology is not one of the modes of DBT therapy. Psychopharmacology may be helpful in some instances. Although these drugs have no effect in direct treatment of personality disorders, some symptomatic relief can be achieved.
3. **Individual psychotherapy is one of the four primary modes of DBT. Weekly sessions address dysfunctional behavioral patterns, personal motivation, and skills strengthening.**
4. **Telephone contact is one of the four primary modes of DBT. Usually on a 24-hour basis, but according to limits set by the therapist, telephone contact gives the client help and support in applying skills in life situations and also aids in finding ways of avoiding self-injury.**
5. **Therapist consultation/team meeting is one of the four primary modes of DBT. Therapists meet regularly to review their work. These meetings are focused specifically on providing effective treatment to their clients.**

TEST-TAKING TIP: Review the four primary modes of dialectal behavior therapy and recognize that it is the treatment of choice for clients diagnosed with borderline personality disorder.

Content Area: Safe and Effective Care Environment: Management of Care;
Integrated Process: Nursing Process: Implementation;
Client Need: Safe and Effective Care Environment: Management of Care;
Cognitive Level: Application;
Concept: Nursing

11. **ANSWERS: 1, 2, 3, 5**
Rationale:
1. **Socially irresponsible, exploitive, and guiltless behaviors are characteristics associated with antisocial personality disorder. These individuals are unconcerned with obeying the law.**
2. **Difficulty in sustaining consistent employment and stable relationships are characteristic behaviors that are associated with antisocial personality disorder. These individuals tend to be argumentative and, at times, cruel and malicious.**
3. **Lacking warmth and compassion and displaying a brusque and belligerent manner are characteristic behaviors that are associated with antisocial personality disorder. When desires are challenged, these individuals are likely to become furious and vindictive.**
4. Attempts at suicide and self-injurious behaviors are characteristics associated with borderline, not antisocial, personality disorder.
5. **Exhibiting low tolerance for frustration and the inability to delay gratification are characteristic behaviors that are associated with antisocial personality disorder. When things go their way, individuals with this disorder act cheerful, even gracious and charming. Because of their low tolerance for frustration, this pleasant exterior can change very quickly.**

TEST-TAKING TIP: Review the clinical picture for antisocial personality disorder in order to recognize characteristic behaviors of this disorder.

Content Area: Safe and Effective Care Environment: Management of Care;
Integrated Process: Nursing Process: Assessment;
Client Need: Safe and Effective Care Environment: Management of Care;
Cognitive Level: Application;
Concept: Self

12. **ANSWER: 1**
Rationale:
1. **Being aloof and isolative while behaving in a bland and apathetic manner is characteristic of schizotypal personality disorder. Individuals with this disorder often cannot orient their thoughts logically and become lost in personal irrelevancies that seem vague and not pertinent to the topic at hand. This feature of their personality only further alienates them from others.**
2. Being overly generous and thoughtful while underplaying one's own worth is characteristic of dependent, not schizotypal, personality disorder.
3. Being overly self-centered while exploiting others to fulfill personal desires is characteristic of narcissistic, not schizotypal, personality disorder.

4. Being extremely sensitive to rejection leading to a socially withdrawn life is characteristic of avoidant, not schizotypal, personality disorder.
TEST-TAKING TIP: Review the definition and clinical picture for schizotypal personality to recognize characteristic behaviors of this disorder.
Content Area: Safe and Effective Care Environment: Management of Care;
Integrated Process: Nursing Process: Evaluation;
Client Need: Safe and Effective Care Environment: Management of Care;
Cognitive Level: Analysis;
Concept: Self

13. **ANSWERS: 1, 3, 4, 5**
Rationale:
1. Explaining acceptable behaviors enlightens the client to the sensitivity of others and promotes self-awareness in an effort to help the client gain insight into his own behavior.
2. There is nothing in the question that indicates that this client intends to harm self or others. A diagnosis of antisocial personality disorder should not automatically be associated with violent behavior.
3. This client must come to understand that certain behaviors will not be tolerated on the unit and that severe consequences will be imposed if the client refuses to comply with the established rules.
4. Charming behavior is a common form of manipulation associated with this disorder. Do not be taken in. Instead, explain to the client that such behavior will not be accepted, and if it continues, consequences will be imposed.
5. Encouraging the client to talk about his past misdeeds might help him understand how he would feel if someone treated him in the manner that he has treated others.
TEST-TAKING TIP: Review the interventions that would be most appropriate for a client diagnosed with antisocial personality disorder.
Content Area: Safe and Effective Care Environment: Management of Care;
Integrated Process: Nursing Process: Implementation;
Client Need: Safe and Effective Care Environment: Management of Care;
Cognitive Level: Application;
Concept: Nursing

14. **ANSWER: 4**
Rationale:
1. OCD symptoms do change in severity over time, whereas OCPD reflects an overly rigid personality style that remains unchanged over a lifetime. This accurate student statement indicates that learning has occurred.
2. OCPD is not associated with the obsessions and compulsions that are prominent in OCD. This accurate student statement indicates that learning has occurred.
3. Clients with OCD want to alleviate their symptoms, whereas clients with OCPD see nothing wrong with their behavior and feel that "other people" are the problem. This

accurate student statement indicates that learning has occurred.
4. OCD and OCPD are different disorders. OCD does not become OCPD, regardless of anxiety levels. In both OCD and OCPD, clients carry out repetitive behaviors, but the underlying motive is very different. Clients with OCD might be compelled to repeatedly write out lists with their motivation being prevention of a catastrophe thereby avoiding excessive anxiety. Clients with OCPD might also write out lists, but their motivation would be to increase efficiency and productivity. This student statement indicates that further instruction is needed.
TEST-TAKING TIP: Review and understand the differences between obsessive-compulsive disorder and obsessive-compulsive personality disorder.
Content Area: Psychosocial Integrity;
Integrated Process: Nursing Process: Evaluation;
Client Need: Psychosocial Integrity;
Cognitive Level: Analysis;
Concept: Nursing Roles

15. **ANSWER: 3**
Rationale:
1. A "helicopter parent" might constantly shadow the child, always playing with and directing his or her behavior by hovering overhead. Hiring drones or an actual helicopter is applying a literal and incorrect meaning to the term "helicopter parent."
2. The behaviors of a "helicopter parent" are generally the product of love and concern. It is not necessarily a sign of parents who are depressed, unhappy, or nastily controlling. It can be a product of good intentions gone awry, the play of culture on natural parental fears.
3. A helicopter parent (also called a "cosseting parent" or simply a "cosseter") is a parent who pays extremely close attention to his or her child's experiences and problems, particularly at educational institutions. Helicopter parents are so named because, like helicopters, they hover overhead.
4. A helicopter parent who, as a child, felt unloved, neglected, or ignored, not overprotected and overcontrolled, often overcompensates with his or her own child. Excessive attention and monitoring are attempts to remedy a deficiency the parents felt in their own upbringing.
TEST-TAKING TIP: Review the key words at the beginning of the chapter to understand the definition of "helicopter parenting."
Content Area: Psychosocial Integrity;
Integrated Process: Nursing Process: Implementation;
Client Need: Psychosocial Integrity;
Cognitive Level: Application;
Concept: Nursing Roles

16. **ANSWER: projection**
Rationale: Individuals using the primary ego defense mechanism of projection are attributing feelings or impulses unacceptable to themselves to another person. This is the primary ego defense mechanism used by individuals diagnosed with antisocial personality disorder.

TEST-TAKING TIP: Review the ego defense mechanisms used by clients diagnosed with various personality disorders. A review of Table 1.1 in Chapter 1 will refresh your memory regarding the ego defense mechanisms.
Content Area: Psychosocial Integrity;
Integrated Process: Nursing Process: Assessment;
Client Need: Psychosocial Integrity;
Cognitive Level: Knowledge;
Concept: Self

17. **ANSWERS: 1, 4**
Rationale:
1. A client diagnosed with borderline personality disorder becomes a master in manipulation. Virtually any behavior is an acceptable means of achieving the desired result; therefore, when faced with a confrontational situation, the nurse would need to employ an intervention that might minimize or prevent this client's possible manipulative behavior.
2. A client diagnosed with avoidant personality disorder is extremely sensitive to rejection and because of this would choose withdrawal rather than manipulation in a confrontational situation.
3. A client diagnosed with schizoid personality disorder has a profound defect in the ability to form personal relationships. In a confrontational situation, this individual would choose social withdrawal rather than manipulative behavior.
4. A client diagnosed with antisocial personality disorder exploits and manipulates others for personal gain; therefore, when faced with a confrontational situation, the nurse would need to employ an intervention to minimize or prevent this client's possible manipulative behavior.
5. A client diagnosed with obsessive-compulsive personality disorder is meticulous and works diligently and patiently at tasks that require accuracy and discipline. In a confrontational situation, this individual would probably revert to rules and regulations rather than resort to manipulation.
TEST-TAKING TIP: Review each of the 10 personality disorders to determine which disorder would most likely employ manipulation.
Content Area: Safe and Effective Care Environment: Management of Care;
Integrated Process: Nursing Process: Implementation;
Client Need: Safe and Effective Care Environment: Management of Care;
Cognitive Level: Application;
Concept: Nursing

18. **ANSWERS: 2, 3, 4**
Rationale:
1. Being suspicious and mistrustful of others is a behavioral characteristic of a paranoid, not a narcissistic, personality disorder.
2. Appearing to lack humility, being overly self-centered, and exploiting others to fulfill their own desires is a behavioral characteristic of individuals diagnosed with narcissistic personality disorder.

3. Feeling entitled to special rights and privileges and viewing themselves as "superior" beings are behavioral characteristics of individuals diagnosed with narcissistic personality disorder.
4. Feeling justified in possessing whatever they seek because they believe they have the inalienable right to receive special consideration is a behavioral characteristic of individuals diagnosed with narcissistic personality disorder.
5. Being indirectly and directly self-destructive is a behavioral characteristic of a borderline, not a narcissistic, personality disorder.
TEST-TAKING TIP: Review the definition and clinical picture for narcissistic personality in order to recognize characteristic behaviors of this disorder.
Content Area: Safe and Effective Care Environment: Management of Care;
Integrated Process: Nursing Process: Assessment;
Client Need: Safe and Effective Care Environment: Management of Care;
Cognitive Level: Application;
Concept: Self

19. **ANSWER: 4**
1. It would not be characteristic of a client diagnosed with dependent personality disorder to seek attention by acts of self-harm. This behavior is more characteristic of a client diagnosed with borderline personality disorder. This nursing diagnosis would not be appropriate to assign to this client.
2. It would not be characteristic of a client diagnosed with dependent personality disorder to exaggerate his or her sense of self. These clients lack self-confidence, which is often apparent in their posture, voice, and mannerisms. This nursing diagnosis would not be appropriate to assign to this client.
3. Clients with dependent personality disorder will do almost anything to earn the acceptance of others and are easily hurt by criticism and disapproval. These traits can lead to problems establishing relationships, but the root of the problem is not typically communication. This nursing diagnosis would not be appropriate to assign to this client.
4. Clients with dependent personality disorder assume a passive and submissive role in relationships. When relationships end, they may hastily and indiscriminately establish another relationship to gain nurturance and guidance. This may lead to inappropriate relationships with others who may take advantage of the client. This nursing diagnosis would be appropriate to assign to this client.
TEST-TAKING TIP: Review the typical problems experienced by clients diagnosed with dependent personality disorder to choose an appropriate nursing diagnosis.
Content Area: Safe and Effective Care Environment: Management of Care;
Integrated Process: Nursing Process: Diagnosis;
Client Need: Safe and Effective Care Environment: Management of Care;
Cognitive Level: Analysis;
Concept: Critical Thinking

20. ANSWER: The correct order is 3, 1, 4, 2
Rationale: Clients diagnosed with antisocial personality disorder disregard the rights of others and ignore rules and regulations. First, all rules and regulations must be reviewed to avoid misunderstanding and potential manipulation. Second, the consequences of rule infractions must be explained. (It is best to provide in writing rules and the consequences of infractions.) Third, it is necessary to immediately set limits on maladaptive behaviors that defy rules to connect the client's action with the infraction. Fourth, it is important to consistently implement the consequences of any rule infraction. Inconsistencies in implementation will open the situation to manipulation.
TEST-TAKING TIP: Understanding that clients diagnosed with antisocial personality disorder ignore the rights of others and discount rules and regulations will lead to the correct ordering of these nursing interventions.
Content Area: Safe and Effective Care Environment: Management of Care;
Integrated Process: Nursing Process: Implementation;
Client Need: Safe and Effective Care Environment: Management of Care;
Cognitive Level: Analysis
Concept: Nursing

21. ANSWERS: 2, 3, 5
Rationale:
1. Colorful, dramatic, and extroverted behavior is a characteristic associated with histrionic, not obsessive-compulsive personality disorder.

2. Efficient, organized, and rigid behavior is associated with obsessive-compulsive personality disorder. These individuals are meticulous and work diligently at tasks that require accuracy and discipline.
3. Being contemptuous of frivolous and impulsive behavior in others is associated with obsessive-compulsive personality disorder. These individuals see themselves as conscientious, loyal, dependable, and responsible. They have little regard for others that do not meet these standards of conduct.
4. Extreme sensitivity to rejection is associated with avoidant, not obsessive-compulsive personality disorder.
5. Being unbending about rules and procedures is a behavior associated with obsessive-compulsive personality disorder. These individuals are especially concerned with matters of organization and tend to be rigid and unbending.
TEST-TAKING TIP: Review the behavioral characteristics of clients diagnosed with obsessive-compulsive personality disorder.
Content Area: Safe and Effective Care Environment: Management of Care;
Integrated Process: Nursing Process: Assessment;
Client Need: Safe and Effective Care Environment: Management of Care;
Cognitive Level: Application;
Concept: Assessment

CASE STUDY: Putting it All Together

After being treated for razor cuts to arms and legs, Emily, age 40, has been admitted to a psychiatric inpatient unit. During the first week of hospitalization, Emily emotionally attaches herself to several staff members. By the end of the week, Emily states that she hates several of the same staff she once adored and attempts to pit one against the other. When Scott, a psychiatric nurse practitioner (PNP), confronts Emily about trying to sneak alcohol onto the unit, Emily seductively says, "Honey, come to my room tonight, and I'll make you forget this incident." History reveals a poor relationship with her mother, and no relationship with her father, who deserted the family when she was a toddler. Angrily, Emily states, "I think she drove him away. My mother only cares about herself." Emily, although well educated, demonstrates poor work ethics. Over the past 10 years, she has been terminated five times for tardiness, absenteeism, and alcohol and drug use during working hours. Emily cannot maintain any friendships on the unit because she's easily bored and becomes angry when not the center of attention. Emily admits to feelings of depression and anxiety and tearfully states that cutting and alcohol somehow make her feel less hollow. She expresses an angry affect and eye contact that vacillates between absent and piercing,

depending on her moment-to-moment mood. Emily's PNP, Scott, begins exploring predisposing factors that may have contributed to her dysfunctional behaviors. He will also explore various behavioral techniques that might help Emily cope more effectively.

1. The PNP would document which tentative medical diagnosis for Emily?
2. What predisposing factors may have contributed to Emily's diagnosis?
3. What subjective symptoms lead the PNP to this diagnosis?
4. What objective symptoms lead the PNP to this diagnosis?
5. What therapy might the PNP use to assist Emily?
6. What NANDA nursing diagnosis would be appropriate for Emily?
7. What short-term outcome would be appropriate for Emily?
8. What long-term outcome would be appropriate for Emily?
9. List the nursing interventions (actions) that will assist Emily to meet these outcomes.
10. List the questions that would determine whether the nursing actions are successful.

Chapter 14

Eating Disorders

KEY TERMS

Amenorrhea—The absence of menstruation; women who have missed at least three menstrual periods in a row have amenorrhea, as do girls who haven't begun menstruation by age 15

Anorexia—Prolonged loss of appetite

Anorexia nervosa—An eating disorder characterized by an abnormally low body weight, intense fear of gaining weight, and a distorted perception of body weight; individuals with this disorder place a high value on controlling their weight and shape, using extreme efforts that tend to significantly interfere with activities of daily living

Bingeing—A period of excessive or uncontrolled indulgence, especially in food or drink

Binge-eating disorder (BED)—This disorder is characterized by a loss of control over eating behaviors; the binge eater compulsively consumes unnaturally large amounts of food in a short time period, but, unlike a bulimic, does not regularly engage in any inappropriate weight-reducing behaviors (e.g., excessive exercise, vomiting, taking laxatives) after the binge episodes

Body image—A subjective concept of one's physical appearance based on the personal perceptions of self and the reactions of others

Bulimia—Excessive, insatiable appetite

Bulimia nervosa—An eating disorder characterized by consuming a large amount of food in a short amount of time (binging), followed by an attempt to rid oneself of the food consumed (purging), typically by vomiting, taking a laxative, diuretic, or stimulant, and/or engaging in excessive exercise, because of an extensive concern for body weight

Calorie—A unit of heat measurement used in nutrition to measure the energy value of foods; a calorie is the amount of heat energy needed to raise the temperature of 1 gram of water 1°C

Emaciation—Extreme weight loss and thinness due to a loss of subcutaneous fat and muscle throughout the body; one who is emaciated could be described as "wasting away" or being "gaunt"; emaciation is caused by severe malnourishment and starvation

Lanugo—A symptom of deep starvation; soft, downy, fine white/light hair that grows mainly on the arms, chest, back, and face of individuals with eating disorders; the body grows lanugo as a means of insulating itself to maintain body temperature as fat stores are depleted

Obesity—A medical condition in which excess body fat has accumulated to the extent that it may have a negative effect on health; in Western countries, people are considered obese when their body mass index (BMI), a measurement obtained by dividing a person's weight in kilograms by the square of the person's height in meters, exceeds 30 kg/m², with the range 25 to 30 kg/m² defined as overweight

Purging—Undergoing or causing an emptying of the bowels or vomiting or forcing oneself to vomit; a symptom of an eating disorder

Nutrition and life sustenance are not the only reasons most people eat food. The hypothalamus contains the appetite regulation center within the brain. This complex neural system regulates the body's ability to recognize when it is hungry and when it is satisfied. But society and culture have a great deal of influence on the social activity of eating and on how people think they should look.

In the late 1960s, the image of super-thin models was propagated by the media, and it remains the ideal today. Eating disorders can be associated with undereating and overeating. Because psychological or behavioral factors play a role in the presentation of these disorders, they fall well within the realm of psychiatry and psychiatric nursing.

I. Epidemiological Factors

A. Anorexia nervosa
1. Increased prevalence in both United States and Western Europe.
2. One percent prevalence rate among young women in the United States.
3. Occurs predominantly in females 12 to 30 years of age.
4. Less than 10% of cases are male.

B. Bulimia nervosa
1. More prevalent than anorexia nervosa.
2. Up to 4% of young women.
3. Onset occurs in late adolescence or early adulthood.

DID YOU KNOW?
Bulimia nervosa occurs primarily in societies that place emphasis on thinness as the model of attractiveness for women and where an abundance of food is available.

C. Obesity
1. A body mass index (BMI; weight/height^2) of 30 or greater.
2. In the United States, among adults 20 years of age or older, 68.5% are overweight and 35% of these are in obese range.
3. Approximately 6.3% of the U.S. adult population may be categorized as *extremely* obese (a BMI greater than 40).
4. Higher rates in African Americans and Latin Americans than whites.
5. Greater rates among lower socioeconomic groups.
6. Greater rates associated with lower levels of education.

II. Predisposing Factors to Development of Anorexia Nervosa and Bulimia Nervosa

A. Biological influences
1. Genetics.
   a. Hereditary predisposition based on family histories.
   b. Approximately 56% of the risk for developing anorexia nervosa is based on genetic factors.
   c. Possible linkage sites for anorexia nervosa on chromosomes 1, 2, and 13.
   d. Anorexia nervosa is more common among sisters and mothers of those with the disorder than among the general population.

DID YOU KNOW?
Higher than expected frequencies of mood and substance use disorders occur among first-degree biological relatives of individuals with eating disorders.

2. Neuroendocrine abnormalities.
   a. Possible primary hypothalamic dysfunction in anorexia nervosa.
   b. Theory supported by:
      i. Elevated cerebrospinal fluid cortisol levels
      ii. Possible impairment of dopaminergic regulation in individuals with anorexia nervosa
      iii. Many people with anorexia nervosa experience amenorrhea (hypothalamic dysfunction) *before* the onset of starvation and significant weight loss
3. Neurochemical influences.
   a. Bulimia nervosa may be associated with the neurotransmitters serotonin and norepinephrine.
   b. Supported by the positive response to selective serotonin reuptake inhibitor (SSRI) therapy.
   c. High levels of endogenous opioids found in spinal fluid of clients with anorexia nervosa (may contribute to denial of hunger).

B. Psychodynamic influences
1. Very early and profound disturbances in mother-infant interactions.
2. Delayed ego development in the child and an unfulfilled sense of separation-individuation.
3. Mother responds to child's physical and emotional needs with food.
4. When the vulnerable ego is threatened, feelings of lack of control over one's body (self) emerge.
5. Behaviors associated with food and eating provide needed control.
6. Psychodynamic influences results in disturbance in body identity and distortion in body image.
7. Influences related to the family include:
   a. Conflict avoidance.
      i. Psychosomatic symptoms (anorexia nervosa) reinforced in an effort to avoid spousal conflict
      ii. Parents deny marital conflict by defining the sick child as the family problem
      iii. Unhealthy involvement (enmeshment) occurs between family members
      iv. Family strives at all costs to maintain "appearances"
      v. Parents retain child in dependent position
      vi. Conflict avoidance may be a strong factor in family dynamics
   b. Elements of power and control.
      i. Predominant in family processes
      ii. Families often consist of a passive father, a domineering mother, and an overly dependent child
      iii. A high value placed on perfectionism
      iv. Parental criticism promotes an increase in obsessive and perfectionistic behavior

---

MAKING THE CONNECTION

A child with an eating disorder who seeks love and approval eventually feels helpless and ambivalent toward the parents. Rebellion in adolescence leads to distorted eating patterns as a means of gaining and remaining in control. Symptoms are often triggered by a stressor related to loss of control.

III. Predisposing Factors to Development of **Obesity**

A. Biological influences
  1. Genetics.
     a. Approximately 80% of offspring of two obese parents are obese.
     b. Twins and adoptees reared by normal and overweight parents support a genetic link to obesity.
     c. Studies show that people differ in their perceptions of hunger and satiety on a genetic basis.
  2. Physiological factors.
     a. Lesions in the appetite and satiety centers in the hypothalamus may contribute to overeating and lead to obesity.
     b. Hypothyroidism interferes with basal metabolism and may lead to weight gain.
     c. Weight gain occurs in response to the decreased insulin production of diabetes mellitus (DM).
     d. Weight gain occurs due to increased cortisone production of Cushing's disease.
     e. Low levels of the neurotransmitter serotonin may play a role in compulsive eating.

DID YOU KNOW?

Weight gain occurs when caloric intake exceeds caloric output related to basal metabolism and physical activity. Many overweight individuals lead sedentary lifestyles, making it difficult to burn off calories.

B. Psychosocial influences
  1. Many obese individuals have unresolved dependency needs.
  2. May be fixed in the oral stage of psychosexual development.
  3. The symptoms of obesity are viewed as attempts to regain "lost" or frustrated nurturance and caring.

🛑 Depression and **binge-eating disorder (BED)** are strongly linked. Half of individuals with BED have a history of depression. Food provides comfort for a despondent mood, but feelings of disgust and despair that occur after episodes of bingeing may lead to further depression.

IV. Nursing Process: Assessment for Anorexia Nervosa

A. Characterized by morbid fear of obesity
B. Symptoms include:
  1. Gross distortion of body image.
  2. Perception of being "fat" when individual is obviously underweight or **emaciated.**
  3. Excessive weight loss accomplished by reduction in food intake and often extensive exercising.
  4. Preoccupation, obsession with food.
     a. Hoard or conceal food.
     b. Talk about food and recipes at great length.
  5. Refusal to eat.
     a. Suffer from pangs of hunger.
     b. Hunger ceases only with food intake less than 200 **calories** per day.
  6. Self-induced vomiting and the abuse of laxatives or diuretics may be present.
  7. Compulsive behaviors (hand washing) may be present.
  8. Hypothermia.
  9. Bradycardia.
  10. Hypotension.
  11. Edema.
  12. **Lanugo.**
  13. A variety of metabolic changes.
  14. **Amenorrhea** usually follows weight loss but can occur early before severe weight loss.
  15. Depression and anxiety often accompany the disorder.
C. Onset usually early to late adolescence
D. Psychosexual development is often delayed

V. Nursing Process: Assessment for Bulimia Nervosa

A. Episodic, uncontrolled, compulsive, rapid ingestion of large quantities of food over a short period of time (**bingeing**), followed by inappropriate compensatory behaviors to rid the body of the excess calories (**purging**)
B. Bingeing
  1. High-calorie, sweet, smooth-textured food that is eaten rapidly, sometimes without being chewed.
  2. Binges often occur in secret and usually are only terminated by abdominal discomfort, sleep, social interruption, or self-induced vomiting.
  3. Binges may bring pleasure during the episode but are followed by self-degradation and depressed mood.

C. Purging (self-induced vomiting or the misuse of laxatives, diuretics, or enemas)
  1. Rids the body of excess calories.
  2. May lead to problems with dehydration and electrolyte imbalance.
  3. Fasting or excessive exercise are other ways to rid body of calories.
  4. Gastric acid in the vomitus contributes to the erosion of tooth enamel.
  5. Weight fluctuations common but most within a normal weight range; some slightly underweight, some slightly overweight.
  6. In rare instances, the individual may experience tears in the gastric or esophageal mucosa.
D. Persistent overconcern with personal appearance and perception of others

🛑 Clients diagnosed with bulimia nervosa may be subject to mood disorders, anxiety disorders, or substance abuse, most frequently involving central nervous system stimulants or alcohol.

VI. Nursing Process: Assessment for Obesity

A. Obesity classified under "Psychological Factors Affecting Medical Condition"
B. Binge-eating disorder (BED) classified as an eating disorder

C. Individual binges on large amounts of food (as in bulimia nervosa) but does *not* engage in behaviors to rid the body of the excess calories
D. The following formula is used to determine extent of obesity in an individual:
$$\text{Metric body mass index} = \frac{\text{Weight (kg)}}{\text{Height (m)}^2} = \underline{\hspace{1cm}}$$
$$\text{US body mass index} = \frac{\text{Weight (lbs)} \times 703}{\text{Height (in)}^2} = \underline{\hspace{1cm}}$$
E. Table 14.1 provides a chart with BMI calculations
F. The BMI range for normal weight is 20 to 24.9
G. Overweight is defined as a BMI of 25.0 to 29.9
H. Obesity is defined as a BMI of 30.0 or greater
I. These definitions markedly increased the number of Americans considered overweight

DID YOU KNOW?
The average American woman has a BMI of 26, and fashion models typically have BMIs of 18.

J. Anorexia nervosa is characterized by a BMI of 17.5 or lower
K. Complications of obesity
  1. Hypertension.
  2. Hyperlipidemia.
  3. Elevated triglyceride and cholesterol levels.
  4. Risk for hyperglycemia.
  5. Risk for developing diabetes mellitus.

Table 14.1 Body Mass Index (BMI) Chart

BMI	19	20	21	22	23	24	25	26	27	28	29	30	31	32	33	34	35	36	37	38	39	40
Height (inches)										Body Weight (pounds)												
58	91	96	100	105	110	115	119	124	129	134	138	143	148	153	158	162	167	172	177	181	186	191
59	94	99	104	109	114	119	124	128	133	138	143	148	153	158	163	168	173	178	183	188	193	198
60	97	102	107	112	118	123	128	133	138	143	148	153	158	163	168	174	179	184	189	194	199	204
61	100	106	111	116	122	127	132	137	143	148	153	158	164	169	174	180	185	190	195	201	206	211
62	104	109	115	120	126	131	136	142	147	153	158	164	169	175	180	186	191	196	202	207	213	218
63	107	113	118	124	130	135	141	146	152	158	163	169	175	180	186	191	197	203	208	214	220	225
64	110	116	122	128	134	140	145	151	157	163	169	174	180	186	192	197	204	209	215	221	227	232
65	114	120	126	132	138	144	150	156	162	168	174	180	186	192	198	204	210	216	222	228	234	240
66	118	124	130	136	142	148	155	161	167	173	179	186	192	198	204	210	216	223	229	235	241	247
67	121	127	134	140	146	153	159	166	172	178	185	191	198	204	211	217	223	230	236	242	249	255
68	125	131	138	144	151	158	164	171	177	184	190	197	203	210	216	223	230	236	243	249	256	262
69	128	135	142	149	155	162	169	176	182	189	196	203	209	216	223	230	236	243	250	257	263	270
70	132	139	146	153	160	167	174	181	188	195	202	209	216	222	229	236	243	250	257	264	271	278
71	136	143	150	157	165	172	179	186	193	200	208	215	222	229	236	243	250	257	265	272	279	286
72	140	147	154	162	169	177	184	191	199	206	213	221	228	235	242	250	258	265	272	279	287	294
73	144	151	159	166	174	182	189	197	204	212	219	227	235	242	250	257	265	272	280	288	295	302
74	148	155	163	171	179	186	194	202	210	218	225	233	241	249	256	264	272	280	287	295	303	311
75	152	160	168	176	184	192	200	208	216	224	232	240	248	256	264	272	279	287	295	303	311	319
76	156	164	172	180	189	197	205	213	221	230	238	246	254	263	271	279	287	295	304	312	320	328

Source: National Heart, Lung, and Blood Institute of the National Institutes of Health (2012).

6. Osteoarthritis due to trauma to weight-bearing joints.
7. Angina or respiratory insufficiency due to increased workload on the heart and lungs.

VII. Nursing Process: Nursing Diagnosis (Analysis)

Table 14.2 presents a list of client behaviors and the NANDA nursing diagnoses that correspond to those behaviors, which may be used in planning care for clients with eating disorders

VIII. Nursing Process: Planning

The following outcomes may be developed to guide the care of a client diagnosed with eating disorders. **The client will:**
A. Achieve and maintain at least 80% of expected body weight (anorexia nervosa)
B. Maintain vital signs, blood pressure, and laboratory serum studies within normal limits
C. Verbalize importance of adequate nutrition
D. Verbalize knowledge regarding consequences of fluid loss caused by self-induced vomiting (or laxative/diuretic abuse) and importance of adequate fluid intake
E. Verbalize events that precipitate anxiety and demonstrate techniques for its reduction
F. Verbalize ways in which he or she may gain more control of the environment and thereby reduce feelings of powerlessness
G. Express interest in welfare of others and less preoccupation with own appearance
H. Verbalize that image of body as "fat" was misperception and demonstrate ability to take control of own life without resorting to maladaptive eating behaviors (anorexia nervosa)
I. Establish a healthy pattern of eating for weight control and weight loss toward a desired goal (obesity)
J. Verbalize plans for future maintenance of weight control (obesity)

IX. Nursing Process: Implementation

DID YOU KNOW?

In most instances, individuals with eating disorders are treated on an outpatient basis, but in some cases, hospitalization becomes necessary. Reasons for hospitalization include malnutrition (less than 85% of expected body weight), dehydration, severe electrolyte imbalance, cardiac arrhythmia, severe bradycardia, hypothermia, hypotension, suicidal ideation, or uncooperative outpatient treatment.

Table 14.2 Assigning Nursing Diagnoses to Behaviors Commonly Associated With Eating Disorders

Behaviors	Nursing Diagnosis
Refusal to eat; abuse of laxatives, diuretics, and/or diet pills; loss of 15% of expected body weight; pale conjunctiva and mucous membranes; poor muscle tone; amenorrhea; poor skin turgor; electrolyte imbalances; hypothermia; bradycardia; hypotension; cardiac irregularities; edema	Imbalanced nutrition: less than body requirements
Decreased fluid intake; abnormal fluid loss caused by self-induced vomiting; excessive use of laxatives, enemas, or diuretics; electrolyte imbalance; decreased urine output; increased urine concentration; elevated hematocrit; decreased blood pressure; increased pulse rate; dry skin; decreased skin turgor; weakness	Deficient fluid volume
Minimizes symptoms; unable to admit effect of disease on life pattern; does not perceive personal relevance of symptoms; does not perceive personal relevance of danger	Ineffective denial
Compulsive eating; excessive intake in relation to metabolic needs; sedentary lifestyle; weight 20% over ideal for height and frame; BMI of 30 or more	Imbalanced nutrition: more than body requirements
Distorted body image; views self as fat, even in the presence of normal body weight or severe emaciation; denies that problem with low body weight exists; difficulty accepting positive reinforcement; self-destructive behavior (self-induced vomiting, abuse of laxatives or diuretics, refusal to eat); preoccupation with appearance and how others perceive it *(anorexia nervosa, bulimia nervosa)* Verbalization of negative feelings about the way he or she looks and the desire to lose weight *(obesity)* Lack of eye contact; depressed mood *(all)*	Disturbed body image/low self-esteem
Increased tension; increased helplessness; overexcited; apprehensive; fearful; restlessness; poor eye contact; increased difficulty taking oral nourishment; inability to learn	Anxiety (moderate to severe)

A. Interventions for clients with imbalanced nutrition: less than body requirements
   1. Monitor ordered nasogastric tube feeding per hospital protocol.
   2. Consult with dietitian to determine appropriate number of calories required to provide adequate nutrition and realistic weight gain.
   3. Discuss contract related to privileges and restrictions based on compliance with treatment and direct weight gain.
   4. Do not focus on food and eating during client interactions.
   5. Weigh client daily.
      a. Immediately on rising and after first voiding.
      b. Use same scale.
   6. Keep strict record of intake and output.
   7. Assess skin turgor and integrity regularly.
   8. Assess moistness and color of oral mucous membranes.
   9. Stay with client during established time for meals (usually 30 min) and for at least 1 hour after meals.

DID YOU KNOW?

Lengthy mealtimes put excessive emphasis on food and eating and provide clients with attention, which reinforces their focus on food. It is important to stay with clients during meals because the hour after meals may be used to discard food stashed from tray or to engage in self-induced vomiting.

   10. If weight loss occurs, enforce restrictions.
   11. Implement interventions and communicate with family in a matter-of-fact, nonpunitive way.
   12. Encourage client to explore and identify true feelings and fears.

B. Interventions for clients with ineffective denial
   1. Establish a trusting relationship.
      a. Be honest, accepting, and available.
      b. Keep all promises.
      c. Convey unconditional positive regard.
   2. Acknowledge client's anger at feelings of loss of control brought about by the established eating regimen.
   3. Avoid arguing or bargaining.

MAKING THE CONNECTION

Restrictions and limits must be established and carried out consistently to avoid power struggles, encourage client compliance with therapy, and ensure client safety.

MAKING THE CONNECTION

The person who is denying a problem and who also has a weak ego will use manipulation to achieve control. Consistency and firmness from staff will decrease the use of these behaviors.

   4. State matter-of-factly which behaviors are unacceptable and how privileges will be restricted for noncompliance.
   5. Encourage client to verbalize feelings regarding the following topics and emphasize how these feelings are related to maladaptive eating behaviors:
      a. Role within the family.
      b. Issues related to dependence/independence.
      c. Intense need for achievement.
      d. Issues related to sexuality.
   6. Discuss ways client can gain control over these problematic areas of life without resorting to maladaptive eating behaviors.

C. Interventions for clients with disturbed body image/low self-esteem
   1. Help client to develop a realistic perception of body image and relationship with food.
   2. Compare specific measurement of the client's body with the client's perceived calculations.
   3. Promote feelings of control within the environment through participation and independent decision-making.
   4. Provide positive feedback to help client learn to accept weaknesses and strengths.
   5. Explore need for perfection and help client realize unrealistic nature of the need.

D. Interventions for clients with imbalanced nutrition: more than body requirements
   1. Encourage client to keep a diary of food intake.
   2. Discuss feelings and emotions associated with eating.
   3. Assess client's usual eating patterns.
   4. With client input, formulate nutritious eating plan that emphasizes low-fat intake.
   5. Identify realistic, weekly weight loss goals.

MAKING THE CONNECTION

There may be a large discrepancy between actual body size and the client's perception of his or her body size. Clients need to recognize that the misperception of body image is unhealthy and that maintaining control through maladaptive eating behaviors is dangerous—even life threatening.

A food diary provides the opportunity for a client to gain a realistic picture of the amount of food ingested and provides a database on which to tailor the dietary program. This helps to identify when a client is eating to satisfy an emotional need rather than a physiological one.

DID YOU KNOW?

Reasonable weight loss (1–2 pounds per week) results in more lasting effects. Excessive, rapid weight loss may result in fatigue and irritability and ultimately lead to failure in meeting goals for weight loss. Motivation is more easily sustained by meeting "stair-step" goals.

6. Plan a progressive exercise program tailored to individual goals and choices.
7. Discuss the probability of reaching plateaus.

DID YOU KNOW?

A weight-loss *plateau* is a period of time when weight remains stable and little weight loss occurs, sometimes for extended periods. Clients should know a plateau is likely to happen as changes in metabolism occur. Plateaus cause frustration, and a client may need additional support during these times to remain on the weight-loss program.

8. Provide instruction about prescribed medications to assist with weight loss.

E. Interventions for clients with disturbed body image/low self-esteem related to obesity
1. Assess client's feelings and attitudes about being obese.
2. Ensure client privacy during self-care activities.
3. Encourage use of previously successful coping patterns related to food.
4. Explore patterns of coping in family of origin and explore how these may affect current situation.
5. Determine client's motivation for weight loss and encourage client to set goals.
6. Help client identify positive self-attributes.
7. Focus on strengths and past accomplishments unrelated to physical appearance.
8. Refer client to support or therapy group.

MAKING THE CONNECTION

The obese individual may harbor repressed feelings of hostility, which may be expressed inward on the self. Because of a poor self-concept, the person often has difficulty with relationships. When the motivation is to lose weight for someone else, successful weight loss is less likely to occur.

X. Nursing Process: Evaluation

Evaluation of the nursing actions for the client diagnosed with eating disorders may be facilitated by gathering information using the following types of questions:
A. For the client with anorexia nervosa or bulimia nervosa:
1. Has the client steadily gained 2 to 3 pounds per week to at least 80% of body weight for age and size?
2. Is the client free of signs and symptoms of malnutrition and dehydration?
3. Does the client consume adequate calories as determined by the dietitian?
4. Have there been any attempts to hide food from the tray to discard later?
5. Have there been any attempts to self-induce vomiting?
6. Has the client admitted that a problem exists and that eating behaviors are maladaptive?
7. Have behaviors aimed at manipulating the environment been discontinued?
8. Is the client willing to discuss the real issues concerning family roles, sexuality, dependence/independence, and the need for achievement?
9. Does the client understand how he or she has used maladaptive eating behaviors in an effort to achieve a feeling of some control over life events?
10. Has the client acknowledged that perception of body image as "fat" is incorrect?
B. For the client with obesity:
1. Has the client shown a steady weight loss since starting the new eating plan?
2. Does the client verbalize a plan to help stay on the new eating plan?
3. Does the client verbalize positive self-attributes not associated with body size or appearance?
C. For the client with anorexia nervosa, bulimia nervosa, or obesity:
1. Has the client been able to develop a more realistic perception of body image?
2. Has the client acknowledged that past self-expectations may have been unrealistic?
3. Does client accept self as less than perfect?
4. Has the client developed adaptive coping strategies to deal with stress without resorting to maladaptive eating behaviors?

XI. Treatment Modalities

The immediate aim of treatment in anorexia nervosa is to restore the client's nutritional status. Complications of emaciation, dehydration, and electrolyte imbalance can lead to death. Once the physical condition is no longer life-threatening, other treatment modalities may be initiated.

A. Behavior modification
1. Goal: to change maladaptive eating behaviors.
2. Must assure that program does not "control" client.
3. Client must perceive that he or she is in control of the treatment.
   a. Contract for privileges based on weight gain.
   b. Client has input into the care plan.
   c. Client can clearly see treatment choices.
   d. Client has ultimate control over eating, over the amount of exercise pursued, and even over whether or not to induce vomiting.
   e. Client and staff set:
      i. Goals of therapy
      ii. Responsibilities for goal achievement
      iii. System of rewards and privileges that can be earned
   f. Client's choices:
      i. Whether to abide by the contract
      ii. Whether to gain weight
      iii. Whether to earn the desired privilege

DID YOU KNOW?
Behavior modification gives a great deal of autonomy to the client. However, these techniques are helpful for weight restoration only. Concomitant individual and/or family psychotherapy are required to prevent or reduce further morbidity.

B. Cognitive therapy
1. Helps client confront irrational thinking.
2. Assists in modifying distorted and maladaptive cognitions about body image and eating behaviors.

C. Cognitive-behavioral therapy (CBT)
1. Incorporates cognitive therapy concepts along with behavior modification techniques.
2. Helpful in treating clients with BED.
3. Beneficial in reducing bingeing.
4. Not consistently helpful in promoting weight loss.

D. Individual psychotherapy
1. Helpful to deal with contributing underlying psychological problems.
2. Client explores unresolved conflicts.
3. Helps client recognize maladaptive eating behaviors as defense mechanisms used to ease emotional pain.
4. Goal to resolve personal issues and establish more adaptive coping strategies.

E. Family therapy

(i) Families are profoundly affected by members diagnosed with eating disorders. The distress generated can cause families to either unite or dissolve. Intervention is critical to prevent family unit breakdown.

1. Eating disorders may be considered *family* disorders.

2. Resolution depends on improvement of family dynamics.
3. Educates family members about the disorder's manifestations, possible etiology, and prescribed treatment.
4. Supports family as they deal with feelings of guilt related to perception that they may have contributed to the onset of the disorder.
5. Supports family to deal with the social stigma related to family member with emotional problems.
6. Referrals to local support groups.

F. Psychopharmacology
1. No medications are specifically indicated for eating disorders other than lisdexamfetamine dimesylate (Vyvanse), which has been approved by the Food and Drug Administration for the treatment of BED.
2. Various medication trials and off-label use research have yielded mixed results based on individual responses.
3. Medications can be prescribed for associated symptoms such as anxiety and depression.
   a. Fluoxetine (Prozac) and clomipramine (Anafranil) used for anorexia nervosa with depression or obsessive-compulsive symptoms.
   b. Cyproheptadine (Periactin) unlabeled use as an appetite stimulant.
   c. Chlorpromazine (Thorazine) prescribed for selected clients diagnosed with anorexia nervosa.
   d. Olanzapine (Zyprexa) is being studied for the treatment of anorexia nervosa.
   e. Fluoxetine (Prozac) useful in the treatment of bulimia nervosa.

MAKING THE CONNECTION

When dysfunctional family dynamics are related to conflict avoidance, the family may be noncompliant with therapy, as they attempt to maintain equilibrium by keeping a member in the sick role. When this occurs, it is essential to focus on the functional operations within the family and to help them manage conflict and create change.

MAKING THE CONNECTION

A dosage of 60 mg/day (triple the usual antidepressant dosage) of fluoxetine (Prozac) was found to be most effective with clients diagnosed with bulimia nervosa. It is possible that fluoxetine, a selective serotonin reuptake inhibitor (SSRI), may decrease the craving for carbohydrates, thereby decreasing the incidence of binge eating, which is often associated with consumption of large amounts of carbohydrates.

G. Other antidepressants, such as imipramine (Tofranil), desipramine (Norpramin), amitriptyline (Elavil), nortriptyline (Aventyl), and phenelzine (Nardil) have been shown to be effective in the treatment of anorexia nervosa

H. The anticonvulsant topiramate (Topamax) has been used with success at high doses for binge-eating disorder with obesity and bulimia nervosa

I. Fluoxetine (Prozac) has been successful in treating obesity

J. **Anorexiants** are used in the treatment of obesity
  1. Anorexia-inducing effects.
  2. Use is limited.
     a. Tolerance develops for the anorectic effects.
     b. High abuse potential.
     c. Withdrawal from anorexiants.
        i. Rebound weight gain
        ii. Lethargy
        iii. Depression

🛑 Two anorexiants that were once widely used, fenfluramine and dexfenfluramine, have been removed from the market because of their association with serious heart and lung disease.

3. The anorexiants phentermine, diethylpropion, benzphetamine, and phendimetrazine are indicated only for short-term weight loss.

4. New weight-loss drugs, lorcaserin (Belviq) and a combined preparation of phentermine and topiramate (Qsymia) in a timed-release capsule, suppress the appetite by altering various 5-HT2C serotonin receptors found within the hypothalamus, which is responsible for appetite and metabolism.

DID YOU KNOW?

Phentermine is a central nervous system stimulant that is thought to suppress appetite by triggering release of the neurotransmitter norepinephrine. Topiramate is an anticonvulsant medication that has weight loss as a side effect. It is also used in migraine prevention.

REVIEW QUESTIONS

1. A subjective concept of one's physical appearance based on the personal perceptions of self and the reactions of others is termed _____ _____.

2. A client diagnosed with anorexia nervosa whose body type could be described as emaciated states, "I don't know what all the fuss is about. I'm just a little underweight." On the basis of this client's statement, which nursing diagnosis would the nurse document?
   1. Altered nutrition: less than body requirements
   2. Ineffective denial
   3. Low self-esteem
   4. Altered coping

3. A client diagnosed with anorexia nervosa has a nursing diagnosis of *disturbed body image.* Which nursing intervention addresses this problem?
   1. Help client to realize that achieving perfection is unrealistic.
   2. Stay with client during mealtime and for at least 1 hour after meals.
   3. Help the client to identify and set weight loss goals.
   4. With client input, determine appropriate privileges and restrictions.

4. A client diagnosed with anorexia nervosa is assigned a nursing diagnosis of disturbed body image. Which assessment information indicates that this client's problem has improved?
   1. The client has gained up to 80% of body weight for age and size.
   2. The client is free of symptoms of malnutrition and dehydration.
   3. The client has not attempted to induce vomiting.
   4. The client has acknowledged that perception of being "fat" is incorrect.

5. From an epidemiological perspective, which of the following factors accurately describe the prevalence of anorexia nervosa? **Select all that apply.**
   1. There is an increased prevalence in both the United States and Western Europe.
   2. There is a 1% prevalence rate among young women in the United States.
   3. This disorder occurs predominantly in females 12 to 30 years of age.
   4. Less than 10% of cases of anorexia nervosa are male.
   5. This disorder is more prevalent than bulimia nervosa.

6. A nursing instructor is teaching about neuroendocrine abnormalities and the possible primary hypothalamic dysfunction related to anorexia nervosa and bulimia nervosa. Which of the following theories support this possibility? **Select all that apply.**
   1. Some studies have found high levels of endogenous opioids in an individual's spinal fluid.
   2. Some individuals have elevated cerebrospinal fluid cortisol levels.
   3. There is possible impairment of dopaminergic regulation with anorexia nervosa.
   4. Many women experience amenorrhea before the onset of starvation and significant weight loss.
   5. There is a positive response to selective serotonin reuptake inhibitors (SSRIs) therapy.

7. Which of the following psychodynamic influences related to anorexia nervosa and bulimia nervosa should a nursing student recognize? **Select all that apply.**
   1. A very early and profound disturbance in mother-infant interactions.
   2. Mother responds to child's physical and emotional needs with food.
   3. Parents deny marital conflict by defining the child with an eating disorder as the family problem.
   4. When the vulnerable ego is threatened, feelings of overcontrol of one's body (self) emerge.
   5. Behaviors associated with food and eating provide needed control.

8. The episodic, uncontrolled, compulsive, rapid ingestion of large quantities of food over a short period of time is termed _____.

9. A client suffering from severe anorexia nervosa has a food intake of less than 200 calories per day. Which symptom would a nurse expect the client to exhibit?
   1. Ravenous hunger
   2. Nausea and vomiting
   3. No hunger sensations
   4. Abnormally heavy menstruation

10. A client in the outpatient clinic is diagnosed with bulimia nervosa. Which medication might the nurse expect the physician to order?
    1. Triple the dosage of fluoxetine (Prozac)
    2. Cyproheptadine (Periactin)
    3. Phentermine (Ionamin)
    4. Lorcaserin (Belviq)

11. A malnourished client diagnosed with anorexia nervosa has mutually developed an eating plan contract with the nursing staff. Which is the most appropriate nursing response when this client refuses to eat lunch?
    1. "You have broken your contract requirements. Your physician might discharge you for nonadherence."
    2. "I see that you have not eaten lunch. Let's review your contract to implement the consequences of your choices."
    3. "We just developed your eating contract yesterday. Why did you not eat your lunch today?"
    4. "You probably have a good reason for not eating lunch. I'm sure you'll do better tomorrow."

12. A client in the outpatient clinic has an assessed BMI of 38. Which medication might the nurse expect the nurse practitioner to order for short-term therapy?
    1. Chlorpromazine (Thorazine)
    2. Diethylpropion (Tenuate)
    3. Fenfluramine (Pondimin)
    4. Low doses of topiramate (Topamax)

13. An obese adolescent's family asks the nurse why their child has been encouraged to keep a diary of food intake. Which of the following responses meets the family's educational needs? **Select all that apply.**
    1. "A food diary provides the opportunity for a client to gain a realistic picture of the amount of food ingested."
    2. "A food diary provides a database on which to tailor the client's dietary program."
    3. "A food diary helps to identify when a client is eating to satisfy an emotional rather than physiological need."
    4. "A food diary can help the client control the cost of a well-balanced diet."
    5. "A food diary can help the client avoid foods with high fat and sodium."

14. Compared with the others presented, which client has the best chance of maintaining his or her weight loss?
    1. A client who has dropped 10 pounds in 1 week on the Atkins diet.
    2. A client on a low-fat diet who has lost 20 pounds in 1 month and who runs five miles a day.
    3. A client who has lost eight pounds in 1 month.
    4. A client who has lost five pounds in 1 month and has started a progressive exercise program.

15. A client asks the nurse how to calculate a body mass index (BMI). What information should the nurse give the client?
    1. Divide your weight in kilograms by your height in inches squared.
    2. Divide your weight in pounds by your height.
    3. Divide your weight in kilograms by your height in meters squared.
    4. Divide your weight in pounds squared by your height in inches.

16. An individual with a BMI of 35 is being admitted to a psychiatric hospital's eating disorder unit. Which NANDA nursing diagnosis would a nurse likely assign?
    1. Disturbed body image
    2. Imbalanced nutrition: Less than body requirements
    3. Fluid volume deficit
    4. Imbalanced nutrition: More than body requirements

17. A client diagnosed with bulimia nervosa has symptoms of bingeing, purging, abdominal discomfort, and depressed mood. Which appropriate client outcome should the nurse assign?
    1. Client will be binge and purge free, have no abdominal discomfort, rate depression on a scale from 1 to 10 as an 8 by day 3.
    2. Client will be binge and purge free, have no abdominal discomfort, rate depression on a scale from 1 to 10 as an 8 by discharge.
    3. Client will be binge and purge free, have no abdominal discomfort, report elevated mood by discharge.
    4. Client will be binge and purge free, rate depression on a scale from 1 to 10 as an 8 and have no abdominal discomfort.

18. A nurse practitioner is performing an admission assessment interview on a client diagnosed with anorexia nervosa. Which client statements describe family dynamics that may influence the family member with this diagnosis? **Select all that apply.**
    1. "My mom always made me feel better with a big dessert."
    2. "I was never really close to my mother. She told dad what to do."
    3. "Dad was in the navy and ran a tight ship when it came to our family."
    4. "I always asked my mom for permission to do what I wanted to do."
    5. "My parents were very laid back. They were easy to please."

19. A client has been diagnosed with bulimia nervosa. The family questions the nurse about their child's binge eating. Which of the following should the nurse teach this family? **Select all that apply.**
    1. "Your child will probably prefer high calorie, sweet, smooth foods."
    2. "Your child will probably binge in secret."
    3. "Binges are followed by self-degradation and depression."
    4. "Clients are guilt-ridden while bingeing."
    5. "Binges are planned to generate a parental reaction."

20. A client is diagnosed with bulimia nervosa. The family is concerned about the complications related to their child's purging. Which of the following information should the nurse teach the family? **Select all that apply.**
    1. "Your child's purging may lead to problems with fluid retention and cardiac overload."
    2. "Your child may not always vomit to purge. Exercise can also purge the body of calories."
    3. "Your child's tooth enamel may erode due to the gastric acid in the vomitus."
    4. "Your child may maintain a normal weight range if bingeing occurs with purging."
    5. "Other ways your child may purge is by the misuse of laxatives, diuretics, or enemas."

21. A client diagnosed with bulimia nervosa presents with dehydration, poor skin turgor, tooth enamel erosion, and depressed mood. Which priority NANDA nursing diagnosis would the nurse assign?
    1. Ineffective coping R/T feelings of helplessness and lack of control over life situations AEB self-induced vomiting
    2. Imbalanced nutrition: less than body requirements R/T refusal to eat AEB dehydration
    3. Fluid volume deficit R/T self-induced vomiting AEB dehydration
    4. Self-care deficit R/T excessive ritualistic behavior AEB tooth enamel erosion

REVIEW ANSWERS

1. ANSWER: Body image

Rationale: *Body image* is a subjective concept of one's physical appearance based on the personal perceptions of self and the reactions of others. Distortion in body image is a symptom of eating disorders and is manifested by the individual's perception of being "fat" when he or she is obviously underweight or even **emaciated.**

TEST-TAKING TIP: Review key terms at the beginning of the chapter.

Content Area: Psychosocial Integrity;
Integrated Process: Nursing Process: Assessment;
Client Need: Psychosocial Integrity;
Cognitive Level: Knowledge;
Concept: Assessment

2. ANSWER: 2

Rationale:

1. Altered nutrition: less than body requirements is a problem experienced by individuals diagnosed with anorexia nervosa, but this diagnosis does not address the client statement presented in the question.

2. The client statement presented in the question indicates that the client is using the defense mechanism of denial to avoid the reality of his or her physiological status. The nursing diagnosis of ineffective denial addresses the clients expressed problem.

3. Low self-esteem is a problem experienced by individuals diagnosed with anorexia nervosa, but this diagnosis does not address the client statement presented in the question.

4. Altered coping is a problem experienced by individuals diagnosed with anorexia nervosa, but this diagnosis does not address the client statement presented in the question.

TEST-TAKING TIP: Remember to read and understand what the question is asking. Although the nursing diagnosis *altered nutrition: less than body requirements* might well be a priority for the safety of this client, the question specifically asks for a nursing diagnosis based on the client's statement.

Content Area: Safe and Effective Care Environment; Management of Care;
Integrated Process: Nursing Process: Diagnosis (Analysis);
Client Need: Safe and Effective Care Environment; Management of Care;
Cognitive Level: Analysis;
Concept: Critical Thinking

3. ANSWER: 1

Rationale:

1. When the nurse helps the client realize that achieving perfection is unrealistic, the nurse is intervening to address a disturbed body image problem. If the client begins to accept certain personal inadequacies, the need for unrealistic achievement and perfectionism should diminish.

2. Staying with the client during mealtime and for at least 1 hour after meals addresses an imbalanced nutrition, not a disturbed body image, problem. Adequate intake must be encouraged and the amount of intake monitored. The client may use time after meals to discard uneaten food, and the presence of the nurse would discourage this behavior.

3. Helping the client to identify and set weight loss goals is inappropriate for a client diagnosed with anorexia nervosa. It is appropriate to set weight gain goals with these clients.

4. With client input, determining that privileges and restrictions will be based on weight gain is an appropriate intervention to address an imbalanced nutrition, not disturbed body image problem. Applying privileges and restrictions based on compliance with treatment and weight gain is a behavioral approach to encourage increased nutritional intake.

TEST-TAKING TIP: Be able to pair the nursing diagnosis presented in the question with the correct nursing intervention. There must always be a correlation between the stated problem and nursing actions to correct the problem.

Content Area: Safe and Effective Care Environment; Management of Care;
Integrated Process: Nursing Process: Implementation;
Client Need: Safe and Effective Care Environment; Management of Care;
Cognitive Level: Application
Concept: Nursing

4. ANSWER: 4

Rationale:

1. Gaining 80% of body weight for age and size indicates that the nursing diagnosis of imbalanced nutrition: less than body requirements, not impaired body image, has been resolved. Normal body weight is an indication of improved nutritional status.

2. Being free of symptoms of malnutrition and dehydration indicates that the nursing diagnosis of imbalanced nutrition: less than body requirement, not impaired body image, has been resolved. Nutritional status has improved when there are no signs of malnutrition and dehydration.

3. Not attempting to induce vomiting indicates that the nursing diagnosis of altered coping, not impaired body image, has been resolved. Not resorting to the maladaptive coping mechanism of self-induced vomiting indicates improvement in the client's ability to cope effectively with stressors.

4. When clients can acknowledge that their perception of being "fat" is incorrect, they perceive a body image that is realistic and not distorted. This is evidence that the client's disturbed body image has improved.

TEST-TAKING TIP: Pair the client problem presented in the question with the assessment data that indicate improvement of this problem. Only Option 4 correlates with the client problem of impaired body image presented in the question.

Content Area: Safe and Effective Care Environment; Management of Care;
Integrated Process: Nursing Process: Evaluation;
Client Need: Safe and Effective Care Environment; Management of Care;
Cognitive Level: Application;
Concept: Critical Thinking

5. ANSWERS: 1, 2, 3, 4

Rationale:

1. Reports have indicated that the prevalence of anorexia nervosa has increased since the mid-20th century in both the United States and Western Europe.
2. Studies indicate that a prevalence rate for anorexia nervosa among young women in the United States is approximately 1%.
3. Anorexia nervosa occurs predominantly in females 12 to 30 years of age.
4. Less than 10% of anorexia nervosa cases are male.
5. Anorexia nervosa is less, not more, prevalent than bulimia nervosa.

TEST-TAKING TIP: Review the epidemiological factors related to anorexia nervosa.

Content Area: Psychosocial Integrity;
Integrated Process: Nursing Process: Assessment;
Client Need: Psychosocial Integrity;
Cognitive Level: Application;
Concept: Nutrition

6. ANSWERS: 2, 3, 4

Rationale:

1. Some studies have found high levels of endogenous opioids in the spinal fluid of clients diagnosed with anorexia, promoting the speculation that these chemicals may contribute to denial of hunger. However, this is related to neurochemical, not neuroendocrine, influences of primary hypothalamic dysfunction.
2. Some speculation has occurred regarding a primary hypothalamic dysfunction in anorexia nervosa. Studies consistent with this theory have revealed elevated cerebrospinal fluid cortisol levels.
3. Studies consistent with this theory suggest a possible impairment of dopaminergic regulation in individuals with anorexia nervosa.
4. Additional evidence in the etiological implication of hypothalamic dysfunction is gathered from the fact that many people with anorexia nervosa experience amenorrhea before the onset of starvation and significant weight loss.
5. Neurochemical influences, not neuroendocrine abnormalities, related to bulimia may be associated with the neurotransmitters serotonin and norepinephrine. This hypothesis has been supported by the positive response these individuals have shown to therapy with the selective serotonin reuptake inhibitors (SSRIs).

TEST-TAKING TIP: Review the theories that support neuroendocrine abnormalities and the possible primary hypothalamic dysfunction related to clients diagnosed with anorexia nervosa or bulimia nervosa. Note that the question is asking for neuroendocrine abnormalities, not neurochemical influences.

Content Area: Psychosocial Integrity;
Integrated Process: Nursing Process: Implementation;
Client Need: Psychosocial Integrity;
Cognitive Level: Application;
Concept: Evidenced-based Practice

7. ANSWERS: 1, 2, 3, 5

Rationale:

1. Psychodynamic theories suggest that eating disorders result from very early and profound disturbances in mother-infant interactions.
2. Eating disorders result from delayed ego development in the child and an unfulfilled sense of separation-individuation. This problem is compounded when the mother responds to the child's physical and emotional needs with food.
3. Parents deny marital conflict by defining the child with an eating disorder as the family problem. This allows for conflict avoidance.
4. When events occur that threaten the vulnerable ego, feelings of lack of control, not overcontrol, of one's body (self) emerge.
5. Behaviors associated with food and eating serve to provide feelings of control over one's life.

TEST-TAKING TIP: Review the predisposing factors of anorexia nervosa and bulimia nervosa as they relate to psychodynamic influences.

Content Area: Psychosocial Integrity;
Integrated Process: Nursing Process: Assessment;
Client Need: Psychosocial Integrity;
Cognitive Level: Application;
Concept: Self

8. ANSWER: Bingeing

Rationale: *Binge eating* is a pattern of disordered eating that consists of episodes of uncontrolled eating. During such binges, a person rapidly consumes an excessive amount of food. Most people who have eating binges try to hide this behavior from others and often feel ashamed about being overweight or depressed about their overeating.

TEST-TAKING TIP: Review key terms at beginning of chapter.

Content Area: Psychosocial Integrity;
Integrated Process: Nursing Process: Assessment;
Client Need: Psychosocial Integrity;
Cognitive Level: Knowledge;
Concept: Assessment

9. ANSWER: 3

Rationale:

1. Research indicates that individuals diagnosed with anorexia nervosa do indeed suffer from pangs of hunger; however, with food intake of less than 200 calories per day, the client's hunger sensations would actually cease.
2. Nausea and vomiting are not typical symptoms of individuals suffering from anorexia nervosa.
3. With a diagnosis of anorexia nervosa and food intake of less than 200 calories a day, hunger sensations cease.
4. Absence of, not abnormally heavy, menstruation usually follows weight loss. It can sometimes happen early on in the disorder, even before severe weight loss has occurred.

TEST-TAKING TIP: Review the assessment data and signs and symptoms of anorexia nervosa.

Content Area: Safe and Effective Care Environment; Management of Care;
Integrated Process: Nursing Process: Assessment;
Client Need: Safe and Effective Care Environment; Management of Care;
Cognitive Level: Application;
Concept: Assessment

10. **ANSWER: 1**
Rationale:
1. A dosage of 60 mg/day (triple the usual antidepressant dosage) of fluoxetine was found to be most effective with clients diagnosed with bulimia nervosa. Binge eating has been associated with consumption of large amounts of carbohydrates. This medication has been found to decrease carbohydrate cravings. The nurse might expect for this medication to be prescribed.
2. Cyproheptadine (Periactin) is used off-label as an appetite stimulant. This type of medication would exacerbate, not improve, the symptoms of bulimia nervosa.
3. The anorexiant phentermine is indicated for short-term weight loss. This would not be an appropriate medication to treat bulimia nervosa.
4. Lorcaserin (Belviq) is a new weight loss drug and would not be an appropriate medication to treat bulimia nervosa.
TEST-TAKING TIP: Review the medications used in the treatment of various eating disorders.
Content Area: Safe and Effective Care Environment; Management of Care;
Integrated Process: Nursing Process: Evaluation;
Client Need: Safe and Effective Care Environment; Management of Care;
Cognitive Level: Application;
Concept: Medication

11. **ANSWER: 2**
Rationale:
1. An eating contract, related to privileges and restrictions based on compliance with treatment and direct weight gain, should be implemented in a matter-of-fact, nonpunitive way. This statement has threatening overtones.
2. This statement implements an eating contract by stating matter-of-factly which behaviors were unacceptable and how privileges will be restricted for nonadherence. This will maintain the client's sense of control while making the client responsible for individual independent choices.
3. By asking the client a "why" question, the nurse has put the client in a defensive position. This will generate conflict versus the cooperation and sense of control needed to overcome an eating disorder.
4. An eating contract should be implemented by stating matter-of-factly which behaviors were unacceptable and how privileges will be restricted for noncompliance. This statement does not hold the client responsible for his or her choices.

TEST-TAKING TIP: Review the behavioral techniques used in the treatment of various eating disorders and how to implement them correctly.
Content Area: Safe and Effective Care Environment; Management of Care;
Integrated Process: Nursing Process: Implementation;
Client Need: Safe and Effective Care Environment; Management of Care;
Cognitive Level: Application
Concept: Communication

12. **ANSWER: 2**
Rationale: A BMI of 38 indicates that the client is obese.
1. Chlorpromazine is an antipsychotic that is prescribed for selected clients diagnosed with anorexia nervosa, not obesity.
2. Diethylpropion (Tenuate) is an anorexiant that can be used as short-term therapy for weight loss. The nurse practitioner may prescribe this medication for an obese client.
3. Fenfluramine is an anorexiant that has been removed from the market because of its association with serious heart and lung disease. The nurse practitioner would not prescribe this medication.
4. The anticonvulsant topiramate (Topamax) has been used with success at high, not low, doses for binge-eating disorder with obesity and bulimia nervosa.
TEST-TAKING TIP: Review the medications used in the treatment of various eating disorders.
Content Area: Safe and Effective Care Environment; Management of Care;
Integrated Process: Nursing Process: Evaluation;
Client Need: Safe and Effective Care Environment; Management of Care;
Cognitive Level: Application;
Concept: Medication

13. **ANSWERS: 1, 2, 3**
Rationale:
1. Keeping a food diary can instantly increase a client's awareness of what and how much is being eaten.
2. A food diary can provide a database based on food preferences from which a practical dietary program can be developed.
3. Keeping a food diary can instantly increase a client's awareness of why he or she is eating. It also assists the client to identify when eating is satisfying an emotional rather than physiological need.
4. Because food prices are not listed in a food diary, it will not assist with the cost control of a nutritious diet.
5. Because the nutritional information of consumed foods is not listed in a food diary, it will not assist the client to avoid high-fat and sodium foods.
TEST-TAKING TIP: Review the appropriate interventions for clients diagnosed with obesity, which include the use of a food diary.
Content Area: Safe and Effective Care Environment; Management of Care;

Integrated Process: Nursing Process: Implementation;
Client Need: Safe and Effective Care Environment;
Management of Care;
Cognitive Level: Application;
Concept: Nursing Roles

14. **ANSWER: 4**
Rationale: Reasonable weight loss (1–2 pounds per week) and a progressive exercise program results in more lasting weight-loss effects.
1. A reasonable weight loss (1–2 pounds per week), rather than rapid weight loss, results in more lasting effects. Also, there is no indication that an exercise program has been developed.
2. Although it is important to begin a progressive exercise program, running 5 miles a day can be considered excessive. A reasonable weight loss is 1 to 2 pounds per week. Excessive, rapid weight loss may result in fatigue and irritability and ultimately lead to failure in meeting goals for weight loss.
3. Losing 8 pounds in 1 month is a reasonable weight loss, but this client has not added an exercise program, which would limit weight loss success.
4. A client who has lost 5 pounds in 1 month and has started a progressive exercise program is both losing weight at a reasonable rate and expending calories on exercise. Compared with the other clients presented, this client has the best chance of maintaining his or her weight loss.
TEST-TAKING TIP: Review the nursing interventions used in the treatment of obesity.
Content Area: Safe and Effective Care Environment;
Management of Care;
Integrated Process: Nursing Process: Evaluation;
Client Need: Safe and Effective Care Environment;
Management of Care;
Cognitive Level: Application;
Concept: Nutrition

15. **ANSWER: 3**
Rationale: To calculate BMI in the metric system, divide weight in kilograms by height in meters squared. To calculate BMI in the U.S. system, divide weight in pounds multiplied by 703 by height in inches squared.
1. This incorrect formula mixes the variables of both the metric and U.S. systems.
2. This incorrect formula doesn't tell what measurement to use for height and omits multiplying weight in pounds by 703.
3. This is the correct formula for calculating BMI in the metric system.
4. This incorrect formula squares the pounds and omits multiplying weight in pounds by 703. Height in inches must also be squared.
TEST-TAKING TIP: Review the formulas for calculating BMI.
Content Area: Safe and Effective Care Environment;
Management of Care;
Integrated Process: Nursing Process: Implementation;
Client Need: Safe and Effective Care Environment;
Management of Care;
Cognitive Level: Application;
Concept: Nutrition

16. **ANSWER: 4**
Rationale:
1. An individual with a BMI of 30 or greater is considered obese and may well have dissatisfaction with appearance. However, it is the individual diagnosed with anorexia nervosa, not obesity, who has a self-mental picture of a distorted body image.
2. A BMI of 30 or greater indicates obesity. This client has imbalanced nutrition: more than body requirements, not less than body requirements.
3. A BMI of 30 or greater indicates obesity. Obesity, in and of itself, would not cause a fluid volume deficit.
4. A BMI of 30 or greater indicates obesity with a problem of imbalanced nutrition: more than body requirements. The BMI range for normal weight is 20 to 24.9, overweight is defined as a BMI of 25.0 to 29.9, and obesity is defined as a BMI of 30.0 or greater.
TEST-TAKING TIP: Review the nursing assessment area for clients diagnosed with obesity, and familiarize yourself with normal, overweight, and obese BMI ranges.
Content Area: Safe and Effective Care Environment;
Management of Care;
Integrated Process: Nursing Process: Diagnosis (Analysis);
Client Need: Safe and Effective Care Environment;
Management of Care;
Cognitive Level: Analysis;
Concept: Critical Thinking

17. **ANSWER: 2**
Rationale: Correctly written outcomes must be client centered, specific, realistic, and measurable and must include a time frame.
1. It is unrealistic to expect a dramatic change by the third day in both behavior and mood in a client diagnosed with an eating disorder.
2. A client being binge and purge free, having no abdominal discomfort, and rating depression on a scale from 1 to 10 as an 8 by discharge is a correctly written realistic outcome. This outcome is client centered, specific, realistic, and measurable and includes a time frame.
3. Reporting an elevated mood is vague and not measurable, and therefore, this outcome is incorrectly written.
4. There is no time frame given; therefore, this outcome is not measureable and is incorrectly written
TEST-TAKING TIP: Match the symptoms presented in the question with the appropriate expected outcome, making sure that all outcomes are written correctly.
Content Area: Safe and Effective Care Environment;
Management of Care;
Integrated Process: Nursing Process: Planning;
Client Need: Safe and Effective Care Environment;
Management of Care;
Cognitive Level: Application;
Concept: Critical Thinking

18. **ANSWERS: 1, 2, 4**
Rationale:
1. The family influences that may predispose a client to anorexia nervosa may include a mother who responds to a child's physical and emotional needs with food.

2. The family influences that may predispose a client to anorexia nervosa may include a delayed ego development in the child and an unfulfilled sense of separation-individuation.

3. Families of clients with anorexia nervosa often consist of a passive father, not a father who runs a "tight ship."

4. In the families of clients with anorexia nervosa, parents usually retain the child in a dependent position. Continually having to ask permission is an example of this dependent relationship.

5. In the families of clients with anorexia nervosa, a high value is placed on perfectionism. Being "laid back" is not an example of this family dynamic.

TEST-TAKING TIP: Review the family dynamics of clients diagnosed with anorexia nervosa.

Content Area: Safe and Effective Care Environment; Management of Care;

Integrated Process: Nursing Process: Evaluation;

Client Need: Safe and Effective Care Environment; Management of Care;

Cognitive Level: Application;

Concept: Assessment

19. **ANSWERS: 1, 2, 3**

Rationale:

1. Bingeing consists of rapidly eating mostly high-calorie, sweet, smooth textured foods, sometimes without even chewing.

2. Binges often occur in secret and are usually only terminated by abdominal discomfort, sleep, social interruption, or self-induced vomiting.

3. Binges may bring pleasure during an episode, but they are followed by self-degradation and depressed mood.

4. Binges may bring pleasure, not guilt, during an episode but are followed by self-degradation and depressed mood.

5. Binges are episodic, uncontrolled, and compulsive, not planned to generate a parental reaction.

TEST-TAKING TIP: Review information related to bingeing that occurs with bulimia nervosa.

Content Area: Safe and Effective Care Environment; Management of Care;

Integrated Process: Nursing Process: Implementation;

Client Need: Safe and Effective Care Environment; Management of Care;

Cognitive Level: Application;

Concept: Nursing Roles

20. **ANSWERS: 2, 3, 4, 5**

Rationale:

1. Purging may lead to problems with dehydration and electrolyte imbalance, not fluid retention and cardiac overload.

2. Besides vomiting, fasting or excessive exercise are other ways to purge the body of calories.

3. Gastric acid in the vomitus during purging contributes to the erosion of tooth enamel.

4. Weight fluctuations are common, but most clients diagnosed with bulimia nervosa are within a normal weight range—some slightly underweight, some slightly overweight.

5. Purging rids the body of excess calories. This can be done by self-induced vomiting or the misuse of laxatives, diuretics, or enemas.

TEST-TAKING TIP: Review the assessment information related to the symptoms of bulimia nervosa.

Content Area: Safe and Effective Care Environment; Management of Care;

Integrated Process: Nursing Process: Implementation;

Client Need: Safe and Effective Care Environment; Management of Care;

Cognitive Level: Application;

Concept: Nursing Roles

21. **ANSWER: 3**

Rationale:

1. This client may have a problem with ineffective coping, but unrecognized and untreated, dehydration can lead to a life-threatening situation. Therefore, the NANDA nursing diagnosis of fluid volume deficit must be prioritized.

2. The client in the question is dehydrated, not underweight or emaciated. Unrecognized and untreated, dehydration can lead to a life-threatening situation. Therefore, the NANDA nursing diagnosis of fluid volume deficit must be prioritized.

3. Presenting with dehydration and poor skin turgor indicates that this client has a fluid volume deficit. Unrecognized and untreated, dehydration can lead to a life-threatening situation; therefore, the NANDA nursing diagnosis of fluid volume deficit would be prioritized.

4. In all probability, this client diagnosed with bulimia nervosa has probably participated in excessive purging with resulting tooth enamel erosion. Although this problem must be addressed, unrecognized and untreated dehydration can lead to a life-threatening situation, and therefore, the NANDA nursing diagnosis of fluid volume deficit must be prioritized.

TEST-TAKING TIP: Match the symptoms in the question with the appropriate NANDA nursing diagnosis and prioritize any problem which may be life threatening.

Content Area: Safe and Effective Care Environment; Management of Care;

Integrated Process: Nursing Process: Diagnosis (Analysis);

Client Need: Safe and Effective Care Environment; Management of Care;

Cognitive Level: Analysis;

Concept: Critical Thinking

CASE STUDY: Putting it All Together

Shannon, age 21, collapsed at a shopping mall and was taken to a hospital, accompanied by her boyfriend, Jack. Shannon presented with less than 85% of expected weight for her height, and a BMI of 17. Initial assessment revealed hypotension and bradycardia; poor skin turgor; dry, pale oral mucosa; dehydration; electrolyte imbalance; and lanugo covering her back, chest, and arms. When offered broth and crackers, she refused saying, "I'm never hungry anymore." As the nurse hung an intravenous bag of fluids, Shannon weakly said, "How many calories are in that bag?" Shannon allowed Jack to answer questions, saying that she was too tired. Jack stated that in the past year, Shannon maintained a very strict diet and exercise routine and, although underweight, always complained of looking fat. When he showed concern about her dramatic weight loss, she always denied its seriousness.

After Shannon was stabilized and admitted to the hospital's eating disorder unit, she was introduced to her assigned psychiatric nurse practitioner (PNP), Sean. With time, Shannon gained strength and openly discussed her family dynamics. Her first memories were of her and her mother at an indoor ice-skating rink taking endless lessons. She said that her mother seemed very proud of her, telling acquaintances that Shannon was training for the Olympics. There was never time for friends, play dates, or outside activities. The problems began during the first competition when Shannon, by then an excellent skater, froze and was unable to perform. This phenomenon continued until she and her mother were told that, although other skating opportunities were available, Shannon was not Olympic material. Shannon confided to Sean, "My world ended. I had no goals, no friends, no interests;

my mother filled this terrible void with comfort food, and I ballooned. At 18 and against my mother's wishes, I moved out, and began to diet and exercise. I lost a lot of weight, but nothing I did ever quite eliminated the image of myself as a fat failure. When Jack came into my life, instead of relaxing and enjoying the relationship, my dieting and exercise escalated. I know things are out of control. I need help. I really don't want to die."

1. On the basis of Shannon's symptoms and client actions, what medical diagnosis would Sean assign to her?
2. What predisposing psychodynamic influences may have been a factor leading to Shannon's disorder?
3. What are Shannon's subjective symptoms that would lead to the determination of this diagnosis?
4. What are Shannon's objective symptoms that would lead to the determination of this diagnosis?
5. What NANDA nursing diagnoses would address Shannon's current problems?
6. On the basis of these nursing diagnoses, what short-term outcomes would be appropriate for Shannon?
7. On the basis of these nursing diagnoses, what long-term outcomes would be appropriate for Shannon?
8. List the psychological treatments the PNP might employ to treat Shannon.
9. What classification of medications might be prescribed for the long-term treatment of Shannon's symptoms?
10. List the nursing interventions (actions) that will assist Shannon in successfully meeting these outcomes.
11. List the questions that should be asked to determine the success of the nursing interventions.

Neurocognitive Disorders

Alzheimer's disease—Alzheimer's disease is an irreversible, progressive brain disease that slowly destroys memory and thinking skills, and eventually even the ability to carry out the simplest tasks

Amnesia—An inability to recall important personal information that is too extensive to be explained by ordinary forgetfulness

Anosmia—The inability to smell

Aphasia—The inability to communicate through speech, writing, or signs, caused by dysfunction of brain centers

Ataxia—A neurological sign consisting of lack of voluntary coordination of muscle movements

Confabulation—A memory disturbance, defined as the production of fabricated, distorted, or misinterpreted memories about oneself or the world, without the conscious intention to deceive

Delirium—A mental state characterized by a disturbance of cognition, which is manifested by confusion, excitement, disorientation, and a clouding of consciousness; hallucinations and illusions are common

Dementia pugilistica—A syndrome affecting boxers that is caused by cumulative cerebral injuries and is characterized by impaired cognitive processes (such as thinking and remembering); parkinsonism; impaired and often slurred speech; and slow, poorly coordinated movements, especially of the legs

Dysarthria—A condition in which problems occur with the muscles that help produce speech, often making it difficult to pronounce words

Dysphagia—Swallowing difficulties that are usually caused by nerve or muscle problems

Hypersomnolence—Also known as *hypersomnia,* a condition characterized by recurrent episodes of excessive daytime sleepiness or prolonged nighttime sleep

Neurocognitive—A term that is used to describe cognitive functions closely linked to particular areas of the brain that have to do with thinking, reasoning, memory, learning, and speaking

Pseudodementia—Symptoms of depression that mimic those of neurocognitive disorder

Reminiscence therapy—A psychosocial intervention used in the care of clients diagnosed with NCD that involves the discussion of past activities, events, and experiences with another person or group of people, usually with the aid of tangible prompts such as photographs, household and other familiar items from the past, or music and archive sound recordings

Sundowning—A term referring to a state of confusion at the end of the day and into the night; sundowning can cause a variety of behaviors, such as confusion, anxiety, aggression, or ignoring directions; it can also lead to pacing or wandering

Neurocognitive disorders (NCD) include those in which a clinically significant deficit in cognition or memory exists, representing a significant change from a previous level of functioning. These disorders are categorized as delirium and mild and major neurocognitive disorders. It is critical to provide individuals with these disorders the dignity and quality of life they deserve, while offering guidance and support to their families or primary caregivers.

I. Delirium

A. Characterized by a disturbance in level of awareness and a change in cognition that develops rapidly over a short period

B. Symptoms begin quite abruptly (e.g., after a head injury or seizure)

DID YOU KNOW?
Symptoms of delirium may be preceded by several hours or days of prodromal symptoms, which may include restlessness, difficulty thinking clearly, insomnia or **hypersomnolence**, and nightmares.

C. Slower onset is more common if the underlying cause is systemic illness or metabolic imbalance
D. Duration is usually brief (e.g., 1 week; rarely more than 1 month)
E. Upon recovery from the underlying determinant, symptoms usually diminish over a 3- to 7-day period
F. May take as long as 2 weeks
G. Age of the client and duration of the delirium influence rate of symptom resolution

🛑 Delirium may transition into a more permanent cognitive disorder (e.g., major neurocognitive disorder) and is also associated with a high mortality rate.

II. Predisposing Factors to Delirium

Most commonly occurs in individuals with serious medical, surgical, or neurological conditions
A. Systemic infections
B. Febrile illness
C. Metabolic disorders (hypoxia, hypercapnia or hypoglycemia)
D. Hepatic encephalopathy
E. Head trauma
F. Seizures
G. Migraine headaches
H. Brain abscess
I. Stroke
J. Postoperative states
K. Electrolyte imbalance

III. Substance-Induced Delirium

A. Characterized by the symptoms of delirium that are attributed to either intoxication or withdrawal from certain substances, side effects of pharmacological agents, or exposure to toxins
B. Medications known to precipitate delirium include:
1. Anticholinergics
2. Antihypertensives
3. Corticosteroids
4. Anticonvulsants
5. Cardiac glycosides
6. Analgesics
7. Anesthetics
8. Antineoplastic agents
9. Antiparkinson drugs
10. H_2-receptor antagonists (e.g., cimetidine [Tagamet])
11. Others

C. Intoxication or withdrawal from substances including:
1. Alcohol
2. Amphetamines
3. Cannabis
4. Cocaine
5. Hallucinogens
6. Inhalants
7. Opioids
8. Phencyclidine-like substances
9. Sedatives
10. Hypnotics
11. Anxiolytics
12. Others
D. Toxins reported to cause delirium include:
1. Organic solvents and fuels
2. Heavy metals, such as lead, mercury, and arsenic
3. Carbon monoxide
4. Insecticides

IV. Neurocognitive Disorders (NCD)

A. Classified as either *mild* or *major,* with the distinction primarily being severity of symptoms
1. Mild NCD can be known as *mild cognitive impairment.*
2. Focus of mild NCD is early intervention to prevent or slow progression.
3. Major NCD previously described as *dementia.*
4. Mild and major NCD may serve to identify earlier and later stages of the same disorder.
B. In the United States, 5.3 million people currently have Alzheimer's disease (AD), the most common form of NCD
C. Prevalence doubles for every 5-year age group beyond age 65
D. Affects 5% of people from aged 71 to 79, 24% of people aged 80 to 89, and 37% of those aged 90 and older
E. After heart disease and cancer, AD is the third most costly disease in the United States, accounting for $100 billion in yearly costs
F. More people now survive into the high-risk period for NCD, which is middle age and beyond

MAKING THE CONNECTION
Major NCD causes can be reversible, or they can be irreversible and progressive. Numerous factors can cause symptoms of this disorder. Potentially reversible symptoms include those caused by depression, stroke, traumatic brain injury, certain medications, and even bladder infections. Irreversible and progressive NCD includes Alzheimer's disease, vascular NCD, Lewy body dementia, and frontotemporal NCD.

G. *Primary NCDs* are those, such as AD, in which the NCD itself is the major sign of some organic brain disease not directly related to any other organic illness

H. *Secondary NCDs* are caused by or related to another disease or condition, such as human immunodeficiency virus (HIV) disease or cerebral trauma

V. Types of Neurocognitive Disorders

Differentiated by etiology and share a common symptom presentation

A. NCD due to AD
B. Vascular NCD
C. Frontotemporal NCD
D. NCD due to traumatic brain injury
E. NCD due to Lewy body dementia
F. NCD due to Parkinson's disease
G. NCD due to HIV infection
H. Substance-induced NCD
I. NCD due to Huntington's disease
J. NCD due to prion disease
K. NCD due to another medical condition
L. NCD not elsewhere classified

VI. Etiology of NCD

A. Alzheimer's disease
1. The exact cause unknown.
2. Several hypotheses supported by varying amounts and quality of data.
   a. Acetylcholine alterations.
      i. Enzyme required to produce acetylcholine is dramatically reduced in brains of AD clients
      ii. Decreased acetylcholine results in cognitive process disruption
      iii. Decreased norepinephrine, serotonin, and dopamine and an increase in the amino acid glutamate implicated in the pathology and clinical symptoms of AD
      iv. Excess glutamate leads to overstimulation of the *N*-methyl-D-aspartate (NMDA) receptors, leading to increased intracellular calcium and subsequent neuronal degeneration and cell death
   b. Plaques and tangles.
      i. Overabundance of structures called *amyloid plaques* and *neurofibrillary tangles* appear in the brains of individuals with AD
         a) Plaques are amyloid beta (Aβ) protein fragments
         b) Neurofibrillary tangles are insoluble twisted fibers of protein called tau
      ii. These structures interfere with the neuronal transport system

      iii. Unknown whether the plaques and tangles cause AD or are a consequence of AD
      iv. Plaques and tangles may contribute to the destruction and death of neurons
   c. Head trauma.
      i. History of head trauma puts clients at risk for AD
      ii. A combination of genetic predisposition and head trauma increases risk
   d. Genetic factors.
      i. There is a familial pattern with some forms of AD
      ii. Pattern of inheritance suggests possible autosomal-dominant gene transmission
      iii. Early-onset cases are more likely to be familial than late-onset cases
      iv. One-third to one-half of all cases may be of the genetic form
      v. Gene mutations found on chromosomes 21, 14, and 1
      vi. Mutations result in an increased amount of the Aβ protein that is a major component of the plaques associated with AD

B. Vascular NCD
1. Directly related to an interruption of blood flow to the brain.
2. Symptoms result from death of nerve cells in regions nourished by diseased vessels.
3. Various diseases and conditions that interfere with blood circulation have been implicated.
   a. Hypertension.
      i. Damage to the lining of blood vessels
      ii. Result in rupture of the blood vessel with subsequent hemorrhage
      iii. Accumulation of fibrin in the vessel with intravascular clotting and inhibited blood flow
   b. Infarcts related to occlusion of blood vessels by particulate matter that travels through the bloodstream to the brain. Emboli may be:
      i. Solid (clots, cellular debris, platelet aggregates)
      ii. Gaseous (air, nitrogen)
      iii. Liquid (fat, after soft tissue trauma or fracture of long bones)
   c. Multiple small infarcts ("silent strokes" or transient ischemic attacks [TIAs]) over time
   d. A single cerebrovascular insult that occurs in a strategic area of the brain
4. Both vascular NCD and AD can occur simultaneously (*mixed* disorder)
5. Prevalence of mixed disorder is likely to increase as the population ages

C. Frontotemporal NCD
1. Cause of frontotemporal NCD is unknown.
2. Genetic factor appears to be involved.
3. Symptoms occur as a result of shrinking of the frontal and temporal anterior lobes of the brain.
4. Previously called Pick's disease.

D. NCD due to traumatic brain injury
1. Caused by an impact to the head.
2. Other mechanisms of rapid movement or displacement of the brain within the skull.

E. NCD due to Lewy body dementia
1. Cause of Lewy body dementia unknown.
2. Related to Alzheimer's or Parkinson's disease.
   a. Lewy bodies contain a protein associated with Parkinson's disease.
   b. Lewy bodies often are present in the brains of people with Parkinson's disease, Alzheimer's disease, and other NCDs.
   c. People who have Lewy bodies in their brains also have the plaques and tangles associated with Alzheimer's disease.

F. NCD due to Parkinson's disease.
1. Cause of Parkinson's disease unknown.
2. Specific genetic mutations and variations can increase risk of Parkinson's disease.
3. Exposure to certain toxins or environmental factors may increase risk of later Parkinson's disease.

G. NCD due to HIV Infection
1. Infection with the human immunodeficiency virus-type 1 (HIV-1) can result in a NCD called *HIV-1-associated cognitive/motor complex.*
2. A less severe form, known as *HIV-1-associated minor cognitive/motor disorder,* also occurs.
3. Immune dysfunction associated with HIV disease can lead to brain infections by other organisms.
4. HIV-1 can cause NCD directly.

H. Substance-induced NCD
1. NCD can occur as the result of substance reactions, overuse, or abuse.
2. Substances that have been associated with the development of NCDs include:
   a. Alcohol
   b. Sedatives
   c. Hypnotics
   d. Anxiolytics
   e. Inhalants
3. Drugs that cause anticholinergic side effects and toxins such as lead and mercury have also been implicated.

I. NCD due to Huntington's disease
1. Huntington's disease is transmitted as a mendelian dominant gene.
2. An autosomal dominant disorder, which means that a person needs only one copy of the defective gene to develop the disorder.

J. NCD due to Prion disease
1. Caused by abnormal versions of a kind of protein called a prion.
2. When misshapen, they become infectious and disrupt normal biological processes.
3. Can be a genetic link, exposure to infected tissue, or there may be no apparent reason.

K. NCD due to another medical condition
1. General medical conditions can cause NCD.
   a. Hypothyroidism.
   b. Hyperparathyroidism.
   c. Pituitary insufficiency.
   d. Uremia.
   e. Encephalitis.
   f. Brain tumor.
   g. Pernicious anemia.
   h. Thiamine deficiency.
   i. Pellagra.
   j. Uncontrolled epilepsy.
   k. Cardiopulmonary insufficiency.
   l. Fluid and electrolyte imbalances.
   m. CNS and systemic infections.
   n. Systemic lupus erythematosus.
   o. Multiple sclerosis.

L. The etiological factors associated with delirium and NCD are summarized in Box 15.1

VII. Nursing Process: Assessment

A. Nursing assessment of the client with delirium or mild or major NCD is based on knowledge of the symptomatology associated with the various disorders

B. Subjective and objective assessment data are gathered using a variety of methods
1. Client history.
   a. Assess specific mental and physical changes that have occurred and the age at which changes began.
   b. If the client is unable to relate information adequately, obtain data from family members or others who would be aware of client's physical and psychosocial history.
   c. Assess type, frequency, and severity of mood swings; personality and behavioral changes; and catastrophic emotional reactions.
   d. Assess cognitive changes, such as problems with attention span, thinking process, problem-solving, and memory (recent and remote).
   e. Assess language difficulties.
   f. Assess orientation to person, place, time, and situation.
   g. Assess appropriateness of social behavior.
   h. Gather information regarding current and past medication usage.

Box 15.1 Etiological Factors Implicated in the Development of Delirium and/or Mild or Major Neurocognitive Disorder

Biological Factors

Hypoxia: any condition leading to a deficiency of oxygen to the brain

Nutritional deficiencies: vitamins (particularly B and C); protein; fluid and electrolyte imbalances

Metabolic disturbances: porphyria; encephalopathies related to hepatic, renal, pancreatic, or pulmonary insufficiencies; hypoglycemia

Endocrine dysfunction: thyroid, parathyroid, adrenal, pancreas, pituitary

Cardiovascular disease: stroke, cardiac insufficiency, atherosclerosis

Primary brain disorders: epilepsy, Alzheimer's disease, Pick's disease, Huntington's chorea, multiple sclerosis, Parkinson's disease

Infections: encephalitis, meningitis, pneumonia, septicemia, neurosyphilis (dementia paralytica), HIV disease, acute rheumatic fever, Creutzfeldt-Jakob disease

Intracranial neoplasms

Congenital defects: prenatal infections, such as first-trimester maternal rubella

Exogenous Factors

Birth trauma: prolonged labor, damage from use of forceps, other obstetric complications

Cranial trauma: concussion, contusions, hemorrhage, hematomas

Volatile inhalant compounds: gasoline, glue, paint, paint thinners, spray paints, cleaning fluids, typewriter correction fluid, varnishes, and lacquers

Heavy metals: lead, mercury, manganese

Other metallic elements: aluminum

Organic phosphates: various insecticides

Substance abuse/dependence: alcohol, amphetamines, caffeine, cannabis, cocaine, hallucinogens, inhalants, nicotine, opioids, phencyclidine, sedatives, hypnotics, anxiolytics

Other medications: anticholinergics, antihistamines, antidepressants, antipsychotics, antiparkinsonians, antihypertensives, steroids, digitalis

---

  i. Assess history of other drug and alcohol use.
  j. Assess possible exposure to toxins.
  k. Assess family history of Huntington's disease, AD, Pick's disease, or Parkinson's disease.
 2. Physical assessment.
  a. Focus on signs of damage to the nervous system.
  b. Look for evidence of diseases of other organs that could affect mental function.
  c. Perform neurological examination.
  d. Assess mental status and alertness, muscle strength, reflexes, sensory perception, language skills, and coordination.
   i. Mental status examination
    a) Assesses general quality of cognitive processing and intellectual functions
    b) Assesses form and content of thought
    c) Is not an intelligence test
    d) Is not a detailed memory test
    e) Is not a fully precise measure of cognition, affect, and behavior
   ii. Important to build rapport in order to obtain the client's cooperation and best effort in responding to the examination
  e. An example of a mental status examination for a client with NCD is presented in Box 15.2.
  f. Results of psychological tests may be used to make a differential diagnosis between NCD and **pseudodementia** (depression).
  g. Cognitive symptoms of depression may mimic NCD.

  h. A comparison of symptoms of NCD and pseudodementia (depression) is presented in Table 15.1.
 3. Diagnostic laboratory evaluations.
  a. Blood and urine samples test for various infections.
  b. Hepatic and renal function tests.
  c. Tests for diabetes or hypoglycemia.
  d. Tests for electrolyte imbalances.
  e. Tests for metabolic and endocrine disorders.
  f. Tests for nutritional deficiencies.
  g. Tests for the presence of toxic substances, including alcohol and other drugs.
  h. Electroencephalogram (EEG) measures and records the brain's electrical activity.
  i. Computed tomography (CT) scanning, to image the size and shape of the brain.
  j. Magnetic resonance imaging (MRI) provides a sharp detailed picture of the tissues of the brain.

MAKING THE CONNECTION

Examination by computerized tomography (CT) scan or magnetic resonance imaging (MRI) reveals a degenerative pathology of the brain that includes atrophy, widened cortical sulci, and enlarged cerebral ventricles (see Fig. 15.1). Various areas of the brain are affected by Alzheimer's disease. The impaired functions of these areas cause the symptoms of the disorder.

Box 15.2 Mental Status Examination for Neurocognitive Disorder

Patient Name _____

Date _____

Age _____ Sex _____

Diagnosis _____

Maximum <u>Client's</u> <u>Score</u>

1. **VERBAL FLUENCY**

   Ask client to name as many animals as he/she can. (Time: 60 seconds)   10 points _____
   (Score 1 point/2 animals)

2. **COMPREHENSION**

   a. Point to the ceiling   1 point _____

   b. Point to your nose and the window   1 point _____

   c. Point to your foot, the door, and ceiling   1 point _____

   d. Point to the window, your leg, the door, and your thumb   1 point _____

3. **NAMING AND WORD FINDING**

   Ask the client to name the following as you point to them:

   a. Watch stem (winder)   1 point _____

   b. Teeth   1 point _____

   c. Sole of shoe   1 point _____

   d. Buckle of belt   1 point _____

   e. Knuckles   1 point _____

4. **ORIENTATION**

   a. Date   2 points _____

   b. Day of week   2 points _____

   c. Month   1 point _____

   d. Year   1 point _____

5. **NEW LEARNING ABILITY**

   Tell the client: "I'm going to tell you four words, which I want you to remember."
   Have the client repeat the four words after they are initially presented, and then
   say that you will ask him/her to remember the words later. Continue with the
   examination, and at intervals of 5 and 10 minutes, ask the client to recall the
   words. Three different sets of words are provided here.   5 min. 10 min.

   a. Brown (Fun) (Grape) 2 points each: _____ _____

   b. Honesty (Loyalty) (Happiness) 2 points each: _____ _____

   c. Tulip (Carrot) (Stocking) 2 points each: _____ _____

   d. Eyedropper (Ankle) (Toothbrush) 2 points each: _____ _____

6. **VERBAL STORY FOR IMMEDIATE RECALL**

   Tell the client: "I'm going to read you a short story, which I want you to   13 points _____
   remember. Listen closely to what I read because I will ask you to tell me
   the story when I finish." Read the story slowly and carefully, but without
   pausing at the slash marks. After completing the paragraph, tell the client
   to retell the story as accurately as possible. Record the number of correct
   memories (information within the slashes) and describe confabulation if it
   is present. (1 point = 1 remembered item [13 maximum points])

Box 15.2 **Mental Status Examination for Neurocognitive Disorder—cont'd**

It was July / and the Rogers family, mom, dad, and four children /
were packing up their station wagon /to go on vacation.
They were taking their yearly trip / to the beach at Gulf Shores.
This year they were making a special 1-day stop / at the aquarium in New Orleans.
After a long day's drive they arrived at the motel / only to discover that in their
excitement / they had left the twins / and their suitcases / in the front yard.

7. VISUAL MEMORY (HIDDEN OBJECTS)

Tell the client that you are going to hide some objects around the
office (desk, bed) and that you want him/her to remember where
they are. Hide four or five common objects (e.g., keys, pen, reflex hammer)
in various places in the client's sight. After a delay of several minutes,
ask the client to find the objects. (1 point per item found)

a. Coin   1 point _____

b. Pen   1 point _____

c. Comb   1 point _____

d. Keys   1 point _____

e. Fork   1 point _____

8. PAIRED ASSOCIATE LEARNING

Tell the client that you are going to read a list of words two at a time.
The client will be expected to remember the words that go together
(e.g., big—little). When he/she is clear on the directions, read the first
list of words at the rate of one pair per second. After reading the first
list, test for recall by presenting the first recall list. Give the first word
of a pair and ask for the word that was paired with it. Correct incorrect responses
and proceed to the next pair. After the first recall has been completed, allow
a 10-second delay and continue with the second presentation and recall lists.

Presentation Lists

1	2
a. High—Low	a. Good—Bad
b. House—Income	b. Book—Page
c. Good—Bad	c. High—Low
d. Book—Page	d. House—Income

Recall Lists

1	2	
a. House _____	a. High _____	2 points _____
b. Book _____	b. Good _____	2 points _____
c. High _____	c. House _____	2 points _____
d. Good _____	d. Book _____	2 points _____

9. CONSTRUCTIONAL ABILITY

Ask client to reconstruct this drawing and to draw the other 2 items:

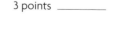

3 points _____

Continued

Box 15.2 Mental Status Examination for Neurocognitive Disorder—cont'd

Draw a daisy in a flowerpot   3 points _____

Draw a clock with all the numbers and set the clock at 2:30.   3 points _____

10. **WRITTEN COMPLEX CALCULATIONS**

   a. Addition 108
      + 79   1 point _____

   b. Subtraction 605
      - 86   1 point _____

   c. Multiplication 108
      x 36   1 point _____

   d. Division $559 \div 43$ 1 point _____

11. **PROVERB INTERPRETATION**

   Tell the client to explain the following sayings. Record the answers.

   a. Don't cry over spilled milk.   2 points _____

   _____

   b. Rome wasn't built in a day.   2 points _____

   _____

   c. A drowning man will clutch at a straw.   2 points _____

   _____

   d. A golden hammer can break down an iron door.   2 points _____

   _____

   e. The hot coal burns, the cold one blackens.   2 points _____

   _____

Box 15.2 Mental Status Examination for Neurocognitive Disorder—cont'd

12. SIMILARITIES

Ask the client to name the similarity or relationship between each of the two items.

a. Turnip .... Cauliflower   2 points _____

b. Car .... Airplane   2 points _____

c. Desk .... Bookcase   2 points _____

d. Poem.. Novel   2 points _____

e. Horse .... Apple   2 points _____

Maximum: 100 points   _____

Age Group	Normal Individuals Mean Score (standard deviation)	Stage	Clients with Alzheimer's Disease Mean Score (standard deviation)
40–49	80.9 (9.7)	I	57.2 (9.1)
50–59	82.3 (8.6)	II	37.0 (7.8)
60–69	75.5 (10.5)	III	13.4 (8.1)
70–79	66.9 (9.1)		
80–89	67.9 (11.0)		

Source: Adapted from Strub, R. I., & Black, F. W. (2000). *The Mental Status Examination in Neurology* (4th ed.). Philadelphia: F.A. Davis. Used with permission.

Table 15.1 A Comparison of Neurocognitive Disorder (NCD) and Pseudodementia (Depression)

Symptom Element	NCD	Pseudodementia (Depression)
Progression of symptoms	Slow	Rapid
Memory	Progressive deficits; recent memory loss greater than remote; may confabulate for memory "gaps;" no complaints of loss	More like forgetfulness; no evidence of progressive deficit; recent and remote loss equal; complaints of deficits; no confabulation (will more likely answer "I don't know")
Orientation	Disoriented to time and place; may wander in search of the familiar	Oriented to time and place; no wandering
Task performance	Consistently poor performance, but struggles to perform	Performance is variable; little effort is put forth
Symptom severity	Worse as the day progresses	Better as the day progresses
Affective distress	Appears unconcerned	Communicates severe distress
Appetite	Unchanged	Diminished
Attention and concentration	Impaired	Intact

    k. A lumbar puncture to examine the cerebrospinal fluid for evidence of central nervous system infection or hemorrhage.

    l. Positron emission tomography (PET) to reveal the metabolic activity of the brain (see Fig. 15-2).

C. Symptoms of delirium include:

1. Difficulty sustaining and shifting attention.
2. Extreme distractibility.
3. Deficits in focused attention.
4. Disorganized thinking.
5. Rambling speech.
6. Irrelevant, pressured, and incoherent speech.
7. Speech unpredictably switches from subject to subject.
8. Impaired reasoning ability and goal-directed behavior.
9. Disorientation to time and place.
10. Impairment of recent memory.
11. Misperceptions of the environment, including illusions and hallucinations.
12. Disturbances in the sleep-wake cycle.
13. State of awareness may range from that of hypervigilance (heightened awareness to environmental stimuli) to stupor or semicoma.

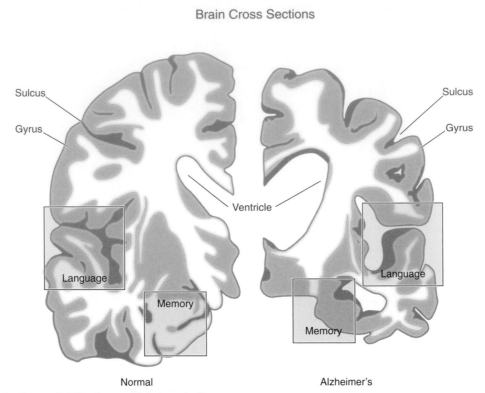

Fig 15.1 Neurobiology of NCD due to Alzheimer's disease.

A decrease in the neurotransmitter *acetylcholine* has been implicated in the etiology of Alzheimer's disease. Cholinergic sources arise from the brainstem and the basal forebrain to supply areas of the basal ganglia, thalamus, limbic structures, hippocampus, and cerebral cortex.

Cell bodies of origin for the *serotonin* pathways lie within the raphe nuclei located in the brainstem. Those for *norepinephrine* originate in the locus ceruleus. Projections for both neurotransmitters extend throughout the forebrain, prefrontal cortex, cerebellum, and limbic system. *Dopamine* pathways arise from areas in the midbrain and project to the frontal cortex, limbic system, basal ganglia, and thalamus. Dopamine neurons in the hypothalamus innervate the posterior pituitary.

Glutamate, an excitatory neurotransmitter, has largely descending pathways with highest concentrations in the cerebral cortex. It is also found in the hippocampus, thalamus, hypothalamus, cerebellum, and spinal cord.

Areas of the Brain Affected
Areas of the brain affected by NCD due to Alzheimer's disease and associated symptoms include the following:
- Frontal lobe: impaired reasoning ability; unable to solve problems and perform familiar tasks; poor judgment; inability to evaluate the appropriateness of behavior; aggressiveness.
- Parietal lobe: impaired orientation ability; impaired visuospatial skills (unable to remain oriented within own environment).
- Occipital lobe: impaired language interpretation; unable to recognize familiar objects.
- Temporal lobe: inability to recall words; inability to use words correctly (language comprehension). In late stages, some clients experience delusions, and hallucinations.
- Hippocampus: impaired memory. Short-term memory is affected initially. Later, the individual is unable to form new memories.
- Amygdala: impaired emotions: depression, anxiety, fear, personality changes, apathy, paranoia.
- Neurotransmitters: alterations in acetylcholine, dopamine, norepinephrine, serotonin and others may play a role in behaviors such as restlessness, sleep impairment, mood, and agitation.

Medications and Their Effects on the Brain
1. Cholinesterase inhibitors (e.g., tacrine, donepezil, rivastigmine, galantamine) act by inhibiting acetylcholinesterase, which slows the degradation of acetylcholine, thereby increasing concentrations of the neurotransmitter in the brain. Most common side effects include dizziness, gastrointestinal upset, fatigue, and headache.
2. *N*-methyl-D-aspartate (NMDA) receptor antagonists (e.g., memantine) act by blocking NMDA receptors from excessive glutamate, preventing continuous influx of calcium into the cells, and ultimately slowing down neuronal degradation. Possible side effects include dizziness, headache, and constipation.

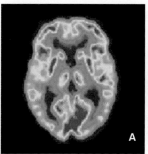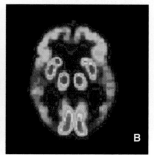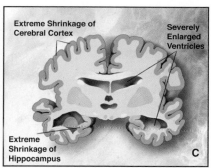

Fig 15.2 Changes in the Alzheimer's brain. (A) Metabolic activity in a normal brain. (B) Diminished metabolic activity in the Alzheimer's diseased brain. (C) Late-stage NCD due to Alzheimer's disease with generalized atrophy and enlargement of the ventricles and sulci. (Source: Alzheimer's Disease Education & Referral Center, A Service of the National Institute on Aging.)

14. Sleep may fluctuate between hypersomnolence (excessive sleepiness) and insomnia.
15. Vivid dreams and nightmares common.
16. Psychomotor activity may fluctuate between agitated, purposeless movements (restlessness, hyperactivity, striking out at nonexistent objects) and a vegetative state resembling catatonic stupor.
17. Various forms of tremor frequently present.
18. Emotional instability.
    a. Fear.
    b. Anxiety.
    c. Depression.
    d. Irritability.
    e. Anger.
    f. Euphoria.
    g. Apathy.
19. Autonomic manifestations.
    a. Tachycardia.
    b. Sweating.
    c. Flushed face.
    d. Dilated pupils (mydriasis).
    e. Elevated blood pressure.
D. Symptoms of NCD include:
1. Impairment in abstract thinking, judgment, and impulse control.
2. Conventional rules of social conduct often disregarded.

MAKING THE CONNECTION

Evidence of emotional instability expressed by individuals diagnosed with NCD may include crying, calls for help, cursing, muttering, moaning, acts of self-harm, fearful attempts to flee, and attacks on others who are falsely viewed as threatening.

---

3. Behavior may be uninhibited and inappropriate.
4. Personal appearance and hygiene neglected.
5. Language may or may not be affected.
6. Difficulty in naming objects.
7. Language may seem vague and imprecise.
8. In severe forms of NCD, individual may not speak at all (**aphasia**).
9. Personality change common in NCD manifested by either an alteration or accentuation of premorbid characteristics.
10. Reversibility of NCD dependent on the basic etiology of the disorder.
11. In most clients, NCD runs a progressive, irreversible course.

DID YOU KNOW?

Truly reversible NCD occurs in only a small percentage of cases and might be more appropriately termed *temporary NCD*. Reversible NCD can occur as a result of cerebral lesions, depression, side effects of certain medications, normal pressure hydrocephalus, vitamin or nutritional deficiencies (especially B$_{12}$ or folate), central nervous system infections, and metabolic disorders.

12. With disease progression, symptoms include:
    a. Apraxia (inability to carry out motor activities despite intact motor function).
    b. Irritability.
    c. Alteration and instability of mood.
    d. Sudden outbursts of temper over trivial issues.
    e. Inability to maintain employment or independently meet personal needs.
    f. Need for constant supervision.
    g. Impaired judgment and high risk for accidents.
    h. Wandering, leading to safety issues.

E. Symptoms of NCD due to Alzheimer's disease (AD)
1. Accounts for 50% to 60% of all cases of NCD.
2. Stages of NCD due to Alzheimer's disease.
   a. Stage 1: no symptoms.
      i. No apparent symptoms
      ii. No apparent decline in memory
   b. Stage 2: forgetfulness.
      i. Begins to lose things
      ii. Forgets people's names
      iii. Short-term memory loss
      iv. Aware of the intellectual decline and may feel ashamed
      v. Anxiety and depression
      vi. Symptoms often not observed by others
   c. Stage 3: mild cognitive decline.
      i. Alterations in work performance, noticeable to coworkers
      ii. May get lost when driving his or her car
      iii. Interrupted concentration
      iv. Difficulty recalling names or words, noticeable to family and close associates
      v. Decline in the ability to plan or organize
   d. Stage 4: mild-to-moderate cognitive decline.
      i. May forget major events in personal history
      ii. Declining ability to perform tasks, such as shopping and managing personal finances
      iii. May be unable to understand current news events
      iv. May deny problem exists
      v. Cover up memory loss with **confabulation** (creating imaginary events to fill in memory gaps)
      vi. Depression and social withdrawal are common
   e. Stage 5: moderate cognitive decline.
      i. Loss of ability to perform some activities of daily living (ADLs) independently (hygiene, dressing, and grooming)
      ii. Requires some assistance with ADLs
      iii. Forgetful of addresses, phone numbers, and names of close relatives
      iv. Disoriented about place and time, but maintain knowledge about themselves
      v. Frustration, withdrawal, and self-absorption are common
   f. Stage 6: moderate-to-severe cognitive decline.
      i. Unable to recall recent major life events or even the name of his or her spouse
      ii. Disorientation to surroundings
      iii. Unable to recall the day, season, or year
      iv. Unable to manage ADLs without assistance
      v. Communication becomes difficult with increasing loss of language skills
      vi. Urinary and fecal incontinence common
      vii. Sleeping problems

viii. Psychomotor symptoms
   a) Wandering
   b) Obsessiveness
   c) Agitation
   d) Aggression

DID YOU KNOW?
Symptoms of NCD due to Alzheimer's disease seem to worsen in the late afternoon and evening, a phenomenon termed sundowning. Being aware of this potential will assist the nurse in anticipating increasing cognitive impairments that may put the client at risk for injury.

   ix. Institutional care usually required
g. Stage 7: severe cognitive decline.
   i. End stage of NCD due to AD
   ii. Unable to recognize family members
   iii. Bedfast and aphasic
   iv. Appetite decreases and **dysphagia** present
   v. Aspiration is common
   vi. Weight loss
   vii. Muscle rigidity
   viii. Primitive reflexes present
   ix. Problems of immobility (decubiti and contractures)
   x. Depressed immune system

🛑 In the late stages of NCD due to Alzheimer's disease, a depressed immune system coupled with immobility may lead to the development of pneumonia, urinary tract infections, sepsis, and pressure ulcers.

   xi. Sleep-wake cycle greatly altered
D. Vascular NCD differs from NCD due to AD in that it has a more abrupt onset and runs a highly variable course
1. More common in men than in women.
2. Prognosis worse than for Alzheimer's clients.

DID YOU KNOW?
The 3-year mortality rate for clients over age 85 years is 67% for vascular NCD, 42% in NCD due to Alzheimer's disease, and 23% in individuals with no NCD. Outcomes are ultimately dependent on the underlying risk factors and mechanism of disease.

3. Memory loss often occurs later in vascular NCD than in NCD due to AD.
4. Memory problems are noticed first in NCD due to AD; people diagnosed with vascular NCD first note problems with reflexes, gait, and muscle weakness.
5. Progression of the symptoms occurs in "steps" rather than as a gradual deterioration.
6. Irregular patterns of decline appear to be an intense source of anxiety.

7. Clients suffer small strokes that destroy many areas of the brain.
8. Pattern of deficits variable, depending on affected regions of the brain.
9. Common neurological signs include:
   a. Weakness of the limbs.
   b. Small-stepped gait.
   c. Difficulty with speech.
E. Frontotemporal NCD
   1. Formerly identified as Pick's disease.
   2. Symptoms tend to fall into two clinical patterns:
      a. Behavioral and personality changes.
         i. Increasingly inappropriate actions
         ii. Lack of judgment and inhibition
         iii. Repetitive compulsive behavior
      b. Speech and language problems.
         i. Marked impairment or loss of speech
         ii. Increasing difficulty in using and understanding written and spoken language
   3. Frontotemporal NCD progresses steadily and often rapidly, ranging from less than 2 years to more than 10 years.
F. NCD due to traumatic brain injury
   1. Symptoms include:
      a. Loss of consciousness.
      b. Posttraumatic amnesia.
      c. Disorientation and confusion.
      d. Neurological signs.
         i. **Amnesia** is the most common neurobehavioral symptom after head trauma
         ii. Neuroimaging demonstrates injury
         iii. New onset of seizures or a marked worsening of a preexisting seizure disorder
         iv. Visual field cuts
         v. **Anosmia**
         vi. Hemiparesis
         vii. Confusion and changes in speech, vision, and personality
   2. Depending on the severity of the injury, symptoms may eventually subside or may become permanent.

DID YOU KNOW?

Repeated head trauma, such as the type experienced by boxers, can result in *dementia pugilistica,* a syndrome characterized by emotional lability, **dysarthria, ataxia,** and impulsivity.

G. NCD due to Lewy body dementia
   1. Twenty-five percent of all NCD cases.
   2. Clinically similar to AD.
   3. Tends to progress more rapidly.
   4. Earlier appearance of visual hallucinations and parkinsonian features.
   5. Presence of Lewy bodies (eosinophilic inclusion bodies) seen in the cerebral cortex and brainstem.

6. Highly sensitive to extrapyramidal effects of antipsychotic medications.
7. Progressive and irreversible.
H. NCD due to Parkinson's disease
   1. Sixty percent of clients with Parkinson's disease acquire NCD.
   2. Loss of nerve cells located in the substantia nigra.
   3. Dopamine activity diminished, resulting in involuntary muscle movements, slowness, and rigidity.
   4. Tremor in the upper extremities.
   5. Cerebral changes closely resemble those of AD.
I. NCD due to HIV infection
   1. The severity of symptoms is correlated to the extent of brain pathology.
   2. In early stages, neuropsychiatric symptoms may be barely perceptible.
   3. In later stages:
      a. Severe cognitive changes.
      b. Confusion.
      c. Changes in behavior.
      d. May have psychotic symptoms.
      e. With antiretroviral therapies, incidence rates of NCD due to HIV infection on decline.
      f. Prolonged life span of HIV-infected clients may increase incidence.
J. Substance-induced NCD
   1. Symptoms are consistent with major or mild NCD.
   2. Symptoms not better explained by substance intoxication, substance withdrawal, or other non–substance use disorder conditions.
K. NCD due to Huntington's disease
   1. Onset of symptoms usually occurs between age 30 and 50 years.
   2. Symptoms include:
      a. Involuntary twitching of the limbs or facial muscles.
      b. Mild cognitive changes.
      c. Depression.
      d. Apathy.
      e. Profound state of cognitive impairment.
      f. Ataxia.
   3. The average duration of the disease is based on age at onset.
   4. Median duration of the disease 21.4 years.
L. NCD due to Prion disease
   1. Evidence from the history, physical examination, or laboratory findings is attributable to prion disease.

DID YOU KNOW?

Prion diseases include Creutzfeldt-Jakob disease or bovine spongiform encephalopathy (mad cow disease).

2. Clinical presentation typical of mild or major NCD.
3. Symptoms include:
   a. Involuntary movements.
   b. Muscle rigidity.
   c. Ataxia.
4. May develop at any age but typically occurs between ages 40 and 60 years.
5. Clinical course extremely rapid.
6. Progression from diagnosis to death in less than 2 years.

M. NCD due to another medical condition
   1. Symptoms are consistent with major or mild NCD.
   2. History of another general medical condition.

VIII. Nursing Process: Diagnosis (Analysis)

Table 15.2 presents a list of client behaviors and the NANDA nursing diagnoses that correspond to those behaviors, which may be used in planning care for the client with a NCD.

IX. Nursing Process: Planning

The following outcomes may be developed to guide the care of a client diagnosed with NCD. **The client will:**

A. Not experienced physical injury
B. Not harm self or others
C. Maintain reality orientation to the best of his or her capability
D. Be able to communicate with consistent caregiver
E. Fulfill activities of daily living with assistance (or for client who is unable: has needs met, as anticipated by caregiver)
F. Discuss positive aspects about self and life

X. Nursing Process: Implementation

A. Interventions for clients at risk for trauma
   1. Arrange furniture and other items in the room to accommodate client's disabilities.
   2. Store frequently used items within easy access.
   3. Maintain bed in low position.
   4. When in bed, keep bed rails up.
   5. Pad side rails and headboard (with history of seizures).
   6. Assign room near nurses' station.
   7. Observe frequently.
   8. Assist client with ambulation.
   9. Keep a dim light on at night.
   10. Frequently orient client to place, time, and situation.
   11. If client is prone to wander, provide an area within which wandering can be carried out safely.
   12. If client is very disoriented and hyperactive, may need soft restraints.
B. Interventions for clients with disturbed thought processes; impaired memory
   1. Frequently orient client to reality.
   2. Use clocks and calendars with large numbers that are easy to read.
   3. Use notes and large, bold signs as reminders.

DID YOU KNOW?

There has been some criticism in recent years about reality orientation of individuals with NCD (particularly those with moderate to severe disease processes), suggesting that constant relearning of material contributes to problems with mood and self-esteem.

   4. Allow client to have personal belongings.
   5. Keep explanations simple.

Table 15.2 Assigning Nursing Diagnoses to Behaviors Commonly Associated With Neurocognitive Disorders

Behaviors	Nursing Diagnoses
Falls, wandering, poor coordination, confusion, misinterpretation of the environment (illusions, hallucinations), lack of understanding of environmental hazards, memory deficits	Risk for trauma
Disorientation, confusion, memory deficits, inaccurate interpretation of the environment, suspiciousness, paranoia	Disturbed thought processes*; impaired memory
Having hallucinations (hears voices, sees visions, feels crawling sensation on skin)	Disturbed sensory perception*
Aggressiveness, assaultiveness (hitting, scratching, or kicking)	Risk for other-directed violence
Inability to name objects/people, loss of memory for words, difficulty finding the right word, confabulation, incoherent, screaming and demanding verbalizations	Impaired verbal communication
Inability to perform activities of daily living (ADLs): feeding, dressing, hygiene, toileting	Self-care deficit (specify)
Expressions of shame and self-degradation, progressive social isolation, apathy, decreased activity, withdrawal, depressed mood	Situational low self-esteem; grieving

*These nursing diagnoses have been resigned from the NANDA-I list of approved diagnoses, but are used for purposes of this text.

6. Use face-to-face interaction.
7. Speak slowly and do not shout.
8. Discourage rumination of delusional thinking.
9. Talk about real events and real people.
10. Appreciate the client's level of reality.
11. Be truthful to the client.
12. Use validation therapy and redirection.
13. Monitor for medication side effects.

🛑 Physiological changes in the elderly can alter the body's response to certain medications. It is critical to monitor the client's responses to medication because toxic effects may intensify altered thought processes.

14. Encourage client to view old photograph albums.
15. Utilize **reminiscence therapy.**
C. Interventions for clients with altered sensory perception
1. Note behaviors indicating the presence of hallucinations.

🛑 Altered sensory perceptions are very real and often very frightening to the client diagnosed with NCD. Unless they are appropriately managed, hallucinations can escalate into disturbing and even hostile behaviors.

2. Assess physical conditions or effects of medications as possible reasons for disturbed perceptions.

DID YOU KNOW?

Physical changes in the elderly result in less ability to metabolize medications, causing an increased risk of side effects. Some infections are also known to cause hallucinations in the elderly.

3. Check to ensure that hearing aids are working properly and that faulty sounds are not being emitted.
4. Check to ensure client is wearing correct eyeglasses.
5. Move or cover an item that might generate visual hallucinations.

MAKING THE CONNECTION

Reality orientation and validation therapy increase a sense of self-worth and personal dignity for clients with NCD. Validation therapy consists of communicating with clients by validating and respecting their feelings in whatever time or place is real to them at the time, even though this may not correspond with "here and now" reality. Validation therapy validates the feelings and emotions of a person with NCD. It often also integrates redirection techniques by steering clients to do something else without them realizing they are actually being redirected.

DID YOU KNOW?

Clients diagnosed with NCD often see faces in patterns on fabrics or in pictures on the wall. A mirror can also be the culprit of false perceptions.

6. Distract the client.
7. Focus on real situations and real people.
8. Use validation therapy if appropriate.
D. Interventions for clients with self-care deficits
1. Provide a simple, structured environment:
   a. Identify self-care deficits and provide assistance as required.
   b. Provide guidance and support to promote independent actions as able.
   c. Allow plenty of time for client to perform tasks.
   d. Talk client through tasks one step at a time.
   e. Provide a structured schedule of activities that is consistent from day to day.
   f. ADLs should follow usual routine as closely as possible.
   g. Provide for consistency in assignment of daily caregivers.
2. Perform ongoing assessment of ability to fulfill nutritional needs.
3. Ensure personal safety.
4. Administer medications and be alert for side effects.
5. For outpatient care:
   a. Assess prospective caregivers' ability to anticipate and fulfill unmet needs.
   b. Teach caregivers how to effectively meet client's needs.
   c. Provide caregivers with information about available community support systems.
      i. Adult day-care centers
      ii. Housekeeping and homemaker services
      iii. Respite-care services
      iv. Local chapter of a national support organization (National Parkinson's Foundation, Alzheimer's Association)

XI. Nursing Process: Evaluation

A. Evaluation is based on a series of short-term rather than long-term goals
B. Resolution of identified problems is unrealistic
C. Outcomes measured in terms of slowing down the process rather than curing the problem
D. Evaluation questions may include the following:
1. Has the client experienced injury?
2. Does the client maintain orientation to time, person, place, and situation most of the time?
3. Is the client able to fulfill basic needs? Have those needs unmet by the client been fulfilled by caregivers?

4. Do familiar objects and structured, routine schedule of activities minimize confusion?
5. Do the prospective caregivers have information regarding the progression of the client's illness?
6. Do caregivers have information regarding where to go for assistance and support in the care of their loved one?
7. Have the prospective caregivers received instruction in how to promote the client's safety, minimize confusion and disorientation, and cope with difficult client behaviors (hostility, anger, depression, agitation)?

XII. Treatment Modalities

A. Delirium
   1. First step is determination and correction of the underlying causes.
   2. Attention to fluid and electrolyte status, hypoxia, anoxia, and diabetic problems.
   3. Remain with client at all times to monitor behavior and provide reorientation and assurance.
   4. Maintain a low level of stimuli.
   5. Medications may compound the syndrome of brain dysfunction.
   6. Agitation and aggression may require chemical and/or mechanical restraint for safety.
      a. Choice of specific therapy based on client's clinical condition and the underlying cause.
      b. Low-dose antipsychotics are the pharmacological treatment of choice in most cases.
      c. Benzodiazepines (e.g., lorazepam [Ativan]) are commonly used when etiology is substance withdrawal.
B. Neurocognitive disorder (NCD)
   1. Primary consideration is the etiology.
   2. Focus directed to the identification and resolution of potentially reversible processes.
   3. Complete a medical and neurological work-up.
   4. Ten to fifteen percent of clients have a potentially reversible condition if treatment is initiated before permanent brain damage.
      a. Hypothyroidism.
      b. Normal pressure hydrocephalus.
      c. Brain tumors.
   5. General supportive care, with provisions for security, stimulation, patience, and nutrition.
   6. Pharmaceutical agents have been tried, with varying degrees of success.
   7. Medications are used for various symptoms.
      a. A summary of medications for clients with NCD is provided in Table 15.3.
      b. Cognitive impairment improves with administration of cholinesterase inhibitors

and *N*-methyl-D-aspartate (NMDA) receptor antagonists (Namenda).
   c. Agitation, aggression, hallucinations, thought disturbances, and wandering improve with administration of antipsychotics.
   d. Depression improves with administration of antidepressants.
      i. Selective serotonin reuptake inhibitors (SSRIs) are the first line drug treatment for depression in the elderly because of favorable side effect profile
      ii. Although still used by some physicians, tricyclic antidepressants are often avoided because of cardiac and anticholinergic side effects
      iii. Trazodone (Desyrel) may be used at bedtime for depression and insomnia
      iv. Dopaminergic agents (e.g., methylphenidate [Ritalin], amantadine [Symmetrel], bromocriptine [Parlodel], and bupropion [Wellbutrin]) helpful in the treatment of severe apathy
      v. The U.S. Food and Drug Administration has ordered black-box warnings on drug labels of all typical and atypical antipsychotics due to an increased risk of death in elderly clients with psychotic behaviors associated with NCD
      vi. Most deaths appeared to be cardiovascular related

🛑 Recognizing the symptoms of depression in individuals experiencing NCD is a challenge. Depression, which affects thinking, memory, sleep, and appetite and interferes with daily life, is sometimes difficult to distinguish from NCD. Clearly, the existence of depression in the client with NCD complicates and worsens the individual's functioning.

   a. Anxiety improves with administration of anxiolytics.
      i. Progressive loss of mental functioning is significant source of anxiety in the early stages of NCD
      ii. Antianxiety medications may be helpful but should not be used routinely or for prolonged periods
      iii. The least toxic and most effective of the antianxiety medications are the benzodiazepines
      iv. Drugs with shorter half-lives (e.g., lorazepam [Ativan] and oxazepam [Serax]) are preferred to longer-acting medications (e.g., diazepam [Valium]), which promote a higher risk of oversedation and falls
      v. Barbiturates are not appropriate as antianxiety agents because they can induce

Table 15.3 Selected Medications Used in the Treatment of Clients With NCD

Medication	Classification	For Treatment of	Daily Dosage Range (mg)	Side Effects
Tacrine (Cognex)	Cholinesterase inhibitor	Cognitive impairment	40–160	Dizziness, headache, GI upset, elevated transaminase
Donepezil (Aricept)	Cholinesterase inhibitor	Cognitive impairment	5–10	Insomnia, dizziness, GI upset, headache
Rivastigmine (Exelon)	Cholinesterase inhibitor	Cognitive impairment	6–12	Dizziness, headache, GI upset, fatigue
Galantamine (Razadyne)	Cholinesterase inhibitor	Cognitive impairment	8–24	Dizziness, headache, GI upset
Memantine (Namenda)	NMDA receptor antagonist	Cognitive impairment	5–20	Dizziness, headache, constipation
Risperidone * (Risperdal)	Antipsychotic	Agitation, aggression, hallucinations, thought disturbances, wandering	1–4 (Increase dosage cautiously)	Agitation, insomnia, headache, insomnia, extrapyramidal symptoms
Olanzapine * (Zyprexa)	Antipsychotic	Agitation, aggression, hallucinations, thought disturbances, wandering	5 (Increase dosage cautiously)	Hypotension, dizziness, sedation, constipation, weight gain, dry mouth
Quetiapine * (Seroquel)	Antipsychotic	Agitation, aggression, hallucinations, thought disturbances, wandering	Initial dose 25 (Titrate slowly)	Hypotension, tachycardia, dizziness, drowsiness, headache, constipation, dry mouth
Haloperidol * (Haldol)	Antipsychotic	Agitation, aggression, hallucinations, thought disturbances, wandering	1–4 (Increase dosage cautiously)	Dry mouth, blurred vision, orthostatic hypotension, extrapyramidal symptoms, sedation
Sertraline (Zoloft)	Antidepressant (SSRI)	Depression	50–100	Fatigue, insomnia, sedation, GI upset, headache, dizziness
Paroxetine (Paxil)	Antidepressant (SSRI)	Depression	10–40	Dizziness, headache, insomnia, somnolence, GI upset
Nortriptyline (Pamelor)	Antidepressant (tricyclic)	Depression	30–50	Anticholinergic, orthostatic hypotension, sedation, arrhythmia
Lorazepam (Ativan)	Antianxiety (benzodiazepine)	Anxiety	1–2	Drowsiness, dizziness, GI upset, hypotension, tolerance, dependence
Oxazepam (Serax)	Antianxiety (benzodiazepine)	Anxiety	10–30	Drowsiness, dizziness, GI upset, hypotension, tolerance, dependence
Temazepam (Restoril)	Sedative/Hypnotic (benzodiazepine)	Insomnia	15	Drowsiness, dizziness, GI upset, hypotension, tolerance, dependence
Zolpidem (Ambien)	Sedative/Hypnotic (nonbenzodiazepine)	Insomnia	5	Headache, drowsiness, dizziness, GI upset
Zaleplon (Sonata)	Sedative/Hypnotic (nonbenzodiazepine)	Insomnia	5	Headache, drowsiness, dizziness, GI upset
Eszopiclone (Lunesta)	Sedative-hypnotic (nonbenzodiazepine)	Insomnia	1–2	Headache, drowsiness, dizziness, GI upset, unpleasant taste
Trazodone (Desyrel)	Antidepressant (heterocyclic)	Depression and Insomnia	50	Dizziness, drowsiness, dry mouth, blurred vision, GI upset
Mirtazapine (Remeron)	Antidepressant (tetracyclic)	Depression and Insomnia	7.5–15	Somnolence, dry mouth, constipation, increased appetite

*Although clinicians may still prescribe these medications in low-risk patients, no antipsychotics have been approved by the Food and Drug Administration for the treatment of patients with NCD-related psychosis. All antipsychotics include black-box warnings about increased risk of death in elderly patients with NCD.

GI, gastrointestinal; NCD, neurocognitive disorder; NMDA, *N*-methyl-D-aspartate.

confusion and paradoxical excitement in the elderly

b. Insomnia improves with administration of sedative-hypnotics.

   i. Because of potential for adverse drug reactions in the elderly, many of whom are already taking multiple medications, pharmacological treatment of insomnia should be considered only after attempts at non-pharmacological strategies have failed

   ii. Behavioral approaches to sleep problems

     a) Rising at the same time each morning

     b) Minimizing daytime sleep

     c) Participating in regular physical exercise (but no later than 4 hours before bedtime)

     d) Getting proper nutrition

     e) Avoiding alcohol, caffeine, and nicotine

     f) Retiring at the same time each night

   iii. Sedative-hypnotic medications may cause:

     a) Daytime sedation and cognitive impairment

     b) Paradoxical agitation.

DID YOU KNOW?

Many antipsychotic, antidepressant, and antihistaminic medications produce anticholinergic side effects, which include confusion, blurred vision, constipation, dry mouth, dizziness, and difficulty urinating. Older people, and especially those with NCD, are particularly sensitive to these effects because of decreased cholinergic reserves. Many elderly individuals are also at increased risk for developing an anticholinergic toxicity syndrome because of the additive anticholinergic effects of multiple medications.

REVIEW QUESTIONS

1. _____ is a mental state characterized by a disturbance of cognition, which is manifested by confusion, excitement, disorientation, and a clouding of consciousness.

2. A nurse is planning a therapeutic interaction with a client diagnosed with NCD due to Alzheimer's disease. At what time during a 24-hour period should a nurse expect this client to have the most difficulty responding appropriately?
   1. When the client first awakens in the morning
   2. When the client abruptly awakens in the morning
   3. When the client awakens from a late afternoon nap
   4. When the client awakens from an early morning nap

3. What facts should be included in an in-service focusing on NCD due to Alzheimer's disease (AD)? **Select all that apply.**
   1. NCD due to AD has a high mortality rate.
   2. NCD due to AD clients have an overabundance of structures called plaques and tangles in the brain.
   3. The brains of NCD due to AD clients contain cellular particles called tau proteins.
   4. Clients diagnosed with NCD due to AD have a rapid onset of signs and symptoms.
   5. Clients diagnosed with NCD due to AD have a dramatic increase in the production of acetylcholine.

4. _____ is the current term used to describe cognitive functions closely linked to particular areas of the brain that have to do with thinking, reasoning, memory, learning, and speaking.

5. An instructor is teaching students about neurocognitive disorders (NCD). Which of the following statements indicate that learning has occurred? **Select all that apply.**
   1. "Vascular NCD is the most common form of NCD."
   2. "After heart disease and cancer, vascular NCD is the third most costly disease to society."
   3. "Prevalence of NCD due to Alzheimer's disease doubles for every 5-year age group beyond age 65."
   4. "NCD due to AD affects 24% of people aged 80 to 89."
   5. "NCD due to Huntington's disease is transmitted as a mendelian dominant gene."

6. The progressive symptoms associated with NCD due to Alzheimer's disease are described in seven stages. Order the symptoms that occur in these stages.
   1. _____ Family begins to notice client has problems recalling names; gets lost when driving.
   2. _____ No apparent decline in memory.
   3. _____ Client begins to forget major events in personal history; can't manage finances; denies a problem and becomes depressed.
   4. _____ Client begins to be aware of short-term memory loss; forgets names; loses things.
   5. _____ Client unable to recognize family members; bedfast and aphasic, only primitive reflexes present.
   6. _____ Client loses ability to perform ADLs independently; disoriented to place/time and is self-absorbed.
   7. _____ Client is disoriented to surroundings; loses language skills, incontinent, wanders, is agitated and aggressive.

7. Which of the following symptoms should a nurse recognize as differentiating a client diagnosed with neurocognitive disorder (NCD) from a client diagnosed with pseudodementia? **Select all that apply.**
   1. Progression of symptoms in NCD is rapid, and in pseudodementia, they are slow.
   2. Memory deficits are progressive in pseudodementia, whereas these deficits are not progressive in NCD.
   3. Wandering frequently occurs with NCD, whereas wandering is infrequent with pseudodementia.
   4. Symptoms of NCD worsen during the day, and symptoms of pseudodementia improve during the day.
   5. Clients diagnosed with NCD appear unconcerned, whereas clients diagnosed with pseudodementia communicate severe distress.

8. A student nurse asks her preceptor, "What can cause reversible neurocognitive disorders (NCD)?" Which response by the preceptor is accurate? **Select all that apply.**
   1. "Reversible NCD can occur as a result of head trauma."
   2. "Reversible NCD can occur as a result of cerebral lesions."
   3. "Reversible NCD can occur as a result of metabolic disorders."
   4. "Reversible NCD can occur as a result of central nervous system infections."
   5. "Reversible NCD can occur as a result of vitamin or nutritional deficiencies."

9. Which symptoms should a nurse recognize that differentiate a client diagnosed with vascular neurocognitive disorder (NCD) from a client diagnosed with NCD due to Alzheimer's disease (AD)? **Select all that apply.**
   1. Clients diagnosed with vascular NCD experience memory loss later in the disease process, whereas clients diagnosed with NCD due to AD experience memory loss earlier.
   2. Clients diagnosed with vascular NCD initially have problems with muscle weakness, whereas clients diagnosed with NCD due to AD initially have problems with memory loss.
   3. Clients diagnosed with vascular NCD have symptoms occurring in steps, whereas clients diagnosed with NCD due to AD have slow, progressive symptoms occurring in stages.
   4. Clients diagnosed with vascular NCD suffer small strokes that destroy many areas of the brain, whereas clients diagnosed with NCD due to AD do not.
   5. Clients diagnosed with vascular NCD have extreme shrinkage of the hippocampus, whereas clients diagnosed with NCD due to AD do not.

10. A nurse is administering a mental status examination to assess for a neurocognitive disorder. What cognitive function is being tested when the nurse asks the client to point to the ceiling?
    1. Comprehension
    2. Orientation
    3. Paired associate learning
    4. New learning ability

11. Choose the correctly matched brain alteration seen in NCD due to Alzheimer's disease with the symptom caused by this alteration?
    1. Alterations in the temporal lobe: anxiety
    2. Alterations in the amygdala: paranoia
    3. Alterations in the frontal lobe: impaired visuospatial skills
    4. Alterations in the hippocampus: inability to use words correctly

12. A client diagnosed with neurocognitive disorder (NCD) has become aggressive toward staff and wanders continuously. Which medication would the nurse expect the physician to order to address these symptoms?
    1. Donepezil (Aricept)
    2. Rivastigmine (Exelon)
    3. Galantamine (Razadyne)
    4. Olanzapine (Zyprexa)

13. A newly admitted client has been prescribed 10 mg of donepezil (Aricept) for the symptoms of neurocognitive disorder (NCD). Which nursing action takes priority related to the care of this client?
    1. Frequently orient the client to objective reality
    2. Keep explanations simple
    3. Assist with ambulation and encourage gradual changes in position
    4. Assess for extrapyramidal symptoms

14. Which symptoms should a nurse recognize as differentiating a client diagnosed with neurocognitive disorder (NCD) from a client diagnosed with delirium?
    1. Depression is common in NCD but much less common in delirium.
    2. Symptoms of delirium develop rapidly, whereas symptoms of NCD develop more slowly.
    3. Disorientation to place and time is common in NCD and limited in delirium.
    4. Impairment of recent memory occurs with NCD but not with delirium.

15. Which symptoms should a nurse recognize as characteristic of a diagnosis of neurocognitive disorder due to prion disease?
    1. The onset of the disease is abrupt and obvious.
    2. Once symptoms present, the progression of the disease slows.
    3. Motor features such as myoclonus and ataxia are characteristic.
    4. Clinical course is chronic, lasting 10 to 20 years.

16. An elderly, hypertensive client, diagnosed with NCD due to Lewy body dementia has been prescribed quetiapine (Seroquel). Why would the nurse question this order?
    1. Quetiapine may increase the production of Lewy bodies in the client's brain.
    2. The client's sensitivity to the extrapyramidal side effects of this medication.
    3. There is a black-box warning related to prescribing quetiapine for elderly clients.
    4. The client's hypertension will be exacerbated by this medication.

17. Which nursing documentation entry accurately describes a client's use of confabulation?
    1. "Attempts to communicate by using rhyming words."
    2. "Nonverbals indicate communication with unseen others."
    3. "Verbalized happiness about trip to park which was not based in fact."
    4. "Rambles about early childhood experiences jumping from topic to topic."

18. A client diagnosed with NCD due to Alzheimer's disease is currently in the sixth stage of the disease process. On the basis of symptoms typical of this stage, which of the following nursing diagnoses would be assigned? **Select all that apply.**
   1. Disturbed body image R/T perceived loss of control over quality of life
   2. Disturbed sleep pattern R/T psychomotor agitation
   3. Risk for other directed violence R/T disorientation and confusion
   4. Impaired verbal communication R/T loss of language skills
   5. Ineffective denial R/T underlying fears and anxieties

19. A postgraduate nursing student is writing a research thesis on medications known to precipitate delirium. Which of the following classifications of medications should be included in this paper? **Select all that apply.**
   1. Anticholinergics
   2. Antivirals
   3. Antihypertensives
   4. Antidiabetics
   5. Anticonvulsants

20. Which of the following stages of NCD due to Alzheimer's disease (AD) is correctly matched with the nursing diagnosis which addresses the problems typical of this stage. **Select all that apply.**
   1. Stage 2: self-care deficit
   2. Stage 3: ineffective role performance
   3. Stage 4: ineffective denial
   4. Stage 5: risk for other-directed violence
   5. Stage 7: risk for altered skin integrity

REVIEW ANSWERS

1. ANSWER: Delirium

Rationale: Delirium is a mental state characterized by a disturbance of cognition that is manifested by confusion, excitement, disorientation, and a clouding of consciousness. Hallucinations and illusions are common. There is a disturbance in the level of awareness and a change in cognition that develops rapidly over a short period.

TEST-TAKING TIP: Review the key words at the beginning of the chapter.

Content Area: *Psychosocial Integrity;*
Integrated Process: *Nursing Process: Assessment;*
Client Need: *Psychosocial Integrity;*
Cognitive Level: *Knowledge;*
Concept: *Cognition*

2. ANSWER: 3

Rationale: Individuals diagnosed with NCD due to Alzheimer's disease (AD) have symptoms that can vary throughout the day. They will have times when they perform well, and others when they will have more difficulty responding appropriately. *Sundowning* is the term used to describe the worsening of symptoms that occurs in the late afternoon and evening.

1. Because of sundowning, the nurse should expect this client to have the most difficulty in responding appropriately when the client awakens from a late afternoon nap, not when the client first awakens in the morning.
2. Because of sundowning, the nurse should expect this client to have the most difficulty in responding appropriately when the client awakens from a late afternoon nap, not when the client awakes abruptly in the morning.
3. The nurse should expect this client to have the most difficulty in responding appropriately when the client awakens from a late afternoon nap. This phenomenon is commonly called sundowning.
4. Because of sundowning, the nurse should expect this client to have the most difficulty in responding appropriately when the client awakens from a late afternoon nap, not when the client awakens from an early morning nap.

TEST-TAKING TIP: Review signs and symptoms of NCD due to AD. Familiarize yourself with the term *sundowning,* and know that interactions should be planned when the client is at his or her cognitive best.

Content Area: *Safe and Effective Care Environment: Management of Care;*
Integrated Process: *Nursing Process: Planning;*
Client Need: *Safe and Effective Care Environment: Management of Care;*
Cognitive Level: *Application;*
Concept: *Assessment*

3. ANSWERS: 1, 2, 3

Rationale:
1. A high mortality rate is associated with NCD due to Alzheimer's disease (AD). This information would be appropriate to include in an in-service about NCD due to AD.

2. An overabundance of structures called plaques and tangles are noted in the brains of clients diagnosed with NCD due to AD. This information would be appropriate to include in an in-service about NCD due to AD.
3. Cellular particles called tau protein are noted in the brains of clients diagnosed with NCD due to AD. This information would be appropriate to include in an in-service about NCD due to AD.
4. There is a slow, not rapid, onset of signs and symptoms associated with NCD due to AD. This information is incorrect and would not be included in an in-service about NCD due to AD.
5. Production of acetylcholine is dramatically decreased, not increased, in clients diagnosed with NCD due to AD. This information is incorrect and would not be included in an in-service about NCD due to AD.

TEST-TAKING TIP: Review facts and information about the diagnosis of NCD due to AD.

Content Area: *Safe and Effective Care Environment: Management of Care;*
Integrated Process: *Nursing Process: Assessment;*
Client Need: *Safe and Effective Care Environment: Management of Care;*
Cognitive Level: *Application;*
Concept: *Nursing Roles*

4. ANSWER: Neurocognitive

Rationale: The current term *neurocognitive* is used to describe cognitive functions closely linked to particular areas of the brain that have to do with thinking, reasoning, memory, learning, and speaking. When there is disruption in these processes, a diagnosis of neurocognitive disorder (NCD) should be considered.

TEST-TAKING TIP: Review the key words at the beginning of the chapter.

Content Area: *Psychosocial Integrity;*
Integrated Process: *Nursing Process: Assessment;*
Client Need: *Psychosocial Integrity;*
Cognitive Level: *Knowledge;*
Concept: *Cognition*

5. ANSWERS: 3, 4, 5

Rationale:
1. NCD due to Alzheimer's disease (AD), not vascular neurocognitive disorder (NCD), is the most common form of NCD. This student's statement indicates that more instruction is needed.
2. After heart disease and cancer, NCD due to AD, not vascular NCD, is the third most costly disease to society. This student's statement indicates that more instruction is needed.
3. It is a fact that the prevalence of NCD due to AD doubles for every 5-year age group beyond age 65. This student's statement indicates that learning has occurred.
4. It is a fact that NCD due to AD effects 24% of people ages 80 to 89. This student's statement indicates that learning has occurred.
5. It is a fact that NCD due to Huntington's disease is transmitted as a mendelian dominant gene. This student's statement indicates that learning has occurred.

TEST-TAKING TIP: Review the epidemiological implications for the various types of NCDs.

Content Area: Safe and Effective Care Environment:
Management of Care;
Integrated Process: Nursing Process: Evaluation;
Client Need: Safe and Effective Care Environment:
Management of Care;
Cognitive Level: Application;
Concept: Assessment

6. **ANSWER: The correct order is 3, 1, 4, 2, 7, 5, 6**
Rationale: The progressive nature of symptoms associated with NCD due to Alzheimer's disease (AD) has been described by the Alzheimer's Association according to the following seven stages:
1. Stage 1: No symptoms—no apparent symptoms and no decline in memory.
2. Stage 2: forgetfulness—begins to lose things; forgets people's names and experiences short-term memory loss. Client is aware of intellectual decline.
3. Stage 3: mild cognitive decline—difficulty recalling names or words, noticeable to family; may get lost when driving his or her car. Experiences interrupted concentration.
4. Stage 4: mild-to-moderate cognitive decline—may forget major events in personal history. Ability to perform tasks such as managing personal finances declines. May deny problem exists and cover up memory loss with confabulation (creating imaginary events to fill in memory gaps). Depression and social withdrawal are common.
5. Stage 5: moderate cognitive decline—loss of ability to perform some activities of daily living independently; disoriented about place and time; and is self-absorbed.
6. Stage 6: moderate-to-severe cognitive decline—disoriented to surroundings; urinary and fecal incontinence common; wanders and can be obsessive, agitated, and aggressive.
7. Stage 7: severe cognitive decline—end stage of NCD due to AD; unable to recognize family members; bedfast and aphasic, aspiration common; weight loss, muscle rigidity, and only primitive reflexes present.
TEST-TAKING TIP: Review the stages that describe the progression of the symptoms of NCD due to Alzheimer's disease.
Content Area: Safe and Effective Care Environment:
Management of Care;
Integrated Process: Nursing Process: Evaluation;
Client Need: Safe and Effective Care Environment:
Management of Care;
Cognitive Level: Analysis;
Concept: Assessment

7. **ANSWERS: 4, 5**
Rationale:
1. Progression of symptoms in pseudodementia, not NCD, is rapid. NCD has a slow progression of symptoms.
2. There is no evidence of a progressive memory deficit in pseudodementia. NCD causes progressive memory deficits.
3. Clients diagnosed with NCD may wander in search of the familiar. Clients diagnosed with pseudodementia rarely wander.
4. **Symptoms of NCD worsen as the day progresses. Symptoms of pseudodementia get better as the day progresses.**

5. **A client diagnosed with NCD appears unconcerned. A client diagnosed with pseudodementia will communicate severe distress.**
TEST-TAKING TIP: Review Table 15.1, "A Comparison of Neurocognitive Disorder and Pseudodementia."
Content Area: Safe and Effective Care Environment:
Management of Care;
Integrated Process: Nursing Process: Evaluation;
Client Need: Safe and Effective Care Environment:
Management of Care;
Cognitive Level: Analysis;
Concept: Cognition

8. **ANSWERS: 2, 3, 4, 5**
Rationale: In most clients, neurocognitive disorder (NCD) runs a progressive and irreversible course. The reversibility of NCD is dependent on the basic etiology of the disorder.
1. Head trauma may increase an individual's risk for an eventual diagnosis of Alzheimer's disease. However, head trauma, in and of itself, does not normally result in a diagnosis of reversible NCD.
2. **Reversible NCD can occur as a result of cerebral lesions.**
3. **Reversible NCD can occur as a result of metabolic disorders.**
4. **Reversible NCD can occur as a result of central nervous system infections.**
5. **Reversible NCD can occur as a result of vitamin or nutritional deficiencies, especially B_{12} or folate.**
TEST-TAKING TIP: Review the factors associated with the etiology of reversible neurocognitive disorders.
Content Area: Safe and Effective Care Environment:
Management of Care;
Integrated Process: Nursing Process: Implementation;
Client Need: Safe and Effective Care Environment:
Management of Care;
Cognitive Level: Application;
Concept: Assessment

9. **ANSWERS: 1, 2, 3, 4**
Rationale:
1. **Clients diagnosed with vascular NCD experience memory loss later in the disease process, whereas clients diagnosed with NCD due to AD have an early-onset memory loss.**
2. **Typically, individuals diagnosed with NCD due to AD notice memory loss first. In contrast, individuals diagnosed with vascular NCD initially experience problems with reflexes, gait, and muscle weakness.**
3. **Clients diagnosed with vascular NCD have progressive symptoms occurring in steps, whereas clients diagnosed with NCD due to AD have symptoms that are slow and insidious and that occur progressively through seven stages.**
4. **In vascular NCD, clients suffer the equivalent of small strokes that destroy many areas of the brain. The pattern of deficits is variable, depending on which regions of the brain have been affected. In NCD due to AD, there are changes in the brain to include enlarged ventricles and shrinkage of the cerebral cortex and hippocampus; however, stroke is not considered a factor.**

5. In NCD due to AD, there are changes in the brain to include enlarged ventricles and shrinkage of the cerebral cortex and hippocampus, whereas with a diagnosis of vascular NCD, shrinkage of the hippocampus is not noted.

TEST-TAKING TIP: Review the facts associated with vascular NCD and NCD due to AD. Be prepared to compare and contrast the signs and symptoms of each.

Content Area: Safe and Effective Care Environment: Management of Care;
Integrated Process: Nursing Process: Evaluation;
Client Need: Safe and Effective Care Environment: Management of Care;
Cognitive Level: Analysis;
Concept: Critical Thinking

10. **ANSWER: 1**

Rationale:

1. Comprehension is the action or capability of understanding. If the client can follow the directions the nurse provides, it indicates understanding and demonstrates intact comprehension.

2. Orientation is a function of the mind involving awareness of three dimensions: time, place, and person. Typically, disorientation occurs first in time, then in place, and finally in person. Asking for the date, day of the week, month, and year will test for orientation.

3. Paired associate learning is an aspect of verbal learning and is the learning of pairs of items, usually words, until the presentation of one leads to the recall of the other. It is an example of associative memory. Presenting a list of paired words and testing the client's recall of the word pairs tests for associative memory.

4. Learning is the ability to comprehend and to understand and profit from experience. A new learning ability test in a mental status examination measures learned recall of three separate words.

TEST-TAKING TIP: Review Box 15.2, "Mental Status Examination for Neurocognitive Disorder (NCD)."

Content Area: Safe and Effective Care Environment: Management of Care;
Integrated Process: Nursing Process: Assessment;
Client Need: Safe and Effective Care Environment: Management of Care;
Cognitive Level: Application;
Concept: Nursing Roles

11. **ANSWER: 2**

Rationale:

1. Alterations in the temporal lobe of the brain can cause the inability to recall words or the inability to use words correctly (language comprehension). In late stages, some clients experience delusions, and hallucinations. Anxiety is not associated with alterations in the temporal lobe.

2. Alterations in the amygdala can cause impaired emotions: depression, anxiety, fear, personality changes, apathy, and paranoia.

3. Alterations in the frontal lobe of the brain can cause impaired reasoning ability, the inability to solve problems and perform familiar tasks, poor judgment, the inability to evaluate the appropriateness of behavior, and

aggressiveness. Impaired visuospatial skills are not associated with alterations in the frontal lobe.

4. Alterations in the hippocampus can cause impaired memory. Short-term memory is affected initially, and later the individual is unable to form new memories. Inability to use words correctly is not associated with alterations in the hippocampus.

TEST-TAKING TIP: Review Figure 15.2 "Neurobiology of NCD due to Alzheimer's Disease."

Content Area: Safe and Effective Care Environment: Management of Care;
Integrated Process: Nursing Process: Assessment;
Client Need: Safe and Effective Care Environment: Management of Care;
Cognitive Level: Application;
Concept: Cognition

12. **ANSWER: 4**

Rationale:

1. Donepezil (Aricept) is a cholinesterase inhibitor that addresses the symptom of cognitive impairment, not aggression and wandering.

2. Rivastigmine (Exelon) is a cholinesterase inhibitor that addresses the symptom of cognitive impairment, not aggression and wandering.

3. Galantamine (Razadyne) is a cholinesterase inhibitor that addresses the symptom of cognitive impairment, not aggression and wandering.

4. Olanzapine (Zyprexa) is an antipsychotic that would address the symptoms of agitation, aggression, hallucinations, thought disturbances, and wandering.

TEST-TAKING TIP: Review Table 15.3, "Selected Medications Used in the Treatment of Clients with Neurocognitive Disorder (NCD)."

Content Area: Safe and Effective Care Environment: Management of Care;
Integrated Process: Nursing Process: Evaluation;
Client Need: Safe and Effective Care Environment: Management of Care;
Cognitive Level: Application;
Concept: Medication

13. **ANSWER: 3**

Rationale:

1. It is important to orient clients diagnosed with neurocognitive disorder (NCD) to reality, but compared with the other nursing actions presented, this intervention does not take priority.

2. It is important to keep explanations simple when interacting with clients diagnosed with NCD, but compared with the other nursing actions presented, this intervention does not take priority.

3. Because one of the side effects of donepezil (Aricept) is dizziness, priority must be given to assisting with ambulation and encouraging gradual changes in position to avoid client injury. Client safety is always prioritized.

4. Extrapyramidal symptoms are a side effect of antipsychotic medications not donepezil, which is a cholinesterase inhibitor.

TEST-TAKING TIP: Review Table 15.3, "Selected Medications Used in the Treatment of Clients with Neurocognitive Disorder."
Content Area: Safe and Effective Care Environment: Management of Care;
Integrated Process: Nursing Process: Implementation;
Client Need: Safe and Effective Care Environment: Management of Care;
Cognitive Level: Analysis
Concept: Medication

14. **ANSWER: 2**
Rationale:
1. In delirium, emotional instability is manifested by fear, anxiety, depression, irritability, anger, euphoria, or apathy. Depression and social withdrawal are common with the mild to moderate cognitive decline of NCD.
2. Symptoms of delirium usually begin quite abruptly and rapidly, over a short period of time. In NCD, symptoms develop slowly over a longer period of time.
3. In delirium, disorientation to time and place is common. Disorientation to time and place is also present in NCD.
4. Impairment of recent memory is evident in both NCD and delirium.
TEST-TAKING TIP: Review the signs and symptoms of both delirium and NCD and be prepared to compare and contrast the two disorders.
Content Area: Safe and Effective Care Environment: Management of Care;
Integrated Process: Nursing Process: Evaluation;
Client Need: Safe and Effective Care Environment: Management of Care;
Cognitive Level: Analysis
Concept: Critical Thinking

15. **ANSWER: 3**
Rationale:
1. Neurocognitive disorder (NCD) due to prion disease is identified by its insidious onset.
2. NCD due to prion disease progresses rapidly.
3. NCD due to prion disease is identified by manifestations of motor features, such as myoclonus or ataxia.
4. The clinical course of NCD due to prion disease is extremely rapid, with the progression from diagnosis to death in less than 2 years.
TEST-TAKING TIP: Review the characteristic of NCD due to prion disease.
Content Area: Safe and Effective Care Environment: Management of Care;
Integrated Process: Nursing Process: Assessment;
Client Need: Safe and Effective Care Environment: Management of Care;
Cognitive Level: Application;
Concept: Assessment

16. **ANSWER: 2**
Rationale:
1. Quetiapine (Seroquel) is an antipsychotic medication sometimes used in neurocognitive disorders (NCD) to address symptoms of agitation, aggression, hallucinations, thought disturbances, and wandering. It does not increase the production of Lewy bodies in the brain.
2. Clients diagnosed with NCD due to Lewy body dementia are highly sensitive to the extrapyramidal side effects of antipsychotic medications.
3. There is no black-box warning related to prescribing quetiapine for elderly clients.
4. Hypotension, not hypertension, is a side effect of quetiapine.
TEST-TAKING TIP: Review the characteristics of Lewy body dementia and note sensitivity to antipsychotic medications.
Content Area: Safe and Effective Care Environment: Management of Care;
Integrated Process: Nursing Process: Evaluation;
Client Need: Safe and Effective Care Environment: Management of Care;
Cognitive Level: Application;
Concept: Medication

17. **ANSWER: 3**
Rationale:
1. The use of rhyming words would be documented as clang associations, not confabulation.
2. Communicating with unseen others is indicative of visual hallucinations, not confabulation.
3. When a client talks about a situation not based in any objective reality, the client is using confabulation. Clients diagnosed with NCD cover up memory loss by the use of confabulation, in which they create imaginary events to fill in memory gaps.
4. Rambling and jumping from topic to topic would be documented as "flight-of-ideas," not confabulation.
TEST-TAKING TIP: Review the key terms at the beginning of this chapter.
Content Area: Safe and Effective Care Environment: Management of Care;
Integrated Process: Nursing Process: Implementation;
Client Need: Safe and Effective Care Environment: Management of Care;
Cognitive Level: Application;
Concept: Communication

18. **ANSWERS: 2, 3, 4**
Rationale:
1. The nursing diagnosis of *disturbed body image* is defined as confusion in a mental picture of one's self. This diagnosis is associated with eating disorders, not with the progressive stages of NCD due to AD.
2. In the sixth stage of the disease process, a client diagnosed with NCD due to AD may have difficulty in sleeping due to psychomotor symptoms, which include wandering, obsessiveness, agitation, and aggression.
3. In the sixth stage of the disease process, a client diagnosed with NCD due to AD may become violent due to disorientation and confusion. Symptoms seem to worsen in the late afternoon and evening. This phenomenon is called *sundowning*.
4. In the sixth stage of the disease process, a client diagnosed with NCD due to AD may experience an increasing loss of language skills leading to *impaired communication*.

5. The nursing diagnosis of *ineffective denial* is defined as a conscious or unconscious attempt to disavow the knowledge or meaning of an event to reduce anxiety. An individual in the sixth stage of the NCD due to AD process would be incapable of employing the defense mechanism of denial.

TEST-TAKING TIP: Review the progression of NCD due to AD and then match the NCD due to AD stage with the appropriate nursing diagnoses that address the problems of that stage.

Content Area: Safe and Effective Care Environment: Management of Care;
Integrated Process: Nursing Process: Diagnosis (Analysis);
Client Need: Safe and Effective Care Environment: Management of Care;
Cognitive Level: Analysis
Concept: Critical Thinking

19. **ANSWERS: 1, 3, 5**
Rationale:
1. Medications that are classified as anticholinergic are known to precipitate delirium and should be included in this thesis paper.
2. Medications that are classified as antivirals are not known to precipitate delirium and should not be included in this thesis paper.
3. Medications that are classified as antihypertensives are known to precipitate delirium and should be included in this thesis paper.
4. Medications that are classified as antidiabetics are not known to precipitate delirium and should not be included in this thesis paper.
5. Medications that are classified as anticonvulsants are known to precipitate delirium and should be included in this thesis paper.

TEST-TAKING TIP: Review medications that can precipitate delirium.

Content Area: Safe and Effective Care Environment: Management of Care;
Integrated Process: Nursing Process: Assessment;

Client Need: Safe and Effective Care Environment: Management of Care;
Cognitive Level: Application;
Concept: Medication

20. **ANSWERS: 2, 3, 5**
Rationale:
1. The diagnosis of *self-care deficit* addresses problems that begin in the sixth, not second, stage of the NCD due to AD process.
2. In the third stage of the NCD due to AD process, clients experience an increasing memory decline, which interferes with work performance. The nursing diagnosis of *ineffective role performance* is correctly matched to this stage of NCD due to AD.
3. In the fourth stage of the NCD due to AD process, clients typically deny that a problem exists and cover up memory loss with confabulation. The nursing diagnosis of *ineffective denial* is correctly matched to this stage of NCD due to AD.
4. The diagnosis of *risk for other-directed violence* addresses problems that begin in the sixth, not the fifth, stage of the NCD due to AD process.
5. In the seventh stage of the NCD due to AD process, clients are typically bedfast. This immobility in combination with poor nutrition and incontinence put the client at high risk for decubiti and contractures. The nursing diagnosis of *risk for altered skin integrity* is correctly matched to this stage of NCD due to AD.

TEST-TAKING TIP: Review the problems associated with the seven stages of NCD due to AD. Consider which nursing diagnoses most accurately describe these problems.

Content Area: Safe and Effective Care Environment: Management of Care;
Integrated Process: Nursing Process: Diagnosis (Analysis);
Client Need: Safe and Effective Care Environment: Management of Care;
Cognitive Level: Analysis
Concept: Critical Thinking

CASE STUDY: Putting it All Together

Jack is a 75-year-old widower of 10 years, who up until 5 years ago was in relatively good physical and mental health. History reveals that Jack owned his own home, has two devoted grown children, and enjoyed a very active social life. After Jack's 70th birthday, his family and close friends began to see progressively more and more forgetfulness and confusion. A time came when his son found his father's front door open, the stove burner on, and Jack not home. The housekeeper reported that Jack was not always taking medication as ordered, dressing bizarrely, and getting lost while driving. With Jack's reluctant agreement, it was decided that an assisted living facility (ALF) might be the safest solution.

During the initial interview with Eve, the psychiatric nurse practitioner, Jack was asked about recent confusion and forgetfulness. He brushed it off saying, "That's nothing but normal aging. This is all a big mistake. I don't belong here. My kids have taken my car away because someone lied and said I was getting lost. That's nonsense!!" After letting Jack vent, Eve administered a mental status examination. Jack scored 57.2. Eve then ordered a complete medical and neurological work-up to include a magnetic resonance tomography (MRI).

During his first year in the ALF, Jack's cognitive abilities began to deteriorate. His appetite declined, he needed reminding to shave and shower, he lost interest in activities, and at times he became belligerent with staff. When Eve questioned him about how he had enjoyed an afternoon activity, he said, "Oh, I met an old friend at the beach, and we watched the dolphins play. It was wonderful." Eve administered another mental status examination. This time Jack's score was 37.0.

1. On the basis of the client symptoms and history, what medical diagnosis would Eve assign to Jack?
2. What might the results from the MRI indicate?
3. What might the results from the two mental status examinations indicate?
4. What should Eve understand about Jack's statement, "Oh, I met an old friend at the beach, and we watched the dolphins play. It was wonderful."
5. Which treatments might Eve employ to assist Jack?
6. What pharmaceutical agents might help Jack?
7. What are Jack's subjective symptoms?
8. What are Jack's objective symptoms?
9. What NANDA nursing diagnosis would address Jack's current problem?
10. Based on this nursing diagnosis, what short-term outcome would be appropriate for Jack?
11. Based on this nursing diagnosis, what long-term outcome would be appropriate for Jack?
12. List the nursing interventions (actions) that will assist Jack in successfully meeting these outcomes.
13. List the questions that should be asked to determine the success of the nursing interventions.

Chapter 16

Somatic Symptom and Dissociative Disorders

KEY TERMS

Amnesia—Pathological loss of memory; a phenomenon in which an area of experience becomes inaccessible to conscious recall; the loss in memory may be organic, emotional, dissociative, or of mixed origin, and may be permanent or limited to a sharply circumscribed period of time

Autogenics—Teaching the body to respond to verbal commands; these commands "tell" the body to relax and control breathing, blood pressure, heartbeat, and body temperature; the goal of autogenics is to achieve deep relaxation and reduce stress

Conversion disorder (Functional neurological symptom disorder)—A disorder, formerly known as *conversion disorder,* that causes clients to suffer from neurological symptoms, such as numbness, blindness, paralysis, or seizures without a definable organic cause; it is thought that symptoms *unconsciously* arise in response to stressful situations affecting a client's mental health

Depersonalization—An anomaly of self-awareness; it consists of a feeling of watching oneself act while having no control over a situation; subjects feel they have changed, and the world has become vague, dreamlike, less real, or lacking in significance

Derealization—An alteration in the perception or experience of the external world so that it seems unreal; other symptoms include feeling as though one's environment is lacking in spontaneity, emotional coloring, and depth

Dissociative fugue—A rare condition in which a person suddenly, without planning or warning, travels far from home or work and leaves behind a past life; the person experiences amnesia and has no conscious understanding or knowledge of the reason for the flight; the condition is usually associated with severe stress or trauma

Dissociative identity disorder (DID)—Previously known as *multiple personality disorder* (MPD); DID is a mental disorder on the dissociative spectrum characterized by at least two distinct and relatively enduring identities or dissociated personality states that alternately control a person's behavior, and is accompanied by memory impairment for important information not explained by ordinary forgetfulness

Dissociation—The splitting off of clusters of mental contents from conscious awareness; a mechanism that is central to hysterical conversion and dissociative disorders

Factitious disorder—A disorder that is not real, genuine, or natural; the symptoms, both physical and psychological, are *consciously* produced by the individual and are under voluntary control; the individual's goal is to assume a "patient" role to seek attention

Illness anxiety disorder (IAD)—Formerly known as *hypochondriasis,* refers to worry about having a serious illness; this debilitating condition is the result of an inaccurate perception of the condition of body or mind despite the absence of an actual medical condition

La belle indifference—A disproportionate degree of indifference to, or complacency about, symptoms such as paralysis or loss of sensation in part of the body; it is characteristic of functional neurological symptom disorder

Munchausen disorder—A type of factitious disorder in which the client may embellish or feign signs and symptoms of illness to gain medical attention

Continued

KEY TERMS—cont'd

Munchausen disorder by proxy—The fabrication of symptoms or physical evidence of another's illness, or the deliberate causing of another's illness, to gain medical attention

Primary gain—Interpersonal, social, or financial advantages from the conversion of emotional stress directly into illness

Pseudocyesis—The appearance of clinical or subclinical signs and symptoms associated with pregnancy when the individual is not actually pregnant

Secondary gain—The social, occupational, or interpersonal advantages obtained as a result of having an illness

Somatic symptom disorder (SSD)— Formerly known as *somatization disorder,* this disorder involves being distressed or having one's life disrupted by concerns involving physical symptoms for which a physical cause cannot be found

Tertiary gain—Those gains sought or attained from a client's illness by someone other than the client.

When severe anxiety has been repressed, it can be expressed in the form of physiological symptoms and dissociative behaviors. Somatic symptom disorders are characterized by physical symptoms suggesting medical disease, but without a demonstrable organic pathology or known pathophysiological mechanism to account for them. They are classified as mental disorders because pathophysiological processes are not demonstrable or understandable by existing laboratory procedures, and there is either evidence or strong presumption that psychological factors are the major cause of the symptoms.

Dissociative disorders are defined by a disturbance of or alteration in the usually integrated functions of consciousness, memory, and identity. **Dissociation** occurs when anxiety becomes overwhelming and the personality becomes disorganized. Defense mechanisms that normally govern consciousness, identity, and memory break down, and behavior occurs with little or no participation on the part of the conscious personality. There are four types of dissociative disorders: depersonalization-derealization disorder, dissociative amnesia, dissociative identity disorder, and dissociative disorder not elsewhere classified.

DID YOU KNOW?

It is well documented that a large proportion of clients in general medical outpatient clinics and private medical offices do not have organic disease requiring medical treatment. It is likely that many of these clients have somatic symptom disorders, but they do not perceive themselves as having a psychiatric problem and thus do not seek treatment from psychiatrists.

I. Epidemiological Statistics

A. Somatic symptom disorder (SSD)
1. One percent in the general population.
2. More common in women than in men.
3. More common in rural areas than in urban.
4. More common in less educated persons.

B. Conversion disorder (functional neurological symptom disorder)
1. Five to thirty percent of general population.
2. Occurs more frequently in women than in men.
3. Occurs more frequently in adolescents and young adults than in other age groups.
4. Higher prevalence in lower socioeconomic groups, rural populations, and among those with less education.

C. Illness anxiety disorder (IAD; formerly *hypochondriasis*)
1. Affects 1% to 5% of general population.
2. Equally common among men and women.
3. Most common age of onset is early adulthood.

D. Factitious disorder
1. Frequency of disorder unknown.
2. May comprise about 0.8% to 1.0% of psychiatry consultation clients.

E. Dissociative disorders
1. Statistically quite rare.
2. Dissociative amnesia.
   a. Relatively rare.
   b. Occurs most frequently during war or natural disasters.
   c. Equally common in men and women.
   d. Can occur at any age but difficult to diagnose in children because it is easily confused with inattention or oppositional behavior.
3. **Dissociative identity disorder** (DID).
   a. Estimates of the prevalence vary widely.
   b. Number of reported cases has grown rapidly.
   c. Occurs from five to nine times more frequently in women than in men.
   d. Onset likely occurs in childhood, although may not be recognized until late adolescence or early adulthood.
   e. More common in first-degree biological relatives of people with the disorder than in the general population.

4. **Depersonalization-derealization disorder.**
   a. Prevalence unknown.
   b. Brief episodes may occur in as many as half of all adults.
   c. Occurs when individual is:
      i. Under severe psychosocial stress
      ii. Sleep deprived
      iii. Traveling to unfamiliar places
      iv. Intoxicated with hallucinogens, marijuana, or alcohol
   d. Symptoms begin in adolescence or early adulthood.
   e. Occurs more often in women than men.
   f. Occurs in the young, rarely occurring in individuals older than 40.
   g. Disorder is chronic, with periods of remission and exacerbation.
   h. Incidence high under conditions of sustained traumatization (military combat, prisoner-of-war camps).
      i. Reported in individuals who endure near-death experiences

II. Predisposing Factors Associated With Somatic Symptom Disorders and Dissociative Disorders

A. **Genetic:** increased incidence of SSD, conversion disorder, and IAD in first-degree relatives, implying a possible inheritable predisposition
B. **Biochemical**
   1. Decreased levels of serotonin and endorphins may play a role, with pain as a predominant symptom.
   2. Serotonin is the main neurotransmitter involved in inhibiting the firing of afferent pain fibers.
   3. Deficiency of endorphins correlates with an increase of incoming sensory (pain) stimuli.
C. **Neuroanatomical**
   1. Brain dysfunction proposed as a factor in factitious disorders.
   2. Impairment in information processing contributes to aberrant behaviors associated with factitious disorders.
   3. No specific electroencephalographic (EEG) abnormalities have been noted.
D. **Psychodynamic**
   1. Some view IAD as an ego defense mechanism.
   2. Physical complaints are expressions of low self-esteem and feelings of worthlessness.
   3. Easier to feel something is wrong with the body than to feel something is wrong with the self.
   4. Some view these disorders as a defense against guilt.
      a. Individual views the self as "bad," based on real or imagined past misconduct.
      b. Views physical suffering as the deserved punishment required for atonement.
   5. In conversion disorder, emotions associated with a traumatic event, which the individual cannot express because of moral or ethical unacceptability, are "converted" into physical symptoms (conversion disorder).
   6. The unacceptable emotions are repressed and converted to a somatic hysterical symptom that is symbolic in some way of the original emotional trauma.
   7. In dissociative identity disorder, severe abuse or neglect that occurs during the personality development of childhood causes the child to develop personalities that can protect him or her from that experienced trauma. The child develops personalities to escape the inflicted emotional and/or physical pain.
E. **Family dynamics**
   1. Some families have difficulty expressing emotions openly and resolving conflicts verbally.
   2. Ill child will shift focus from the open family conflict to the child's illness.
   3. Child's illness brings some stability to the family, as harmony replaces discord and the child's welfare becomes the common concern.
   4. Child receives positive reinforcement for the illness.
F. **Learning theory**
   1. Somatic complaints are reinforced when the sick role relieves the individual from the need to deal with a stressful situation
   2. The sick person learns that he or she may avoid stressful obligations, postpone unwelcome challenges, and be excused from troublesome duties (**primary gain**).
   3. The sick person becomes the prominent focus of attention because of the illness (**secondary gain**).
   4. Conflict within the family is relieved as concern is shifted to the ill person and away from the real issue (**tertiary gain**).
   5. Positive reinforcements virtually guarantee repetition of the response.
   6. Past experience with serious or life-threatening physical illness, either personal or that of close family members, can predispose an individual to IAD.
   7. Develop a fear of recurrence of a threat to biological integrity.
   8. Generates an exaggerated response to minor physical changes.
   9. Leads to excessive anxiety and health concerns.

III. Nursing Process: Assessment

A. Somatic symptoms disorder (SSD)
  1. Multiple somatic symptoms that cannot be explained medically.
  2. Symptoms associated with psychosocial distress and long-term seeking of assistance from health-care professionals.
  3. Symptoms may be vague, dramatized, or exaggerated in their presentation, and an excessive amount of time and energy is devoted to worry and concern about the symptoms.
  4. Convinced that their symptoms are related to organic pathology.
  5. Adamantly reject, and are often irritated by, any implication that stress or psychosocial factors play any role in their condition.
  6. Chronic, with symptoms beginning before age 30.
  7. Anxiety and depression frequently manifested.
  8. Suicidal threats and attempts not uncommon.
  9. Runs a fluctuating course, with periods of remission and exacerbation.

🚫 Because clients diagnosed with SSD are convinced that their symptoms are related to organic pathology, they often receive medical care from several physicians, sometimes concurrently, leading to the possibility of dangerous combinations of treatments. They have a tendency to seek relief through overmedicating with prescribed analgesics or antianxiety agents. Drug abuse and dependence are common complications of SSD. When suicide results, it is usually in association with substance abuse.

  10. Personality characteristics and features can be associated with histrionic personality disorder.
    a. Heightened emotionality.
    b. Impressionistic thought and speech.
    c. Seductiveness.
    d. Strong dependency needs.
    e. Preoccupation with symptoms and oneself.
B. Illness anxiety disorder (IAD); formerly *hypochondriasis*
  1. An unrealistic or inaccurate interpretation of physical symptoms or sensations, leading to preoccupation and fear of having a serious disease.
  2. Fear becomes disabling and persists despite appropriate reassurance that no organic pathology can be detected.
  3. Symptoms may be minimal or absent, but the individual is highly anxious about and suspicious of the presence of an undiagnosed, serious medical illness.

DID YOU KNOW?
Individuals with IAD are extremely conscious of bodily sensations and changes; they may become convinced that a rapid heart rate indicates they have heart disease or that a small sore is skin cancer. They are profoundly preoccupied with their bodies and are totally aware of even the slightest change in feeling or sensation. Their response to these small changes, however, is usually unrealistic and exaggerated.

  4. "Doctor shopping" is common.
    a. Will not accept that problems are psychological in nature.
    b. Convinced that they are not receiving the proper care.
  5. Others avoid seeking medical assistance because to do so would increase their anxiety to intolerable levels.
  6. Depression is common.
  7. Obsessive-compulsive traits frequently present.
  8. Symptoms may interfere with social or occupational functioning.
C. Conversion disorder (functional neurological symptom disorder)
  1. A loss of or change in body function which cannot be explained by any known medical disorder or pathophysiological mechanism.
  2. A psychological component involved in the initiation, exacerbation, or perpetuation of the symptom (may or may not be obvious or identifiable).
  3. Individuals have a naive, inappropriate lack of concern about the seriousness or implications of their physical symptoms (**la belle indifference**).
  4. Symptoms affect voluntary motor or sensory functioning suggestive of neurological disease.
    a. Paralysis.
    b. Aphonia (inability to produce voice).
    c. Seizures.
    d. Coordination disturbance.
    e. Difficulty swallowing.
    f. Urinary retention.
    g. Akinesia (muscle weakness).
    h. Blindness.
    i. Deafness.
    j. Diplopia (double vision).
    k. Anosmia (inability to perceive odor).
    l. Loss of pain sensation.
    m. Hallucinations.

DID YOU KNOW?
Pseudocyesis (false pregnancy) is a conversion disorder resulting from anxiety generated by a strong desire to become pregnant.

  5. Most symptoms resolve within a few weeks.
  6. About 20% of individuals have a relapse within 1 year.

7. Good outcomes associated with:
   a. Acute onset.
   b. A precipitating stressful event.
   c. Good premorbid adjustment.
   d. Absence of medical or neurological comorbidity.
D. Psychological factors affecting other medical conditions
   1. Psychological or behavioral factors are implicated in the development, exacerbation, or delayed recovery from a medical condition.
   2. There is objective evidence of a general medical condition that has been precipitated by or is being perpetuated by psychological or behavioral circumstances.
E. Factitious disorder
   1. Involves conscious, intentional feigning of physical or psychological symptoms.
   2. Individuals pretend to be ill to receive emotional care and support commonly associated with the role of "patient."
   3. Behaviors are conscious, deliberate, and intentional.
   4. May be an associated compulsive element that diminishes personal control.
   5. May aggravate existing symptoms, induce new ones, or even inflict painful injuries on themselves.
   6. May be identified as **Munchausen disorder.**
   7. Symptoms may be psychological, physical, or a combination of both.
   8. May be imposed on oneself or on another person under the care of the perpetrator (**Munchausen disorder by proxy**).
   9. Diagnosis can be difficult, as individuals become very inventive in their quest to produce symptoms.
      a. Self-inflicted wounds.
      b. Injection or insertion of contaminated substances.

MAKING THE CONNECTION

Historically, in Western medical practice, mind and body have been viewed as two distinct entities, each subject to different laws of causality. Indeed, in many instances—particularly in highly specialized areas of medicine—the biological and psychological components of disease remain separate. However, current medical research findings are questioning this theory. Research associated with biological functioning is being expanded to include the psychological and social determinants of health and disease. This psychobiological approach to illness reflects a more holistic perspective and one that promotes concern for helping clients achieve optimal functioning.

   c. Manipulating a thermometer to feign a fever.
   d. Urinary tract manipulation.
   e. Surreptitious use of medications.
F. Dissociative amnesia
   1. Inability to recall important personal information, usually of a traumatic or stressful nature, that is too extensive to be explained by ordinary forgetfulness and is not due to the direct effects of substance use or a neurological or other medical condition.
   2. Types of **amnesia.**
      a. Localized.
         i. Related to a specific stressful event
         ii. Unable to recall all incidents associated with the stressful event for a specific time period following the event (few hours to a few days)
      b. Selective.
         i. Related to a specific stressful event
         ii. Can recall only certain incidents associated with a stressful event for a specific period after the event
      c. Generalized: Cannot recall his or her identity and total life history
   3. Usually individual appears alert with no indication that anything is wrong.
   4. Some clients may present with alterations in consciousness, with conversion disorders, or in trance states.
   5. Onset usually follows severe psychosocial stress.
   6. Termination typically abrupt and followed by complete recovery.
   7. Recurrences are unusual.
G. Dissociative amnesia with **dissociative fugue**
   1. Characterized by a sudden, unexpected travel away from customary place of daily activities.
   2. Bewildered wandering, with the inability to recall some or all of one's past.
   3. May not be able to recall personal identity and sometimes assumes a new identity.
H. Dissociative identity disorder (DID; formerly *multiple personality disorder*)
   1. Characterized by the existence of two or more personalities in a single individual.
   2. Only one personality is evident at any given moment.
   3. One personality is dominant most of the time over the course of the disorder.
   4. Each personality is unique and composed of a complex set of memories, behavior patterns, and social relationships that surface during the dominant interval.
   5. Transition from one personality to another may be sudden or gradual, and is sometimes quite dramatic.

MAKING THE CONNECTION

Client's diagnosed with DID experience personality transitions. Personality switches can occur during stressful situations, disputes among the alters, and psychological conflicts. A sudden disruption in the individual's train of thought may generate a personality switch. There may be rapid eye blinking and changes in voice or facial expression.

6. Before therapy, the original personality usually has no knowledge of the other personalities.
7. Subpersonalities have different names, but they may be unnamed and may be of a different gender, race, and age than the original personality.

DID YOU KNOW?
Personalities that emerge when a client is diagnosed with DID are usually quite different from and may be the exact opposite of the original personality. For example, a normally shy, socially withdrawn, faithful husband may become a gregarious womanizer and heavy drinker with the emergence of another personality.

8. Generally, there is amnesia for the events that took place when another personality was in the dominant position.
9. Clients may experience "gaps" in memory or "lost time" or blackouts when other subpersonalities are dominant.
10. Clients may "wake up" in unfamiliar situations with no idea where they are, how they got there, or of the identities of the people around them.
11. Some individuals with DID maintain responsible positions, complete graduate degrees, and are successful spouses and parents before diagnosis and while in treatment.
12. Many individuals are misdiagnosed with depression, borderline and antisocial personality disorders, schizophrenia, epilepsy, or bipolar disorder.
I. Depersonalization-derealization disorder
   1. Characterized by a temporary change in the quality of self-awareness, which often takes the form of feelings of unreality, changes in body image, feelings of detachment from the environment, or a sense of observing oneself from outside the body.
   2. Depersonalization is a disturbance in the perception of oneself.
   3. Derealization is an alteration in the perception of the external environment.
   4. Both also occur in schizophrenia, depression, anxiety states, and neurocognitive disorders.

5. Diagnosis is made only if symptoms cause significant distress or impairment in functioning.
6. With depersonalization, a client experiences a mechanical or dreamlike feeling or a belief that the body's physical characteristics have changed.
7. With derealization, objects in the environment are perceived as altered in size or shape, and other people in the environment may seem automated or mechanical.
8. Distorted perceptions are disturbing.
9. Perceptions often accompanied by anxiety, depression, fear of going insane, obsessive thoughts, somatic complaints, and an alteration in the subjective sense of time.

IV. Nursing Process: Diagnosis (Analysis)

Table 16.1 presents a list of client behaviors and the NANDA nursing diagnoses that correspond to those behaviors, which may be used in planning care for the client with somatic symptom and dissociative disorders.

V. Nursing Process: Planning.

The following outcomes may be developed to guide the care of a client with somatic symptom and dissociative disorder. **The client will:**
A. Effectively use adaptive coping strategies during stressful situations without resorting to physical symptoms (*somatic symptom disorder*)
B. Verbalize relief from pain and demonstrate adaptive coping strategies during stressful situations to prevent the onset of pain (*somatic symptom disorder*)
C. Interpret bodily sensations rationally; verbalize understanding of the significance the irrational fear held for him or her; and decrease the number and frequency of physical complaints (*illness anxiety disorder*)
D. Be free of physical disability and able to verbalize understanding of the possible correlation between the loss of or alteration in function and extreme emotional stress (*conversion disorder*)
E. Recall events associated with a traumatic or stressful situation (*dissociative amnesia*)
F. Recall all events of past life (*dissociative amnesia*)
G. Verbalize the extreme anxiety that precipitated the dissociation (*depersonalization-derealization disorder*)
H. Demonstrate more adaptive coping strategies to avert dissociative behaviors in the face of severe anxiety (*depersonalization-derealization disorder*)
I. Verbalize understanding of the existence of multiple personalities and the purposes they serve (*dissociative identity disorder*)
J. Be able to maintain a sense of reality during stressful situations (*depersonalization-derealization disorder*)

Table 16.1 Assigning Nursing Diagnoses to Behaviors Commonly Associated With Somatic Symptom and Dissociative Disorders

Behaviors	Nursing Diagnoses
Verbalization of numerous physical complaints in the absence of any pathophysiological evidence; focus on the self and physical symptoms (*Somatic symptom disorder*)	Ineffective coping; chronic pain
History of "doctor shopping" for evidence of organic pathology to substantiate physical symptoms; statements such as, "I don't know why the doctor put me on the psychiatric unit. I have a physical problem." (*Somatic symptom disorder*)	Deficient knowledge (psychological causes for physical symptoms)
Preoccupation with and unrealistic interpretation of bodily signs and sensations (*Illness Anxiety Disorder*)	Fear (of having a serious disease)
Loss or alteration in physical functioning without evidence of organic pathology (*Conversion disorder*)	Disturbed sensory perception*
Need for assistance to carry out self-care activities such as eating, dressing, maintaining hygiene, and toileting due to alteration in physical functioning (*Conversion disorder*)	Self-care deficit
History of numerous exacerbations of physical illness; inappropriate or exaggerated behaviors; denial of emotional problems (*Psychological factors affecting medical condition*)	Deficient knowledge (psychological factors affecting medical condition)
Loss of memory (*Dissociative amnesia*)	Impaired memory
Verbalizations of frustration over lack of control and dependence on others (*Dissociative amnesia*)	Powerlessness
Unresolved grief; depression; self-blame associated with childhood abuse (*DID*)	Risk for suicide
Presence of more than one personality within the individual (*DID*)	Disturbed personality identity
Alteration in the perception or experience of the self or the environment (*Depersonalization disorder*)	Disturbed sensory perception (visual/kinesthetic)*

*This diagnosis has been resigned from the NANDA-I list of approved diagnoses. It is used in this instance because it is most compatible with the identified behaviors.

VI. Nursing Process: Implementation

A. Interventions for clients who are experiencing ineffective coping/chronic pain
 1. Monitor physician's ongoing assessments, laboratory reports, and other data to maintain assurance that possibility of organic pathology is clearly ruled out. Review findings with client.
 2. Recognize and accept that the physical complaint is real to the client, even though no organic etiology can be identified.
 3. Provide pain medication as prescribed by physician.
 4. Identify gains that the physical symptoms are providing for the client: increased dependency, attention, distraction from other problems.

MAKING THE CONNECTION

It can be frustrating to work with a client who has physical complaints without any organic etiology for the complaints. But the nurse must recognize that these complaints are real to the client and the main source of the client's distress. Denial of the client's feelings is nontherapeutic and interferes with establishment of a trusting relationship.

 5. Initially, fulfill the client's most urgent dependency needs, but gradually withdraw attention to physical symptoms. Minimize time given in response to physical complaints.
 6. Explain to client that any new physical complaints will be referred to the physician and give no further attention to them. Ensure physician's assessment of the complaint.

🛈 The possibility of organic pathology must always be considered when dealing with clients diagnosed with somatic symptom disorder. Failure to explore any new physical complaints could jeopardize client safety.

 7. Encourage client to verbalize fears and anxieties. Explain that attention will be withdrawn if rumination about physical complaints begins. Follow through.
 8. Discuss possible alternative coping strategies client may use in response to stress.
    a. Relaxation exercises.
    b. Physical activities.
    c. Assertiveness skills.
 9. Give positive reinforcement for use of these alternatives.
 10. Help client identify ways to achieve recognition from others without resorting to physical symptoms.

B. Interventions for clients who are experiencing fear (of having a serious illness)

1. Monitor physician's ongoing assessments and laboratory reports.
2. Refer all new physical complaints to physician.
3. Assess the function that client's excessive concern is fulfilling for him or her (unfulfilled needs for dependency, nurturing, caring, attention, or control).
4. Identify times during which preoccupation with physical symptoms is worse.
5. Determine extent of correlation of physical complaints with times of increased anxiety.
6. Convey empathy. Let client know that you understand how a specific symptom may conjure up fears of previous life-threatening illness.
7. Initially allow client a limited amount of time (10 minutes each hour) to discuss physical concerns.
8. Help client determine what techniques may be most useful for him or her to implement when fear and anxiety are exacerbated.
   a. Relaxation techniques.
   b. Mental imagery.
   c. Thought-stopping techniques.
   d. Physical exercise.
9. Gradually increase the limit on amount of time spent each hour in discussing physical concerns. If client violates the limits, withdraw attention.
10. Allow client to discuss feelings associated with fear of serious illness.
11. Role-play the client's plan for dealing with the fear the next time it assumes control and before anxiety becomes disabling.

C. Interventions for clients who are experiencing disturbed sensory perception

1. Monitor physician's ongoing assessments, laboratory reports, and other data to ensure that

---

MAKING THE CONNECTION

Because the discussion of and focus on physical concerns has been the client's primary method of coping for so long, complete prohibition of this activity would likely raise the client's anxiety level significantly. Increased anxiety will further exacerbate the client's behavior.

MAKING THE CONNECTION

Verbalization of feelings in a nonthreatening environment facilitates the expression and resolution of disturbing emotional issues. When the client can express feelings directly, there is less need to express them through physical symptoms.

---

possibility of organic pathology is clearly ruled out.

2. Identify primary or secondary gains that the physical symptom may be providing for the client (increased dependency, attention, protection from experiencing a stressful event).
3. Do not focus on the disability, and encourage client to be as independent as possible. Intervene only when client requires assistance.
4. Maintain nonjudgmental attitude when providing assistance to the client. The physical symptom is not within the client's conscious control and is very real to him or her.
5. Do not allow the client to use the disability as a manipulative tool to avoid participation in therapeutic activities. Withdraw attention if client continues to focus on physical limitation.
6. Encourage the client to verbalize fears and anxieties. Help identify physical symptoms as a coping mechanism that is used in times of extreme stress.
7. Help client identify coping mechanisms that he or she could use when faced with stressful situations, rather than retreating from reality with a physical disability.
8. Give positive reinforcement for identification or demonstration of alternative, more adaptive, coping strategies.

D. Interventions for clients who are experiencing deficient knowledge

1. Assess client's level of knowledge regarding effects of psychological problems on the body.
2. Assess client's level of anxiety and readiness to learn.
3. Discuss physical examinations and laboratory tests that have been conducted. Explain purpose and results of each.
4. Explore client's feelings and fears. Go slowly. These feelings may have been suppressed or repressed for so long that their disclosure may be a painful experience. Be supportive.
5. Have client keep a diary of appearance, duration, and intensity of physical symptoms. A separate record of situations that the client finds especially stressful should also be kept.
6. Help client identify needs that are being met through the sick role. Together, formulate more

---

MAKING THE CONNECTION

Positive reinforcement for physical complaints will encourage the client to continue to use the maladaptive response for secondary gains, such as dependency. Lack of reinforcement may help to extinguish the maladaptive response.

MAKING THE CONNECTION

Comparison of the incidents of physical symptoms and the client's experience of stressful situations may provide objective data from which to observe the relationship between physical symptoms and stress.

---

adaptive means for fulfilling these needs. Practice by role-playing.

7. Provide instruction in assertiveness techniques, especially the ability to recognize the differences among passive, assertive, and aggressive behaviors and the importance of respecting the rights of others while protecting one's own basic rights.

8. Discuss adaptive methods of stress management.
   a. Relaxation techniques.
   b. Physical exercise.
   c. Meditation.
   d. Breathing exercises.
   e. **Autogenics.**

E. Interventions for clients who are experiencing impaired memory

1. Obtain as much information as possible about the client from family and significant others, if possible. Consider likes, dislikes, important people, activities, music, and pets.

2. Do not flood client with data regarding his or her past life.

🛑 Individuals who are exposed to painful information from which amnesia is providing protection may decompensate even further into a psychotic state if quickly flooded with overwhelming information.

3. Instead, expose client to stimuli that represent pleasant experiences from the past.
   a. Smells associated with enjoyable activities.
   b. Beloved pets.
   c. Music known to have been pleasurable.

4. As memory begins to return, engage client in activities that may provide additional stimulation.

5. Encourage client to discuss situations that have been especially stressful and to explore the feelings associated with those times.

6. Identify specific conflicts that remain unresolved, and assist client to identify possible solutions.

7. Provide instruction regarding more adaptive ways to respond to anxiety.

F. Interventions for clients who are experiencing disturbed personal identity

1. Develop a trusting relationship with the original personality and with each of the subpersonalities.

2. Help client understand the existence of the subpersonalities and the need each serves in the personal identity of the individual.

3. Help client identify stressful situations that precipitate transition from one personality to another. Carefully observe and record these transitions.

4. Use therapeutic communication to deal with maladaptive behaviors associated with individual subpersonalities.

🛑 A client diagnosed with DID may have numerous subpersonalities with various traits. One personality may be suicidal. Precautions must be taken to guard against the client's self-harm. If another personality exhibits physical hostility, precautions must be taken to protect others. It may be possible to seek assistance from one of the personalities. For example, a strong-willed personality may be able to help control the behaviors of a "suicidal" personality.

5. Help subpersonalities understand that their "being" will not be destroyed but rather integrated into a unified identity within the individual.

6. Provide support during disclosure of painful experiences and reassurance when client becomes discouraged with lengthy treatment.

G. Interventions for clients who are experiencing disturbed sensory perception (visual/kinesthetic)

1. Provide support and encouragement during times of depersonalization. Clients manifesting these symptoms may express fear and anxiety at experiencing such behaviors. They do not understand the response and may express a fear of going insane.

2. Explain the depersonalization behaviors and the purpose they usually serve.

3. Explain the relationship between severe anxiety and depersonalization behaviors.

4. Help relate depersonalization behaviors to times of severe psychological stress.

5. Explore past experiences and possibly repressed painful situations, such as trauma or abuse.

6. Discuss these painful experiences with client and encourage him or her to deal with the feelings associated with these situations. Work to resolve the conflicts these repressed feelings have nurtured.

7. Discuss ways the client may more adaptively respond to stress.

8. Use role-play to practice using adaptive responses.

VII. Nursing Process: Evaluation

A. Evaluation of the nursing actions for the client diagnosed with *somatic symptom disorder* may be facilitated by gathering information using the following types of questions:

1. Can the client recognize signs and symptoms of escalating anxiety?

2. Can the client intervene with adaptive coping strategies to interrupt the escalating anxiety before physical symptoms are exacerbated?

3. Can the client verbalize an understanding of the correlation between physical symptoms and times of escalating anxiety?

4. Does the client have a plan for dealing with increased stress to prevent exacerbation of physical symptoms?

5. Does the client demonstrate a decrease in ruminations about physical symptoms?

6. Have fears of serious illness diminished?

7. Does the client demonstrate full recovery from previous loss or alteration of physical functioning?

B. Evaluation of the nursing actions for the client diagnosed with *dissociative disorder* may be facilitated by gathering information using the following types of questions:

1. Has the client's memory been restored?

2. Can the client connect occurrence of psychological stress to loss of memory?

3. Does the client discuss fears and anxieties with members of the staff in an effort toward resolution?

4. Can the client discuss the presence of various personalities within the self?

5. Can he or she verbalize why these personalities exist?

6. Can the client verbalize situations that precipitate transition from one personality to another?

7. Can the client maintain a sense of reality during stressful situations?

8. Can the client verbalize a correlation between stressful situations and the onset of depersonalization behaviors?

9. Can the client demonstrate more adaptive coping strategies for dealing with stress without resorting to dissociation?

VIII. Treatment Modalities

A. Somatic symptom disorders

1. Individual psychotherapy.
   a. Goal to help clients develop healthy and adaptive behaviors, encourage them to move beyond their somatic symptoms, and manage their lives more effectively.
   b. Focus on personal and social difficulties and achievement of practical solutions.
   c. Advocate for complete physical examination to rule out organic pathology.
   d. Focus attention on social and personal problems and away from somatic complaints.

MAKING THE CONNECTION

The treatment of choice for both somatic symptoms disorder and illness anxiety disorder is group psychotherapy. During group therapy, clients can learn to verbalize thoughts and feelings and can be confronted by group members and leaders when they reject responsibility for maladaptive behaviors.

---

2. Group psychotherapy.
   a. Provides needed social support and social interactions.
   b. Provides a setting where clients can share their experiences of illness.

3. Behavior therapy.
   a. Likely successful when secondary gain is prominent.
   b. Teaches that negative outcomes come from perpetuating physical symptoms when these symptoms are rewarded with passivity and dependency and when others are overly solicitous and helpful toward the client.
   c. Focuses on rewarding the client's autonomy, self-sufficiency, and independence.

4. Psychopharmacology.
   a. Antidepressants often used with somatic symptom disorder when predominant symptom is pain.
   b. Antidepressants relieve pain, independent of influences on mood.
   c. The tricyclic antidepressants (TCAs) have also been used extensively in relieving pain.
   d. TCA side effects may make use problematic.
   e. Norepinephrine reuptake inhibitors (SNRIs) venlafaxine (Effexor) and duloxetine (Cymbalta) have been used as analgesic agents with less side effect profile.
   f. Selective serotonin reuptake inhibitors (SSRIs) have not exhibited the consistent analgesic efficacy demonstrated by the TCAs and SNRIs.
   g. Anticonvulsants such as phenytoin (Dilantin), carbamazepine (Tegretol), and clonazepam (Klonopin) have been reported to be effective short term in treating neuropathic and neuralgic pain.
   h. Anticonvulsants seem effective in other somatic symptom (pain) disorders.

B. Dissociative amnesia

1. Removal from stressful situation can resolve problem spontaneously.

2. For more refractory conditions, intravenous administration of amobarbital useful in the retrieval of lost memories.

3. Supportive psychotherapy is recommended.
   i. Reinforce adjustment to the psychological effect of the retrieved memories
   ii. Help deal with emotions associated with memories
4. Psychotherapy may be primary treatment.
5. Techniques of persuasion and free or directed association are used to help the client remember.

DID YOU KNOW?
When a client has refractory amnesia, hypnosis may be required to mobilize the memories. Hypnosis is sometimes facilitated by the use of pharmacological agents, such as amobarbital sodium. Once the memories have been obtained through hypnosis, supportive psychotherapy or group psychotherapy may be employed to help the client integrate the memories into his or her conscious state.

C. Dissociative identity disorder
   1. Goal is to optimize the client's potential and ability to function.
   2. Achievement of integration (a blending of all the personalities into one) is desirable but lengthy.
   3. Smooth collaboration among the subpersonalities may be all that is realistic.
   4. Intensive, long-term psychotherapy goals:
      a. Uncovering underlying psychological conflicts.
      b. Helping client gain insight into these conflicts.
      c. Striving to synthesize the various identities into one integrated personality.
   5. Assisted to recall past traumas in detail.
   6. Mentally reexperience the abuse that caused their illness.

DID YOU KNOW?
The process of mentally reexperiencing the abuse that caused DID is called *abreaction,* or "remembering with feeling." It is so painful that clients may actually cry, scream, and feel the pain that they felt at the time of the abuse.

   7. Each personality is actively explored and encouraged to become aware of the other personalities.
   8. Traumatic memories, especially those related to childhood abuse, are examined.
   9. When aggressive or suicidal personalities are in the dominant role, brief periods of hospitalization may be necessary.
   10. When integration is achieved, the individual becomes a total of all the feelings, experiences, memories, skills, and talents that were previously in the command of the various personalities.
   11. Integration may take years of intense psychotherapy, and even then, recovery is often incomplete.

D. Depersonalization-derealization disorder
   1. Treatment is inconclusive.
   2. Various psychiatric medications have been tried, both independently and in combination: antidepressants, mood stabilizers, anticonvulsants, and antipsychotics with mixed results.
   3. The antidepressant clomipramine (Anafranil) shown to be promising in treatment of primary depersonalization-derealization disorder.
   4. Psychotherapy may be useful for clients with evident intrapsychic conflicts.
   5. Hypnotherapy or cognitive-behavioral therapy (CBT) may be helpful.
   6. With CBT, clients learn to confront distorted thoughts and challenge feelings of unreality.

REVIEW QUESTIONS

1. A factitious disorder in which an individual fabricates symptoms to obtain medical attention and secondary gains can be identified as _____ disorder.

2. A client is exhibiting symptoms of depersonalization-derealization disorder. Which of the following symptoms would the nurse expect to assess, and what predisposing factor may be associated with these symptoms? **Select all that apply.**
   1. Objects in the environment are perceived as altered; severe psychosocial stress
   2. A belief that his or her body's physical characteristics have changed; near-death experience
   3. Feels detached from his or her body; extreme social anxiety
   4. Alteration in bodily functioning; client is intoxicated with marijuana
   5. An exaggerated belief that the body is deformed or defective; medication side effect

3. After 11 visits to the emergency department in less than a year, a client has been admitted to a psychiatric unit with a diagnosis of factitious disorder. Which physician's progress note would the nurse recognize as supporting this diagnosis?
   1. "Client continually worries about an undiagnosed, serious medical illness."
   2. "Client insists that she is 6 months pregnant without any medical evidence."
   3. "Client has history of sexual abuse and has developed multiple personalities."
   4. "Client purposefully overmedicates self to gain medical attention."

4. Which of the following would be classified by the *Diagnostic and Statistical Manual of Mental Disorders* (DSM-5) as dissociative disorders? **Select all that apply.**
   1. Munchausen disorder by proxy
   2. Illness anxiety disorder
   3. Dissociative amnesia
   4. Depersonalization-derealization disorder
   5. Dissociative identity disorder

5. A client with a history of conversion disorder asks the nurse about prognosis. Which is the most accurate nursing response?
   1. "The symptoms of conversion disorder resolve within a few weeks, and about 50% of individuals relapse within 1 year."
   2. "The symptoms of conversion disorder resolve within a few months, and about 20% of individuals relapse within 1 year."
   3. "The symptoms of conversion disorder resolve within a few weeks, and about 20% of individuals relapse within 1 year."
   4. "The symptoms of conversion disorder resolve within a few months, and about 50% of individuals relapse within 1 year."

6. A newly admitted client is diagnosed with illness anxiety disorder. Which short-term outcome is appropriate?
   1. The client will rate anxiety as 3 out of 10 by discharge.
   2. The client will note a link between anxiety and somatic symptoms by day 2.
   3. The client will participate in group therapy activities by discharge.
   4. The client will recognize behaviors that generate secondary gains by day 2.

7. A female client has missed six menstrual cycles and has a protuberant abdomen. She tells the nurse, "I don't care if my pregnancy test is negative. My baby is due in 3 months." The nurse recognizes that this client is suffering from which condition?
   1. Depersonalization
   2. Derealization
   3. Pseudocyesis
   4. Illness anxiety disorder

8. During an assessment interview, a female client tells the nurse that she has traveled to a new location but has no memory of where she came from or who she is. Which medical diagnosis will the nurse expect the psychiatrist to assign?
   1. Factitious disorder
   2. La belle indifference
   3. Illness anxiety disorder
   4. Dissociative fugue

9. An instructor is teaching students about factitious disorder (FD). Which of the following student statements indicate that learning has occurred? **Select all that apply.**
   1. "Onset of FD symptoms usually follows severe psychosocial stress."
   2. "In FD, behaviors are conscious, deliberate, and intentional."
   3. "Clients may experience "gaps" in memory or "lost time.""
   4. "Clients diagnosed with FD may inflict painful injuries on themselves."
   5. "Clients often have a history of frequent childhood hospitalizations."

10. Which of the following symptoms should a nurse recognize that differentiates a client diagnosed with illness anxiety disorder (IAD) from a client diagnosed with dissociative identity disorder (DID)? **Select all that apply.**
   1. Clients diagnosed with IAD go "doctor shopping," whereas clients diagnosed with DID do not.
   2. Clients diagnosed with IAD may experience "gaps" in memory or "lost time," whereas clients diagnosed with DID do not.
   3. Clients diagnosed with IAD have an unrealistic interpretation of physical symptoms, whereas clients diagnosed with DID do not.
   4. Clients diagnosed with IAD are anxious about an undiagnosed, serious medical illness, whereas clients diagnosed with DID are not.
   5. Clients diagnosed with IAD are extremely conscious of bodily sensations and changes, whereas clients diagnosed with DID are not.

11. Feelings of detachment from, and an alteration in, the perception of the external environment is called _____.

12. A psychiatric nurse practitioner documents that a client recently in a severe car crash is experiencing localized amnesia. Which client behavior would support this documentation?
   1. The client is unable to recall all events associated with the crash.
   2. The client traveled unexpectedly and lost all personal memories.
   3. The client cannot recall his or her identity and total life history.
   4. The client can recall everything before the crash but nothing after the crash.

13. A client is diagnosed with somatic symptom disorder with a predominant symptom of pain. Compared with the following medications, which medication would a nurse practitioner choose as a first-line treatment for this client?
   1. Meperidine (Demerol)
   2. Clomipramine (Anafranil)
   3. Venlafaxine (Effexor)
   4. Fluvoxamine (Luvox)

14. Which of the following symptoms should a nurse recognize as characteristic of a diagnosis of dissociative identity disorder (DID)? **Select all that apply.**
   1. Most individuals are totally debilitated by the disorder.
   2. Transition from one personality to another may be sudden or gradual.
   3. Clients usually have a history of severe abuse or neglect.
   4. Clients experience "gaps" in memory or "lost time" when personalities emerge.
   5. Before therapy, the original personality is acutely aware of the other personalities.

15. Which characteristic does the nurse understand is common to all somatic symptom disorders?
   1. Delusions
   2. Pain
   3. Paranoia
   4. Physical symptoms

16. Which of the following nursing documentation entries accurately describe the behaviors of a client suspected of having Munchausen disorder by proxy? **Select all that apply.**
   1. "Attempts to simulate fever by placing son's thermometer under hot water."
   2. "Attempts to injure self by purposely falling off examination table."
   3. "Attempts to inject self with contaminated saline."
   4. "Attempts to self-medicate with high doses of Tylenol."
   5. "Attempts to intentionally administer son an overdose of laxatives."

17. Which of the following principles of learning theory relate to the etiology of the diagnosis of somatic symptom disorder? **Select all that apply.**
   1. The client's symptoms are reinforced when the sick role relieves stress.
   2. Symptoms are expressions of low self-esteem and feelings of worthlessness.
   3. Symptoms make the sick person the prominent focus of attention.
   4. Positive reinforcements virtually guarantee repetition of the response.
   5. It is easier to feel something is wrong with the body than with the self.

18. A client developed paralysis of the lower extremities after experiencing severe psychological trauma. Which medical intervention would the nurse expect to take priority?
    1. Individual psychotherapy
    2. Neurological testing
    3. Consultation with physical therapy
    4. Autogenic therapy

19. Which of the following client behaviors associated with somatic symptom disorder are correctly matched with the nursing diagnosis that addresses the behavior? **Select all that apply.**
    1. History of "doctor shopping": deficient knowledge
    2. Alteration in the experience of the self: disturbed sensory perception
    3. Feigning of physical symptoms: ineffective coping
    4. Preoccupation with bodily symptoms: fear of having a serious illness
    5. Inability to accept psychological etiology of symptoms: ineffective denial

20. On the basis of epidemiological statistics, which of the following clients would a nurse recognize as most likely to be diagnosed with depersonalization-derealization disorder?
    1. A 50-year-old male veteran of the Gulf War
    2. An 89-year-old woman Holocaust survivor
    3. An adolescent girl who suffered a near death experience
    4. An 20-year-old man who saw a friend killed in a drive-by shooting

REVIEW ANSWERS

1. ANSWER: Munchausen

Rationale: The diagnosis of factitious disorder can also be identified as Munchausen syndrome. The syndrome of fabricating symptoms for emotional gain was first described by Richard Asher in 1951. He described a pattern of behavior in which individuals fabricated or embellished their histories and signs and symptoms of illness. He termed this condition "Munchausen syndrome," after Baron Friedrich Hieronymus Freiherr von Munchhausen, a German cavalry officer and nobleman who was known for his fabricated stories and fanciful exaggerations about himself.

TEST-TAKING TIP: Review the key terms at the beginning of the chapter.

Content Area: Psychosocial Integrity;
Integrated Process: Nursing Process: Assessment;
Client Need: Psychosocial Integrity;
Cognitive Level: Knowledge;
Concept: Assessment

2. ANSWERS: 1, 2, 3

Rationale: Depersonalization-derealization disorder is characterized by a temporary change in the quality of self-awareness, which often takes the form of feelings of unreality, changes in body image, feelings of detachment from the environment, or a sense of observing oneself from outside the body.

1. Derealization describes an alteration in the perception of the external environment. By perceiving objects in the environment as altered, the client is experiencing derealization symptoms of depersonalization-derealization disorder (DDD). DDD, a dissociative disorder, occurs when anxiety becomes overwhelming. Severe psychosocial stress would be a predisposing factor for this disorder.

2. DDD is characterized by a temporary change in the quality of self-awareness including body image misinterpretation. A belief that the body's physical characteristics have changed is indicative of DDD. DDD, a dissociative disorder, occurs when anxiety becomes overwhelming. A near-death experience would be a predisposing factor for this disorder.

3. DDD is characterized by feelings of detachment from the body. DDD, a dissociative disorder, occurs when anxiety becomes overwhelming. Extreme social anxiety would be a predisposing factor for this disorder.

4. True alteration in bodily functioning is not a typical characteristic of DDD. Also, the symptoms of DDD should not be attributable to the direct physiological effects of a substance (a drug of abuse or a medication) such as marijuana.

5. An exaggerated belief that the body is deformed or defective is not a typical characteristic of DDD. This symptom is more typical of body dysmorphic disorder. Also, the symptoms of DDD should not be attributable to the direct physiological effects of a substance (a drug of abuse or a medication) or to medication side effects.

TEST-TAKING TIP: Review the cause and typical symptoms of DDD.

Content Area: Safe and Effective Care Environment;
Management of Care;
Integrated Process: Nursing Process: Assessment;
Client Need: Safe and Effective Care Environment;
Management of Care;
Cognitive Level: Analysis;
Concept: Assessment

3. ANSWER: 4

Rationale:

1. Continually worrying about an undiagnosed, serious medical illness is indicative of illness anxiety disorder (IAD), not a factitious disorder. IAD may be defined as an unrealistic or inaccurate interpretation of physical symptoms or sensations, leading to preoccupation and fear of having a serious disease.

2. Insisting that she is 6 months pregnant without any medical evidence is indicative of the somatic symptom disorder (SSD) pseudocyesis, not a factitious disorder. SSD is a syndrome of multiple somatic symptoms that cannot be explained medically.

3. Developing multiple personalities is indicative of dissociative identity disorder (DID), not a factitious disorder. DID is characterized by the existence of two or more personalities in a single individual. The predisposing factor for this disorder is a history of severe abuse in early childhood

4. Overmedicating self to gain medical attention is indicative of a factitious disorder, often termed Munchausen syndrome. Factitious disorders involve conscious, intentional feigning of physical or psychological symptoms. Individuals with factitious disorder pretend to be ill to receive emotional care and support commonly associated with the role of "patient." Individuals become very inventive in their quest to produce symptoms. Examples include self-inflicted wounds, injection or insertion of contaminated substances, manipulating a thermometer to feign a fever, urinary tract manipulation, and surreptitious use of medications.

TEST-TAKING TIP: Review the characteristics typical of factitious disorder.

Content Area: Safe and Effective Care Environment;
Management of Care;
Integrated Process: Nursing Process: Evaluation;
Client Need: Safe and Effective Care Environment;
Management of Care;
Cognitive Level: Application;
Concept: Assessment

4. ANSWERS: 3, 4, 5

Rationale: Dissociative disorders are conditions that involve disruptions or breakdowns of memory, awareness, identity, or perception. People with dissociative disorders use dissociation, a defense mechanism, pathologically and involuntarily. Dissociative disorders are thought to be caused primarily by psychological trauma.

1. Munchausen disorder by proxy is defined as a behavior pattern in which a caregiver fabricates, exaggerates, or induces mental or physical health problems in those who are under his or her care. This disorder is classified by the DSM-5 as a factitious disorder, not a dissociative disorder.

2. Illness anxiety disorder may be defined as an unrealistic or inaccurate interpretation of physical symptoms or sensations, leading to preoccupation and fear of having a serious disease. This disorder is classified by the DSM-5 as a somatic symptom disorder, not a dissociative disorder.

3. Dissociative amnesia may be defined as an inability to recall important personal information, usually of a traumatic or stressful nature, that is too extensive to be explained by ordinary forgetfulness and is not due to the direct effects of substance use or a neurological or other medical condition. This disorder is classified by the DSM-5 as a dissociative disorder.

4. Depersonalization-derealization disorder is character-ized by a temporary change in the quality of self-awareness, which often takes the form of feelings of unreality, changes in body image, feelings of detachment from the environment, or a sense of observing oneself from outside the body. This disorder is classified by the DSM-5 as a dissociative disorder.

5. Dissociative identity disorder was formerly called multiple personality disorder. This disorder is character-ized by the existence of two or more personalities in a single individual. Each personality is unique and composed of a complex set of memories, behavior patterns, and social relationships that surface during the dominant interval. This disorder is classified by the DSM-5 as a dissociative disorder.

TEST-TAKING TIP: Review the characteristics associated with dissociative disorder, and differentiate between the various disorder classifications.
Content Area: Psychosocial Integrity;
Integrated Process: Nursing Process: Evaluation;
Client Need: Psychosocial Integrity;
Cognitive Level: Comprehension;
Concept: Cognition

5. **ANSWER: 3**
Rationale:
1. The symptoms of conversion disorder resolve within a few weeks, but about 20%, not 50%, of individuals relapse within 1 year.
2. The symptoms of conversion disorder resolve within a few weeks, not months, and about 20% of individuals re-lapse within 1 year.
3. The most accurate nursing response is to teach the client that the symptoms of conversion disorder resolve within a few weeks, and about 20% of individuals relapse within 1 year.
4. The symptoms of conversion disorder resolve within a few weeks, not months, and about 20%, not 50%, of individ-uals relapse within 1 year.
TEST-TAKING TIP: Review information about conversion disorder and the possible prognosis for the disease.
Content Area: Safe and Effective Care Environment; Management of Care;
Integrated Process: Nursing Process: Implementation;
Client Need: Safe and Effective Care Environment; Management of Care;
Cognitive Level: Application;
Concept: Assessment

6. **ANSWER: 1**
Rationale: Illness anxiety disorder is defined as an individual's preoccupation with, fear of contracting, or the belief of having a serious disease.
1. Anxiety is experienced by a client diagnosed with illness anxiety disorder because of an unfounded fear of contracting disease. Expecting the client to rate anxiety as 3 out of 10 is an appropriate short-term outcome for clients diagnosed with this disorder.
2. It is unrealistic to expect a client to recognize the link between anxiety and somatic symptoms by day 2. Because of the potential for client denial and the need for ego defense, this insight may take considerably longer than 2 days to develop.
3. The outcome of client participation in group therapy activities does not address the underlying problem of anxiety experienced by clients diagnosed with illness anxiety disorder.
4. A newly admitted client diagnosed with illness anxiety disorder is not likely to understand the link between anxiety and somatic symptoms. It would be unrealistic to expect recognition of attention-seeking behaviors (secondary gains) this early in treatment.
TEST-TAKING TIP: Understand that clients diagnosed with illness anxiety disorder have little recognition of the link between anxiety and the symptoms that are experiencing. This lack of client insight would affect the formulation of realistic outcomes by the nurse.
Content Area: Safe and Effective Care Environment; Management of Care;
Integrated Process: Nursing Process: Planning;
Client Need: Safe and Effective Care Environment; Management of Care;
Cognitive Level: Application;
Concept: Critical Thinking

7. **ANSWER: 3**
Rationale:
1. Depersonalization is a condition in which there is an alteration in the perception or experience of the self so that the feeling of one's own reality is lost. The symptoms presented in the question are not indicative of depersonalization.
2. Derealization is a condition in which an alteration in the perception or experience of the external world seems unreal. Other symptoms include feeling as though one's environment is lacking in spontaneity, emotional coloring, and depth. The symptoms presented in the question are not indicative of derealization.
3. The client in the question is suffering from pseudocye-sis. Pseudocyesis is a condition in which an individual has nearly all the signs and symptoms of pregnancy but is not actually pregnant. This condition is considered a conversion disorder.
4. Illness anxiety disorder, formerly known as hypochon-driasis, refers to worry about having a serious illness. This debilitating condition is the result of an inaccurate percep-tion of the condition of body or mind despite the absence of an actual medical condition. The symptoms presented in the question are not indicative of illness anxiety disorder.

TEST-TAKING TIP: Review the key terms at the beginning of the chapter.
Content Area: Safe and Effective Care Environment;
Management of Care;
Integrated Process: Nursing Process: Assessment;
Client Need: Safe and Effective Care Environment;
Management of Care;
Cognitive Level: Application;
Concept: Assessment

8. **ANSWER: 4**
Rationale:
1. Factitious disorder is a disorder that is not real, genuine, or natural. The symptoms, physical and psychological, are *consciously* produced by the individual and are under voluntary control. The individual's goal is to assume a "patient" role to seek attention. The symptoms presented in the question are not indicative of factitious disorder.
2. La belle indifference is a disproportionate degree of indifference to, or complacency about symptoms, such as paralysis or loss of sensation in part of the body. It is characteristic of functional neurological symptom disorder. The symptoms presented in the question are not indicative of la belle indifference.
3. Illness anxiety disorder, formerly known as hypochondriasis, refers to worry about having a serious illness. This debilitating condition is the result of an inaccurate perception of the condition of body or mind despite the absence of an actual medical condition. The symptoms presented in the question are not indicative of illness anxiety disorder.
4. **The client in the question is suffering from dissociative fugue. Dissociative fugue is a rare condition in which a person suddenly, without planning or warning, travels far from home or work and leaves behind a past life. He or she experiences amnesia and has no conscious understanding or knowledge of the reason for the flight. The condition is usually associated with severe stress or trauma.**
TEST-TAKING TIP: Review the key terms at the beginning of the chapter.
Content Area: Safe and Effective Care Environment;
Management of Care;
Integrated Process: Nursing Process: Evaluation;
Client Need: Safe and Effective Care Environment;
Management of Care;
Cognitive Level: Application;
Concept: Nursing

9. **ANSWERS: 2, 4, 5**
Rationale:
1. Severe psychological stress does not typically precipitate a factitious disorder (FD). This student's statement indicates that further instruction is needed.
2. **Behaviors that are conscious, deliberate, and intentional are associated with FD, whereas behaviors associated with somatic symptom disorder are unconscious in nature. This student's statement indicates that learning has occurred.**

3. "Gaps" in memory or episodes of "lost time" are associated with dissociative identity disorder, not FD. This student's statement indicates that further instruction is needed.
4. **Clients diagnosed with FD may inflict painful injuries on themselves. Other client behaviors may include aggravating existing symptoms and/or inducing new ones. This student's statement indicates that learning has occurred.**
5. **Clients diagnosed with FD often have a history of frequent childhood hospitalizations. These hospitalizations may provide a reprieve from a traumatic home situation and a loving and caring environment that was absent in the child's family. This student's statement indicates that learning has occurred.**
TEST-TAKING TIP: Review the characteristics associated with FD.
Content Area: Safe and Effective Care Environment;
Management of Care;
Integrated Process: Nursing Process: Implementation;
Client Need: Safe and Effective Care Environment;
Management of Care;
Cognitive Level: Application;
Concept: Nursing Roles

10. **ANSWER: 1, 3, 4, 5**
Rationale:
1. **Clients diagnosed with illness anxiety disorder (IAD) do not appreciate the role that anxiety plays in their symptom profile and are convinced that they are not receiving proper care. This leads to "doctor shopping." Doctor shopping is not a characteristic associated with dissociative identity disorder (DID).**
2. Clients diagnosed with DID, not IAD, experience "gaps" in memory or "lost time" or blackouts during domination by subpersonalities. Symptoms of IAD do not include the presence of subpersonalities.
3. **Clients diagnosed with IAD do have an unrealistic, inaccurate interpretation of physical symptoms or sensations. This interpretation of symptoms and sensations is not a characteristic associated with DID.**
4. **It is true that clients diagnosed with IAD are highly anxious about and suspicious of the presence of an undiagnosed serious medical illness. High anxiety concerning medical illness is not a characteristic associated with DID.**
5. **It is true that clients diagnosed with IAD are extremely conscious of bodily sensations and changes and may become convinced that a rapid heart rate indicates that they have heart disease. This extreme consciousness regarding bodily sensations is not a characteristic associated with DID.**
TEST-TAKING TIP: Review the symptoms associated with IAD and DID, and be able to differentiate one from the other.
Content Area: Safe and Effective Care Environment;
Management of Care;
Integrated Process: Nursing Process: Evaluation;
Client Need: Safe and Effective Care Environment;
Management of Care;

Cognitive Level: Application;
Concept: Critical Thinking

11. **ANSWER: derealization**
Rationale: Derealization is characterized by feelings of detachment from and an alteration in the perception of the external environment. The symptom of derealization is associated with depersonalization-derealization disorder and can also occur in a variety of psychiatric illnesses such as schizophrenia, depression, anxiety states, and neurocognitive disorders.
TEST-TAKING TIP: Review the key terms at the beginning of the chapter.
Content Area: Psychosocial Integrity;
Integrated Process: Nursing Process: Assessment;
Client Need: Psychosocial Integrity;
Cognitive Level: Knowledge;
Concept: Assessment

12. **ANSWER: 1**
Rationale:
1. **When this client is unable to recall all events associated with the crash, the client is experiencing localized amnesia.**
2. If this client traveled unexpectedly and lost all personal memories, the client would be experiencing dissociative amnesia with dissociative fugue, not localized amnesia.
3. When the client cannot recall his or her identity and total life history, the client is experiencing generalized, not localized, amnesia.
4. When the client can recall everything before the crash but nothing after the crash, the client is recalling only certain incidents associated with a stressful event. This behavior is indicative of selective, not localized, amnesia.
TEST-TAKING TIP: Review the characteristics of the various types of amnesia.
Content Area: Safe and Effective Care Environment;
Management of Care;
Integrated Process: Nursing Process: Assessment;
Client Need: Safe and Effective Care Environment;
Management of Care;
Cognitive Level: Application;
Concept: Assessment

13. **ANSWER: 3**
Rationale:
1. Because there is no organic cause for the pain experienced in a somatic symptom disorder, meperidine (Demerol), an analgesic, is not the treatment of choice.
2. Tricyclic antidepressants (TCA) such as clomipramine (Anafranil) have been used extensively in relieving pain in somatic symptom disorders, but TCA side effects may make their use problematic. Compared with the other medications presented, this medication would not be chosen as a first line treatment.
3. **Serotonin-Norepinephrine reuptake inhibitors (SNRI), such as venlafaxine (Effexor), have been used as analgesic agents in the treatment of somatic symptom disorder with fewer side effects. Compared with the**

other medications presented, this medication would be chosen as a first line treatment.
4. Selective serotonin reuptake inhibitors, such as fluvoxamine (Luvox), have not exhibited the consistent analgesic efficacy demonstrated by the TCAs and SNRIs. Compared with the others presented, this medication would not be chosen as a first line treatment.
TEST-TAKING TIP: Review the medications used in the treatment of somatic symptom disorder when the prominent symptom is pain.
Content Area: Safe and Effective Care Environment;
Management of Care;
Integrated Process: Nursing Process: Implementation;
Client Need: Safe and Effective Care Environment;
Management of Care;
Cognitive Level: Application;
Concept: Medication

14. **ANSWERS: 2, 3, 4**
Rationale:
1. Some individuals with dissociative identity disorder (DID) maintain responsible positions, complete graduate degrees, and are successful spouses and parents before diagnosis and while in treatment.
2. **In DID, transition from one personality to another may be sudden or gradual and is sometimes quite dramatic.**
3. **Severe abuse or neglect that occurs during the personality development of childhood causes the child to develop personalities that can protect him or her from that experienced trauma. The child develops personalities to escape, or dissociate, from the inflicted emotional and/or physical pain, which leads to DID.**
4. **In DID, clients may experience "gaps" in memory or "lost time" or blackouts when other subpersonalities are dominant.**
5. Before therapy for DID, the original personality usually has no knowledge of the other personalities.
TEST-TAKING TIP: Review the characteristics associated with a diagnosis of dissociative identity disorder.
Content Area: Safe and Effective Care Environment;
Management of Care;
Integrated Process: Nursing Process: Assessment
Client Need: Safe and Effective Care Environment;
Management of Care;
Cognitive Level: Application;
Concept: Assessment

15. **ANSWER: 4**
Rationale:
1. Delusions are not a typical symptom of somatic symptom disorders.
2. Pain is present in some, but not all, somatic symptom disorders.
3. Paranoia is not a typical symptom of somatic symptom disorders.
4. **Somatic symptom disorders are characterized by physical symptoms suggesting medical disease but without demonstrable organic pathology. Physical symptoms are common to all somatic symptom disorders.**

TEST-TAKING TIP: Review the typical symptoms of somatic symptom disorders.
Content Area: Safe and Effective Care Environment; Management of Care;
Integrated Process: Nursing Process: Assessment;
Client Need: Safe and Effective Care Environment; Management of Care;
Cognitive Level: Application
Concept: Assessment

16. **ANSWERS: 1, 5**
Rationale: Munchausen disorder is a factitious disorder, which involves the conscious, intentional feigning of physical or psychological symptoms. Munchausen disorder by proxy is a factitious disorder in which a perpetrator imposes physical harm on a dependent individual under their care.
1. When a client puts his or her son's thermometer under hot water to simulate a fever, the client is intentionally imposing symptoms on a person under his or her care. This is indicative of Munchausen disorder by proxy.
2. It is indicative of Munchausen disorder, not Munchausen disorder by proxy, when a client inflicts painful injuries on self.
3. It is indicative of Munchausen disorder, not Munchausen disorder by proxy, when a client purposefully injures self by injecting a contaminated substance.
4. It is indicative of Munchausen disorder, not Munchausen disorder by proxy, when a client purposefully injures self by self-medicating with high doses of Tylenol.
5. It is indicative of Munchausen disorder by proxy when a client intentionally gives his or her son an overdose of laxatives.
TEST-TAKING TIP: Review the characteristics of both Munchausen disorder and Munchausen disorder by proxy and be able to differentiate the two disorders.
Content Area: Safe and Effective Care Environment; Management of Care;
Integrated Process: Nursing Process: Implementation;
Client Need: Safe and Effective Care Environment; Management of Care;
Cognitive Level: Application;
Concept: Communication

17. **ANSWERS: 1, 3, 4**
Rationale:
1. Somatic complaints are reinforced when the sick role relieves the individual from the need to deal with a stressful situation. The sick person learns that symptoms may help him or her to avoid stressful obligations, postpone unwelcome challenges, and be excused from troublesome duties.
2. From a psychodynamic, not a learning, perspective, the symptoms of somatic symptom disorder are viewed as expressions of low self-esteem and feelings of worthlessness.
3. In somatic symptom disorder, the client learns that symptoms make him or her the prominent focus of attention, which provides secondary gains.

4. Learning theory postulates that positive reinforcements virtually guarantee repetition of the response. Both the primary and secondary gains achieved reinforce the "sick role" behavior.
5. From a psychodynamic, not learning, perspective, physical symptoms are embraced because it is easier to feel something is wrong with the body than with the self.
TEST-TAKING TIP: Review the predisposing factors that explain the etiology of somatic symptom disorder with a focus on a learning perspective.
Content Area: Psychosocial Integrity;
Integrated Process: Nursing Process: Assessment;
Client Need: Psychosocial Integrity;
Cognitive Level: Application;
Concept: Evidenced-based Practice

18. **ANSWER: 2**
Rationale:
1. The causative agent of the paralysis must first be identified before initiating any psychotherapy. Physical cause must be ruled out before assuming psychological involvement.
2. The initial medical intervention is to rule out any organic factors contributing to the paralysis. Once a physical cause has been ruled out, a treatment plan can be effectively established.
3. Consultation with physical therapy will be meaningless if the cause of the paralysis is psychological in nature. Physical cause must be ruled out before assuming psychological involvement.
4. Autogenic therapy teaches the body to respond to verbal commands. These commands "tell" the body to relax and control breathing, blood pressure, heartbeat, and body temperature. The goal of autogenics is to achieve deep relaxation and reduce stress, but if the cause of the paralysis is neurological, reducing stress will not relieve the symptoms.
TEST-TAKING TIP: Understand that ruling out organic causes for physical symptoms must take priority before any treatment is initiated.
Content Area: Safe and Effective Care Environment; Management of Care;
Integrated Process: Nursing Process: Evaluation;
Client Need: Safe and Effective Care Environment; Management of Care;
Cognitive Level: Application;
Concept: Critical Thinking

19. **ANSWERS: 1, 4, 5**
Rationale:
1. Clients diagnosed with the somatic symptom disorder of illness anxiety often "doctor shop" because they are convinced that they are not receiving proper care. These clients have a deficient knowledge of the true cause of their symptoms, which is psychological, not physical, in nature.
2. Clients diagnosed with depersonalization-derealization disorder experience a temporary change in the quality of self-awareness. Disturbed sensory perception is correctly

matched with this symptom; but depersonalization-derealization disorder is classified as a dissociative disorder, not a somatic symptom disorder.

3. Ineffective coping is a nursing diagnosis that reflects the behavior of consciously feigning physical symptoms to gain attention. But this behavior is a characteristic of a factitious disorder, not a somatic symptom disorder.

4. Preoccupation with bodily symptoms is characteristic of illness anxiety disorder. Illness anxiety disorder, a somatic symptom disorder, may be defined as an unrealistic or inaccurate interpretation of physical symptoms, leading to preoccupation and fear of having a serious disease. Fear is an appropriately matched nursing diagnosis with the behaviors presented.

5. Ineffective denial is correctly matched with a client's inability to accept the psychological etiology of symptoms. When diagnosed with a somatic symptom disorder, the connection between physical symptoms and anxiety is unconscious; therefore, clients have difficulty accepting the psychological etiology of their symptoms.

TEST-TAKING TIP: Match the diagnosis with the client behavior that indicates a somatic symptom disorder. Other types of disorders should not be considered.

Content Area: Safe and Effective Care Environment; Management of Care;
Integrated Process: Nursing Process: Diagnosis (Analysis);
Client Need: Safe and Effective Care Environment; Management of Care;
Cognitive Level: Analysis;
Concept: Critical Thinking

20. **ANSWER: 3**
    Rationale:
    1. Depersonalization-derealization disorder (DDD) occurs more frequently in the young, rarely occurring in individuals older than 40. Incidence of the disorder is high under conditions of sustained traumatization like military combat; it also occurs more often in women than in men. Compared with the others presented, this client would not have the highest chance of being diagnosed with depersonalization-derealization disorder.

    2. Depersonalization-derealization disorder occurs in the young, rarely occurring in individuals older than 40. Even though the client has experienced conditions of sustained traumatization, this client's age of 89 years would decrease her chance of being diagnosed with depersonalization-derealization disorder.

    3. Symptoms of depersonalization-derealization disorder begin in adolescence or early adulthood and occur more often in women than men. The disorder has been reported in individuals who endure near-death experiences. Compared with the others presented, this client would have the highest chance of being diagnosed with depersonalization-derealization disorder.

    4. Symptoms of depersonalization-derealization disorder do begin in adolescence or early adulthood, but the incidence of the disorder is higher under conditions of sustained traumatization. Also the disorder occurs more often in women than men. Compared with the others presented, this client would not have the highest chance of being diagnosed with depersonalization-derealization disorder.

    TEST-TAKING TIP: Review the epidemiological statistics for the diagnosis of depersonalization-derealization disorder.

    Content Area: Safe and Effective Care Environment; Management of Care;
    Integrated Process: Nursing Process: Evaluation;
    Client Need: Safe and Effective Care Environment; Management of Care;
    Cognitive Level: Application;
    Concept: Assessment

CASE STUDY: Putting it All Together

Megan, a 25-year-old ballerina who collapsed after a sudden onset of paralysis involving both legs, was examined in the emergency department and admitted to the hospital's neurological unit. Assessment revealed a well-nourished, attractive young woman, whose only complaint was "My legs gave way just before my ballet performance, and now I can't move them at all." During the neurological work-up, Megan remained unconcerned about her condition and the potential impact on her dancing career. When she was told that all the neurological tests were within normal limits, she seemed indifferent to the news and agreed to a transfer to the psychiatric unit.

After psychiatric nurse practitioner (PNP) Jessie and Megan make introductions, he shows her around the unit and purposely does not offer to push Megan's wheelchair as she maneuvers her way through the day area. Jessie documents Megan's flat, sad affect as 2 out of 10 and notes her apathetic disinterest in her surroundings. During the assessment interview, Jessie asks Megan to tell him what's going on. Megan states, "This is the second time my legs have been paralyzed. A year ago, when I was about to audition for a very important part, I collapsed, couldn't move my legs, and didn't recover for 3 weeks. By then, I'd lost the part to someone else. I worked all year to regain my reputation. I got the starring role in *Swan Lake,* and at the debut, 10 days ago, it happened again! This role would have landed me a major ballet award that few ever receive."

Jessie responds by saying, "Sounds like you were under a great deal of stress."

"Yes, that's true. I'm an only child and my parents have very high expectations of me. I love them both so much, and I never want to disappoint them. In their eyes, my success is their success. They call me their prima ballerina. I guess they'll have to figure out a new pet name for me now."

1. Based on the client's symptoms and actions, what medical diagnosis would Jessie assign to Megan?
2. How does paralyzing illness meet Megan's needs?
3. What is the purpose of Jessie not offering to push Megan's wheelchair?
4. Why is Megan unconcerned about her paralysis and the effect it might have on her career?
5. What are Megan's subjective symptoms that would lead to the determination of this diagnosis?
6. What are Megan's objective symptoms that would lead to the determination of this diagnosis?
7. What NANDA nursing diagnosis would address Megan's current problem?
8. On the basis of this nursing diagnosis, what short-term outcome would be appropriate for Megan?
9. On the basis of this nursing diagnosis, what long-term outcome would be appropriate for Megan?
10. List the psychological treatments the PNP might employ to treat Megan.
11. List the nursing interventions (actions) that will assist Megan in successfully meeting these outcomes.
12. List the questions that should be asked to determine the success of the nursing interventions.

Chapter 17

Children and Adolescents

KEY TERMS

Autism spectrum disorder—A disorder that is characterized by impairment in social interaction skills and interpersonal communication and a restricted repertoire of activities and interests

Aversive stimulus—An unpleasant or punishing stimulus that causes avoidance of a thing, situation, or behavior, as in techniques of behavior modification

Conduct disorder—A psychological disorder diagnosed in childhood or adolescence that presents through a repetitive and persistent pattern of behavior in which the basic rights of others or major age-appropriate norms are violated; it is often seen as the precursor to antisocial personality disorder, which is not diagnosed until age 18 (not to be confused with *oppositional defiant disorder*)

Hyperactivity—Excessive psychomotor activity that may be purposeful or aimless, accompanied by physical movements and verbal utterances that are usually more rapid than normal; inattention and distractibility are common with hyperactive behavior

Impulsiveness—The trait of acting without reflection and without thought to the consequences of the behavior; an abrupt inclination to act (and the inability to resist acting) on certain behavioral urges

Intellectual developmental disorder (formerly known as *mental retardation*)—A generalized neurodevelopmental disorder characterized by

significantly impaired intellectual and adaptive functioning; it is defined by an IQ score below 70 in addition to deficits in two or more adaptive behaviors that affect everyday, general living.

Oppositional defiant disorder—A condition in which a child displays an ongoing pattern of uncooperative, defiant, hostile, and annoying behavior toward people in authority (not to be confused with *conduct disorder*)

Palilalia—Repeating one's own sounds or words (a type of vocal tic associated with Tourette's disorder)

Separation anxiety disorder—A condition in which a child becomes fearful and nervous when away from home or separated from a loved one— usually a parent or other caregiver—to whom the child is attached. Separation anxiety is normal in very young children (those between 8 and 14 months old)

Temperament—Personality characteristics that define an individual's mood and behavioral tendencies, that are evident very early in life and may be present at birth; the sum of physical, emotional, and intellectual components that affect or determine a person's actions and reactions

Tourette's disorder—An inherited neuropsychiatric disorder with onset in childhood, characterized by multiple physical (motor) tics and at least one vocal (phonic) tic

This chapter examines various disorders in which the symptoms first become evident during infancy, childhood, or adolescence. All nurses working with children or adolescents should be knowledgeable about "normal" stages of growth and development. Behavioral responses are individual and idiosyncratic. Whether a child's behavior indicates emotional problems is often difficult to determine. Guidelines for making such a determination should consider appropriateness of the behavior regarding age and cultural norms and whether the behavior interferes with adaptive functioning. This chapter focuses on the nursing process in

care of clients with intellectual developmental disorder, autism spectrum disorder, attention deficit-hyperactivity disorder, conduct disorder, oppositional defiant disorder, Tourette's disorder, and separation anxiety disorder.

I. Neurodevelopmental Disorders

A. Intellectual developmental disorder (IDD)
  1. Onset before age 18 years.
  2. Impairments in general intellectual functioning by measured intellectual performance on IQ tests.

3. Impairments in adaptive skills across multiple domains.

DID YOU KNOW?

Adaptive skills are an individual's ability to adapt to the requirements of daily living and the expectations of his or her age and cultural group.

4. Predisposing factors.
   a. Etiology may be primarily biological, primarily psychosocial, a combination of both, or in some instances, unknown.
   b. Genetic factors.
      i. Implicated in 5% of cases
      ii. Inborn errors of metabolism (Tay-Sachs disease, phenylketonuria, and hyperglycinemia)
      iii. Chromosomal disorders (Down syndrome, Klinefelter syndrome)
      iv. Single-gene abnormalities (tuberous sclerosis and neurofibromatosis)
   c. Disruptions in embryonic development.
      i. Thirty percent of cases due to early alterations in embryonic development
      ii. Response to toxicity associated with maternal ingestion of alcohol or other drugs
      iii. Maternal illnesses and infections during pregnancy (rubella, cytomegalovirus)
      iv. Complications of pregnancy (toxemia, uncontrolled diabetes)
   d. Pregnancy and perinatal factors.
      i. Ten percent of cases are the result of circumstances that occur during pregnancy
      ii. Fetal malnutrition
      iii. Viral and other infections
      iv. Prematurity
   e. Result of circumstances that occur during the birth process.
      i. Trauma to the head during delivery
      ii. Placenta previa
      iii. Premature separation of the placenta
      iv. Prolapse of the umbilical cord
   f. General medical conditions acquired in infancy or childhood.
      i. Implicated in 5% of cases
      ii. Infections
         a) Meningitis
         b) Encephalitis
      iii. Poisonings
         a) Insecticides
         b) Medications
         c) Lead
      iv. Physical trauma
         a) Head injuries
         b) Asphyxiation
         c) Hyperpyrexia
   g. Sociocultural factors and other mental disorders.
      i. Fifteen to twenty percent of cases attributed to deprivation of nurturance and social stimulation
      ii. Impoverished environments
      iii. Poor prenatal and perinatal care
      iv. Inadequate nutrition
   h. Severe mental disorders (autism spectrum disorder) can result in IDD.
5. Nursing Process: Assessment for intellectual developmental disorder (IDD).
   a. Severity measured by client's IQ level.
      i. Mild
      ii. Moderate
      iii. Severe
      iv. Profound
   b. Various behavioral manifestations and abilities associated with each of these levels of severity are outlined in Table 17.1.
   c. Critical to assess and focus on client's strengths and abilities.
      i. Level of independence
      ii. Ability to perform self-care activities
6. Nursing Process: Diagnosis (Analysis)—based on data collected during the nursing assessment, the degree of severity of the condition, and the client's capabilities, possible nursing diagnoses for the client diagnosed with intellectual developmental disorder (IDD) include:
   a. Risk for injury R/T altered physical mobility or aggressive behavior.
   b. Self-care deficit R/T altered physical mobility or lack of maturity.
   c. Impaired verbal communication R/T developmental alteration.
   d. Impaired social interaction R/T speech deficiencies or difficulty adhering to conventional social behavior.
   e. Delayed growth and development R/T isolation from significant others; inadequate environmental stimulation; genetic factors.
   f. Anxiety (moderate to severe) R/T hospitalization and absence of familiar surroundings.

MAKING THE CONNECTION

Recognition of the cause and period of inception of IDD provides information regarding what to expect from the child in terms of behavior and potential. However, each child is different, and consideration must be given on an individual basis in every case.

Table 17.1 **Developmental Characteristics of Intellectual Developmental Disorder by Degree of Severity**

Level (IQ)	Ability to Perform Self-Care Activities	Cognitive/Educational Capabilities	Social/Communication Capabilities	Psychomotor Capabilities
Mild (50–70)	Capable of independent living, with assistance during times of stress.	Capable of academic skills to sixth-grade level. As adult can achieve vocational skills for minimum self-support.	Capable of developing social skills. Functions well in a structured, sheltered setting.	Psychomotor skills usually not affected, although may have some slight problems with coordination.
Moderate (35–49)	Can perform some activities independently. Requires supervision.	Capable of academic skill to second-grade level. As adult may be able to contribute to own support in sheltered workshop.	May experience some limitation in speech communication. Difficulty adhering to social convention may interfere with peer relationships.	Motor development is fair. Vocational capabilities may be limited to unskilled gross motor activities.
Severe (20–34)	May be trained in elementary hygiene skills. Requires complete supervision.	Unable to benefit from academic or vocational training. Profits from systematic habit training.	Minimal verbal skills. Wants and needs often communicated by acting-out behaviors.	Poor psychomotor development. Only able to perform simple tasks under close supervision.
Profound (below 20)	No capacity for independent functioning. Requires constant aid and supervision.	Unable to profit from academic or vocational training. May respond to minimal training in self-help if presented in the close context of a one-to-one relationship.	Little, if any, speech development. No capacity for socialization skills.	Lack of ability for both fine and gross motor movements. Requires constant supervision and care. May be associated with other physical disorders.

Adapted from Black & Andreasen (2011); Sadock & Sadock (2007); Ursano, Kartheiser, & Barnhill (2008).

    g. Defensive coping R/T feelings of powerlessness and threat to self-esteem.

    h. Ineffective coping R/T inadequate coping skills secondary to developmental delay.

7. Nursing Process: Planning—the following outcomes may be developed to guide the care of a client diagnosed with IDD.

    a. **The client will**

       i. Experience no physical harm

       ii. Have self-care needs fulfilled

       iii. Interact with others in a socially appropriate manner

       iv. Maintain anxiety at a manageable level

       v. Accept direction without becoming defensive

       vi. Demonstrate adaptive coping skills in response to stressful situations

    b. Essential that family members or primary caregivers participate in planning and implementing the ongoing care of the client with IDD. Need information related to:

       i. Scope of condition

       ii. Realistic expectations

       iii. Client potentials

       iv. Methods for modifying behavior as required

       v. Community resources for assistance and support

8. Nursing Process: Implementation for clients diagnosed with intellectual developmental disorder (IDD)

    a. Interventions for clients who are experiencing risk for injury.

       i. Create a safe environment

       ii. Ensure that small items are removed from area where client will be ambulating and that sharp items are out of reach

       iii. Store items that client uses frequently within easy reach

       iv. Pad side rails and headboard of client with history of seizures

       v. Prevent physical aggression and acting out behaviors by learning to recognize signs of increased agitation

    b. Interventions for clients who are experiencing a self-care deficit.

       i. Identify aspects of self-care that may be within the client's capabilities

       ii. Work on one aspect of self-care at a time

       iii. Provide simple, concrete explanations

       iv. Offer positive feedback for efforts

       v. When one aspect of self-care has been mastered to the best of the client's ability, move on to another

       vi. Encourage independence but intervene when client is unable to perform

c. Interventions for clients who are experiencing impaired verbal communication.
   i. Maintain consistency of staff assignment
   ii. Anticipate and fulfill client's needs until satisfactory communication patterns are established
   iii. Learn (from family) special words client uses that are different from the norm
   iv. Identify nonverbal gestures or signals that client may use to convey needs
   v. Practice communication skills repeatedly

DID YOU KNOW?

Some children with IDD, particularly at the severe level, can only learn through behavior modification techniques. The goal of behavior modification is to modify maladaptive behavior patterns by reinforcing more adaptive behaviors.

d. Interventions for clients who are experiencing impaired social interaction.
   i. Remain with client during initial interactions with others
   ii. Explain to other clients the meaning behind some of the client's nonverbal gestures and signals
   iii. Use simple language to explain to client which behaviors are acceptable and which are not
   iv. Establish a procedure for behavior modification with rewards for appropriate behaviors and aversive reinforcement for inappropriate behaviors
9. Nursing Process: Evaluation of the nursing actions for the client diagnosed with IDD may be facilitated by gathering information using the following types of questions:
  a. Have nursing actions provided for the client's safety been sufficient to prevent injury?

MAKING THE CONNECTION

Consistency of staff assignments facilitates trust and the ability to understand client's actions and unique communications.

MAKING THE CONNECTION

Positive, negative, and aversive reinforcements can contribute to desired changes in behavior. An **aversive stimulus** is an unpleasant event that is intended to decrease the probability of a behavior when it is presented as a consequence. Privileges and penalties are individually determined as staff learns the likes and dislikes and abilities of the client.

b. Have all of the client's self-care needs been fulfilled? Can he or she fulfill some of these needs independently?
c. Has the client been able to communicate needs and desires so that he or she can be understood?
d. Has the client learned to interact appropriately with others?
e. When regressive behaviors surface, can the client accept constructive feedback and discontinue the inappropriate behavior?
f. Has anxiety been maintained at a manageable level?
g. Has the client learned new coping skills through behavior modification?
h. Does the client demonstrate evidence of increased self-esteem because of the accomplishment of new skills and adaptive behaviors?
i. Have primary caregivers been taught realistic expectations of the client's behavior and methods for attempting to modify unacceptable behaviors?
j. Have primary caregivers been given information regarding various resources from which they can seek assistance and support within the community?

B. Autism spectrum disorder (ASD)

DID YOU KNOW?

ASD encompasses a broad spectrum of diagnoses that included autistic disorder, Rett's disorder, childhood disintegrative disorder, pervasive developmental disorder not otherwise specified, and Asperger's disorder.

1. Adapted to each individual by clinical specifiers (level of severity, verbal abilities) and associated features (known genetic disorders, epilepsy, intellectual disability).
2. Characterized by a withdrawal into the self and into a fantasy world of his or her own creation.
3. Markedly abnormal or impaired development in social interaction and communication.
4. Markedly restricted repertoire of activities and interests some of which may be considered somewhat bizarre.

DID YOU KNOW?

Children diagnosed with ASD and functioning at a high level on the autism spectrum were previously categorized with "Asperger's syndrome." These children do not typically have language development delays but have difficulty picking up on social cues and lack social skills. They have trouble interpreting verbal and nonverbal signals, often take abstract comments literally, and lack a sense of empathy.

5. Epidemiology.
   a. Prevalence of ASD in the United States is 11.3 per 1,000 (one in 88) children.
   b. Occurs about 4.5 times more often in boys than in girls.
   c. Onset of the disorder occurs in early childhood.
   d. Runs a chronic course, with symptoms persisting into adulthood.
6. Predisposing factors.
   a. Neurological implications.
      i. Number of alterations in major brain structures
      ii. Disproportionate enlargement in temporal lobe white matter
      iii. Increase in surface area in the temporal, frontal, and parieto-occipital lobes
      iv. Overall impairment in brain connectivity networks associated with attention, consciousness, and self-awareness
      v. Role of neurotransmitters (serotonin, dopamine, and epinephrine) under investigation
   b. Physiological implications.
      i. Medical conditions may be implicated in the predisposition to ASD
         • Tuberous sclerosis
         • Fragile X syndrome
         • Congenital hypothyroidism
         • Phenylketonuria
         • Down's syndrome
         • Neurofibromatosis
         • Angelman's syndrome
      ii. Ninety percent of cases have no readily identifiable cause
   c. Genetics.
      i. Genetic factors play a significant role in the etiology
      ii. Parents who have one child with ASD are at increased risk for having another child with the disorder
      iii. Monozygotic and dizygotic twin studies have provided evidence of genetic involvement
      iv. Involvement of chromosomes 2, 7, 15, 16, and 17
      v. Region on chromosome 11 may be implicated
      vi. Aberrations in a brain-development gene called *neurexin 1* may contribute
   d. Perinatal influences.
      i. Women who suffer with asthma and allergies during the second trimester have a greater than twofold elevated risk of having an affected child
      ii. May be due to maternal immune response during pregnancy

      iii. Asthma and allergy may share environmental risk factors with ASD
      iv. Maternal rubella
7. Nursing Process: Assessment for autism spectrum disorder (ASD)
   a. Impairment in social interaction.
      i. Difficulty forming interpersonal relationships with others
      ii. Show little interest in people
      iii. Often do not respond to others' attempts at interaction
      iv. As infants, may have an aversion to affection and physical contact
      v. As toddlers, attachment to a significant adult may be either absent or manifested as exaggerated adherence behaviors
      vi. In childhood, there is failure to develop cooperative play, imaginative play, and friendships
      vii. With minimal handicaps, may eventually progress to the point of passively recognizing other children as part of their environment
   b. Impairment in communication and imaginative activity
      i. Both verbal and nonverbal skills affected
      ii. Language may be absent

DID YOU KNOW?

The language of children diagnosed with ASD may be characterized by immature structure or idiosyncratic utterances, the meaning of which is clear only to those who are familiar with the child's past experiences.

      iii. Nonverbal communication (facial expression, gestures) often absent or socially inappropriate
      iv. Unable to interpret verbal cues during interactions
      v. Pattern of imaginative play often restricted and stereotypical
   c. Restricted activities and interests.
      i. Even minor changes in environment can be met with resistance or sometimes hysterical responses
      ii. Lower-functioning children may show an attachment to, or extreme fascination with, objects that move or spin (fans)

MAKING THE CONNECTION

ASD is a spectrum disorder; therefore, symptomatology would be observed on a degree-of-gravity continuum from mild to more severe.

iii. Higher-functioning children often display intense interests almost to the point of obsession

iv. Routine may become an obsession, with minor alterations in routine leading to marked distress

v. Stereotyped body movements (hand-clapping, rocking, whole-body swaying)

vi. Verbalizations (repetition of words or phrases)

vii. Diet abnormalities
- Eating only a few specific foods
- Consuming an excessive amount of fluids

🛇 Behaviors that are self-injurious such as head banging and/or biting the hands or arms may be evident in children diagnosed with ASD. Nurses must be alert to protect the child from these injurious behaviors.

8. Nursing Process: Diagnosis (Analysis)—on the basis of data collected during the nursing assessment, possible nursing diagnoses for the client diagnosed with autism spectrum disorder (ASD) include:

a. Risk for self-mutilation R/T neurological alterations; history of self-mutilative behaviors; hysterical reactions to changes in the environment.

b. Impaired social interaction R/T inability to trust; neurological alterations AEB lack of responsiveness to, or interest in, people.

c. Impaired verbal communication R/T withdrawal into the self; neurological alterations AEB inability or unwillingness to speak; lack of nonverbal expression; misinterpretation of verbal cues.

d. Disturbed personal identity R/T neurological alterations; delayed developmental stage AEB difficulty separating own physiological and emotional needs and personal boundaries from those of others.

9. Nursing Process: Planning—the following outcomes may be developed to guide the care of a client diagnosed with ASD. **The client will**

a. Exhibit no evidence of self-harm.

b. Interact appropriately with at least one staff member.

c. Demonstrate trust in at least one staff member.

d. Be able to communicate so that he or she can be understood by at least one staff member.

e. Demonstrate behaviors that indicate he or she has begun the separation/individuation process.

10. Nursing Process: Implementation for clients diagnosed with ASD.

a. Interventions for clients who are experiencing risk for self-mutilation.

i. Work with the child on one-to-one basis

ii. Determine whether self-mutilative behavior occurs in response to increasing anxiety

iii. Determine to what the anxiety may be attributed

iv. Intervene with diversion or replacement activities

v. Offer self to the child as anxiety level rises

vi. Protect the child (use helmet, padded hand mitts, or arm covers)

b. Interventions for clients who are experiencing impaired social interactions.

i. Assign a limited number of caregivers

ii. Convey warmth, acceptance, and availability

iii. Provide child with familiar objects (toys, blanket)

iv. Support child's attempts to interact with others

v. Give positive reinforcement for eye contact with something acceptable to the child (food, familiar object)

DID YOU KNOW?

When the nurse is working with children diagnosed with ASD, it is essential to recognize the importance of reinforcing the child's ability to establish eye contact. This interpersonal skill is essential to a child's ability to form satisfactory interpersonal relationships.

vi. Gradually replace with social reinforcement (touch, smiling, hugging)

c. Interventions for clients who are experiencing impaired verbal communication.

i. Maintain consistent caregiver assignment

ii. Anticipate and fulfill the child's needs until communication can be established

iii. Seek clarification and validation

iv. Give positive reinforcement when eye contact is used to convey nonverbal expressions

d. Interventions for clients who are experiencing disturbed personal identity.

i. Assist child to recognize separateness during self-care activities (dressing and feeding)

DID YOU KNOW?

One of the ways to help a child with ASD recognize their separateness is by assisting the child in learning to name his or her own body parts. This can be facilitated by the use of mirrors, drawings, and pictures of the child.

ii. Encourage appropriate touching of, and being touched by, others

11. Nursing Process: Evaluation—evaluation of nursing actions for the client diagnosed with ASD may be facilitated by gathering

information using the following types of questions:

a. Has the child been able to establish trust with at least *one* caregiver?

b. Have the nursing actions directed toward preventing mutilative behaviors been effective in protecting the client from self-harm?

c. Has the child attempted to interact with others? Has he or she received positive reinforcement for these efforts?

d. Has eye contact improved?

e. Has the child established a means of communicating his or her needs and desires to others?

f. Have all self-care needs been met?

g. Does the child demonstrate an awareness of self as separate from others?

h. Can he or she name own body parts and body parts of caregiver?

i. Can he or she accept touch from others?

j. Does he or she willingly and appropriately touch others?

12. Psychopharmacological interventions used for clients diagnosed with ASD.

a. Risperidone (Risperdal) and aripiprazole (Abilify) are used for the following behavior symptoms:

i. Aggression

ii. Deliberate self-injury

iii. Temper tantrums

iv. Quickly changing moods

b. Risperidone (Risperdal) is used in children and adolescents 5 to 16 years.

i. Dosage is based on weight of child and clinical response

ii. Most common side effects

a) Drowsiness

b) Mild to moderate increase in appetite

c) Nasal congestion

d) Fatigue

e) Constipation

f) Drooling

g) Dizziness

h) Weight gain

iii. Less common but more serious possible side effects

a) Neuroleptic malignant syndrome

b) Tardive dyskinesia

c) Hyperglycemia

d) Diabetes

iv. "Abnormal movements" but no cases of tardive dyskinesia reported

c. Aripiprazole (Abilify) used in children and adolescents 6 to 17 years

i. Most common side effects

a) Sedation

b) Fatigue

c) Weight gain

d) Vomiting

e) Somnolence

f) Tremor

ii. Common reasons for discontinuation

a) Sedation

b) Drooling

c) Tremor

d) Vomiting

e) Extrapyramidal symptoms (EPS)

iii. Maintenance therapy has not been evaluated

iv. Clients should be periodically reassessed to determine the need for continued treatment

C. Attention deficit-hyperactivity disorder (ADHD)

1. Difficult to diagnose in children younger than 4 years of age.

2. Characteristic behavior of younger children much more variable.

3. Frequently not recognized until the child enters school.

4. Epidemiology.

a. More common in boys than girls by a ratio of 3:1.

b. Prevalence as high as 9% of school-age children.

c. Sixty to seventy percent of the cases persist into young adulthood.

d. Twenty-five percent will meet criteria for antisocial personality disorder as adults.

5. Predisposing factors.

a. Biological influences.

i. Genetics

a) Large number of parents of hyperactive children were themselves hyperactive

b) Siblings tend to also be hyperactive

c) When one identical twin has the disorder, the other is also likely to have it

d) Variants found on specific region of chromosome 16

e) Variation in chromosomal regions previously linked to ASD and schizophrenia

ii. Biochemical: abnormal levels of dopamine, norepinephrine, and possibly serotonin are involved in producing symptoms

iii. Anatomical influences: specific brain area alterations implicated including prefrontal lobes, basal ganglia, caudate nucleus, globus pallidus, and cerebellum. See Figure 17.1

iv. Prenatal, perinatal, and postnatal factors

a) Maternal smoking during pregnancy

b) Intrauterine exposure to toxic substances, including alcohol

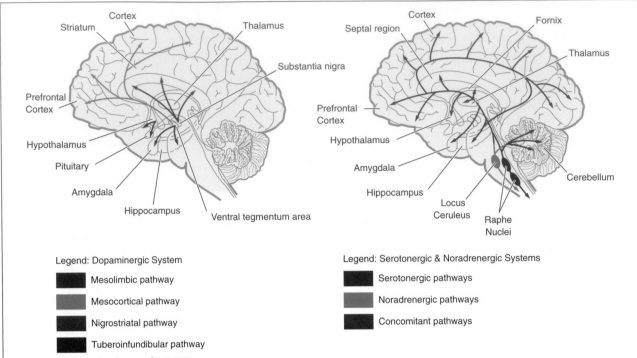

Legend: Dopaminergic System
- Mesolimbic pathway
- Mesocortical pathway
- Nigrostriatal pathway
- Tuberoinfundibular pathway

Legend: Serotonergic & Noradrenergic Systems
- Serotonergic pathways
- Noradrenergic pathways
- Concomitant pathways

Fig 17.1 Neurobiology of ADHD.

Neurotransmitters

The major neurotransmitters implicated in the pathophysiology of ADHD are dopamine, norepinephrine, and possibly serotonin. Dopamine and norepinephrine appear to be depleted in ADHD. Serotonin in ADHD has been studied less extensively, but recent evidence suggests that it also is reduced in children with ADHD.

Neurotransmitter Functions

- Norepinephrine is thought to play a role in the ability to perform executive functions, such as analysis and reasoning, and in the cognitive alertness essential for processing stimuli and sustaining attention and thought (Hunt, 2006).
- Dopamine is thought to play a role in sensory filtering, memory, concentration, controlling emotions, locomotor activity, and reasoning.
- Deficits in both norepinephrine and dopamine have been implicated in the inattention, impulsiveness, and hyperactivity associated with ADHD.
- Serotonin appears to play a role in ADHD, although possibly less significant than norepinephrine and dopamine. It has been suggested that alterations in serotonin may be related to the disinhibition and impulsivity observed in children with ADHD. It may play a role in mood disorders, particularly depression, which is a common comorbid disorder associated with ADHD.

Functional Areas of the Brain Affected

- **Prefrontal cortex:** Associated with maintaining attention, organization, and executive function. Also serves to modulate behavior inhibition, with serotonin as the predominant central inhibiting neurotransmitter for this function.
- **Basal ganglia** (particularly the caudate nucleus and globus pallidus): Involved in the regulation of high-level movements. In association with its connecting circuits to the prefrontal cortex, may also be important in cognition. Interruptions in these circuits may result in inattention or impulsivity.
- **Hippocampus:** Plays an important role in learning and memory.
- **Limbic System** (composed of the amygdala, hippocampus, mammillary body, hypothalamus, thalamus, fornix, cingulate gyrus and septum pellucidum): regulation of emotions. A neurotransmitter deficiency in this area may result in restlessness, inattention, or emotional volatility.
- **Reticular activating system** (composed of the reticular formation [located in the brainstem] and its connections): this is the major relay system among the many pathways that enter and leave the brain. It is thought to be the center of arousal and motivation and is crucial for maintaining a state of consciousness.

Medications for ADHD

Central Nervous System Stimulants

- Amphetamines (dextroamphetamine, lisdexamfetamine, methamphetamine, and mixtures): cause the release of norepinephrine from central noradrenergic neurons. At higher doses, dopamine may be released in the mesolimbic system.
- Methylphenidate and dexmethylphenidate: block the reuptake of norepinephrine and dopamine into the presynaptic neuron and increase the release of these monoamines into the extraneuronal space.
  Side effects of central nervous system stimulants include restlessness, insomnia, headache, palpitations, weight loss, suppression of growth in children (with long-term use), increased blood pressure, abdominal pain, anxiety, tolerance, and physical and psychological dependence.

Others

- Atomoxetine: selectively inhibits the reuptake of norepinephrine by blocking the presynaptic transporter. Side effects include headache, upper abdominal pain, nausea and vomiting, anorexia, cough, dry mouth, constipation, increase in heart rate and blood pressure, and fatigue.
- Bupropion: inhibits the reuptake of norepinephrine and dopamine into presynaptic neurons. Side effects include headache, dizziness, insomnia or sedation, tachycardia, increased blood pressure, dry mouth, nausea and vomiting, weight gain or loss, and seizures (dose dependent).
- Alpha agonists (clonidine, guanfacine): stimulate central alpha-adrenoreceptors in the brain, resulting in reduced sympathetic outflow from the CNS. Side effects include palpitations, bradycardia, constipation, dry mouth, and sedation.

c) Fetal alcohol syndrome includes hyperactivity, impulsivity, and inattention, as well as physical anomalies
d) Prematurity or low birth weight
e) Signs of fetal distress
f) Precipitated or prolonged labor
g) Perinatal asphyxia
h) Low Apgar scores
i) Cerebral palsy
j) Seizures
k) Other central nervous system abnormalities, for example, trauma, infections, other neurological disorders

b. Environmental influences.
 i. Environmental lead
 ii. Diet factors
  a) Food dyes
  b) Additives (artificial flavorings and preservatives)
  c) Dye and additive studies remain controversial
  d) Research results strongly suggest that sugar plays no role in hyperactivity

c. Psychosocial influences.
 i. Disorganized or chaotic environments
 ii. Disruption in family equilibrium
 iii. High degree of psychosocial stress
 iv. Maternal mental disorder
 v. Paternal criminality
 vi. Low socioeconomic status
 vii. Living in poverty

viii. Growing up in an institution
 ix. Unstable foster care

6. Nursing Process: Assessment for attention deficit-hyperactivity disorder (ADHD).
 a. The essential behavior pattern is of inattention and/or hyperactivity and **impulsivity**.
 b. Specified according to clinical presentation.
  i. Combined presentation (inattention and hyperactivity/impulsivity)
  ii. Predominantly inattentive presentation
  iii. Predominantly hyperactive/impulsive presentation
 c. Highly distractible.
 d. Extremely limited attention spans.
 e. Excessive motor activity.
 f. Random and impulsive movements.
 g. Difficulties in performing age-appropriate tasks.
 h. Often shift from one uncompleted activity to another.
 i. Impulsive with a deficit in inhibitory control.
 j. Difficulty forming satisfactory interpersonal relationships.
 k. Behaviors inhibit acceptable social interaction.
 l. Disruptive and intrusive in group endeavors.
 m. Difficulty complying with social norms.
 n. May be very aggressive or oppositional.
 o. May exhibit more regressive and immature behaviors.
 p. Low frustration tolerance.
 q. Outbursts of temper.
 r. Have boundless energy.

🛑 Children diagnosed with ADHD are restless, continuously running, jumping, wiggling, or squirming. They experience a greater-than-average number of accidents, from minor mishaps to more serious incidents that may lead to physical injury or the destruction of property.

   s. Eighty-four percent have comorbid psychiatric disorders.
      i. Oppositional defiant disorder
      ii. Conduct disorder
      iii. Anxiety
      iv. Depression
      v. Bipolar disorder
      vi. Substance abuse
   u. Anxiety and depression may be treated concurrently with bupropion (Wellbutrin) or atomoxetine (Strattera)
   v. Coexisting anxiety may benefit from treatment with atomoxetine
   w. With coexisting substance use disorders, priority is to stabilize addiction before treating ADHD
   x. With coexisting bipolar disorder, medication for ADHD should be initiated only after bipolar symptoms are controlled with a mood stabilizer (stimulants can exacerbate mania)
   y. Types of conditions often seen with ADHD and their rate of comorbidity are presented in Table 17.2.
7. Nursing Process: Diagnosis (Analysis)—on the basis of data collected during the nursing assessment, possible nursing diagnoses for the client diagnosed with ADHD include:
   a. Risk for injury R/T impulsive and accident-prone behavior and the inability to perceive self-harm.
   b. Impaired social interaction R/T intrusive and immature behavior.
   c. Low self-esteem R/T dysfunctional family system and negative feedback.

Table 17.2 Type and Frequency of Comorbidity With ADHD

Comorbidity	Rates
Oppositional defiant disorder	Up to 50%
Conduct disorder	~33%
Learning disorders	20%–30 %
Anxiety	25%–35%
Depression	~26%
Bipolar disorder	11%–20 %
Substance use	13%–26 %

Sources: Dopheide & Pliszka (2009); Ferguson-Noyes & Wilkinson (2008); Jenson (2005); Robb (2006).[CE4]

   d. Noncompliance with task expectations R/T low frustration tolerance and short attention span.
8. Nursing Process: Planning—the following outcomes may be developed to guide the care of a client diagnosed with ADHD. **The client will:**
   a. Experience no physical harm.
   b. Interact with others appropriately.
   c. Verbalize positive aspects about self.
   d. Demonstrate fewer demanding behaviors.
   e. Cooperate with staff in an effort to complete assigned tasks.
9. Nursing Process: Implementation for ADHD.
   a. Interventions for clients who are experiencing risk for injury.
      i. Ensure a safe environment
      ii. Remove objects from immediate area to avoid client injury due to random, hyperactive movements

🛑 Normal living situations and environments can be hazardous to the child diagnosed with ADHD, whose motor activities are out of control. Client safety is always a nursing priority.

      iii. Identify deliberate behaviors that put the child at risk for injury to self or others
      iv. Institute consequences for repetition of unsafe behavior
      v. Assess for situations during therapeutic activities that could lead to client injury
      vi. Provide adequate supervision and assistance during therapeutic activities
      vii. Limit client's participation in therapeutic activities if adequate supervision is not possible
   b. Interventions for clients who are experiencing impaired social interaction.
      i. Convey acceptance of the child separate from the unacceptable behavior
      ii. Discuss with client those behaviors that are and are not acceptable
      iii. Describe in a matter-of-fact manner the consequences of unacceptable behavior
      iv. Follow through with consequences
      v. Provide group situations for client

MAKING THE CONNECTION

Appropriate social behavior is often learned from the positive and negative feedback of peers. Providing situations that allow for interactions with peers can assist the client to observe and imitate appropriate behavior.

c. Interventions for clients who are experiencing low self-esteem.
 i. Ensure that goals are realistic
 ii. Plan activities that provide opportunities for success
 iii. Convey unconditional acceptance and positive regard
 iv. Offer recognition of successful endeavors and positive reinforcement for attempts made
 v. Give immediate positive feedback for acceptable behavior
d. Interventions for clients who are experiencing nonadherence (with task expectations).
 i. Provide an environment for task efforts that is free of distractions
 ii. Provide assistance on a one-to-one basis
 iii. Provide simple, concrete instructions
 iv. Ask client to repeat instructions to you
 v. Establish goals that allow client to complete a part of the task, rewarding each step-completion with a break for physical activity

DID YOU KNOW?

Because clients diagnosed with ADHD have short attention spans, it is important to help them set short-term goals. These goals are less likely to overwhelm the client. Giving positive reinforcement for partial goal completion increases self-esteem and provides incentive for clients to complete tasks.

 vi. Gradually decrease the amount of assistance given
 vii. Assure client that assistance is still available
10. Nursing process: evaluation—evaluation of nursing actions for the client diagnosed with ADHD may be facilitated by gathering information using the following types of questions:
a. Have the nursing actions directed at client safety been effective in protecting the child from injury?
b. Has the client been able to establish a trusting relationship with the primary caregiver?
c. Is the client responding to limits set on unacceptable behaviors?
d. Is the client able to interact appropriately with others?

MAKING THE CONNECTION

Assisting clients to set realistic goals is important to help them maintain their self-esteem. Unrealistic goals often precipitate failure, diminishing self-worth. Self-esteem can be improved by successful experiences coupled with affirmation of the client as a worthwhile human being.

e. Is the client able to verbalize positive statements about self?
f. Is the client able to complete tasks independently or with a minimum of assistance?
g. Can the client follow through after listening to simple instructions?
h. Is the client able to apply self-control to decrease motor activity?
11. Psychopharmacological interventions for ADHD
a. Examples of commonly used agents for ADHD are presented in Table 17.3.
b. The exact mechanism by which the medications (stimulant and nonstimulant) produce a therapeutic effect is unclear.
c. Stimulants.
 i. Central nervous system (CNS) stimulants increase levels of neurotransmitters (probably norepinephrine, dopamine, and serotonin)

DID YOU KNOW?

Previously, it was accepted that stimulant medications such as amphetamine and dextroamphetamine (Adderall) and methylphenidate (Ritalin) work one way in people diagnosed with ADHD, but a different way in people without ADHD. Current research is showing that this concept is a myth. It is now known that low doses of stimulants increase levels of neurotransmitters in the brain, focus attention, and improve executive function in both subjects diagnosed with ADHD and those without the disorder.

 ii. CNS stimulants produce:
 a) CNS and respiratory stimulation
 b) Dilated pupils
 c) Increased motor activity
 d) Mental alertness
 e) Diminished sense of fatigue
 f) Brighter spirits
d. Nonstimulant drugs:
 i. Atomoxetine (Strattera) inhibits the reuptake of norepinephrine
 ii. Bupropion (Wellbutrin) blocks the neuronal uptake of serotonin, norepinephrine, and dopamine
 iii. Clonidine (Catapres) and guanfacine (Tenex) stimulate central alpha-adrenoreceptors resulting in reduced sympathetic outflow from the CNS
 iv. Exact mechanism by which these nonstimulant drugs produce the therapeutic effect in ADHD is unclear
e. Contraindications to/precautions with pharmacological interventions for ADHD.
 i. CNS stimulants
 a) Contraindicated with hypersensitivity to sympathomimetic amines

Table 17.3 Medications for Attention Deficit-Hyperactivity Disorder

Chemical Class	Generic (Trade) Name	Daily Dosage Range (mg)	Controlled Categories	Pregnancy Categories/ Half-life (hr)
CNS Stimulants	Dextroamphetamine sulfate (Dexedrine; DextroStat)	2.5–40	CII	C/~12
Amphetamines	Methamphetamine (Desoxyn)	5–25	CII	C/4–5
	Lisdexamfetamine (Vyvanse)	20–70	CII	C/<1
Amphetamine Mixtures	Dextroamphetamine/ amphetamine	2.5–40	CII	C/9–13
	(Adderall; Adderall XR)	10–60	CII	C/2–4
Miscellaneous	Methylphenidate (Ritalin; Ritalin-SR; Ritalin LA; Methylin; Methylin ER; Metadate ER; Metadate CD; Concerta; Daytrana)	5–20	CII	C/ 2.2
ALPHA AGONISTS	Dexmethylphenidate (Focalin)	0.05–0.3	—-	C/ 12–16
	Clonidine (Catapres)	1–4		B/ 10–30
	Guanfacine (Tenex; Intuniv)	>70 kg: 40–100;	—-	
MISCELLANEOUS	Atomoxetine (Strattera)	≤70 kg: 0.5–1.4 mg/kg (or 100 mg, whichever is less)	—	C/5.2 (metabolites 6–8)
	Bupropion (Wellbutrin; Wellbutrin SR; Wellbutrin XL)	3 mg/kg (ADHD); 100–300 (depression)	—	C/8–24

b) Do not use in advanced arteriosclerosis, cardiovascular disease, hypertension, hyperthyroidism, glaucoma, agitated or hyperexcitability states
c) Do not use for clients with a history of:
- Drug abuse
- Within 14 days of receiving monoamine oxidase inhibitors (MAOIs)
- In children younger than 3 years of age
- During pregnancy and lactation
d) Caution advised in:
- Children with psychosis
- Clients diagnosed with Tourette's disorder
- Clients diagnosed with anorexia or insomnia
- Elderly, debilitated, or weak clients

- Clients with a history of suicidal or homicidal tendencies
ii. CNS nonstimulants
a) Atomoxetine and bupropion contraindicated in clients with hypersensitivity to the drugs or their components
b) Do not use atomoxetine and bupropion during lactation
c) Do not use atomoxetine and bupropion during or within 14 days of receiving monoamine oxidase inhibitors (MAOIs)
d) Atomoxetine and bupropion should be used cautiously for:
- Clients with urinary retention
- Clients experiencing hypertension and/or hepatic, renal, or cardiovascular disease
- Suicidal clients

- Pregnant clients
- Elderly and debilitated clients

e) Atomoxetine contraindicated in clients with narrow-angle glaucoma

f) Bupropion contraindicated with known or suspected seizure disorder

g) Bupropion contraindicated during acute phase of myocardial infarction

h) Bupropion contraindicated for clients diagnosed with bulimia or anorexia nervosa

iii. Alpha agonists

a) Use is contraindicated in clients with known hypersensitivity to the drugs

b) Use is contraindicated in clients with coronary insufficiency, recent myocardial infarction, or cerebrovascular disease

c) Use is contraindicated in clients with chronic renal or hepatic failure

d) Use is contraindicated in the elderly

e) Use is contraindicated in pregnant and lactating clients

DID YOU KNOW?

Prolonged use of CNS stimulants may result in tolerance and physical or psychological dependence.

f. Interactions.

i. CNS stimulants (amphetamines):

a) Effects increased with furazolidone or urinary alkalinizers

🛑 Hypertensive crisis may occur when CNS stimulants are used concurrently with (and up to several weeks after discontinuing) MAOIs.

b) Increased risk of serotonin syndrome occurs with coadministration of selective serotonin reuptake inhibitors (SSRIs)

c) Decreased effects of amphetamines occur with urinary acidifiers

d) Decreased hypotensive effects of guanethidine occur with amphetamines

ii. Dexmethylphenidate and methylphenidate:

a) Decreased effects of antihypertensive agents and pressor agents (dopamine, epinephrine, phenylephrine) with concomitant use of the methylphenidates

b) Increased effects of coumarin anticoagulants, anticonvulsants (phenobarbital, phenytoin, primidone), tricyclic antidepressants, and SSRIs with the methylphenidates

iii. Atomoxetine:

a) Increased effects with concomitant use of cytochrome P450 isozyme 2D6 (CYP2D6) inhibitors (paroxetine, fluoxetine, quinidine)

🛑 When atomoxetine is used concurrently (or within 2 weeks of discontinuation of) MAOIs, a potentially fatal reaction may occur. Always review a client's medications to avoid this risk.

b) Increased risk of cardiovascular effects with concomitant use of albuterol or vasopressors

iv. Bupropion:

a) Increased effects when used with amantadine, levodopa, or ritonavir

b) Decreased effects with carbamazepine

c) Increased risk of acute toxicity with MAOIs

d) Increased risk of hypertension with nicotine replacement agents

e) Adverse neuropsychiatric events with alcohol

f) Increased anticoagulant effects of warfarin

g) Increased effects of drugs metabolized by CYP2D6 (nortriptyline, imipramine, desipramine, paroxetine, fluoxetine, sertraline, haloperidol, risperidone, thioridazine, metoprolol, propafenone, and flecainide).

v. Alpha agonists:

🛑 Synergistic pharmacological and toxic effects, possibly causing atrioventricular (AV) block, bradycardia, and severe hypotension, may occur with concomitant use of calcium channel blockers or beta blockers with alpha agonists.

a) Additive sedation occurs with CNS depressants (alcohol, antihistamines, opioid analgesics, and sedative/hypnotics)

b) Decreased effects of clonidine with concomitant use of tricyclic antidepressants and prazosin

c) Decreased effects of levodopa when used with clonidine

d) Decreased effects of guanfacine when used with barbiturates or phenytoin.

g. Side effects of medications used for ADHD and their nursing implications:

i. Overstimulation, restlessness, insomnia (with CNS stimulants)

a) Assess mental status for changes in mood, level of activity, degree of stimulation, and aggressiveness

b) Ensure that the client is protected from injury

c) Keep stimuli low and environment as quiet as possible

d) Administer the last dose at least 6 hours before bedtime to prevent insomnia.

Administer sustained-release forms in the morning.

ii. Palpitations, tachycardia (with CNS stimulants; atomoxetine; bupropion; clonidine) or bradycardia (with clonidine; guanfacine)
   a) Monitor and record vital signs at regular intervals (two or three times a day) throughout therapy
   b) Report significant changes to the physician immediately

The Food and Drug Administration has issued warnings associated with CNS stimulants and atomoxetine for the risk of sudden death in clients who have cardiovascular disease. A careful personal and family history of heart disease, heart defects, or hypertension should be obtained before these medications are prescribed. Careful monitoring of cardiovascular function during administration must be ongoing.

iii. Anorexia, weight loss (with CNS stimulants; atomoxetine; bupropion)
   a) To reduce anorexia, administer medication immediately after meals
   b) Weigh client regularly (at least weekly) when receiving therapy with CNS stimulants, atomoxetine, or bupropion

iv. Tolerance, physical and psychological dependence (with CNS stimulants)
   a) Tolerance develops rapidly
   b) In children with ADHD, a drug "holiday" should be attempted periodically under the supervision of the physician to determine the effectiveness of the medication and the need for continuation
   c) The drug should not be withdrawn abruptly. May cause:
      • Nausea and vomiting
      • Abdominal cramping
      • Headache
      • Fatigue
      • Weakness
      • Mental depression
      • Suicidal ideation
      • Increased dreaming
      • Psychotic behavior

v. Nausea and vomiting (with atomoxetine and bupropion): may be taken with food to minimize gastrointestinal upset

vi. Constipation (with atomoxetine; bupropion; clonidine; guanfacine: increase fiber and fluid in diet, if not contraindicated

vii. Dry mouth (with clonidine and guanfacine)
   a) Offer client sugarless candy, ice, frequent sips of water
   b) Strict oral hygiene

viii. Sedation (with clonidine and guanfacine)
   a) Warn client that this effect is increased by concomitant use of alcohol and other CNS drugs
   b) Warn clients to refrain from driving or performing hazardous tasks until response has been established

ix. Potential for seizures (with bupropion)
   a) Protect client from injury if seizure should occur
   b) Instruct family and significant others how to protect client during a seizure
   c) Ensure that doses of the immediate-release medication are administered at least 4 to 6 hours apart
   d) Ensure that doses of the sustained-release medication are administered at least 8 hours apart

x. Severe liver damage (with atomoxetine): monitor for the following side effects and report immediately:
   a) Itching
   b) Dark urine
   c) Right upper quadrant pain
   d) Yellow skin or eyes
   e) Sore throat
   f) Fever
   g) Malaise

xi. New or worsened psychiatric symptoms (with CNS stimulants and atomoxetine)
   a) Monitor for psychotic symptoms (hearing voices, paranoid behaviors, delusions)
   b) Monitor for manic symptoms (to include aggressive and hostile behaviors)

The Food and Drug Administration has issued a black box warning associated with atomoxetine for an increased risk of suicidal ideation in children or adolescents. Clients should be monitored for suicidality, clinical worsening, and unusual changes in behavior.

xii. Rebound syndrome (with clonidine and guanfacine)
   a) Client should be instructed not to discontinue therapy abruptly
   b) May result in symptoms of:
      • Nervousness
      • Agitation
      • Headache
      • Tremor
      • Rapid rise in blood pressure
   c) Dosage should be tapered gradually under supervision of physician.

D. Tourette's disorder
1. Characterized by presence of multiple motor tics and one or more vocal tics, which may appear simultaneously or at different periods during the illness.
2. Symptoms cause marked distress or interfere with social, occupational, or other important areas of functioning.
3. Age of onset can be as early as 2 years, but most commonly occurs during childhood (age 6–7 years).
4. Prevalence is estimated at from 1 to 10 per 10,000 individuals between the ages of 6 and 17.
5. More common in boys than girls.
6. Can be lifelong, but symptoms usually diminish during adolescence and adulthood and may disappear altogether by early adulthood.
7. Predisposing factors.
   a. Biological factors.
      i. Genetics
         a) Tics noted in two-thirds of relatives of Tourette's disorder clients
         b) Twin studies with both monozygotic and dizygotic twins suggest inheritance
         c) May be transmitted in an autosomal pattern intermediate between dominant and recessive
      ii. Biochemical factors
         a) Abnormalities in levels of dopamine, serotonin, dynorphin, gamma-aminobutyric acid (GABA), acetylcholine, and norepinephrine
         b) Neurotransmitter pathways through the basal ganglia, globus pallidus, and subthalamic regions appear to be involved
      iii. Structural factors
         a) Neuroimaging brain studies find dysfunction in area of the basal ganglia
         b) Smaller size of corpus callosum
         c) Larger volumes in subregions of the hippocampus and amygdala
      iv. Environmental factors related to nongenetic Tourette's
         a) Complications during pregnancy (severe nausea and vomiting or excessive stress)
         b) Low birth weight
         c) Head trauma
         d) Carbon monoxide poisoning
         e) Encephalitis
         f) Post infection autoimmune phenomenon induced by childhood streptococcal infection
8. Nursing process: assessment for Tourette's disorder.
   a. Motor tics may involve the head, torso, and upper and lower limbs.
      b. May begin with a single motor tic, most commonly eye blinking, or with multiple symptoms.
      c. Simple motor tics include:
         i. Eye blinking
         ii. Neck jerking
         iii. Shoulder shrugging
         iv. Facial grimacing
      d. Complex motor tics include:
         i. Squatting
         ii. Hopping
         iii. Skipping
         iv. Tapping
         v. Retracing steps
      e. Vocal tics include:
         i. Squeaks
         ii. Grunts
         iii. Barks
         iv. Sniffs
         v. Snorts
         vi. Coughs

DID YOU KNOW?

In rare instances, a complex vocal tic involves the uttering of obscenities. Vocal tics may include repeating certain words or phrases out of context, repeating one's own sounds or words (**palilalia**), or repeating what others say (echolalia). The movements and vocalizations are experienced as compulsive and irresistible, but they can be suppressed for varying lengths of time. They are exacerbated by stress and attenuated during periods in which the individual becomes totally absorbed by an activity. In most cases, tics are diminished during sleep.

      f. Comorbid disorders:
         i. ADHD
         ii. Obsessive-compulsive disorder
         iii. Depression
         iv. Anxiety
         v. Episodic outbursts
         vi. School difficulties
         vii. Self-injurious behaviors (in severe cases)
9. Nursing Process: Diagnosis (Analysis)—on the basis of data collected during the nursing assessment, possible nursing diagnoses for the client diagnosed with Tourette's disorder include:
   i. Risk for self-directed or other-directed violence R/T low tolerance for frustration
   ii. Impaired social interaction R/T impulsiveness, oppositional and aggressive behavior
   iii. Low self-esteem R/T embarrassment associated with tic behaviors
10. Nursing Process: Planning—the following outcomes may be developed to guide the care of a

client diagnosed with Tourette's disorder. **The client will:**

a. Not harm self or others.
b. Interact appropriately with staff and peers.
c. Demonstrate self-control by managing tic behavior.
d. Follow rules of unit without becoming defensive.

9. Nursing Process: Implementation for Tourette's disorder.
   a. Interventions for clients who are experiencing risk for self-directed or other-directed violence.
      i. Observe client's behavior frequently through routine activities and interactions
      ii. Note behaviors that indicate a rise in agitation

Stress commonly increases both tic and agitated behavior. Recognition of behaviors that precede the onset of aggression in clients diagnosed with Tourette's disorder may provide the opportunity to intervene before violence occurs.

      iii. Monitor for self-destructive behavior and impulses
      iv. Stay with client to prevent self-mutilation
      v. Provide hand coverings and other restraints that prevent self-mutilative behaviors
      vi. Redirect frustration and violent behavior to physical activities
   b. Interventions for clients who are experiencing impaired social interaction
      i. Develop a trusting relationship
      ii. Convey acceptance of the person separate from any unacceptable behavior
      iii. Discuss with client behaviors which are acceptable and which are not
      iv. Describe in matter-of-fact manner the consequences of unacceptable behavior; follow through
      v. Provide group situations for client

DID YOU KNOW?
Appropriate social behavior is often learned from the positive and negative feedback of peers. This feedback can occur in both formal and informal group settings.

   c. Interventions for clients who are experiencing low self-esteem.
      i. Convey unconditional acceptance and positive regard
      ii. Spend time interacting with client
      iii. Set limits on manipulative behavior
      iv. Do not reinforce manipulative behaviors by providing desired attention
      v. Identify the consequences of manipulation
      vi. When manipulation occurs, administer consequences matter-of-factly

      vii. Help client understand that he or she uses manipulative behavior to try to increase own self-esteem

10. Nursing Process: Evaluation—evaluation of nursing actions for the client diagnosed with Tourette's disorder may be facilitated by gathering information using the following types of questions:
   a. Has the client refrained from causing harm to self or others during times of increased tension?
   b. Has the client developed adaptive coping strategies for dealing with frustration to prevent resorting to self-destruction or aggression toward others?
   c. Is the client able to interact appropriately with staff and peers?
   d. Is the client able to suppress tic behaviors when he or she chooses to do so?
   e. Does the client set a time for "release" of the suppressed tic behaviors?
   f. Does the client verbalize positive aspects about self, particularly as they relate to his or her ability to manage the illness?
   g. Does the client comply with treatment in a nondefensive manner?

11. Psychopharmacological intervention for clients with Tourette's disorder.
   a. Pharmacotherapy not recommended unless there is significant functional impairment or physical discomfort, or if there is interference with overall quality of life or psychological adjustment.
   b. Pharmacotherapy most effective when it is combined with psychosocial therapy (behavioral therapy, individual counseling or psychotherapy, family therapy).

c. Medications used in treatment include antipsychotics and alpha agonists.
 i. Antipsychotics
   a) Haloperidol (Haldol) and pimozide (Orap), approved by the Food and Drug Administration (FDA) for control of tics and vocal utterances
   b) These drugs often not first-line choice of therapy due to potential for severe adverse effects (extrapyramidal symptoms [EPS], neuroleptic malignant syndrome, tardive dyskinesia, electrocardiographic changes)
   c) Haloperidol not recommended for children younger than 3 years
   d) Pimozide should not be administered to children younger than 12 years
   e) Atypical antipsychotics, such as risperidone (Risperdal), olanzapine (Zyprexa), or ziprasidone (Geodon) not approved by FDA but shown to be effective and used off-label, due to favorable side-effect profiles
   f) Atypical antipsychotics have lower incidence of neurological side effects; common side effects include weight gain and sedation
   g) EPS have been observed with risperidone
   h) Ziprasidone associated with increased risk of QTc interval prolongation
   i) Hyperglycemia reported when taking atypical antipsychotics
 ii. Alpha agonists
   a) Clonidine (Catapres) and guanfacine (Tenex; Intuniv) extended-release forms are first-line treatment of Tourette's disorder because of favorable side-effect profile
   b) Often effective for comorbid symptoms of ADHD, anxiety, and insomnia
   c) Common side effects:
     • Dry mouth
     • Sedation
     • Headaches
     • Fatigue
     • Dizziness
     • Postural hypotension
   d) Guanfacine is longer lasting and less sedating than clonidine
   e) Should not be prescribed for children and adolescents with preexisting cardiac or vascular disease

Alpha agonists should not be discontinued abruptly. Stopping the medication abruptly could result in symptoms of nervousness, agitation, tremor, and a rapid rise in blood pressure.

II. Disruptive Behavior Disorders

A. Oppositional defiant disorder (ODD)
 1. Characterized by a persistent pattern of angry mood and defiant behavior that occurs more frequently than is usually observed in individuals of comparable age and developmental level and interferes with social, educational, or vocational activities.
 2. Typically begins by 8 years of age, usually not later than early adolescence.
 3. Prevalence of 2% to 12%.
 4. Common comorbid disorders:
   a. ADHD
   b. Anxiety disorders
   c. Mood disorders
 5. More prevalent in boys than in girls before puberty.
 6. Prevalence rates more closely equal after puberty.
 7. Some cases progress to conduct disorder.
 8. Predisposing factors.
   a. Biological influences.
     i. Still under investigation
     ii. Potential alteration in genes for metabolism of dopamine, serotonin, and norepinephrine
   b. Family influences.
     i. Opposition normal during various developmental stages
       a) First exhibited 10 or 11 months of age
       b) Toddlers between 18 and 36 months of age
       c) During adolescence
     ii. Pathology considered when:
       a) Developmental phase is prolonged
       b) There is parental overreaction to the child's behavior
     iii. Combination of a strong-willed child with a reactive and high-energy temperament and parents who are authoritarian can lead to ODD
     iv. The parents become frustrated with the strong-willed child who does not obey and increase their attempts to enforce authority
     v. The child reacts to the excessive parental control with anger and increased self-assertion
     vi. Both parties become angry and increasingly rigid in their stances as they try to defend their self-esteem
     vii. Child's negative behavior may be inadvertently rewarded by desired attention (even negative attention)
 9. Nursing Process: Assessment for ODD.

DID YOU KNOW?

Unlike children with conduct disorder, children diagnosed with oppositional defiant disorder are not aggressive toward people or animals, do not destroy property, and do not show a pattern of theft or deceit. A diagnosis of ODD cannot be given if the child presents with conduct disorder.

   a. Characterized by passive-aggressive behaviors:
      i. Stubbornness
      ii. Procrastination
      iii. Disobedience
      iv. Carelessness
      v. Negativism
      vi. Testing of limits
      vii. Resistance to directions
      viii. Deliberately ignoring the communication of others
      ix. Unwillingness to compromise
   b. Other symptoms:
      i. Running away
      ii. School avoidance
      iii. School underachievement
      iv. Temper tantrums
      v. Fighting
      vi. Argumentativeness
   c. Initially, oppositional attitude directed toward the parents.
   d. In time, relationships with peers and teachers are affected.
   e. Social impairments lead to:
      i. Depression
      ii. Anxiety
      iii. Additional problematic behavior
   f. Do not see themselves as being oppositional but view the problem as arising from others who make unreasonable demands.
   g. Often friendless, perceiving human relationships as negative and unsatisfactory.
   h. School performance usually poor because of their refusal to participate and their resistance to external demands.
10. Nursing Process: Diagnosis (Analysis)—on the basis of data collected during the nursing assessment, possible nursing diagnoses for the client diagnosed with ODD include:
   a. Nonadherence with therapy R/T negative temperament, denial of problems, underlying hostility.
   b. Defensive coping R/T retarded ego development, low self-esteem, unsatisfactory parent/child relationship.
   c. Low self-esteem R/T lack of positive feedback, retarded ego development.
   d. Impaired social interaction R/T negative temperament, underlying hostility, manipulation of others.
11. Nursing Process: Planning—the following outcomes may be developed to guide the care of a client diagnosed with ODD. **The client will:**
   a. Comply with treatment by participating in therapies without negativism.
   b. Accept responsibility for his or her part in the problem.
   c. Take direction from staff without becoming defensive.
   d. Not manipulate other people.
   e. Verbalize positive aspects about self.
   f. Interact with others in an appropriate manner.
12. Nursing Process: Implementation for ODD
   a. Interventions for clients who are experiencing nonadherence with therapy.
      i. Set structured plan of therapeutic activities
      ii. Start with minimum expectations and increase as client begins to manifest evidence of adherence
      iii. Establish a system of rewards for adherence with therapy and consequences for nonadherence
      iv. Ensure that the rewards and consequences are concepts of value to the client
   b. Interventions for clients who are experiencing defensive coping.
      i. Help client recognize that feelings of inadequacy provoke defensive behaviors (blaming others for problems, needing to "get even")
      ii. Provide immediate, nonthreatening feedback for passive-aggressive behavior

---

MAKING THE CONNECTION

Structure provides security. Participation in one or two activities may not seem as overwhelming as a whole schedule of activities. Taking small, realistic steps can provide an opportunity for the client to succeed and recognize the benefits of adhering to expectations.

MAKING THE CONNECTION

The nurse should convey acceptance of the client separate from the undesirable behaviors being exhibited. Statements like. "It is not *you*, but your *behavior*, that is unacceptable" can be used as positive reinforcement.

      iii. Help identify situations that provoke defensiveness

      iv. Role-play appropriate responses

      v. Provide immediate positive feedback for acceptable behaviors

  c. Interventions for clients who are experiencing low self-esteem.

      i. Encourage setting realistic goals

DID YOU KNOW?

Creating unrealistic client goals can precipitate failure, further diminishing self-esteem. A successful experience driven by a realistic goal enhances self-esteem.

      ii. Plan activities that provide opportunities for success

      iii. Convey unconditional acceptance and positive regard

      iv. Set limits on manipulative behavior

      v. Do not reinforce manipulative behaviors with desired attention

      vi. Identify the consequences of manipulation

      vii. Administer consequences matter of factly when manipulation occurs

      viii. Help client understand that he or she uses manipulative behavior to try to increase own self-esteem

  d. Interventions for clients who are experiencing impaired social interaction.

      i. Develop trusting relationship

      ii. Convey acceptance of the person separate from the unacceptable behavior

      iii. Define and explain passive-aggressive behavior

      iv. Discuss how passive-aggressive behaviors are perceived by others

      v. Describe which behaviors are not acceptable and role-play more adaptive responses

      vi. Give positive feedback for acceptable behaviors

      vii. Provide peer group situations for client participation

DID YOU KNOW?

Appropriate social behavior is often learned from the positive and negative feedback of peers that

---

MAKING THE CONNECTION

Positive feedback encourages repetition of acceptable and appropriate behaviors; and immediacy is significant for children diagnosed with oppositional defiant disorder, who readily respond to immediate gratification.

---

can occur in both formal and informal group settings. Groups also provide a context for using the acceptable and appropriate behaviors rehearsed in role-play.

  13. Nursing Process: Evaluation—evaluation of nursing actions for the client diagnosed with ODD may be facilitated by gathering information using the following types of questions:

    a. Is the client cooperating with schedule of therapeutic activities? Is level of participation adequate?

    b. Is the client's attitude toward therapy less negative?

    c. Is the client accepting responsibility for problem behavior?

    d. Is the client verbalizing the unacceptability of his or her passive-aggressive behavior?

    e. Is he or she able to identify which behaviors are unacceptable and substitute more adaptive behaviors?

    f. Is the client able to interact with staff and peers without defending behavior in an angry manner?

    g. Is the client able to verbalize positive statements about self?

    h. Is increased self-worth evident with fewer manifestations of manipulation?

    i. Is the client able to make compromises with others when issues of control emerge?

    j. Is anger and hostility expressed in an appropriate manner? Can the client verbalize ways of releasing anger adaptively?

    k. Is he or she able to verbalize true feelings instead of allowing them to emerge through use of passive-aggressive behaviors?

B. Conduct disorder

  1. A pattern of behavior that is repetitive and persistent in which the basic rights of others or major age-appropriate societal norms or rules are violated.

  2. Prevalence is 1% to 10% of general population.

  3. Male predominance ranging from 2:1 to 4:1.

  4. Comorbidities include:

    a. ADHD

    b. Mood disorders

    c. Learning disorders

    d. Substance use disorders

  5. If symptoms begin in childhood:

    a. Likely to be a history of oppositional defiant disorder.

    b. Greater likelihood of antisocial personality disorder developing in adulthood; 40% of boys and 25% of girls with disorder will develop adult antisocial personality disorder.

6. Predisposing factors.
   a. Biological influences.
      i. Genetics
         a) Family, twin, and adoptive studies reveal significantly higher incidence among those who have family members with the disorder
         b) Studies have found alterations in chromosomes 19 and 2
         c) Same region on chromosome 2 also linked to alcohol dependence
         d) Childhood conduct disorder is associated with future alcohol problems
      ii. Temperament
         a) Personality traits that become evident very early in life and may be present at birth
         b) May be a genetic component
         c) May be associated with behavioral problems later in life
         d) Without appropriate intervention, difficult temperament at age 3 is linked to the diagnosis of conduct disorder and leads to outpatient treatment or institutionalization by age 17
      iii. Biochemical factors
         a) May be alterations in the neurotransmitters norepinephrine and serotonin
         b) Association of testosterone with violence, social dominance, and association with deviant peers
   b. Psychosocial influences.
      i. Peer relationships
         a) Social groups have significant effect on a child's development
         b) Peers play essential role in the socialization of interpersonal competence
         c) Skills acquired through peer relationships affects long-term adjustment
         d) Poor peer relations during childhood consistently implicated in the etiology of later deviance
         e) Aggression usually the cause of peer rejection, leading to a cycle of maladaptive behavior
      ii. Family influences:
         a) Parental rejection
         b) Inconsistent management with harsh discipline
         c) Early institutional living
         d) Frequent shifting of parental figures
         e) Large family size
         f) Absent father
         g) Parents with antisocial personality disorder and/or alcohol dependence
         h) Marital conflict and divorce
         i) Inadequate communication patterns
         j) Parental permissiveness
7. Nursing Process: Assessment for conduct disorder.
   a. Classic characteristic is the use of physical aggression in the violation of the rights of others.
   b. Behaviors fall into four main groupings:
      i. Aggressive conduct that causes or threatens physical harm to other people or animals
      ii. Nonaggressive conduct that causes property loss or damage
      iii. Deceitfulness or theft
      iv. Repeated serious violations of rules
   c. Peer relationships disturbed.
   d. Behavior patterns manifest in virtually all areas of the child's life (home, school, peers, community).
   e. Stealing, lying, and truancy are common problems.
   f. Lacks feelings of guilt or remorse.
   g. The use of tobacco, liquor, or nonprescribed drugs, and participation in sexual activities, occurs earlier than at the expected age for the peer group.
   h. Projection is a common defense mechanism.
   i. Low self-esteem is manifested by a "tough guy" image.
   j. Poor frustration tolerance.
   k. Irritability.
   l. Frequent temper outbursts.
   m. Symptoms of anxiety and depression common.
   n. Level of academic achievement may be low in relation to age and IQ.
   o. Symptoms associated with ADHD (attention difficulties, impulsiveness, and hyperactivity) common.
8. Nursing Process: Diagnosis (Analysis)—on the basis of data collected during the nursing assessment, possible nursing diagnoses for the client diagnosed with conduct disorder include:
   a. Risk for other-directed violence R/T characteristics of temperament, peer rejection, negative parental role models, dysfunctional family dynamics.
   b. Impaired social interaction R/T negative parental role models, impaired peer relations leading to inappropriate social behaviors.
   c. Defensive coping R/T low self-esteem and dysfunctional family system.
   d. Low self-esteem R/T lack of positive feedback and unsatisfactory parent/child relationship.
9. Nursing Process: Planning—the following outcomes may be developed to guide care of a client diagnosed with conduct disorder. **The client will:**
   a. Not harm self or others.
   b. Interact with others in a socially appropriate manner.

    c. Accept direction without becoming defensive.

    d. Demonstrate evidence of increased self-esteem by discontinuing exploitative and demanding behaviors toward others.

10. Nursing Process: Implementation for conduct disorder.

    a. Interventions for clients who are experiencing a risk for other-directed violence.

      i. Observe client's behavior frequently through routine activities and interactions

      ii. Be alert to behaviors that indicate an increase in agitation

🛑 Recognition of behaviors that precede the onset of aggression in clients diagnosed with conduct disorder may provide the opportunity to intervene before violence occurs.

      iii. Redirect violent behavior with physical outlets for suppressed anger and frustration

      iv. Encourage client to express anger and act as a role model for appropriate expression of anger

      v. Ensure that a sufficient number of staff members are available to indicate a show of strength if necessary

      vi. Administer tranquilizing medication, if ordered, or use mechanical restraints and/or isolation room only if situation cannot be controlled with less restrictive means

    b. Interventions for clients who are experiencing impaired social interaction.

      i. Develop a trusting relationship

      ii. Convey acceptance of the person separate from the unacceptable behavior

      iii. Discuss with client which behaviors are and are not acceptable

      iv. Describe in matter-of-fact manner the consequence of unacceptable behavior; follow through

      v. Provide opportunities for group interactions

DID YOU KNOW?

Appropriate social behavior is often learned from the positive and negative feedback of peers. Group settings provide this opportunity.

    c. Interventions for clients who are experiencing defensive coping.

      i. Explain correlation between feelings of inadequacy and need for acceptance from others

      ii. Discuss how these feelings provoke defensive behaviors (blaming others for own behaviors)

      iii. Provide immediate, matter-of-fact, non-threatening feedback for unacceptable behaviors

MAKING THE CONNECTION

Client recognition of the problem is the first step in the change process toward resolution.

      iv. Help identify situations that provoke defensiveness

      v. Practice more appropriate responses through role-play

      vi. Provide immediate positive feedback for acceptable behaviors

    d. Interventions for clients who are experiencing low self-esteem.

      i. Assist with setting realistic goals

      ii. Plan activities that provide opportunities for success

      iii. Convey unconditional acceptance and positive regard

      iv. Set limits on manipulative behavior

      v. Avoid providing attention when client is exhibiting manipulative behavior

      vi. Identify the consequences of manipulation

      vii. Administer consequences matter-of-factly when manipulation occurs

      viii. Help client understand that he or she uses manipulation to seek attention in an attempt to increase self-esteem

11. Nursing Process: Evaluation—evaluation of the nursing actions for the client diagnosed with conduct disorder may be facilitated by gathering information using the following types of questions:

    a. Have the nursing actions directed toward managing the client's aggressive behavior been effective?

    b. Have interventions prevented harm to others or others' property?

    c. Is the client able to express anger in an appropriate manner?

    d. Has the client developed more adaptive coping strategies to deal with anger and feelings of aggression?

    e. Does the client demonstrate the ability to trust others? Is he or she able to interact with staff and peers in an appropriate manner?

    f. Is the client able to accept responsibility for his or her own behavior? Is there less blaming of others?

MAKING THE CONNECTION

Unrealistic goals can precipitate failure, diminishing self-esteem. Success enhances self-esteem.

g. Is the client able to accept feedback from others without becoming defensive?

h. Is the client able to verbalize positive statements about self?

i. Is the client able to interact with others without engaging in manipulation?

II. Anxiety Disorders: Separation Anxiety Disorder

A. Characterized by excessive fear or anxiety concerning separation from those to whom the individual is attached

B. Anxiety is beyond that which would be expected for the individual's developmental level

C. Anxiety interferes with social, academic, occupational, or others areas of functioning

D. Onset any time before age 18 years

E. Commonly diagnosed around age 5 or 6, when the child goes to school

F. Prevalence 4% in children and young adults

G. More common in girls than in boys

H. Most children grow out of it (but can persist into adulthood)

I. Can be a precursor to adult panic disorder

J. Predisposing factors
   1. Biological influences.
      a. Genetics.
         i. Greater number of children with relatives who manifest anxiety problems develop anxiety disorders
         ii. Hereditary influence toward anxiety leading to heightened levels of arousal, emotional reactivity, and increased negative affect
         iii. Mode of genetic transmission has not been determined
      b. Temperament
         i. Irritable as an infant
         ii. Unusually shy and fearful as a toddler
         iii. Quiet, cautious, and withdrawn in the preschool and early school age years, with marked behavioral restraint and physiological arousal in unfamiliar situations

DID YOU KNOW?
Parent-child attachment may combine with temperament to increase the risk for the development of childhood anxiety disorders.

   2. Environmental influences: stressful life events.
      a. There is a relationship between life events and the development of anxiety disorders.
      b. Vulnerable or predisposed children may be affected significantly by stressful life events.
   3. Family influences.
      a. Theories of overattachment to the mother.

b. Parental overprotection or exaggeration of the dangers of the present or future.

DID YOU KNOW?
Parents may transfer their fears and anxieties to their children through role modeling. For example, a parent who becomes fearful in the presence of a small, harmless dog and retreats with dread and apprehension teaches the young child by example that this is an appropriate response.

K. Nursing Process: Assessment for separation anxiety disorder
   1. Age at onset as early as preschool age.
   2. Rarely begins as late as adolescence.
   3. Anticipation of separation may result in tantrums, crying, screaming, complaints of physical problems, and clinging behaviors.
   4. Reluctance or refusal to attend school especially common in adolescent clients diagnosed with separation anxiety.
   5. During middle childhood or adolescence, they may refuse to sleep away from home (friend's house, camp).
   6. No problem with interpersonal peer relationships.
   7. Generally well liked by peers and reasonably socially skilled.
   8. Tend to exhibit perfectionistic behaviors.
   9. Anxiety relates to the possibility of harm coming to self or attachment figure.
   10. Younger children may have nightmares related to harm coming to self or attachment figure.
   11. Specific phobias are common (fear of the dark, ghosts, animals).

DID YOU KNOW?
In separation anxiety disorder, depressed mood is frequently present and often precedes the onset of the anxiety symptoms, which commonly occur following a major stressor.

L. Nursing Process: Diagnosis (Analysis)—based on data collected during the nursing assessment, possible nursing diagnoses for the client diagnosed with separation anxiety disorder include:
   1. Anxiety (severe) R/T family history, temperament, overattachment to parent, negative role modeling.

MAKING THE CONNECTION

In most cases of separation anxiety disorder, the child has difficulty separating from the mother. Occasionally the separation reluctance is directed toward the father, a sibling, or another significant individual to whom the child is attached.

2. Ineffective coping R/T unresolved separation conflicts and inadequate coping skills AEB numerous somatic complaints.
3. Impaired social interaction R/T reluctance to be away from attachment figure.

M. Nursing Process: Planning—the following outcomes may be developed to guide care of a client diagnosed with separation anxiety disorder. **The client will:**
1. Be able to maintain anxiety at manageable level.
2. Demonstrate adaptive coping strategies for dealing with anxiety when separation from attachment figure is anticipated.
3. Interact appropriately with others and spend time away from attachment figure to do so.

N. Nursing Process: Implementation for clients diagnosed with separation anxiety disorder
1. Interventions for clients who are experiencing anxiety (severe).
   a. Establish an atmosphere of calmness, trust, and genuine positive regard.
   b. Assure client of his or her safety and security.
   c. Explore the child or adolescent's fears of separating from the attachment figure.
   d. Explore with the parents possible fears they may have of separation from the child.
   e. Help parents and child initiate realistic goals.
   f. Give, and encourage parents to give, positive reinforcement for desired behaviors.
2. Interventions for clients who are experiencing ineffective coping.
   a. Encourage child or adolescent to discuss specific situations in life that produce the most distress and describe his or her response to these situations. Include parents in the discussion.
   b. Help the child or adolescent who is perfectionistic to recognize that self-expectations may be unrealistic.
   c. Connect times of unmet self-expectations to the exacerbation of symptoms.
   d. Encourage parents and child to identify more adaptive coping strategies that the child could use in the face of overwhelming anxiety.
   e. Practice adaptive coping skills through role-play.

MAKING THE CONNECTION

Some realistic goals for children diagnosed with separation anxiety could be:
• Child to stay with sitter for 2 hours with minimal anxiety
• Child to stay at friend's house without parents until 9:00 p.m. without experiencing panic anxiety

---

3. Interventions for clients who are experiencing impaired social interaction.
   a. Develop a trusting relationship with client.
   b. Attend groups with the child and support efforts to interact with others. Give positive feedback.
   c. Convey to the child the acceptability of his or her not participating in groups in the beginning. Gradually encourage small contributions until client is able to participate more fully.
   d. Help client set small personal goals ("Today I will speak to one person I don't know without my mother present").

O. Nursing Process: Evaluation—evaluation of nursing actions for the client diagnosed with separation anxiety disorder may be facilitated by gathering information using the following types of questions:
1. Is the client able to maintain anxiety at a manageable level (without temper tantrums, screaming, or "clinging")?
2. Have complaints of symptoms diminished?
3. Has the client demonstrated the ability to cope in more adaptive ways in the face of escalating anxiety?
4. Have the parents identified their role in the separation conflict? Are they able to discuss more adaptive coping strategies?
5. Does the client verbalize an intention to return to school?
6. Have nightmares and fears of the dark subsided?
7. Is the client able to interact with others away from the attachment figure?
8. Has the precipitating stressor been identified?
9. Have strategies for coping more adaptively to similar stressors in the future been established?

III. General Treatment Modalities for Children and Adolescents

A. Behavior therapy
1. Based on the concepts of classical and operant conditioning.
2. Common and effective treatment for disruptive behavior disorders.
3. System of rewards and consequences.
4. Consistency is essential component.
5. Rewards are given for appropriate behaviors.
6. Rewards withheld when behaviors are disruptive or inappropriate.
7. Positive reinforcements encourage repetition of desirable behaviors.
8. Aversive reinforcements (punishments) discourage repetition of undesirable behaviors.
9. Behavior modification techniques can be taught to parents for use in home environment.

B. Family therapy
1. Basis for the use of family therapy.
   a. Family dynamics identified as affecting disruptive behavior disorders.
   b. Disruptive behavior disorders affect family dynamics.
   c. Children should not be separated from their families if possible.
   d. Family coping becomes severely compromised by the chronic stress of dealing with a child with a behavior disorder.
   e. Therapy for children and adolescents must be family centered and involve entire family.
2. Parents should be involved in designing and implementing treatment plan.
3. Parents should be involved in all aspects of treatment process.
4. Genograms can be used to identify areas of family problems.
   a. Provides an overall picture of the life of the family over several generations.
   b. Includes roles that various family members play.
   c. Includes emotional distance between specific individuals.
   d. Helps to easily identify areas for change.
5. The client's treatment plan should be instituted within the context of family centered care.

C. Group therapy
1. Provides opportunity to interact within an association of peers.
2. Benefits include:
   a. Appropriate social behavior learned from the positive and negative feedback of peers.
   b. Opportunity is provided to learn to tolerate and accept differences of others.
   c. Opportunity to learn that it is acceptable to disagree.
   d. Opportunity to learn to offer and receive support from others.
   e. Opportunity to practice new skills in a safe environment.
   f. Opportunity to learn from the experiences of others.

MAKING THE CONNECTION

Children's play therapy can be compared with adult psychotherapy. Through play, children can express their inner worlds and by the use of toys symbolically represent their anxieties, fears, fantasies, and guilt. Play therapy provides a safe environment for the child to express feelings without judgmental reactions and to learn more adaptive skills.

---

3. Types of group therapy with children and adolescents.
   a. Music therapy: allows clients to express feelings through music.
   b. Art and activity/craft therapy: allows individual expression through artistic means.
   c. Group play therapy: the treatment of choice for 3- to 9-year-olds.
   d. Psychoeducational groups: very beneficial for adolescents.
      i. Should be closed-ended (no new members added)
      ii. Members are allowed to propose discussion topics
      iii. Leader serves as teacher
      iv. Leader facilitates discussion
      v. Members may be presenters and serve as discussion leaders
      vi. May evolve into traditional therapy discussion groups

D. Psychopharmacology
1. Child and adolescent disorders can be treated with medications.
2. Medications improve quality of family life.
3. Medications should *never* be the sole method of treatment.
4. Most effective is combination of medication and psychosocial therapy.
5. Medications promote improved coping ability, which enhances the effectiveness of the psychosocial therapy.

REVIEW QUESTIONS

1. A personality trait that becomes evident very early in life and may be present at birth is called_____.

2. Which nursing intervention should be employed when caring for a child diagnosed with moderate intellectual developmental disorder (IDD)?
   1. Encourage the parents to prioritize all the needs of the child.
   2. Modify the child's environment to promote independence and encourage impulse control.
   3. Encourage parents to meet client needs that require gross motor skills.
   4. Provide one-on-one tutorial education in a private setting to decrease overstimulation.

3. Which of the following interventions should a nurse anticipate when planning care for a child diagnosed with oppositional defiant disorder (ODD)? **Select all that apply.**
   1. Behavior therapy
   2. Cognitive therapy
   3. Aversion therapy
   4. Group therapy
   5. Family therapy

4. A client has been diagnosed with an IQ level of 60. Which client social/communication capability would the nurse expect to observe?
   1. The client has almost no speech development and no socialization skills.
   2. The client may experience some limitation in speech and social convention.
   3. The client may have minimal verbal skills, with acting-out behavior.
   4. The client is capable of developing social and communication skills.

5. A child diagnosed with severe intellectual disability becomes aggressive with staff members when faced with the inability to complete simple tasks. Which nursing diagnosis would reflect this client's problem?
   1. Ineffective coping R/T inability to deal with frustration
   2. Anxiety R/T feelings of powerlessness and threat to self-esteem
   3. Social isolation R/T unconventional social behavior
   4. Risk for injury R/T altered physical mobility

6. From an epidemiological perspective, which of the following factors accurately describe the prevalence of autism spectrum disorder (ASD)? **Select all that apply.**
   1. In the United States, about 11.3 per 1,000 (1 in 88) children are diagnosed with ASD.
   2. ASD may be initially diagnosed in as many as 9% of school-age children.
   3. ASD occurs about 4.5 times more often in boys than in girls.
   4. In most cases, ASD runs a chronic course, with symptoms persisting into adulthood.
   5. ASD can be a precursor to adult panic disorder.

7. A disorder that is characterized by impairment in social interaction skills and interpersonal communication and a restricted repertoire of activities and interests is called_____ _____ disorder.

8. From a genetic perspective, which of the following factors would the nurse recognize as being associated with the etiology of autism spectrum disorder (ASD)? **Select all that apply.**
   1. ASD may be transmitted in an autosomal pattern somewhere between dominant and recessive.
   2. Parents who have one child diagnosed with ASD are at increased risk for having another child with the disorder.
   3. Both monozygotic and dizygotic twin studies have provided evidence of genetic involvement.
   4. Chromosomes 2, 7, 15, 16, and 17 are linked in the development of ASD.
   5. Studies suggest that alterations in genes for metabolism of neurotransmitters may be contributing factors in the development of ASD.

9. An 8-year-old girl has been diagnosed with separation anxiety disorder and screams, cries, and complains of stomachaches when faced with separating from her mother. Which nursing diagnosis would the nurse consider a priority?
   1. Disturbed body image
   2. Self-care deficit
   3. Dysfunctional family process
   4. Impaired social interaction

10. Which of the following factors support a genetic predisposition to attention deficit hyperactivity disorder (ADHD)? **Select all that apply.**
    1. Evidence suggests that ADHD may be transmitted in an autosomal pattern intermediate between dominant and recessive.
    2. Researchers found that copy number variants overlap with chromosomal regions previously linked to autism spectrum disorder and schizophrenia.
    3. Studies suggest that the genes for metabolism of dopamine, serotonin, and norepinephrine may be contributing factors to the development of ADHD.
    4. Research has indicated that a large number of parents of hyperactive children showed signs of hyperactivity during their own childhood.
    5. Evidence supports that hyperactive children are more likely to have siblings who are also hyperactive.

11. A child with a history of violence directed at others has a diagnosis of conduct disorder (CD). Which priority nursing intervention should be implemented?
    1. Set limits on manipulative behavior and administer consequences matter-of-factly when manipulation occurs.
    2. Help identify situations that provoke defensiveness and practice through role-play more appropriate responses.
    3. Discuss with the client the consequences of behaviors that are not acceptable.
    4. Observe client's behavior frequently for signs of escalating agitation.

12. A child diagnosed with attention deficit disorder is being intrusive with staff and acting immaturely by whirling and falling down. Which of the following short-term outcomes would be appropriate for this client? **Select all that apply.**
    1. The child will interact in age-appropriate manner with a nurse in one-to-one relationship within 1 week.
    2. The child will not harm self or others.
    3. The child will begin to behave normally within 2 days.
    4. The child will observe limits set on intrusive actions by exhibiting fewer attention-seeking behaviors.
    5. The child will be free of injury during hospitalization.

13. Which of the following factors support a genetic predisposition to Tourette's disorder? **Select all that apply.**
    1. The disorder is observed in one-third of relatives of Tourette's disorder clients.
    2. Twin studies with both monozygotic and dizygotic twins suggest an inheritable component.
    3. Evidence suggests that Tourette's disorder may be transmitted in an autosomal pattern intermediate between dominant and recessive.
    4. The precise gene and mechanism of inheritance remain undetermined.
    5. Abnormalities in levels of dopamine, serotonin, and norepinephrine have been associated with Tourette's disorder.

14. An 8-year-old girl has an IQ of 69. Understanding the problems caused by this degree of disability, which client outcome would the nurse prioritize?
    1. The client will have all self-care needs met.
    2. The client will remain free from injury.
    3. The client will socially interact with others.
    4. The client will demonstrate adaptive coping skills in response to stress.

15. Family dynamics have been implicated as contributing to the etiology of conduct disorder (CD). On reviewing the history of a client diagnosed with CD, which of the following factors might the nurse expect to recognize? **Select all that apply.**
    1. Parental rejection
    2. Parental expectation of child to live up to imposed standards of conduct
    3. Inconsistent parental management with harsh discipline
    4. Absent father
    5. Parental permissiveness

16. A child diagnosed with autism spectrum disorder does not make eye contact, does not communicate, repeatedly bangs his head on the wall, and constantly claps his hands. Which nursing diagnosis would the nurse consider a priority?
    1. Impaired social interaction
    2. Impaired verbal communication
    3. Risk for self-mutilation
    4. Risk for other-directed violence

17. A child diagnosed with separation anxiety disorder has a nursing diagnosis of ineffective coping. Which of the following nursing interventions address this problem? **Select all that apply.**
    1. Encourage child to discuss specific situations in life that produce the most stress.
    2. Provide a variety of meaningful sensory stimulation.
    3. Help the perfectionist child to recognize that self-expectations may be unrealistic.
    4. Set limits on manipulative behavior.
    5. Help the child recognize that feelings of inadequacy provoke defensive behavior.

18. A nursing instructor is teaching about the differences between clients diagnosed with conduct disorder (CD) and those diagnosed with oppositional defiant disorder (ODD). Which student statement indicates that learning has occurred?
    1. "Clients diagnosed with ODD exhibit an angry mood and defiant behavior, whereas clients diagnosed with CD violate of the rights of others."
    2. "Clients diagnosed with ODD may exhibit cruelty toward animals, whereas clients diagnosed with CD do not typically exhibit this behavior."
    3. "Clients diagnosed with ODD may set fires with intention to do harm, whereas clients diagnosed with CD do not typically exhibit this behavior."
    4. "Clients diagnosed with ODD may have a comorbid diagnosis of attention deficit-hyperactivity disorder, whereas clients diagnosed with CD do not."

19. When providing care to a client diagnosed with autism spectrum disorder, the nurse would recognize that which of the following nursing diagnoses and nursing interventions address the documented problem? **Select all that apply.**
    1. Impaired verbal communication: *Seek clarification and validation*
    2. Impaired social interaction: *Positively reinforce maintaining eye contact*
    3. Risk for other directed violence: *Restrain when aggressive toward others*
    4. Disturbed personal identity: *Assist the client to name own body parts*
    5. Altered body image: *Present and challenge the client's perception of reality*

20. A child is diagnosed with Tourette's disorder and is withdrawn, refuses to participate in group therapy, and initiates little or no communication with peers. On the basis of the symptoms presented, which nursing diagnosis should the nurse assign to this child?
    1. Risk for self-directed or other-directive violence
    2. Impaired social interaction
    3. Low self-esteem
    4. Anxiety (severe)

REVIEW ANSWERS

1. **ANSWER: temperament**
   Rationale: *Temperament* refers to those aspects of an individual's personality, such as mood and behavioral tendencies. Temperament is the sum of physical, emotional, and intellectual components that affect or determine a person's actions and reactions.
   TEST-TAKING TIP: Review the key terms at the beginning of the chapter.
   Content Area: Psychosocial Integrity;
   Integrated Process: Nursing Process: Assessment;
   Client Need: Psychosocial Integrity;
   Cognitive Level: Knowledge;
   Concept: Development

2. **ANSWER: 2**
   Rationale:
   1. The child in the question has been diagnosed with moderate intellectual developmental disorder (IDD) and is therefore capable of performing some tasks independently. Although it is important to have the child's self-care needs met, it is equally important to have the child independently meet as many of these needs as possible; therefore, this intervention would not be a priority.
   2. The nurse should prioritize modifying that child's environment to promote independence and encourage impulse control. This intervention is related to the nursing diagnosis *self-care deficit*. Positive reinforcement can serve to increase self-esteem and encourage repetition of behavior.
   3. Motor development at the moderate level of IDD is fair. Vocational capabilities may be limited to unskilled gross motor activities. Therefore, the child can meet his or her own needs related to gross motor skill performance. At this level, parents may have to assist with fine motor skills.
   4. A child diagnosed with moderate IDD is capable of academic skills to the second-grade level and, as an adult, may be able to contribute to his or her own support in a sheltered workshop. Therefore, the intervention of providing one-on-one tutorial education in a private setting would not be appropriate.
   TEST-TAKING TIP: Review the developmental characteristics of intellectual disability by degree of severity, and match the nursing interventions with the appropriate level of individual capability.
   Content Area: Safe and Effective Care Environment; Management of Care;
   Integrated Process: Nursing Process: Implementation;
   Client Need: Safe and Effective Care Environment; Management of Care;
   Cognitive Level: Application;
   Concept: Nursing

3. **ANSWERS: 1, 4, 5**
   Rationale:
   1. Behavior therapy is a form of psychotherapy, the goal of which is to modify maladaptive behavior patterns by reinforcing more adaptive behaviors. The nurse should anticipate employing behavior therapy when planning care for a child diagnosed with ODD.
   2. Cognitive therapy is a type of therapy in which the client is taught to control thought distortions. Thought distortion is not a symptom of ODD; therefore, this therapy would not be appropriate for a client diagnosed with ODD.
   3. Aversion therapy is a type of conditioning intended to cause the client to associate a stimulus with unpleasant sensations to stop a specific behavior, such as placing unpleasant-tasting substances on the fingernails to discourage nail chewing. This therapy would not be appropriate for a client diagnosed with ODD.
   4. Group therapy provides a number of benefits. Appropriate social behavior is often learned from the positive and negative feedback of peers. The nurse should anticipate employing group therapy when planning care for a child diagnosed with ODD.
   5. Family therapy is a type of therapy in which the focus is on relationships within the family. The family is viewed as a system in which the members are interdependent, and a change in one creates a change in all. The nurse should anticipate employing group therapy when planning care for a child diagnosed with ODD.
   TEST-TAKING TIP: Review general therapeutic approaches that treat various child and adolescent disorders.
   Content Area: Safe and Effective Care Environment; Management of Care;
   Integrated Process: Nursing Process: Planning;
   Client Need: Safe and Effective Care Environment; Management of Care;
   Cognitive Level: Application;
   Concept: Nursing

4. **ANSWER: 4**
   Rationale: An IQ level of 60 in within the range of mild intellectual disability.
   1. A client with profound intellectual disability (IQ level <20), not a mild level of intellectual disability, would have little, if any, speech development and no capacity for socialization skills.
   2. A client with moderate intellectual disability (IQ level 35–49), not a mild level of intellectual disability, may experience some limitation in speech and social communication. The client also may have difficulty adhering to social convention, which would interfere with peer relationships.
   3. A client with severe intellectual disability (IQ level 20–34), not a mild level of intellectual disability, would have minimal verbal skills. Because of this deficit, wants and needs are often communicated by acting-out behaviors.
   4. A client with mild intellectual disability (IQ level 50–70) would be capable of developing social and communication skills. The client would function well in a structured, sheltered setting.
   TEST-TAKING TIP: Review Table 17.1, "Developmental Characteristics of Intellectual Disability by Degree of Severity."
   Content Area: Safe and Effective Care Environment; Management of Care;
   Integrated Process: Nursing Process: Assessment;
   Client Need: Safe and Effective Care Environment; Management of Care;
   Cognitive Level: Application;
   Concept: Development

5. ANSWER: 1
Rationale:

1. A child diagnosed with severe intellectual disability (IQ level 20–34) who strikes out at staff members when not being able to complete simple tasks is using aggression to deal with frustration. *Ineffective coping related to inability to deal with frustration* is the appropriate nursing diagnosis for this child.

2. A child diagnosed with severe intellectual disability probably would not have the cognitive ability to experience feelings of powerlessness or have the insight to experience deficits in self-esteem. Also, the aggressive behavior described in the question is not reflective of the nursing diagnosis of anxiety.

3. A child diagnosed with severe intellectual disability probably would not have the cognitive awareness to isolate self from others. Also, the aggressive behavior described in the question is not reflective of the nursing diagnosis of social isolation.

4. A child diagnosed with severe intellectual disability may be at risk for injury because of altered physical mobility. However, the actual aggressive behavior presented in the question is indicative of ineffective coping, not risk for injury.

TEST-TAKING TIP: Pair the client symptoms described in the question with the problem statement, or nursing diagnosis, that relates to these symptoms. Although Option 4 is a safety priority, it is not reflective of the immediate client problem of aggression with staff members.
Content Area: Safe and Effective Care Environment; Management of Care;
Integrated Process: Nursing Process: Diagnosis (Analysis);
Client Need: Safe and Effective Care Environment; Management of Care;
Cognitive Level: Analysis;
Concept: Critical Thinking

6. ANSWERS: 1, 3, 4
Rationale:

1. It has been determined that the prevalence of autism spectrum disorder (ASD) in the United States is about 11.3 per 1,000 or (1 in 88) children.

2. ASD is diagnosed in early childhood before, not after, the child reaches school age.

3. ASD does occur about 4.5 times more often in boys than in girls.

4. In most cases ASD does run a chronic course, with symptoms persisting into adulthood.

5. The diagnosis of separation anxiety disorder, not ASD, can be a precursor to adult panic disorder.

TEST-TAKING TIP: Review the epidemiological section of ASD in the outline.
Content Area: Safe and Effective Care Environment; Management of Care;
Integrated Process: Nursing Process: Assessment;
Client Need: Safe and Effective Care Environment; Management of Care;
Cognitive Level: Application;
Concept: Development

7. ANSWER: autism spectrum
Rationale: Autism spectrum disorder is characterized, in varying degrees, by difficulties in social interaction, verbal and nonverbal communication, and repetitive behaviors.
TEST-TAKING TIP: Review the key terms at the beginning of the chapter.
Content Area: Psychosocial Integrity;
Integrated Process: Nursing Process: Assessment;
Client Need: Psychosocial Integrity;
Cognitive Level: Knowledge;
Concept: Development

8. ANSWERS: 2, 3, 4
Rationale:

1. Tourette's disorder, not autism spectrum disorder (ASD), may be transmitted in an autosomal pattern somewhere between dominant and recessive.

2. Studies have shown that parents who have one child with ASD are at increased risk for having more than one child with the disorder.

3. Studies with both monozygotic and dizygotic twins have provided evidence of a genetic involvement. Research into how genetic factors influence the development of ASD is ongoing.

4. A number of linkage studies have implicated areas on several chromosomes to the development of the disorder, most notably chromosomes 2, 7, 15, 16, and 17.

5. Studies suggest that the genes for the metabolism of dopamine, serotonin, and norepinephrine may be a contributing factor to the development of oppositional defiant disorder, not a factor associated with ASD.

TEST-TAKING TIP: Review the predisposing factors to the diagnosis of ASD in the genetic section of the outline.
Content Area: Safe and Effective Care Environment; Management of Care;
Integrated Process: Nursing Process: Assessment;
Client Need: Safe and Effective Care Environment; Management of Care;
Cognitive Level: Application;
Concept: Development

9. ANSWER: 4
Rationale:

1. Disturbed body image is defined as confusion and/or dissatisfaction in the mental picture of one's physical self. There is nothing presented in the question that would indicate that this child has a disturbed body image.

2. Self-care deficit is defined as the impaired ability to perform activities to meet self-care needs. There is nothing presented in the question that would indicate that this child has a deficit in her ability to perform self-care activities.

3. Dysfunctional family process is defined as chronically disorganized psychosocial, spiritual, and physiological functions of the family unit that leads to conflict, denial of problems, resistance to change, ineffective problem-solving, and a series of self-perpetuating crises. Even though the behaviors of children diagnosed with separation anxiety disorder could strain the family, there is nothing presented in the question that would indicate that this child herself has a dysfunctional family process.

4. Impaired social interaction is defined as insufficient or excessive quantity or ineffective quality of social exchange. The fear of being separated from the attachment figure, which is a major symptom of separation anxiety disorder, prevents this child from establishing effective social exchanges within her peer group.

TEST-TAKING TIP: Look closely at the behaviors and symptoms presented in the question and match the nursing diagnosis with the client behavior presented.

Content Area: Safe and Effective Care Environment; Management of Care;
Integrated Process: Nursing Process: Diagnosis (Analysis);
Client Need: Safe and Effective Care Environment; Management of Care;
Cognitive Level: Analysis;
Concept: Critical Thinking

10. **ANSWERS: 2, 4, 5**
Rationale:
1. There is evidence suggesting that Tourette's disorder, not attention deficit-hyperactivity disorder (ADHD), may be transmitted in an autosomal pattern intermediate between dominant and recessive.
2. A number of ADHD studies have found that copy number variants overlap with chromosomal regions previously linked to autism spectrum disorder and schizophrenia.
3. Studies suggest that the genes for metabolism of dopamine, serotonin, and norepinephrine may be contributing factors to the development of oppositional defiant disorder, not ADHD.
4. A number of ADHD studies have found that a large number of parents of hyperactive children showed signs of hyperactivity during their own childhood.
5. A number of ADHD studies support the premise that hyperactive children are more likely to have siblings who are also hyperactive.

TEST-TAKING TIP: Review genetic influences associated with ADHD.

Content Area: Safe and Effective Care Environment; Management of Care;
Integrated Process: Nursing Process: Assessment;
Client Need: Safe and Effective Care Environment; Management of Care;
Cognitive Level: Application;
Concept: Development

11. **ANSWER: 4**
Rationale:
1. Setting limits on manipulative behavior may be helpful in decreasing unacceptable behaviors. However, observing a client's behavior frequently for signs of escalating agitation may provide an opportunity to intervene before violence occurs. Because safety is the first concern, observing for signs of escalating agitation is the intervention that takes priority.
2. Working through situations that provoke defensiveness may provide confidence in dealing with situations when they actually occur. However, safety is the first concern; therefore, observing for signs of escalating agitation is the intervention that takes priority.

3. Discussing consequences for unacceptable behavior is an important component of behavioral therapy that works to extinguish undesirable behaviors. However, safety is the first concern; therefore, observing for signs of escalating agitation is the intervention that takes priority.
4. Client safety is always a nurse's first consideration. When dealing with a client who has a history of violence, a nurse must continually observe the client's behavior and become aware of conduct that indicates a rise in agitation. Recognition of behaviors that precede the onset of aggression may provide the opportunity to intervene before violence occurs. This intervention, above all other interventions mentioned, takes priority.

TEST-TAKING TIP: Note the client behaviors presented in the question and match them with the appropriate intervention that addresses these behaviors. Remember that safety issues are always prioritized.

Content Area: Safe and Effective Care Environment; Management of Care;
Integrated Process: Nursing Process: Implementation;
Client Need: Safe and Effective Care Environment; Management of Care;
Cognitive Level: Analysis;
Concept: Nursing

12. **ANSWERS: 1, 5**
Rationale: Correctly written outcomes must be client centered, specific, realistic, and must also include a time frame.
1. *The child will interact in age-appropriate manner with a nurse in one-to-one relationship within 1 week* meets the criteria for a correctly written outcome.
2. There is nothing to indicate that the child in the question is inflicting harm on self or others. There is also no inclusion of a time frame; therefore, this outcome is inappropriate and, without a time frame, is incorrectly written.
3. Behaving *normally* is an arbitrary term that cannot be measured; therefore, this outcome is incorrectly written.
4. This outcome does not include a time frame; therefore, this outcome is incorrectly written.
5. The child will be free of injury during hospitalization meets the criteria for a correctly written outcome.

TEST-TAKING TIP: Review criteria for a correctly written client outcome and identify and select outcomes that are based on client behaviors described in the question.

Content Area: Safe and Effective Care Environment; Management of Care;
Integrated Process: Nursing Process: Planning;
Client Need: Safe and Effective Care Environment; Management of Care;
Cognitive Level: Application;
Concept: Critical Thinking

13. **ANSWERS: 2, 3, 4, 5**
Rationale:
1. The disorder is observed in two-thirds, not one-third, of relatives of clients with Tourette's disorder.
2. Twin studies with both monozygotic and dizygotic twins do suggest an inheritable component associated with Tourette's disorder.

3. According to studies, Tourette's disorder may be transmitted in an autosomal pattern intermediate between dominant and recessive.

4. It is true that the precise gene and mechanism of inheritance in Tourette's disorder remains undetermined.

5. Research has found abnormalities in levels of dopamine, serotonin, and norepinephrine associated with Tourette's disorder.

TEST-TAKING TIP: Review the predisposing genetic factors associated with Tourette's disorder.
Content Area: Safe and Effective Care Environment; Management of Care;
Integrated Process: Nursing Process: Assessment;
Client Need: Safe and Effective Care Environment; Management of Care;
Cognitive Level: Application;
Concept: Development

14. **ANSWER: 4**
Rationale: An IQ of 69 indicates mild intellectual disability

1. Clients with profound, not mild, intellectual disability lack the ability for both fine and gross motor movements and require constant supervision and care. Clients with mild intellectual disability should be encouraged to meet as many of their own needs as possible. This outcome would not be prioritized.

2. Clients with mild intellectual disability have intact psychomotor skills. Even though they may experience some slight alterations in coordination, this would not limit their activities and put them at risk for injury. This outcome would not be prioritized.

3. Clients with mild intellectual disability are capable of developing social skills and function well in a structured, sheltered setting. Their intellectual disability would not severely limit their social interaction. This outcome would not be prioritized.

4. **Clients with mild intellectual disability are capable of independent living, with assistance during times of stress. The outcome of demonstrating adaptive coping skills under times of stress will focus the client on developing these skills to meet the challenges of life and should be prioritized.**

TEST-TAKING TIP: You must first determine the client's severity of intellectual disability and then choose the outcome that addresses the needs of that level of disability.
Content Area: Safe and Effective Care Environment; Management of Care;
Integrated Process: Nursing Process: Planning;
Client Need: Safe and Effective Care Environment; Management of Care;
Cognitive Level: Analysis;
Concept: Critical Thinking

15. **ANSWERS: 1, 3, 4, 5**
Rationale:

1. **Parental rejection is often a factor that has been implicated as a family dynamic contributing to the etiology of conduct disorder (CD).**

2. A family dynamic that imposes parental expectations of conduct standards is observed in the families of children diagnosed with obsessive-compulsive personality disorder, not CD.

3. **Inconsistent parental management with harsh discipline is a family dynamic that contributes to the etiology of CD.**

4. **Having an absent father is a family dynamic that contributes to the etiology of CD.**

5. **Parental permissiveness happens when the parents abdicate all authority in favor of taking the "easy" road, which then results in the child becoming out of control. This is family dynamic that contributes to the etiology of CD.**

TEST-TAKING TIP: Review the family dynamics that are associated with the diagnosis of CD.
Content Area: Safe and Effective Care Environment; Management of Care;
Integrated Process: Nursing Process: Assessment;
Client Need: Safe and Effective Care Environment; Management of Care;
Cognitive Level: Application;
Concept: Assessment

16. **ANSWER: 3**
Rationale:

1. The child's impaired social interaction will need to be addressed. However, the child's safety is always the first consideration. Therefore, risk for self-mutilation, not impaired social interaction, takes priority.

2. The child's impaired verbal communication will need to be addressed. However, the child's safety is always the first consideration. Therefore, risk for self-mutilation, not impaired verbal communication, takes priority.

3. **Risk for self-mutilation would take priority. Client safety is always a nurse's first consideration.**

4. There is nothing in the question that indicates that this child is at risk for harming others; therefore, this nursing diagnosis would be inappropriate for this child.

TEST-TAKING TIP: Match the nursing diagnosis with the presented client behavior, and remember that client safety always takes priority.
Content Area: Safe and Effective Care Environment; Management of Care;
Integrated Process: Nursing Process: Diagnosis (Analysis);
Client Need: Safe and Effective Care Environment; Management of Care;
Cognitive Level: Analysis;
Concept: Critical Thinking

17. **ANSWERS: 1, 3**
Rationale:

1. **Encouraging a child to discuss specific situations in life that produce the most stress is an appropriate intervention for a child diagnosed with separation anxiety disorder. The child and family may be unaware of the correlation between stressful situations and the exacerbation of client symptoms. Promoting this awareness can assist the client to cope.**

2. Providing a variety of meaningful sensory stimulation is an intervention that addresses a client's problem with disturbed sensory perception, not ineffective coping. Also, sensory deficits are not typically associated with separation anxiety disorder.

3. **Helping the perfectionist child to recognize that self-expectations may be unrealistic is an appropriate**

intervention for a child diagnosed with separation anxiety disorder. Recognition of maladaptive behavior patterns, such as perfectionism, is the first step toward adaptive change.

4. Manipulative behavior is an attempt to gain attention and therefore increase self-esteem. Setting limits on this behavior addresses low self-esteem, not ineffective coping. Also, there is nothing in the question that indicates that this child is exhibiting low self-esteem.

5. Defensive behavior can be generated by feelings of inadequacy. Helping the child recognize the relationship between feelings of inadequacy and defensive behavior is an intervention that addresses a client's defensive coping, not ineffective coping. Also, there is nothing in the question that indicates that this child is exhibiting defensive coping.

TEST-TAKING TIP: Match the appropriate nursing intervention with the nursing diagnosis presented in the question.

Content Area: Safe and Effective Care Environment; Management of Care;
Integrated Process: Nursing Process: Implementation;
Client Need: Safe and Effective Care Environment; Management of Care;
Cognitive Level: Application;
Concept: Nursing

18. **ANSWER: 1**
Rationale:
1. **A client diagnosed with oppositional defiant disorder (ODD) exhibits a persistent pattern of angry mood and defiant behavior that occurs more frequently than is usually observed in individuals of comparable age and developmental level. This behavior interferes with social, educational, or vocational activities. Clients diagnosed with conduct disorder (CD) exhibit a repetitive and persistent pattern of behavior in which the basic rights of others or major age-appropriate societal norms or rules are violated. This student statement indicates that learning has occurred.**
2. Clients diagnosed with CD, not ODD, often exhibit aggression toward animals. This student statement indicates that further instruction is needed.
3. Clients diagnosed with CD, not ODD, often set fires with intention to do harm. Destruction of property is characteristic of clients diagnosed with CD. This student statement indicates that further instruction is needed.
4. Clients diagnosed with both CD and ODD have attention deficit-hyperactivity disorder as a common comorbid disorder.

TEST-TAKING TIP: Review clinical findings, epidemiology, and course of ODD and CD to be able to compare and contrast the two disorders.

Content Area: Safe and Effective Care Environment; Management of Care;
Integrated Process: Nursing Process: Evaluation;
Client Need: Safe and Effective Care Environment; Management of Care;
Cognitive Level: Analysis;
Concept: Nursing Roles

19. **ANSWERS: 1, 2, 4**
Rationale:
1. **Clients diagnosed with autism spectrum disorder (ASD) can experience impaired verbal communication. They can withdraw into themselves, be unable or unwilling to speak, and lack nonverbal expressions. Seeking clarification and validation ensures that the client's intended message has been conveyed. This nursing diagnosis and nursing intervention are correctly matched.**
2. **Clients diagnosed with ASD can experience impaired social interaction. This may be due to their lack of responsiveness to, or interest in, people. Giving positive reinforcement for maintaining eye contact will encourage the client to acquire a skill essential to the ability to form satisfactory interpersonal relationships. This nursing diagnosis and nursing intervention are correctly matched.**
3. Clients diagnosed with ASD may be at risk for self-directed violence or self-mutilation but are usually not prone to violence toward others. Also, restraints should only be used when injury is imminent and all other avenues of intervention have been exhausted.
4. **Clients diagnosed with ASD can experience disturbed personal identity. This may be due to their difficulty separating their own physiological and emotional needs and personal boundaries from those of others. Assisting the client in naming his or her own body parts may help increase the client's awareness of self as separate from others. This nursing diagnosis and nursing intervention are correctly matched.**
5. Clients diagnosed with ASD can experience disturbed personal identity but are not so out of touch with reality to experience altered body image. Also, a client's perception of reality should not be challenged. When caring for clients experiencing altered perceptions, the nurse should assess the client's perception of reality, present objective reality, and redirect the client to a neutral stimulus.

TEST-TAKING TIP: You must first determine the nursing diagnoses that would apply to a client diagnosed with ASD. Then you should evaluate the appropriateness of the nursing intervention presented.

Content Area: Safe and Effective Care Environment; Management of Care;
Integrated Process: Nursing Process: Diagnosis (Analysis);
Client Need: Safe and Effective Care Environment; Management of Care;
Cognitive Level: Analysis;
Concept: Critical Thinking

20. **ANSWER: 2**
Rationale:
1. There is nothing in the question that indicates that this child has any intention of harming self or others; therefore, this nursing diagnosis is inappropriate and would not be assigned.
2. **Impaired social interaction is defined as an insufficient or excessive quantity or ineffective quality of social exchange. The nurse would assign this diagnosis to a child diagnosed with Tourette's disorder, who is withdrawn, refuses to participate in group therapy, and initiates little or no communication with peers.**

3. Although this child may well have a low self-esteem, which will need addressing, the child in the question is exhibiting behaviors that indicate impaired social interaction, not low-self-esteem.

4. Although this child may experience anxiety related to Tourette's disorder and fear of embarrassment, there is nothing in the question that indicates that this child is experiencing severe anxiety. This nursing diagnosis is inappropriate and would not be assigned.

TEST-TAKING TIP: Pair the child's symptoms described in the question with the nursing diagnosis that relates to these symptoms.
Content Area: Safe and Effective Care Environment; Management of Care;
Integrated Process: Nursing Process: Diagnosis (Analysis);
Client Need: Safe and Effective Care Environment; Management of Care;
Cognitive Level: Analysis
Concept: Critical Thinking

CASE STUDY: Putting it All Together

With both 15-year-old Elise and Elise's mother sitting in the conference room, psychiatric nurse practitioner (PNP) Tessa asks Elise to help her understand what is going on. Elise glares and says, "My mother thinks I have a problem."

Tessa leans forward and says, "Go on."

Elise frowns and snarls, "That's just it. I don't have the problem—she does! I want you to know I'm here against my will." Elise furiously jumps out of her seat and with clenched fist, yells, "Big deal. So I skipped school? So what? That's it! I'm not answering any more stupid questions. My bitchy mother has all the answers anyway."

To get a history, Tessa continues the assessment interview with the mother after Elise is dismissed to the day area with a staff member. Elise's mother begins, "Problems started in second grade when Elise became disruptive and refused to do class work. The behavior has continued and progressed through the years. Now, she is more often absent from school than in attendance. At home, Elise is sullen, belligerent, strong-willed, and defiant. Elise has had several run-ins with the authorities for vandalism and disrespectful behavior. We've been through family therapy, psychological testing, and school counseling for years, but nothing seems to make a difference. The latest problem is that Elise sneaks out at night and doesn't return until the next day. Her father and I are terrified for her safety. This behavior is so out of character for our family. My husband is in the military, and with the exception of

Elise, we're all conscientious rule followers. We just don't know what to do."

Later, when Tessa approaches Elise, Elise sneers and says, "I bet you got an earful from my holier-than-thou mother. Did she tell you what an embarrassment I am to the family? Well, I plan to live my life my way, and just as soon as I'm old enough, I'm out of there. Now, what's it going to take for me to get out of *this* nut house?"

1. On the basis of the preceding symptoms and client actions, what medical diagnosis would Tessa assign to Elise?
2. What predisposing factors might have led to Elise's behavior?
3. What are Elise's subjective symptoms that would lead to the determination of this diagnosis?
4. What are Elise's objective symptoms that would lead to the determination of this diagnosis?
5. What NANDA nursing diagnosis would address Elise's current problem?
6. On the basis of this nursing diagnosis, what short-term outcome would be appropriate for Elise?
7. On the basis of this nursing diagnosis, what long-term outcome would be appropriate for Elise?
8. List the nursing interventions (actions) that will assist Elise in successfully meeting these outcomes.
9. List the psychological treatments Tessa might employ to treat Elise.
10. List the questions that should be asked to determine the success of the nursing interventions.

Chapter 18

Issues Related to Human Sexuality and Gender Dysphoria

KEY TERMS

Anorgasmia—A type of sexual dysfunction in which a person cannot achieve orgasm despite adequate stimulation

Bisexuality—Romantic or sexual feelings toward both men and women; one of the three main classifications of sexual orientation along with heterosexuality and homosexuality

Exhibitionistic disorder—A mental health condition that centers on a need to expose one's genitals to other people (typically strangers caught off guard) to gain sexual satisfaction

Fetishistic disorder—A mental health condition that centers on the employment of inanimate objects as a source of sexual satisfaction or the fulfillment of sexual fantasies or urges

Frotteuristic disorder—A mental health condition that centers on achieving sexual stimulation or orgasm by touching and rubbing against a person, usually in a public place, without the person's consent

Gender—The condition of being either male or female

Gender identity—The sense of knowing whether one is male or female; the awareness of one's masculinity or femininity

Gender dysphoria—The experience of significant discontent with the sex and gender assigned at birth; evidence suggests that people who identify with a gender different from the one they were assigned at birth may do so not just due to psychological or behavioral causes but also biological ones related to their genetics, the makeup of their brains, or prenatal exposure to hormones

Homosexuality—Romantic attraction, sexual attraction, or sexual behavior between members of the same sex or gender; as a sexual orientation, is an enduring pattern of emotional, romantic, and/or sexual attraction primarily or exclusively to people of the same sex

Lesbianism—Homosexual relations between women

Orgasm—The sudden discharge of accumulated sexual excitement during the sexual response cycle, resulting in rhythmic muscular contractions in the pelvic region characterized by sexual pleasure

Paraphilic disorders—Sexual behaviors that society may view as distasteful, unusual, or abnormal: In descending order, the most common are pedophilic disorder (sexual activity with a child usually 13 years old or younger), exhibitionistic disorder (exposure of genitals to strangers), voyeuristic disorder (observing private activities of unaware victims), and frotteuristic disorder (touching, rubbing against a nonconsenting person); fetishistic disorder (use of inanimate objects), sexual masochistic disorder (being humiliated or forced to suffer), sexual sadistic disorder (inflicting humiliation or suffering), and transvestic disorder (cross-dressing) are far less common

Pedophilic disorder—A mental health condition in which an adult has sexual fantasies about or engages in sexual acts with a prepubescent child of the same or opposite sex

Sensate focus—A set of specific sexual exercises for couples or individuals to increase personal and

Continued

KEY TERMS—cont'd

interpersonal awareness of self and partner's needs; each participant is encouraged to focus on his or her own varied sense experience rather than to see orgasm as the sole goal of sex

Sexuality—The constitution and life of an individual relative to characteristics regarding intimacy; reflects the totality of the person and does not relate exclusively to the sex organs or sexual behavior

Transvestic disorder—The urge or desire to dress in the clothes of the opposite sex, or cross-dress, to achieve sexual excitement or arousal; cross-dressing must be the preferred or exclusive means of achieving sexual gratification

Voyeuristic disorder—A mental health condition in which a person derives sexual pleasure and gratification from looking at the naked bodies and genital organs or observing the sexual acts of others

---

Sexuality is a basic human need and an innate part of the total personality. It influences our thoughts, actions, and interactions and is involved in aspects of physical and mental health. Nurses can readily integrate information on sexuality into their client care by focusing on preventive, therapeutic, and educational interventions to assist individuals to attain, regain, or maintain sexual wellness. This chapter focuses on disorders associated with sexual functioning and gender dysphoria. Primary consideration is given to the categories of paraphilic disorders and sexual dysfunctions.

I. Human Sexuality Development

A. Birth through age 12 years
  1. **Gender identity** is determined before birth by chromosomal factors and physical appearance of the genitals.
  2. Postnatal factors can greatly influence the way developing children perceive themselves sexually.
  3. Masculinity, femininity, and gender roles are culturally defined.

DID YOU KNOW?
Differentiation of gender roles may be initiated at birth by painting a child's room pink or blue and by clothing the child in frilly, delicate dresses or tough, sturdy rompers.

  1. Common for infants to touch and explore their genitals.
  2. Both male and female infants are capable of sexual arousal and **orgasm.**
  3. By age 2 or 2.5 years:
     a. Children know what **gender** they are.
     b. They know they are like the parent of the same gender and different from the parent of the opposite gender and from other children of the opposite gender.
     c. Children become acutely aware of anatomical gender differences.
  4. By age 4 or 5 years:
     a. Children engage in heterosexual play.
     b. Through this play, they form a concept of marriage to a member of the opposite gender.

c. "Playing doctor" can be a popular game.
d. Children increasingly gain experience with masturbation.

DID YOU KNOW?
Although not all children masturbate by the age of 4 or 5 years, most children begin self-exploration and genital self-stimulation as soon as they gain sufficient control over their physical movements.

  5. Late childhood and preadolescence:
     a. Characterized by heterosexual or homosexual play.
     b. Activity usually involves no more than touching the other's genitals.
     c. May include a wide range of sexual behaviors.
     d. Girls become interested in menstruation.
     e. Both genders are interested in learning about fertility, pregnancy, and birth.
     f. Interest in the opposite gender increases.
     g. Become self-conscious about their bodies.
     h. Concerned with physical attractiveness.
     i. Preoccupied with pubertal changes and the beginnings of romantic sexual attraction.
     j. Boys may engage in group sexual activities such as genital exhibition or group masturbation.
     k. Homosexual sex play is common.
     l. Girls may engage in some genital exhibition but are not as preoccupied with the genitalia as boys.
B. Adolescence
  1. Acceleration occurs in terms of biological changes and psychosocial and sexual development.
  2. New set of psychosocial tasks to undertake.
     a. How to deal with new or more powerful sexual feelings.
     b. Whether to participate in various types of sexual behavior.
     c. How to recognize love.
     d. How to prevent unwanted pregnancy.
     e. How to define age-appropriate gender roles.
  3. Masturbation is common sexual activity among males and females.

4. Biological changes.
    a. Puberty for females begins with:
        i. Breast enlargement
        ii. Widening of the hips
        iii. Growth of pubic and ancillary hair
        iv. Onset of menstruation (usually occurs between 11 and 13 years of age)
    b. Puberty for males begins with:
        i. Growth of pubic hair and enlargement of the testicles (12–16 years of age)
        ii. Penile growth and the ability to ejaculate (13–17 years of age)
        iii. Marked growth of the body (11–17 years of age)
        iv. Increased growth of body and facial hair
        v. Increased muscle mass
        vi. Deeper voice
    c. Male sexual drive remains high through young adulthood.
    d. Experience with sexual intercourse.
        i. More adolescents are engaging in premarital intercourse
        ii. Incidence of premarital intercourse for girls has increased
        iii. Average age of first intercourse has decreased
        iv. Trend is toward safer sex with condom use
5. Rise in sexually transmitted disease (STD) cases, some of which are life threatening, contributes to fears associated with unprotected sexual activity in all age-groups.
6. Cervical cancer kills 3,700 American women every year.
7. Gardasil, first vaccine developed to prevent cervical cancer and other diseases caused by certain strains of human papillomavirus (HPV).
8. Cervarix, vaccine if administered before exposure can protect women from ultimately developing cervical cancer caused by specific strains of HPV.
9. Centers for Disease Control and Prevention (CDC) recommends routine administration of three doses of either vaccine to all girls aged 11 or 12 years.
10. Also recommended for girls and women aged 13 through 26 years who have not already received the complete vaccine series.
11. CDC recommends routine administration of Gardasil in males aged 11 or 12 years.
12. Also recommended for males aged 13 through 21 years who have not already received the complete vaccine series.
13. Males aged 22 through 26 years may also be vaccinated.
14. Some state legislatures have proposed making HPV vaccine mandatory for girls aged 9 to 12 years.
    a. Some parents believe these laws circumvent their rights.
    b. May send message of promoting promiscuity by offering unrealistic protection.
    c. Some believe that prevention of premarital sex should be the priority.
    d. Recent studies indicate that the HPV vaccination in the recommended age-group was not associated with increased sexual activity.

C. Adulthood
1. This period of the life cycle begins at approximately age 20 years and continues to age 65.
2. Marital sex.
    a. Choosing a marital partner or developing a sexual relationship with another individual is one of the major tasks in the early years of this life-cycle stage.
    b. Eighty percent to 90% of all people in the United States marry.
    c. Of those who divorce, a high percentage remarry.
    d. Intimacy in marriage is one of the most common forms of sexual expression for adults.
    e. The average American couple has coitus about two or three times per week when they are in their 20s.
    f. Frequency gradually declines to about weekly for those age 45 years and over.
    g. Many adults continue to masturbate even though they are married and have ready access to heterosexual sex.
    h. Masturbation is perfectly normal.
    i. Masturbation often evokes feelings of guilt and may be kept secret.
3. Extramarital sex.
    a. About one-third of married men and one-fourth of married women have engaged in extramarital sex at some time during their marriages.
    b. Incidence of extramarital sex for men is holding constant.
    c. Evidence suggests that extramarital sex is increasing for women.
    d. Attitudes toward extramarital sex remain relatively stable.
    e. Most individuals believe goal in marriage should be sexual exclusivity.

MAKING THE CONNECTION

Sexuality is slower to develop in females than in the males. Women show a steady increase in sexual responsiveness that peaks in their middle 20s or early 30s. Sexual maturity for men is usually reached in late teens. Women stabilize at the same level of sexual activity as at the previous stage in the life cycle and often have a greater capacity for orgasm in middle adulthood.

f. Increased ambivalence toward consequences of infidelity.

g. Twenty percent of all divorces are caused by infidelity or adultery.

4. Sex and the single person.

a. Attitudes about sexual intimacy among singles (never married, divorced, or widowed) vary.

b. Some single people will settle for any kind of relationship (casual or committed).

c. Others deny any desire for marriage or sexual intimacy.

d. Others cherish independence of being "unattached."

e. Others may search desperately for a spouse, with increasing desperation.

f. Most divorced men and women return to an active sex life after separation.

g. More widowed men than widowed women return to an active sex life after the loss.

h. Widows outnumber widowers by more than four to one.

5. The "middle" years—ages 40 to 65.

a. Decrease in hormonal production initiates changes in the sex organs, as well as the rest of the body.

b. Average age of onset of menopause for woman is around 50 (changes due to menopause can be noted from about 40–60).

c. One percent of women experience symptoms of menopause as early as age 35.

d. Decreased estrogen can result in:

i. Loss of vaginal lubrication, making intercourse painful

ii. Insomnia

iii. "Hot flashes"

iv. Headaches

v. Heart palpitations

vi. Depression

DID YOU KNOW?

Hormonal supplements may alleviate some of the symptoms of menopause, although controversy currently exists within the medical community regarding the safety of hormone replacement therapy.

6. Decreased androgen can result in:

a. Sexual changes.

b. Decreased amount of ejaculate.

c. Less forceful ejaculation.

d. Decreased size of testes.

e. Less frequent and less rigid erections.

f. By age 50, refractory period increases, and men may require 8 to 24 hours after orgasm before achieving another erection.

g. Biological drives decrease.

h. Most men continue to produce viable sperm well into old age.

DID YOU KNOW?

By age 50, male interest in sexual activity may decrease. They need a longer period of stimulation to reach orgasm, and the intensity of pleasure may decrease. On the other hand, women stabilize at the same level of sexual activity as at the previous stage in the life cycle and often have a greater capacity for orgasm in middle adulthood than in young adulthood. For women, enjoyment rather than frequency is a key factor to the continuance of sexual activity. Frequency and enjoyment are both important to men.

D. Sexuality and aging

1. Negative stereotyped notions are common.

a. Older people have no sexual interests or desires.

b. They are sexually undesirable.

c. They are too fragile or too ill to engage in sexual activity.

2. Cultural stereotypes play a large part in misperception.

3. Reinforced by tendency of young to deny the inevitability of aging.

DID YOU KNOW?

With reasonable good health and an interesting and interested partner, there is no inherent reason why individuals should not enjoy an active sexual life well into late adulthood.

4. Sexual behavior in the elderly.

a. Interest and behavior do appear to decline somewhat.

b. Significant numbers of elderly men and women have active and satisfying sex lives well into their 80s.

II. Sexual Disorders

A. Paraphilic disorders

1. *Paraphilia* identifies repetitive or preferred sexual fantasies or behaviors that involve:

a. Nonhuman objects.

b. Suffering or humiliation of oneself or one's partner.

c. Nonconsenting persons.

MAKING THE CONNECTION

Sexuality and the sexual needs of elderly people are frequently misunderstood, condemned, stereotyped, ridiculed, repressed, and ignored. Americans have grown up in a society that has liberated sexual expression for all other age-groups but still retains certain Victorian standards regarding sexual expression by the elderly. Some people even believe it is disgusting or comical to consider elderly individuals as sexual beings.

2. Behaviors are recurrent over a period of at least 6 months.
3. Cause the individual clinically significant distress or impairment in social, occupational, or other important areas of functioning.

DID YOU KNOW?

Historically, some restrictions on human sexual expression have always existed. Under the code of Orthodox Judaism, masturbation was punishable by death. In ancient Catholicism, it was considered a carnal sin. In the late 19th century, masturbation was viewed as a major cause of insanity. The sexual exploitation of children was condemned in ancient cultures, as it continues to be today. Incest remains the one taboo that crosses cultural barriers. It was punishable by death in Babylonia, Judea, and ancient China, and offenders were given the death penalty as late as 1650 in England.

4. Historically, oral-genital, anal, homosexual, and animal sexual contacts were viewed as unnatural.
5. Today, among these acts, only sex with animals (zoophilic disorder) retains its classification as a paraphilia.
6. Few individuals with paraphilic disorders experience personal distress from their behavior.
7. Treatment initiated as result of pressure from partners or authorities.
8. Seek outpatient treatment for:
   a. Pedophilic disorder (45%).
   b. Exhibitionistic disorder (25%).
   c. Voyeuristic disorder (12%).
9. Most individuals with a paraphilic disorder are men.
10. Behavior generally established in adolescence.
11. Behavior peaks between ages 15 and 25.
12. Behavior gradually declines.
13. By age 50, the occurrence of paraphilic acts is very low.
14. Some individuals experience multiple paraphilic disorders.
15. Types of paraphilic disorders.
    a. **Exhibitionistic disorder.**
       i. Characterized by recurrent and intense sexual arousal (manifested by fantasies, urges, or behaviors of at least a 6-month duration) from the exposure of one's genitals to an unsuspecting individual
       ii. Masturbation may occur during the exhibitionism
       iii. In most cases, perpetrators are men, and the victims are women
       iv. Urges for genital exposure intensify when:
          a) Exhibitionist has excessive free time
          b) Exhibitionist is under significant stress

c) Most exhibitionists have rewarding sexual relationships with adult partners but concomitantly expose themselves to others
   b. **Fetishistic disorder.**
      i. Involves recurrent and intense sexual arousal (manifested by fantasies, urges, or behaviors for at least 6 months) from the use of either nonliving objects or specific nongenital body parts
      ii. Onset usually occurs during adolescence
      iii. Sexual focus commonly on objects intimately associated with the human body (shoes, gloves, stockings)
      iv. The fetish object is usually used during masturbation or incorporated into sexual activity with another person to produce sexual excitation

DID YOU KNOW?

Requirement of the fetish object for sexual arousal may become so intense in clients diagnosed with a fetishistic disorder that to be without it may result in impotence.

      v. Disorder is chronic
      vi. Complications arise when the individual becomes progressively more intensely aroused by sexual behaviors that exclude a sexual partner
      vii. Person with the fetish and his or her partner may become distant, and the partner terminates the relationship
   c. **Frotteuristic disorder.**
      i. Recurrent and intense sexual arousal (manifested by urges, behaviors, or fantasies for at least 6 months) involving touching and rubbing against a nonconsenting person
      ii. Almost without exception, gender of the frotteur is male
      iii. Sexual excitement is derived from the actual touching or rubbing, not from the coercive nature of the act
      iv. Act usually committed in crowded places (buses, subways during rush hour)
         a) Can provide rationalization for behavior
         b) Can more easily escape arrest
      v. Fantasizes a relationship with victim
   d. **Pedophilic disorder.**
      i. Essential feature is sexual arousal from prepubescent or early pubescent children equal to or greater than that derived from physically mature persons
      ii. Disorder has lasted for at least 6 months and is manifested by fantasies or sexual urges on which the individual has acted, or which

cause significant distress or impairment in social, occupational, or other important areas of functioning

iii. Onset usually occurs during adolescence, and disorder often runs a chronic course

iv. Most common of sexual assaults

v. Age of molester at least 18

vi. He or she at least 5 years older than the child

vii. Most child molestations involve genital fondling or oral sex

viii. Vaginal or anal penetration of the child is most common in cases of incest

ix. Sexual abuse of a child may include:
a) Speaking to child in a sexual manner
b) Indecent exposure and masturbation in the presence of the child
c) Inappropriate touching or acts of penetration (oral, vaginal, anal)

e. Sexual masochism disorder.

i. Recurrent and intense sexual arousal (manifested by urges, behaviors, or fantasies for at least 6 months) of being humiliated, beaten, bound, or otherwise made to suffer

ii. Masochistic activities may be:
a) Fantasized (being raped)
b) Performed alone (self-inflicted pain)
c) Performed with a partner (being restrained, spanked, or beaten by the partner)

iii. Some masochistic activities have resulted in death (sexual arousal by oxygen deprivation)

iv. Usually chronic and can progress to the point that the individual cannot achieve sexual satisfaction without masochistic fantasies or activities

f. Sexual sadism disorder.

i. Recurrent and intense sexual arousal (manifested by urges, behaviors, or fantasies for at least 6 months) from the physical or psychological suffering of another individual

ii. Sadistic activities may be:
a) Fantasized
b) Acted on with a consenting partner
c) Acted on with nonconsenting partner

iii. Examples of sadistic acts:
a) Restraint
b) Beating
c) Burning
d) Rape
e) Cutting
f) Torture
g) Killing

iv. Course is usually chronic

v. Severity of sadistic acts often increase over time

vi. Activities with nonconsenting partners usually terminated by legal apprehension

g. **Transvestic disorder.**

i. Recurrent and intense sexual arousal (as manifested by fantasies, urges, or behaviors for at least 6 months) from dressing in the clothes of the opposite gender

ii. Individual commonly a heterosexual man

iii. Keeps women's clothing that he intermittently dresses in when alone

iv. Sexual arousal may be produced by an accompanying fantasy of the individual as a woman with female genitalia

v. Sexual arousal may be produced by the view of himself fully clothed as a woman without attention to the genitalia

h. **Voyeuristic disorder.**

i. Recurrent and intense sexual arousal (manifested by urges, behaviors, or fantasies for at least 6 months) involving the act of observing an unsuspecting individual who is naked, in the process of disrobing, or engaging in sexual activity

ii. Sexual excitement is achieved through the act of looking

iii. No contact with the person is attempted

iv. Masturbation usually accompanies the "window peeping" but may occur later as the individual fantasizes about the voyeuristic act

v. Onset of voyeuristic behavior usually before age 15

vi. Disorder is often chronic

DID YOU KNOW?

Most voyeurs enjoy satisfying sexual relationships with an adult partner. There is little apprehension of these individuals because most targets of voyeurism are unaware that they are being observed.

16. Predisposing factors to paraphilic disorders.
a. Biological factors.

i. Destruction of parts of the limbic system in animals has caused hypersexual behavior

ii. Temporal lobe diseases (psychomotor seizures, temporal lobe tumors) are implicated

iii. Abnormal levels of androgens may contribute to inappropriate sexual arousal

DID YOU KNOW?

The majority of studies on biological factors that may predispose to paraphilic disorders have involved violent sex offenders. The results of these studies cannot accurately be generalized.

b. Psychoanalytic theory.
   i. Postulated that clients have failed the normal developmental process toward heterosexual adjustment
   ii. Failure to resolve the Oedipal crisis
      a) Identifies with the parent of the opposite gender
      b) Selects an inappropriate object for libido fulfillment
      c) Severe castration anxiety leads to the substitution of a symbolic object (inanimate or an anatomic part) for the mother, as in fetishistic and transvestic disorders
      d) Anxiety over arousal to the mother leads to the choice of "safe," inappropriate sexual partners, as in pedophilic and zoophilic disorders
      e) Anxiety over arousal to the mother leads to *safe* sexual behaviors in which there is no sexual contact, as in exhibitionistic and voyeuristic disorders
c. Behavioral theory.
   i. Whether or not an individual engages in paraphilic behavior depends on the type of reinforcement he or she receives following the behavior
   ii. The initial act may be committed for various reasons:
      a) Recalling memories of experiences from an individual's early life (especially the first shared sexual experience)
      b) Modeling behavior of others who have carried out paraphilic acts
      c) Mimicking sexual behavior depicted in the media
      d) Recalling past trauma such as one's own molestation
   iii. Once the initial act has been committed, the individual consciously evaluates the behavior and decides whether to repeat it
   iv. Behavior may be extinguished by:
      a) Fear of punishment
      b) Perceived harm or injury to the victim
      c) Lack of pleasure derived from the experience
   v. Activity more likely repeated when:
      a) Negative consequences do not occur
      b) The act itself is highly pleasurable
      c) Negative consequences are avoided by escape
      d) There is no knowledge of harm experienced by the victim
17. Treatment modalities for paraphilic disorders.
   a. Biological treatment.
      i. Focused on blocking or decreasing the level of circulating androgens

   ii. Antiandrogenic medications include progestin derivatives that block testosterone synthesis or block androgen receptors
   iii. Antiandrogenic medications do not influence the direction of sexual drive toward appropriate adult partners
   iv. They act to decrease libido and thus break the individual's pattern of compulsive deviant sexual behavior
   v. Work best when given in conjunction with participation in individual or group psychotherapy
   b. Psychoanalytic therapy.
      i. Therapist helps client to identify unresolved conflicts and traumas from early childhood
      ii. Focuses on helping the individual resolve early conflicts
   c. Behavioral therapy.
      i. Aversion techniques
         a) Diminishes impulse by pairing it with noxious stimuli (electric shocks, bad odors)
         b) Skills training and cognitive restructuring can be used to change maladaptive beliefs
      ii. Covert sensitization: individual combines inappropriate sexual fantasies with aversive, anxiety-provoking scenes under the guidance of the therapist
      iii. Satiation: individual repeatedly fantasizes deviant behaviors to the point of saturation with the deviant stimuli, making the fantasies and behavior unexciting
18. Role of the nurse
   a. Focus is to diagnose and treat the problem as early as possible to minimize difficulties (secondary prevention).

MAKING THE CONNECTION

Psychoanalytic therapy focuses on helping the individual resolve early conflicts, thus relieving the anxiety that prevents him or her from forming appropriate sexual relationships. In turn, the individual has no further need for paraphilic fantasies.

MAKING THE CONNECTION

Treatment of the person with a paraphilic disorder is frustrating for both the client and therapist. Most individuals with paraphilic disorders deny that they have a problem and seek psychiatric care only after their inappropriate behavior comes to the attention of others. These individuals should be referred to specialists who are accustomed to working with this special population.

b. Focus of nursing care is to intervene in home life or other facets of childhood in an effort to prevent problems from developing (primary prevention).

c. Assist in the development of adaptive coping strategies to deal with stressful life situations.

d. Nurses can evaluate developmental components to ensure healthy development as children mature.

e. Major components of sexual development.
   i. Gender identity (one's sense of maleness or femaleness)
   ii. Sexual responsiveness (arousal to appropriate stimuli)
   iii. Ability to establish relationships with others

f. A disturbance in one or more of these components may lead to a variety of sexual deviations.
   i. Gender identity may be disturbed in transvestic disorder
   ii. Sexual responsiveness to appropriate stimuli, may be disturbed in fetishistic disorder
   iii. Ability to form relationships may be disturbed in exhibitionistic or frotteuristic disorders

g. Accurate nursing assessment and early intervention can contribute toward primary prevention of sexual disorders.

III. Sexual Dysfunctions

A. Sexual response cycle

DID YOU KNOW?

Sexual dysfunctions can occur as disturbances in any of the phases of the sexual response cycle; therefore, an understanding of anatomy and physiology is a prerequisite to considerations of pathology and treatment.

1. Phase I—Desire: desire to have sexual activity occurs in response to verbal, physical, or visual stimulation, or sexual fantasies.

2. Phase II—Excitement: the phase of sexual arousal and erotic pleasure.
   a. Male responds with penile tumescence and erection.
   b. Female changes include vasocongestion in the pelvis, vaginal lubrication, and swelling of the external genitalia.

3. Phase III—Orgasm: a peaking of sexual pleasure, with release of sexual tension and rhythmic contraction of the perineal muscles and reproductive organs.
   a. In women, marked by simultaneous rhythmic contractions of the uterus, the lower third of the vagina, and the anal sphincter.
   b. In men, marked by a forceful emission of semen occurring in response to rhythmic spasms of the prostate, seminal vesicles, vas, and urethra.

4. Phase IV—Resolution:
   a. If orgasm is achieved, characterized by disgorgement of blood from the genitalia, creating a sense of general relaxation and well-being.
   b. If orgasm is not achieved, resolution may take several hours, producing pelvic discomfort and a feeling of irritability.
   c. After orgasm:
      i. Men experience a refractory period lasting from a few minutes to many hours, during which they cannot be stimulated to further orgasm
      ii. Length of the refractory period increases with age
      iii. Women have no refractory period and may be capable of multiple and successive orgasms

B. Sexual dysfunction consists of an impairment or disturbance in any of the phases of the sexual response cycle

C. Data related to prevalence of sexual problems in the United States are presented in Table 18.1

D. This survey included a total of 1,491 men and women aged 40 to 80

E. Less than 25% had sought help for their sexual problem(s) from a health professional

F. Types of sexual dysfunction
   1. Erectile disorder.
      a. Characterized by marked difficulty in obtaining or maintaining an erection during sexual activity, or a decrease in erectile rigidity that interferes with sexual activity.
      b. The problem has persisted for at least 6 months and causes the individual significant distress.
      c. *Primary erectile disorder* refers to cases in which the man has never been able to have intercourse.

Table 18.1 Prevalence of Sexual Problems in Sexually Active Men and Women in the United States

Disorder	Men (%)	Women (%)
Lack of sexual interest	18.1	33.2
Inability to reach orgasm	12.4	20.7
Pain during sex	3.1	12.7
Premature ejaculation	26.2	—
Erectile difficulties	22.5	—
Lubrication difficulties	—	21.5

Source: Adapted from Laumann, Glasser, Neves, and Moreira (2009).

d. *Secondary erectile disorder* refers to cases in which the man has difficulty getting or maintaining an erection but has been able to have vaginal or anal intercourse at least once.

2. Female orgasmic disorder (anorgasmia).
   a. A marked delay in, infrequency of, or absence of orgasm during sexual activity.
   b. May also be characterized by a reduced intensity of orgasmic sensation.
   c. Condition has lasted at least 6 months and causes the individual significant distress.
   d. Women who can achieve orgasm through non-coital clitoral stimulation but are not able to experience it during coitus in the absence of manual clitoral stimulation are not necessarily categorized as anorgasmic.
   c. *Primary orgasmic disorder* refers to cases when the women has never experienced orgasm by any kind of stimulation.
   f. *Secondary orgasmic disorder* exists if the woman has experienced at least one orgasm, regardless of the means of stimulation, but no longer does so.

3. Delayed ejaculation.
   a. Characterized by marked delay in ejaculation or marked infrequency or absence of ejaculation during partnered sexual activity.
   b. Condition has lasted for at least 6 months and causes the individual significant distress.
   c. The male is unable to ejaculate even though he has a firm erection and has had more than adequate stimulation.
   d. *Secondary disorder* when the male only occasionally has problems ejaculating.
   e. *Primary disorder* when the male has never experienced an orgasm.
   f. Most common version, the male cannot ejaculate during coitus but may be able to ejaculate as a result of other types of stimulation.

4. Early ejaculation.
   a. Persistent or recurrent ejaculation occurring within 1 minute of beginning partnered sexual activity and before the person wishes it.
   b. Condition has lasted at least 6 months and causes the individual significant distress.
   c. Factors that affect the duration of the excitement phase:
      i. Person's age
      ii. Uniqueness of the sexual partner
      iii. Frequency of sexual activity
   d. Early ejaculation is the most common sexual disorder for which men seek treatment.
   e. Common among young men who have a high sex drive and have not yet learned to control ejaculation.

5. Female sexual interest/arousal disorder.
   a. Characterized by reduced or absent frequency or intensity of interest or pleasure in sexual activity.
   b. Condition has lasted for at least 6 months and causes the individual significant distress.
   c. Individual typically does not initiate sexual activity and is commonly unreceptive to partner's attempts to initiate.
   d. Absence of sexual thoughts or fantasies.
   e. Absent or reduced arousal in response to sexual or erotic cues.

6. Male hypoactive sexual desire disorder.
   a. A persistent or recurrent deficiency or absence of sexual fantasies and desire for sexual activity.
   b. Factors that affect sexual functioning:
      i. Age
      ii. Circumstances of the person's life
   c. Condition has persisted for at least 6 months and causes the individual significant distress.
   d. Important to differentiate the disorder from a discrepancy between the partners' levels of desire.

7. Genito-pelvic pain/penetration disorder.
   a. Individual experiences considerable difficulty with vaginal intercourse and attempts at penetration.
   b. Pain is felt in the vagina, around the vaginal entrance and clitoris, or deep in the pelvis.
   c. There is fear and anxiety associated with anticipation of pain or vaginal penetration.
   d. A tensing and tightening of the pelvic floor muscles occurs during attempted vaginal penetration.
   e. Condition may be generalized (ongoing) or situational (occurs only in specific circumstances).
   f. Condition has persisted for at least 6 months and causes the individual clinically significant distress.

8. Substance/medication-induced sexual dysfunction.
   a. Sexual dysfunction developed after:
      i. Beginning a substance/medication
      ii. A dosage increase
      iii. After withdrawal from a substance/medication
   b. Dysfunction may involve:
      i. Pain
      ii. Impaired desire
      iii. Impaired arousal
      iv. Impaired orgasm
   c. Some substances/medications that can interfere with sexual functioning include:
      i. Alcohol
      ii. Amphetamines

      iii. Cocaine
      iv. Opioids
      v. Sedatives
      vi. Hypnotics
      vii. Anxiolytics
      viii. Antidepressants
      ix. Antipsychotics
      x. Antihypertensives

G. Predisposing factors to sexual dysfunction
  1. Biological factors.
    a. Sexual desire disorders.
      i. Correlated with decreased levels of serum testosterone with hypoactive sexual desire disorder in men
      ii. Relationship between serum testosterone levels and increased female libido
      iii. Diminished libido observed in both men and women with elevated levels of serum prolactin
      iv. Various medications implicated in the etiology of hypoactive sexual desire disorder
        a) Antihypertensives
        b) Antipsychotics
        c) Antidepressants
        d) Anxiolytics
        e) Anticonvulsants
        f) Alcohol and cocaine (chronic use)
    b. Sexual arousal disorders.
      i. Postmenopausal women require longer period of stimulation for lubrication to occur
      ii. Generally less vaginal transudate after menopause
      iii. Medications, particularly those with anti-histaminic and anticholinergic properties, contribute to decreased ability for arousal in women
      iv. Arteriosclerosis is a common cause of male erectile disorder due to arterial insufficiency
      v. Neurological disorders can contribute to erectile dysfunctions
        a) Most common cause: diabetes (men at high risk for neuropathy)
        b) Temporal lobe epilepsy
        c) Multiple sclerosis
      vi. Trauma (spinal cord injury, pelvic cancer surgery) can also result in erectile disorder
      vii. Medications have been implicated in the etiology
        a) Antihypertensives
        b) Antipsychotics
        c) Antidepressants
        d) Anxiolytics
        e) Chronic alcohol use

    c. Orgasmic disorders.
      i. Reports of decreased ability to achieve orgasm after hysterectomy
      ii. Other reports of increased sexual activity and decreased sexual dysfunction after hysterectomy
      iii. Some medications (selective serotonin reuptake inhibitors) may inhibit orgasm
      iv. Medical conditions may cause decreased sexual arousal and orgasm:
        a) Depression
        b) Hypothyroidism
        c) Diabetes mellitus
      v. Factors associated with delayed male orgasm include:
        a) Surgery of the genitourinary tract (prostatectomy)
        b) Neurological disorders (Parkinson's disease)
        c) Other diseases (diabetes mellitus)
        d) Medications that have been implicated include:
          • Opioids
          • Antihypertensives
          • Antidepressants
          • Antipsychotics
          • Transient cases may occur with excessive alcohol intake
      vi. Early ejaculation commonly caused by psychological factors
      vii. General medical conditions or substance use may also play a role particularly in cases of secondary dysfunction
        1) Local infection (prostatitis)
        2) Degenerative neural disorder (multiple sclerosis)
    d. Sexual pain disorder.
      i. Painful intercourse is termed dyspareunia
      ii. Organic factors in women:
        a) Intact hymen
        b) Episiotomy scar
        c) Vaginal or urinary tract infection
        d) Ligament injuries
        e) Endometriosis
        f) Ovarian cysts or tumors
        g) Allergic reaction to vaginal spermicides
        h) Irritation caused by vaginal infections
      iii. Organic factors in men:
        1) Infection caused by poor hygiene under the foreskin of an uncircumcised man
        2) Phimosis, a condition in which the foreskin cannot be pulled back
        3) Allergic reaction to vaginal spermicides
        4) Irritation caused by vaginal infections
        5) Prostate problems may cause pain on ejaculation

2. Psychosocial factors.
   a. Sexual desire disorders: factors that may contribute to hypoactive sexual desire disorder.
      i. Religious orthodoxy
      ii. Sexual identity conflicts
      iii. Past sexual abuse
      iv. Financial, family, or job problems
      v. Depression
      vi. Aging-related concerns (changes in physical appearance)
      vii. Relationship problems
         a) Interpersonal conflicts
         b) Current physical, verbal, or sexual abuse
         c) Extramarital affairs
         d) Desire or practices that differ from those of the partner
   b. Sexual arousal disorders.
      i. Psychological factors implicated as possible impediments to female arousal
         a) Doubt
         b) Guilt
         c) Fear
         d) Anxiety
         e) Shame
         f) Conflict
         g) Embarrassment
         h) Tension
         i) Disgust
         j) Irritation
         k) Resentment
         l) Grief
         m) Hostility toward partner
         n) Puritanical or moralistic upbringing
         o) Sexual abuse (significant risk factor)
      ii. Problems with male sexual arousal may be related to:
         a) Chronic stress
         b) Anxiety
         c) Depression
         d) Developmental factors that hinder the ability to be intimate
         e) Inability to be intimate can lead to a feeling of inadequacy or distrust
         f) May develop a sense of being unloving or unlovable leading to impotence
      iii. Relationship factors that may affect erectile functioning include:
         a) Lack of attraction to one's partner
         b) Anger toward one's partner
         c) Having an unfaithful partner
      iv. Once erectile dysfunction occurs, the man's performance anxiety may increase, which perpetuates the problem

   c. Orgasmic disorders.
      i. Psychological factors are associated with inhibited female orgasm include:
         a) Fears of becoming pregnant
         b) Fear of damage to the vagina
         c) Rejection by the sexual partner
         d) Hostility toward men
         e) Feelings of guilt regarding sexual impulses

DID YOU KNOW?
Negative cultural conditioning ("nice girls don't enjoy sex") may influence the adult female's sexual response.

      ii. Developmental factors also have relevance to orgasmic dysfunction
         a) Childhood exposure to rigid religious orthodoxy
         b) Negative family attitudes toward nudity and sex
         c) Traumatic sexual experiences during childhood or adolescence (incest, rape)
      iii. Psychological factors associated with inhibited male orgasm
         a) In primary disorder (male has never experienced orgasm)
            • Rigid, puritanical background
            • Perceives sex as sinful
            • Perceives genitals as dirty
            • May have conscious or unconscious incest wishes and guilt
         b) In secondary disorder (previously experienced orgasms that have now stopped)
            • Ambivalence about commitment
            • Fear of pregnancy
            • Unexpressed hostility
      iv. Premature (early) ejaculation may be related to a lack of physical awareness on the part of a sexually inexperienced man
      v. Contributing factors to premature ejaculation
         a) Relationship problems such as a stressful marriage
         b) Negative cultural conditioning
         c) Anxiety over intimacy
         d) Lack of comfort in the sexual relationship
   d. Sexual pain disorders.
      i. May be due to organic causes
      ii. Involuntary constriction within the vagina occurs in response to anticipatory pain, making intercourse impossible
      iii. Diagnosis does not apply if etiology is due to another medical condition
      iv. Psychosocial factors have been implicated
         a) Negative childhood conditioning of sex as dirty, sinful, and shameful

b) Early traumatic sexual experiences (rape, incest)

c) Homosexual orientation

d) Traumatic experience with an early pelvic examination

e) Pregnancy phobia

f) STD phobia

g) Cancer phobia

H. Treatment modalities for sexual dysfunctions

1. Hypoactive sexual desire disorder is treated with:

a. Administration of testosterone.

b. Cognitive therapy.

c. Behavioral therapy.

d. Relationship therapy.

2. Female sexual interest/arousal disorder is treated with **sensate focus** exercises.

a. Object is to reduce the goal-oriented demands of intercourse on both man and woman.

b. Goal to reduce performance pressures and anxiety associated with possible failure.

DID YOU KNOW?

Sensate focus exercises are highly structured touching activities designed to increase comfort with physical intimacy and help overcome performance anxiety. The couple agrees not to have intercourse or experience genital stimulation until the end of treatment. New patterns of relating are established and performance anxiety is decreased.

3. Erectile disorder.

a. Senate focus used effectively.

b. Group therapy.

c. Hypnotherapy.

d. Systematic desensitization.

e. Various medications.

i. Testosterone

ii. Yohimbine

iii. Penile injections of papaverine or prostaglandin

iv. Avanafil (Stendra)

v. Sildenafil (Viagra)

vi. Tadalafil (Cialis)

vii. Vardenafil (Levitra)

f. Implantation of penile prostheses (when refractory to other treatments).

4. Female orgasmic disorder.

a. Goal to maximize stimulation and minimize inhibition.

b. Sensate focus therapy.

c. Masturbation.

d. Vibrator use.

e. Muscle control exercises.

f. Relationship therapy.

5. Delayed ejaculation.

a. Sensate focus therapy.

b. Masturbatory training.

c. Therapy almost always includes sexual partner.

6. Early ejaculation.

a. Senate focus therapy.

b. "Squeeze" technique (pressure applied at base of penis).

c. No medication approved for this disorder.

7. Genito-pelvic pain/penetration disorder.

a. Thorough physical and gynecological examination to eliminate organic pathology.

b. Investigate underlying fears and anxieties.

c. Systematic desensitization.

d. Muscle exercises to gain pelvic relaxation.

e. Use of dilators.

I. Nursing process: assessment for sexual disorders

1. Nurse may be uncomfortable with subject matter.

2. Sexual health is an integral part of physical and emotional well-being.

3. Accurate data must be collected if problems are to be identified and resolutions attempted.

4. Nurses usually need to gather basic data related to sexual history.

5. Certain clients may need a more extensive sexual history.

a. Medical or surgical conditions that may affect sexuality.

b. Infertility problems.

c. STDs.

d. Complaints of sexual inadequacy.

e. Pregnancy.

f. Gynecological problems.

g. Clients seeking information on abortion or family planning.

h. Individuals in premarital, marital, and psychiatric counseling

i. Best to use nondirective approach.

j. Use sexual history as an outline.

DID YOU KNOW?

A nondirective approach while taking a sexual history allows time for the client to interject information related to feelings or concerns about his or her sexuality.

k. Use understandable terms.

l. Clarify any unfamiliar terminology client may use.

m. Take into consideration level of education and cultural influences.

n. Convey warmth, openness, honesty, and objectivity.

o. Personal feelings, attitudes, and values should be clarified and should not interfere with acceptance of the client.

p. Remain nonjudgmental.
  i. Listen in an interested, matter-of-fact manner
  ii. Do not overreact to any presented information
q. Outline for a sexual history presented in Box 18.1 (use as guideline).
r. Outline should be individualized according to client needs.

J. Nursing process: diagnosis (analysis)—Based on data collected during the nursing assessment, possible nursing diagnoses for clients diagnosed with sexual disorders include:

1. Sexual dysfunction R/T depression and conflict in relationship or certain biological or psychological contributing factors to the disorder AEB loss of sexual desire or ability to perform.
2. Ineffective sexuality pattern R/T conflicts with sexual orientation or variant preferences AEB expressed dissatisfaction with sexual behaviors.

Box 18.1 **Sexual History: Content Outline**

I. Identify data
  A. Client
    1. Age
    2. Gender
    3. Marital status
  B. Parents
    1. Ages
    2. Dates of death and ages at death
    3. Birthplace
    4. Marital status
    5. Religion
    6. Education
    7. Occupation
    8. Congeniality
    9. Demonstration of affection
    10. Feelings toward parents
  C. Siblings (same information as for parents)
  D. Marital partner (same information as for parents)
  E. Children
    1. Ages
    2. Gender
    3. Strengths
    4. Identified problems
II. Childhood sexuality
  A. Family attitudes about sex
    1. Parents' openness about sex
    2. Parents' attitudes about nudity
  B. Learning about sex
    1. Asking parents about sex
    2. Information volunteered by parents
    3. At what age and how did client learn about: pregnancy, birth, intercourse, masturbation, nocturnal emissions, menstruation, homosexuality, STDs
  C. Childhood sex activity
    1. First sight of nude body:
      a. Same gender
      b. Opposite gender
    2. First genital self-stimulation
      a. Age
      b. Feelings
      c. Consequences
    3. First sexual exploration at play with another child
      a. Age (of self and other child)
      b. Gender of other child
      c. Nature of the activity
      d. Feelings and consequences
    4. Sexual activity with older persons
      a. Age (of self and other person)
      b. Gender of other person
      c. Nature of the activity

    d. Client willingness to participate
    e. Feelings and consequences
  D. Did you ever see your parents (or others) having intercourse? Describe your feelings.
  E. Childhood sexual theories or myths:
    1. Thoughts about conception and birth.
    2. Roles of male/female genitals and other body parts in sexuality
III. Onset of adolescence
  A. In girls:
    1. Information about menstruation:
      a. How received; from whom
      b. Age received
      c. Feelings
    2. Age:
      a. Of first period
      b. When breasts began to develop
      c. At appearance of ancillary and pubic hair
    3. Menstruation
      a. Regularity; discomfort; duration
      b. Feelings about first period
  B. In boys:
    1. Information about puberty:
      a. How received; from whom
      b. Age received
      c. Feelings
    2. Age
      a. Of appearance of ancillary and pubic hair
      b. Change of voice
      c. First orgasm (with or without ejaculation); emotional reaction
IV. Orgastic experiences
  A. Nocturnal emissions (male) or orgasms (female) during sleep.
    1. Frequency
  B. Masturbation
    1. Age begun; ever punished?
    2. Frequency; methods used
    3. Marital partner's knowledge
    4. Practiced with others? Spouse?
    5. Emotional reactions
    6. Accompanying fantasies
  C. Necking and petting ("making out")
    1. Age when begun
    2. Frequency
    3. Number of partners
    4. Types of activity
  D. Premarital intercourse
    1. Frequency
    2. Relationship with and number of partners

Continued

Box 18.1 **Sexual History: Content Outline—cont'd**

3. Contraceptives used
4. Feelings
E. Orgasmic frequency
1. Past
2. Present
V. Feelings about self as masculine/feminine
A. The male client:
1. Does he feel masculine?
2. Accepted by peers?
3. Sexually adequate?
4. Feelings/concerns about body:
a. Size
b. Appearance
c. Function
B. The female client:
1. Does she feel feminine?
2. Accepted by peers?
3. Sexually adequate?
4. Feelings/concerns about body:
a. Size
b. Appearance
c. Function
VI. Sexual fantasies and dreams
A. Nature of sex dreams
B. Nature of fantasies
1. During masturbation
2. During intercourse.
VII. Dating
A. Age and feelings about:
1. First date
2. First kissing
3. First petting or "making out"
4. First going steady
VIII. Engagement
A. Age
B. Sex activity during engagement period:
1. With fiancée
2. With others
IX: Marriage
A. Date of marriage
B. Age at marriage: Spouse:
C. Spouse's occupation
D. Previous marriages: Spouse:
E. Reason for termination of previous marriages:
Client: Spouse:
F. Children from previous marriages:
Client: Spouse:
G. Wedding trip (honeymoon):
1. Where? How long?
2. Pleasant or unpleasant?
3. Sexual considerations?
H. Sex in marriage:
1. General satisfaction/dissatisfaction.
2. Thoughts about spouse's general satisfaction/dissatisfaction
I. Pregnancies
1. Number: Ages of couple:
2. Results (normal birth; cesarean delivery; miscarriage; abortion)
3. Planned or unplanned.
4. Effects on sexual adjustment.
5. Sex of child wanted or unwanted.

X. Extramarital sex
A. Emotional attachments
1. Number; frequency; feelings
B. Sexual intercourse
1. Number; frequency; feelings
C. Postmarital masturbation
1. Frequency; feelings
D. Postmarital homosexuality
1. Frequency; feelings
E. Multiple sex ("swinging")
1. Frequency; feelings
XI. Sex after widowhood, separation, or divorce:
A. Outlet
1. Orgasms in sleep
2. Masturbation
3. Petting
4. Intercourse
5. Homosexuality
6. Other
B. Frequency; feelings
XII. Variation in sexual orientation:
A. Homosexuality
1. First experience; describe circumstances.
2. Frequency since adolescence
XIII. Paraphilias
A. Sexual contact with animals
1. First experience; describe nature of contact
2. Frequency and recent contact.
3. Feelings
B. Voyeurism
1. Describe types of observation experienced
2. Feelings
C. Exhibitionism
1. To whom? When?
2. Feelings
D. Fetishes; transvestitism
1. Nature of fetish
2. Nature of transvestite activity
3. Feelings
E. Sadomasochism
1. Nature of activity
2. Sexual response
3. Frequency; recency
4. Consequences
F. Seduction and rape
1. Has client seduced/raped another?
2. Has client ever been seduced/raped?
G. Incest
1. Nature of the sexual activity
2. With whom?
3. When occurred? Frequency; recency
4. Consequences
XIV. Prostitution
A. Has client ever accepted/paid money for sex?
B. Type of sexual activity engaged in
C. Feelings about prostitution
XV. Certain effects of sex activities
A. STDs
1. Age at learning about STDs
2. Type of STD contracted
3. Age and treatment received

Box 18.1 Sexual History: Content Outline—cont'd

B. Illegitimate pregnancy
  1. At what age(s)
  2. Outcome of the pregnancy(ies)
  3. Feelings
C. Abortion
  1. Why performed?
  2. At what age(s)?
  3. How often?
  4. Before or after marriage?
  5. Circumstance: who, where, how?

  6. Feelings about abortion: at the time; in retrospect; anniversary reaction.
XVI. Use of erotic material
  A. Personal response to erotic material
    1. Sexual pleasure—arousal
    2. Mild pleasure
    3. Disinterest; disgust
  B. Use in connection with sexual activity
    1. Type and frequency of use
    2. To accompany what type of sexual activity

Adapted from an outline prepared by the Group for Advancement of Psychiatry, based on the Sexual Performance Evaluation Questionnaire of the Marriage Council of Philadelphia. Used with permission.

K. Nursing process: planning—The following outcomes may be developed to guide the care of a client diagnosed with a sexual disorder: **The client will:**
  1. Correlate stressful situations that decrease sexual desire.
  2. Communicate with partner about sexual situation without discomfort.
  3. Verbalize ways to enhance sexual desire.
  4. Verbalize resumption of sexual activity at level satisfactory to self and partner.
  5. Correlate variant behaviors with times of stress.
  6. Verbalize fears about abnormality and inappropriateness of sexual behaviors.
  7. Express desire to change variant sexual behaviors.
  8. Participate and cooperate with extended plan of behavior modification.
  9. Express satisfaction with own sexuality pattern.
L. Nursing process: implementation for clients diagnosed with sexual disorders
  1. Interventions for clients who are experiencing sexual dysfunction.
    a. Assess client's sexual history and previous level of satisfaction in sexual relationships.
    b. Assess client's perception of the problem.
    c. Help client determine time dimension associated with the onset of the problem and discuss what was happening in life situation at that time.
    d. Assess client's level of energy.
    e. Review medication regimen; observe for side effects.
    f. Encourage the client to discuss the disease process that may be contributing to sexual dysfunction.
    g. Ensure that client is aware that alternative methods of achieving sexual satisfaction exist and can be learned through sex counseling if he or she and the partner desire to do so.
    h. Provide information regarding sexuality and sexual functioning.
    i. Refer for additional counseling or sex therapy if required.

  2. Interventions for clients who are experiencing ineffective sexuality pattern.
    a. Take sexual history, noting client's expression of areas of dissatisfaction with sexual pattern.
    b. Assess areas of stress in client's life and examine relationship with sexual partner.
    c. Note cultural, social, ethnic, racial, and religious factors that may contribute to conflicts regarding variant sexual practices.
    d. Be accepting and nonjudgmental.
    e. Assist the therapist to develop a plan of behavior modification to help the client who desires to decrease variant sexual behaviors.
    f. If altered sexuality patterns are related to illness or medical treatment, provide information to the client and partner regarding the correlation between the illness and the sexual alteration.
    g. Explain possible modifications in usual sexual pattern that the client and partner may try in an effort to achieve a satisfying sexual experience despite limitations.
    h. Teach client that sexuality is a normal human response and not synonymous with any one sexual act.
    i. Teach that sexuality reflects the totality of the person and does not relate exclusively to the sex organs or sexual behavior.
    j. Assist client to understand that sexual feelings are human feelings.
M. Nursing process: evaluation
  1. Evaluation of the nursing actions for the client diagnosed with sexual dysfunction may be facilitated by gathering information using the following types of questions:
    a. Has the client identified life situations that promote feelings of depression and decreased sexual desire?
    b. Can he or she verbalize ways to deal with this stress?
    c. Can the client satisfactorily communicate with sexual partner about the problem?

d. Have the client and sexual partner identified ways to enhance sexual desire and the achievement of sexual satisfaction for both?

e. Are client and partner seeking assistance with relationship conflict?

f. Do both partners agree on what the major problem is? Do they have the motivation to attempt change?

g. Do client and partner verbalize an increase in sexual satisfaction?

2. Evaluation of the nursing actions for the client diagnosed with variant sexual behaviors may be facilitated by gathering information using the following types of questions:

a. Can the client correlate an increase in variant sexual behavior to times of severe stress?

b. Has the client been able to identify those stressful situations and verbalize alternative ways to deal with them?

c. Does the client express a desire to change variant sexual behavior and a willingness to cooperate with extended therapy to do so?

d. Does the client express an understanding about the normalcy of sexual feelings, aside from the inappropriateness of his or her behavior?

e. Are expressions of increased self-worth evident?

IV. Gender Dysphoria in Children

A. Occurs when there is incongruence between biological/assigned gender and one's experienced/expressed gender

B. Types of diagnoses
1. Gender dysphoria in children.
2. Gender dysphoria in adolescents or adults.

C. Most cases begin in childhood

D. Any age can present clinically with gender dysphoria

E. Treatment aimed at reversal in behavior, if it is desired by the client

F. Treatment considered cautiously optimistic if initiated in childhood

DID YOU KNOW?

After establishment of a core gender identity, it is difficult later in life to instill attributes of an opposite identity. Most commonly, individuals do not desire this change.

G. Epidemiology
1. Prevalence is estimated at 1 in 30,000 men and 1 in 100,000 women.
2. Among persons experiencing gender dysphoria, 75% are biological males desiring reassignment to female gender (MTF).
3. Twenty-five percent are biological females desiring to be male (FTM).

DID YOU KNOW?

Some individuals choose to find ways of living with their transgender identity without altering their bodies. Others have a strong desire to change their physical body to reflect their core gender identity. Sometimes gender dysphoria dissipates after early childhood. However, if it persists into adolescence, it appears to be irreversible.

H. Predisposing factors
1. Biological influences.
a. May be a relation between high levels of prenatal androgens and gender dysphoria.
b. Decreased levels of testosterone found in male transgendered individuals.
c. Abnormally high levels of testosterone were found in female transgendered individuals.
d. Research results have been inconsistent.
e. Twins studies revealed that the similarity for transgender behavior was greater in monozygotic (identical) than in dizygotic (nonidentical) twin pairs, suggesting a possible genetic link.
f. The red nucleus of the stria terminalis (a region of the hypothalamus) in male-to-female transsexuals corresponded to that of typical females, rather than of typical males.

2. Family dynamics.
a. Gender roles are culturally determined.
b. Parents encourage masculine or feminine behaviors in their children.
c. Temperament may play a role with certain behavioral characteristics being present at birth.
d. Mothers usually foster a child's pride in his or her gender.
e. Presence of father helps the separation–individuation process.
f. Without a father, mother and child may remain overly close.
g. Father is normally the prototype of future love (girls).
h. Father is a model for male identification (boys).
i. Psychopathology and dysfunction noted in families of children with gender dysphoria.
   i. Maternal depression and bipolar disorder
   ii. Fathers often exhibited depression and substance abuse disorders

3. Psychoanalytic theory.
a. Gender identity problems may begin during the struggle of the Oedipal conflict.
b. Conflicts interfere with the child's ability to love the opposite-gender parent.
c. Conflicts interfere with the child's ability to identify with the same-gender parent.
d. This may lead to problems developing normal gender identity.

I. Nursing process: assessment for gender dysphoria in children
  1. Not a common disorder.
  2. Occurs more frequently in boys than girls.
  3. Insistence on being the opposite gender.
  4. Disgust with one's own genitals.
  5. Belief that one will grow up to become the opposite gender.
  6. Refusal to wear clothing of the assigned gender.
  7. Desirous of having the genitals of the opposite gender.
  8. Refusal to participate in the games and activities culturally associated with the assigned gender.
  9. May be teased and rejected by peers.
  10. Rejection hampers interpersonal relationships.
  11. May receive disapproval from family members.
  12. Symptoms occur early in childhood for boys.
  13. Symptoms may not occur before adolescence in girls.

DID YOU KNOW?

Gender dysphoria may not be recognized before adolescence in girls because masculine behavior in girls is more culturally acceptable than feminine behavior in boys.

J. Nursing process: diagnosis (analysis)—Based on data collected during the nursing assessment, possible nursing diagnoses for the child diagnosed with gender dysphoria include:
  1. Disturbed personal identity R/T biological factors or parenting patterns that encourage culturally unacceptable behaviors for assigned gender.
  2. Impaired social interaction R/T socially and culturally unacceptable behaviors.
  3. Low self-esteem R/T rejection by peers.
K. Nursing process: planning—The following outcomes may be developed to guide the care of a child diagnosed with gender dysphoria. **The client will:**
  1. Demonstrate trust in a therapist of the same gender.
  2. Demonstrate development of a close relationship with the parent of the same gender.
  3. Demonstrate a diminishment in the excessively close relationship with the parent of the opposite gender.
  4. Demonstrate behaviors that are culturally appropriate for assigned gender.
  5. Verbalize and demonstrate comfort in, and satisfaction with, assigned gender role.
  6. Interact appropriately with others demonstrating culturally acceptable behaviors.
  7. Verbalize and demonstrate self-satisfaction with assigned gender role.

L. Nursing process: implementation for the child diagnosed with gender dysphoria
  1. Interventions for a child who is experiencing disturbed personal identity.
    a. Spend time with the child and show positive regard.
    b. Be aware of personal feelings and attitudes toward this child and his or her behavior.
    c. Allow the child to describe his or her perception of the problem.
    d. Discuss with the child the types of behaviors that are more culturally acceptable.
    e. Practice culturally acceptable behaviors through role-playing or with play therapy strategies (male and female dolls).
    f. Give positive reinforcement or social attention for use of appropriate behaviors.
    g. Withhold response for stereotypical opposite-gender behaviors.
  2. Interventions for a child who is experiencing impaired social interaction.
    a. Once the child feels comfortable with the new behaviors in role-playing or one-to-one nurse–client interactions, encourage trying the new behaviors in group situations.
    b. Remain with the child during initial interactions with others.
    c. Observe child's behaviors and the responses elicited from others.
    d. Give social attention (smile, nod) to desired behaviors.
    e. Follow up these "practice" sessions with one-to-one processing of the interaction.
    f. Give positive reinforcement for efforts.
    g. Offer support if client is feeling hurt from peer ridicule.
    h. Matter-of-factly discuss the behaviors that elicited the ridicule.
    i. Offer no personal reaction to the behavior.

MAKING THE CONNECTION

Attitudes influence behavior. The nurse must not allow negative attitudes to interfere with the effectiveness of interventions when caring for a child diagnosed with gender dysphoria.

MAKING THE CONNECTION

The objective in working for behavioral change in a child who has gender dysphoria is to enhance culturally appropriate same-gender behaviors but not necessarily to extinguish all coexisting opposite-gender behaviors.

    j. The goal is to create a trusting, nonthreatening atmosphere for the child in an attempt to change behavior and improve social interactions.

  3. Interventions for a child who is experiencing low self-esteem.

    a. Encourage the child to engage in activities in which he or she is likely to achieve success.

    b. Help the child focus on aspects of his or her life for which positive feelings exist.

    c. Discourage rumination about situations that are perceived as failures or over which the child has no control. Give positive feedback for these behaviors.

    d. Help the child identify behaviors or aspects of life he or she would like to change.

    e. Assist the child to problem solve realistic ways to bring about change.

    f. Offer to be available for support to the child when he or she is feeling rejected by peers.

M. Nursing process: evaluation of the nursing actions for the child diagnosed with gender dysphoria may be facilitated by gathering information using the following types of questions:

  1. Does the child perceive that a problem existed that requires a change in behavior for resolution?

  2. Does the child demonstrate use of behaviors that are culturally accepted for his or her assigned gender?

  3. Can the child use these culturally accepted behaviors in interactions with others?

  4. Is the child accepted by peers when same-gender behaviors are used?

  5. If the child is refusing to change behaviors, what is the peer reaction?

  6. What is the child's response to negative peer reaction?

  7. Can the child verbalize positive statements about self?

  8. Can the child discuss past accomplishments without dwelling on perceived failures?

  9. Has the child shown progress toward accepting self as a worthwhile person regardless of others' responses to his or her behavior?

N. Treatment issues

  1. Goals of treatment.

    a. Accepting a culturally appropriate self-image.

    b. Increasing support and acceptance by peers.

    c. Treating co-occurring mental health concerns.

    d. Reducing the likelihood of gender dysphoria in adulthood.

    e. Reducing the likelihood of mental health concerns coming from discomfort associated with the assigned gender.

  2. Treatment initiated when behaviors cause significant distress and when the client desires it.

  3. Should be encouraged to become satisfied with his or her assigned gender.

  4. Behavior modification therapy helps the child embrace the games and activities of his or her assigned gender and promotes development of friendships with same gender peers.

DID YOU KNOW?

  5. Alternate treatment theories suggest that children should be accepted as they see themselves—different from their assigned gender.

  6. Children should be supported in their efforts to live as the gender in which they feel most comfortable.

  7. Some professionals are recommending pubertal delay for:

    a. Adolescents aged 12 to 16 years.

    b. Those who have suffered with extreme, lifelong gender dysphoria.

    c. Those with supportive parents who encourage the child to pursue a desired change in gender.

  8. A gonadotropin-releasing hormone agonist is administered, which suppresses pubertal changes.

  9. Treatment is reversible if adolescent later decides not to pursue the gender change.

    a. Medication is withdrawn.

    b. External sexual development proceeds.

    c. Permanent surgical intervention has been avoided.

10. Treatment should include interventions for any depression, anxiety, social isolation, anger, self-esteem, and parental conflict that might exist.
11. With resolution of these issues, the gender dysphoria may dissipate.
12. Behavior therapy for children with gender dysphoria typically occurs in outpatient clinics.

V. Gender Dysphoria in Adolescents or Adults

A. Despite having the anatomical characteristics of a given gender, the adult or adolescent has the self-perception of being of the opposite gender
B. Individuals do not feel comfortable wearing the clothes of their assigned gender and often engage in cross-dressing
C. May find their own genitals repugnant
D. May repeatedly submit requests to the health-care system for hormonal and surgical gender reassignment
E. Depression and anxiety are common and are often attributed by the individual to his or her inability to live in the desired gender role
F. Adolescents rarely have the desire or motivation to alter their cross-gender roles
G. Disruptive behaviors are common among adolescents
H. Treatment issues
   1. Intervention with adolescents and adults is a difficult, complex process.
   2. Some adults seek therapy to learn how to cope with their altered sexual identity.
   3. Others have direct and immediate requests for hormonal therapy and surgical sex reassignment.
   4. Must undergo extensive psychological testing and counseling.
   5. Must live in the role of the desired gender for up to 2 years before surgery.
   6. Hormonal treatment initiated during this period.
      a. Male clients receive estrogen.
         i. Redistribution of body fat in a more "feminine" pattern
         ii. Enlargement of the breasts
         iii. Softening of the skin
         iv. Reduction in body hair
      b. Women receive testosterone.
         i. Redistribution of body fat
         ii. Growth of facial and body hair
         iii. Enlargement of the clitoris
         iv. Deepening of the voice
         v. Amenorrhea occurs within a few months
   7. Surgical treatment for male-to-female transgender reassignment.
      a. Removal of the penis and testes.
      b. Creation of an artificial vagina.
      c. Care is taken to preserve sensory nerves in the area so that the individual may continue to experience sexual stimulation.

8. Surgical treatment for female-to-male transgender reassignment.
   a. More complex.
   b. Mastectomy and sometimes a hysterectomy.
   c. Penis and scrotum are constructed from tissues in the genital and abdominal area.
   d. Vaginal orifice is closed.
   e. Penile implant is used to attain erection.
9. Both men and women continue maintenance hormone therapy after surgery.
10. Satisfaction with the results is highest among clients.
    a. Who are emotionally healthy.
    b. Have adequate social support.
    c. Attain reasonable cosmetic results.
11. Continued psychotherapy helps clients adjust to their new gender role.
12. Nursing care of the post–gender-reassignment surgical client.
    a. Similar to most other postsurgical clients.
    b. Maintaining comfort.
    c. Preventing infection.
    d. Preserving integrity of surgical site.
    e. Maintaining elimination.
    f. Meeting nutritional needs.
    g. Meeting psychosocial needs related to:
       i. Body image
       ii. Fears and insecurities about relating to others
       iii. Anxiety about being accepted in the new gender role
    h. Providing nonthreatening, nonjudgmental healing atmosphere

VI. Variations in Sexual Orientation

A. Homosexuality
   1. Sexual preference for individuals of the same gender.
      a. May be applied to homosexuals of both genders.
      b. Often used to specifically denote male homosexuality.
      c. **Lesbianism** identifies female homosexuality.
      d. Most homosexuals prefer the term "gay" because it is less derogatory in its lack of emphasis on the sexual aspects of the orientation.
      e. A heterosexual is referred to as "straight."
   2. At one time, nearly all states had sodomy laws that forbade any sexual behavior that could not result in reproduction.
   3. In 2003, the U.S. Supreme Court issued a broad-scoped decision that essentially invalidated all sodomy laws.
   4. Americans' attitudes toward homosexuals can best be described as homophobic.
      a. *Homophobia* is defined as a negative attitude toward or fear of homosexuality or homosexuals.

412 Chapter 18 Issues Related to Human Sexuality and Gender Dysphoria

b. It may be indicative of a deep-seated insecurity about one's own gender identity.

c. Homophobic behaviors include:

    i. Extreme prejudice against, abhorrence of, and discomfort around homosexuals

    ii. Rationalized by religious, moral, or legal considerations

5. Relationship patterns are as varied among homosexuals as they are among heterosexuals.

a. Some may remain with one partner for an extended period of time, even for a lifetime.

b. Others prefer not to make a commitment and "play the field."

6. No one knows for sure why people become homosexual or heterosexual.

7. Predisposing factors.

a. Biological theories:

    i. Fifty-two percent concordance for homosexual orientation in monozygotic twins

    ii. Twenty-two percent in dizygotic twins

    iii. Possible heritable trait

    iv. Gay men have more brothers who are gay than heterosexual men

    v. Thirty-three of 40 pairs of gay brothers shared a genetic marker on the bottom half of the X chromosome

    vi. Hypothesized that levels of testosterone may be lower and levels of estrogen higher in homosexual men than in heterosexual men

    vii. Hypothesized that exposure to inappropriate levels of androgens during the critical fetal period of sexual differentiation may contribute to homosexual orientation

    viii. Results have been inconsistent

b. Psychosocial theories.

    i. Freud believed that all humans are inherently bisexual, with the capacity for both heterosexual and homosexual behavior

    ii. Freud theorized all individuals go through a homoerotic phase of psychosexual development as children

    iii. Homosexuality is due to an arrest of normal psychosexual development

    iv. Homosexuality could occur as a result of pathological family relationships in which the child forms a sexualized attachment to the parent of the same gender and identification with the parent of the opposite gender

    v. Some theories suggest that a dysfunctional parent–child relationship, most specifically, the relationship with the same-gender parent family pattern may be implicated

    vi. These theorists believe that gay men often have a dominant, supportive mother and a weak, remote, or hostile father

    vii. These theorists believe that lesbians may have had a dysfunctional mother–daughter relationship

    viii. Both subsequently try to meet their unmet same-gender needs through sexual relationships

    ix. Others believe that family dynamics have very little influence on the outcome of their children's sexual-partner orientation

    x. Others suggest there is no one single answer—that sexual orientation may result from a complex interaction between biological and psychosocial factors, shaping the individual at an early age

8. Special concerns.

a. Considerations of attractiveness, finding a partner, and concerns about sexual adequacy are common to both heterosexual and homosexual individuals.

b. STDs, including AIDS, are epidemic among sexually active individuals of all sexual orientations.

c. AIDS was initially considered a "gay disease."

d. Fear of the discovery of their sexual orientation.

e. Fear of being rejected by parents and significant others.

f. Issue of gay marriage.

    i. Opponents

        a) Define marriage as an institution between one man and one woman

        b) A gay relationship is not an optimal environment in which to raise children

        c) It goes against the traditional American value system

        d) Oppose based on their religious beliefs:

            • Homosexuality is wrong because it involves sex that doesn't create life

            • Homosexuality is "unnatural" (that God created men and women with the innate capacities for sexual relations that are distinctly absent from a same-sex relationship)

            • Homosexuality is discouraged (or forbidden) by the Bible

    ii. Proponents

        a) Believe issue has to do with equality

        b) Believe all loving, consenting adult couples have the same rights under the law

        c) Cite the real nature of marriage as a binding commitment (legally, socially, and personally) between two people

        d) Believe that individuals of the same gender have an equal right to make such a commitment to each other as heterosexual couples

e) Cite research suggesting that having a gay or lesbian parent does not affect a child's social adjustment, school success, or sexual orientation

B. Bisexuality
1. Not exclusively heterosexual or homosexual.
2. Engages in sexual activity with members of both genders.
3. Also sometimes referred to as ambisexual.
4. More common than exclusive homosexuality.
5. Seventy-five percent of men are exclusively heterosexual.
6. Two percent of men are exclusively homosexual.
7. Twenty-three percent of men have engaged in sexual activity with both men and women.
8. Some individuals prefer men and women equally.
9. Others prefer one gender but also accept sexual activity with the other gender.
10. Some may alternate between homosexual and heterosexual activity for long periods.
11. Others may have both a male and a female lover at the same time.
12. Some maintain their bisexual orientation throughout life.
13. Others may become exclusively homosexual or heterosexual
14. Predisposing factors.
    a. Freud believed that all humans are inherently bisexual with the capacity for both heterosexual and homosexual interactions.
    b. Theorists believe sexual preference determined by pathological conditions in childhood.
    c. Heterosexuals may have their first homosexual encounter later in life, making childhood pathological conditions an unlikely cause.

DID YOU KNOW?
Some homosexual encounters are based on circumstances. A heterosexual man may engage in homosexual behavior while in prison, for example, and then return to heterosexuality following his release.

MAKING THE CONNECTION

Nurses must examine their personal attitudes and feelings about homosexuality to ensure that homosexual clients receive care with dignity. Nurses who have come to terms with their own feelings about homosexuality are better able to separate the person from the behavior.

15. Gender identity (determining whether one is male or female) is usually established by age 2 to 3 years.
16. Sexual identity (determining whether one is heterosexual or homosexual or both) may continue to evolve throughout one's lifetime.

VII. Sexually Transmitted Diseases

A. Infections that are contracted primarily through sexual activities or intimate contact with the genitals, mouth, or rectum of another individual
B. May be transmitted through heterosexual or homosexual contact
C. External genital evidence of pathology may or may not be manifested
D. At epidemic levels in the United States
E. Individuals are beginning an active sex life at an earlier age
F. More women are sexually active than ever before
G. Contributing social changes to increase in STDs
   1. Permissiveness.
   2. Promiscuity.
      a. Availability of antibiotics.
      b. Availability of oral contraceptives.
   3. Acceptance of oral contraceptives pill.
H. Primary nursing responsibility is early education aimed at disease prevention
   1. Teach in hospitals and clinics.
   2. Outreach to communities.
I. Information needed for this teaching
   1. Which diseases are most prevalent.
   2. How they are transmitted.
   3. Signs and symptoms.
   4. Available treatment.
   5. Consequences of avoiding treatment.
   6. See Table 18.2 for this information.
J. STDs generate sensitive issues
   1. Connotations of illicit sex.
   2. Social stigma.
   3. Potentially disastrous medical consequences.
   4. Feelings of overwhelming guilt.
   5. Clients need strong support to overcome physical and emotional difficulties.
K. Goal is prevention
L. Realistic objective: early detection and appropriate treatment

Table 18.2 **Sexually Transmitted Diseases**

Disease	Organism of Transmission	Method of Transmission	Signs and Symptoms	Treatment	Potential Complications
Gonorrhea	*Neisseria gonorrhoeae* (bacterium)	Vaginal sex, anal sex, genital-oral sex, via hand moistened with infected secretions and placed in contact with mucous membranes (e.g., the eyes)	Men: urethritis; dysuria, purulent discharge from urethra; proctitis; pharyngitis Women: initially asymptomatic; progression to infection of cervix, urethra, and fallopian tubes	Combination therapy with ceftriaxone and azithromycin or doxycycline (CDC, 2012c)	Men: sterility from orchitis or epididymitis Women: chronic pelvic inflammatory disease, infertility, ectopic pregnancy, blindness from gonococcal conjunctivitis
Syphilis	*Treponema pallidum* (spirochete)	Vaginal sex, anal sex, genital-oral sex, via contact of infected secretions with intact mucous membranes or abraded skin	Primary stage: painless chancre on penis, vulva, vagina, mouth, anus, or other point of contact with mucous membranes or abraded skin Secondary stage: rash, headache, anorexia, weight loss, fever, sore throat, body aches, anemia	Long-acting penicillin G, tetracycline, erythromycin	Latent stage: lasts many years; no symptoms, but can be passed on to fetus Tertiary stage: blindness; heart disease; insanity; ulcerated lesions on skin, mucous membranes, or internal organs
Chlamydial infection	*Chlamydia trachomatis* (intracellular bacterium)	Vaginal sex, anal sex, via hand moistened with infected secretions and placed in contact with mucous membranes	Men: urethral discharge and dysuria Women: cervicitis (either asymptomatic or may have discharge, dysuria, soreness, bleeding)	Tetracycline; erythromycin; azithromycin	Scarring in the fallopian tubes, ectopic pregnancy, infertility
Genital herpes	Herpes simplex virus, type 1 or type 2	Vaginal sex, anal sex, genital-oral sex; skin-to-skin contact with infected areas, to newborn through vaginal delivery	Blistery lesions in the genital area causing pain, itching, burning; also vaginal or urethral discharge, fever, headache, malaise, and myalgias	No cure; treatment is palliative with acyclovir, valacyclovir, or famciclovir	Recurrences are possible; potential complications include: meningitis, encephalitis, urethral strictures; possible risk of cervical cancer
Genital warts	*Condyloma acuminatum* (human papilloma virus)	Vaginal sex, anal sex, skin-to-skin contact with infected areas	Cauliflower-like warts that appear on penis or scrotum in men, and labia, vaginal walls, or cervix in women; mild itching may occur	Application of podofilox or podophyllin; cryotherapy; electrocautery; surgical removal	Recurrences possible; potential increased risk of cervical cancer
Hepatitis B	Hepatitis B virus	Vaginal sex, anal sex, genital-oral sex, contact with infectious blood or blood products, contact of infectious secretions with mucous membranes or abraded skin	Malaise, anorexia, nausea/vomiting, fever, headache, mild pain in right upper quadrant of abdomen, jaundice	No cure; treatment involves supportive care, bedrest for extended period; medications generally have not been found to be useful	Chronic hepatitis; cirrhosis; liver cancer
AIDS	Human immunodeficiency virus (HIV)	Exchange of body fluids via anal sex, vaginal sex, genital-oral sex Shared use of needles during drug use or accidental needle	May be asymptomatic for 10 years or longer after infection with HIV Early signs of AIDS include severe weight loss, diarrhea, fever, night sweats or the presence	No cure; antiretroviral medication used to slow growth of the virus Other medications given for	Regardless of treatment, AIDS is eventually fatal; new medications have dramatically increased the time from diagnosis to

Table 18.2 Sexually Transmitted Diseases—cont'd

Disease	Organism of Transmission	Method of Transmission	Signs and Symptoms	Treatment	Potential Complications
		stick with infected needle Skin-to-skin contact when there are open sores on the skin Transfusion with contaminated blood Perinatal transmission: during delivery and through breast milk	of a persistent opportunistic infection (e.g., herpes or candidiasis)	symptomatic relief and to treat opportunistic infections The drug Truvada can be used as a preventive measure for people at high risk of acquiring HIV	death, and research continues in drug treatments and vaccine development

REVIEW QUESTIONS

1. The result of incongruence between biological/assigned gender and one's experienced/expressed gender is termed _____ _____.

2. A nurse is admitting a client with a diagnosis of gender dysphoria. On review of past history, which of the following would the nurse expect to find? **Select all that apply.**
   1. The client's father was diagnosed with a substance abuse disorder.
   2. The client experienced dyspareunia.
   3. The client's mother was diagnosed with major depressive disorder.
   4. The client has been unable to achieve satisfactory orgasm.
   5. The client has been insisting that he or she is the opposite gender.

3. At an outpatient clinic, a nurse is about to administer an ordered Gardasil vaccination to a client. Which of the following client information alerts the nurse that the physician's order is appropriate? **Select all that apply.**
   1. The client is a 12-year-old girl.
   2. The client is a 20-year-old woman who has not completed the Gardasil vaccination series.
   3. The client is a 30-year-old man who is beginning the vaccine series.
   4. The client is a 10-year-old boy and has not completed the Gardasil vaccination series.
   5. The client is an 8-year-old girl who is beginning the vaccine series.

4. A nursing student is writing a paper that focuses on current trends related to intimate relationships. Which of the following information should the student include? **Select all that apply.**
   1. Men typically choose mature women 2 to 3 years older than themselves.
   2. Divorced individuals often avoid remarriage.
   3. Intimacy in marriage is one of the most common forms of sexual expression for adults.
   4. The average American couple has coitus about two or three times per week when they are in their 20s.
   5. Sexual activity typically ceases after age 65.

5. A mother asks the nurse what signs would determine the onset of puberty for her preadolescent daughter? Which of the following would be appropriate nursing responses? **Select all that apply.**
   1. "Breast enlargement is an indication of the onset of puberty in females."
   2. "The growth of pubic hair is an indication of the onset of puberty in females."
   3. "The widening of the hips is an indication of the onset of puberty in females."
   4. "The onset of menstruation is an indication of the onset of puberty in females."
   5. "Loss of ancillary hair is an indication of the onset of puberty in females."

6. At her yearly physical, a 35-year-old women complains of insomnia, hot flashes, and headaches. She asks the nurse practitioner if she is going through menopause. Which is the most appropriate nursing response?
   1. "Menopause doesn't begin until 50. We'll need to investigate these symptoms."
   2. "One percent of women can experience menopause symptoms as early as 35 years of age."
   3. "Menopause can start as early as age 40; we'll have to rule out other causes."
   4. "Yes, probably because you are within the typical age range."

7. A nursing instructor is teaching about the differences between male and female interest in sex throughout the life span. Which of the following student statements indicates that learning has occurred? **Select all that apply.**
   1. "By age 50, male interest in sexual activity may decrease, whereas women of the same age stabilize at the same level of sexual activity."
   2. "By age 50, female interest in sexual activity may decrease, whereas men of the same age stabilize at the same level of sexual activity."
   3. "Women continue sexual activity based on enjoyment rather than frequency, whereas frequency and enjoyment are both important to men."
   4. "Men continue sexual activity based on enjoyment rather than frequency, whereas frequency and enjoyment are both important to women."
   5. "As men age, they need a longer period of stimulation to reach orgasm, whereas older women often have a greater capacity for orgasm."

8. Paraphilia identifies repetitive or preferred sexual fantasies or behaviors that may involve which of the following? **Select all that apply.**
1. Shoes
2. The suffering of oneself or one's partner
3. A consenting 20-year-old
4. The humiliation of oneself or one's partner
5. Two adult concurrent consenting sexual contacts

9. Which diagnosis would the nurse recognize as being currently classified as a paraphilic disorder?
1. Zoophilic disorder
2. Oral-genital sexual disorder
3. Sodomistic disorder
4. Homosexualistic disorder

10. Which of the presented paraphilic disorders is correctly matched with its characteristic symptom?
1. Exhibitionistic disorder: sexual arousal from prepubescent children
2. Frotteuristic disorder: sexual arousal from being humiliated, beaten, bound, or otherwise made to suffer
3. Fetishistic disorder: sexual arousal from the use of nonliving objects
4. Pedophilic disorder: sexual arousal involving touching and rubbing against a nonconsenting person

11. Which of the following behaviors toward a child would the nurse recognize as sexual abuse? **Select all that apply.**
1. Speaking to a child in a sexual manner
2. Masturbation in the presence of a child
3. Using profanity in the presence of a child
4. Inappropriate touching
5. Exposing a child to parental alcohol and tobacco use

12. Which of the following are nursing care challenges when intervening with clients diagnosed with paraphilic disorders? **Select all that apply.**
1. Clients deny that they have a problem.
2. Clients only seek treatment after behavior comes to the attention of others.
3. Specialists are needed to work with this special population.
4. Clients tend to be suicidal or at risk for injury.
5. Clients are usually nonadherent to medications prescribed for these disorders.

13. Which of the following components of sexual development is correctly matched with the paraphilic disorder that may result from a disturbance in this phase? **Select all that apply.**
1. Disturbed development of gender identity: transvestic disorder
2. Disturbed development of gynecomastia: homosexuality
3. Disturbed development of sexual responsiveness to appropriate stimuli: fetishistic disorder
4. Disturbed development of the ability to form relationships: exhibitionistic disorder
5. Disturbed development of the knowledge of appropriate moral behaviors: frotteuristic disorders

14. Which of the following types of sexual dysfunction is correctly matched with its characteristic symptom? **Select all that apply.**
1. *Primary erectile disorder:* A man has difficulty getting or maintaining an erection but has been able to have vaginal or anal intercourse at least once.
2. *Secondary erectile disorder:* A man has never been able to have intercourse.
3. *Delayed ejaculation:* Persistent or recurrent ejaculation occurring within 1 minute of beginning partnered sexual activity and before the person wishes it.
4. *Male hypoactive sexual desire disorder:* A persistent or recurrent deficiency or absence of sexual fantasies and desire for sexual activity.

15. A woman is experiencing anorgasmia. Which nursing diagnosis would the nurse consider appropriate to assign?
1. Impaired social interaction
2. Sexual dysfunction
3. Risk for self-mutilation
4. Disturbed personal identity

16. A man is experiencing phimosis. Which nursing diagnosis would the nurse consider appropriate to assign?
1. Impaired social interaction
2. Risk for self-mutilation
3. Acute pain
4. Disturbed personal identity

17. A client diagnosed with female sexual interest/arousal disorder is despondent and tearful. Which short-term outcome would be appropriate for this client?
1. The client will verbalize an understanding of sensate focus exercises by day 2.
2. The client will be adherent to prescribed medications for this disorder.
3. The client will recognize husband's primary role in the disorder's etiology.
4. The client will feel better about herself by day 3.

18. A 28-year-old man has been diagnosed with gonorrhea. Understanding the problems associated with
this disease, which client outcome would the nurse
prioritize?
    1. The client will identify all sexual contacts by day 2.
    2. The client will understand the consequences if the
    gonorrhea goes untreated.
    3. The client will agree to refrain from unprotected
    sexual activity until laboratory work indicates that
    no gonorrhea is present.
    4. The client will verbalize an understanding of the
    need to complete full course of medication treat-
    ment by day 3.

19. When providing care to a client diagnosed with
gender dysphoria, the nurse would recognize which
appropriate nursing diagnosis that is matched with
the nursing intervention that addresses the documented problem?
    1. Impaired social interaction: *Positively reinforce
    maintaining eye contact*
    2. Risk for other directed violence: *Restrain when
    aggressive toward others*
    3. Disturbed personal identity: *Role play gender
    appropriate behaviors*
    4. Altered body image: *Present and challenge the
    client's perception of reality*

20. The condition of experiencing sexual arousal in
response to the extreme pain, suffering, or humiliation
of others is termed sexual _____ disorder.

REVIEW ANSWERS

1. ANSWER: Gender dysphoria

Rationale: Gender identity is the sense of knowing whether one is male or female—that is, the awareness of one's masculinity or femininity. Gender dysphoria can result when there is incongruence between biological/assigned gender and one's experienced/expressed gender.

TEST-TAKING TIP: Review the key terms at the beginning of the chapter.
Content Area: Psychosocial Integrity;
Integrated Process: Nursing Process: Assessment;
Client Need: Psychosocial Integrity;
Cognitive Level: Knowledge;
Concept: Sexuality

2. ANSWERS: 1, 3, 5
Rationale:
1. Fathers of children diagnosed with gender dysphoria often exhibit depression and substance abuse disorders.
2. *Dyspareunia* is the term for painful intercourse. This is not a symptom of gender dysphoria.
3. Maternal depression and bipolar disorder are frequently demonstrated by mothers of children diagnosed with gender dysphoria.
4. The inability to achieve satisfactory orgasm is a symptom of both female and male orgasmic disorder, not gender dysphoria.
5. Symptoms of gender dysphoria include the following: the insistence of being of the opposite gender, disgust with one's own genitals, belief that one will grow up to become the opposite gender, refusal to wear clothing of the assigned gender, having a desire for the genitals of the opposite gender, and refusal to participate in the games and activities culturally associated with the assigned gender.

TEST-TAKING TIP: Review the symptoms of gender dysphoria.
Content Area: Safe and Effective Care Environment: Management of Care;
Integrated Process: Nursing Process: Assessment;
Client Need: Safe and Effective Care Environment: Management of Care;
Cognitive Level: Application;
Concept: Sexuality

3. ANSWERS: 1, 2
Rationale:
1. The Centers for Disease Control and Prevention (CDC) recommends routine administration of three doses of Gardasil vaccine to all girls age 11 or 12 years. Because this client is 12, the physician's order is appropriate.
2. Gardasil vaccination is recommended for girls and women aged 13 through 26 years who have not already received the complete vaccine series. Because this client meets these criteria, the physician's order is appropriate.
3. Men aged 22 through 26 years may also begin the Gardasil vaccine series, but a 30 year-old man would be too old to receive the vaccine, making the physician's order inappropriate.
4. Boys can be vaccinated from age 11 to age 26. A 10-year-old male client would be too young to receive the vaccine, making the physician's order inappropriate.

5. It is recommended that females receive the Gardasil vaccine series from ages 11 to 26. An 8-year-old girl would be too young to receive the vaccine, making the physician's order inappropriate.
TEST-TAKING TIP: Review the CDC recommendation for administration of the Gardasil vaccine.
Content Area: Safe and Effective Care Environment: Management of Care;
Integrated Process: Nursing Process: Implementation;
Client Need: Safe and Effective Care Environment: Management of Care;
Cognitive Level: Application;
Concept: Medication

4. ANSWERS: 3, 4
Rationale:
1. Men typically choose women partners younger, not older, than themselves. This inaccurate information should not be included in the student's paper.
2. Of those individuals who divorce, a high percentage remarries. This inaccurate information should not be included in the student's paper.
3. Intimacy in marriage is one of the most common forms of sexual expression for adults. This is accurate information and should be included in the student's paper.
4. The average American couple has coitus about two or three times per week when they are in their 20s. This is accurate information and should be included in the student's paper.
5. Frequency of sexual activity gradually declines to about weekly for those 45 years of age and over. However, with reasonable good health and an interesting and interested partner, there is no inherent reason why individuals should not enjoy sexual activity throughout the life span.
TEST-TAKING TIP: Review current trends related to normal sexual activity throughout the life span.
Content Area: Psychosocial Integrity;
Integrated Process: Nursing Process: Assessment;
Client Need: Psychosocial Integrity;
Cognitive Level: Application;
Concept: Sexuality

5. ANSWERS: 1, 2, 3, 4
Rationale:
1. Puberty for females begins with enlargement of the breasts.
2. Puberty for females begins with the growth of pubic hair.
3. Puberty for females begins with widening of the hips.
4. Puberty for females begins with the onset of menstruation.
5. Puberty for females begins with growth, not loss, of ancillary hair.
TEST-TAKING TIP: Review the changes that herald the onset of puberty in females.
Content Area: Safe and Effective Care Environment: Management of Care;
Integrated Process: Nursing Process: Implementation;
Client Need: Safe and Effective Care Environment: Management of Care;
Cognitive Level: Application;
Concept: Assessment

6. **ANSWER: 2**
   Rationale:
   1. The average age of onset of menopause for woman is around 50, but changes due to menopause can be noted from about 40 to 60. One percent of women experience symptoms of menopause as early as age 35. This response does not take into consideration the potential for this client to be in the 1% of women that experience symptoms at an early age.
   2. **One percent of women can experience symptoms of menopause as early as age 35. This is an accurate and appropriate nursing response.**
   3. Menopause symptoms can begin as early as 35 in 1% of women. This response does not take into consideration the potential for this client to be in the 1% of women that experience symptoms at an early age.
   4. The average age of onset of menopause for woman is around 50, but changes due to menopause can be noted from about 40 to 60. Only 1% of women experience menopause as early as 35. This client may be in the 1%, but her age is not *typical* for the onset of the symptoms of menopause.
   TEST-TAKING TIP: Note the key word *typical* in Option 4. This word makes the option incorrect. Review information about the symptoms and onset of menopause.
   Content Area: *Safe and Effective Care Environment: Management of Care;*
   Integrated Process: *Nursing Process: Implementation;*
   Client Need: *Safe and Effective Care Environment: Management of Care;*
   Cognitive Level: *Application;*
   Concept: *Assessment*

7. **ANSWERS: 1, 3, 5**
   Rationale:
   1. **By age 50, male interest in sexual activity may decrease, whereas women stabilize at the same level of sexual activity as at the previous stage in the life cycle. This student statement indicates that learning has occurred.**
   2. By age 50, male, not female, interest in sexual activity may decrease, whereas women, not men, stabilize at the same level of sexual activity as at the previous stage in the life cycle. This student statement indicates a need for further instruction.
   3. **For women, enjoyment rather than frequency is a key factor to the continuance of sexual activity. Frequency and enjoyment are both important to men. This student statement indicates that learning has occurred.**
   4. For women, not men, enjoyment rather than frequency is a key factor to the continuance of sexual activity. Frequency and enjoyment are both important to men, not women. This student statement indicates a need for further instruction.
   5. **Older men need a longer period of stimulation to reach orgasm, and the intensity of pleasure may decrease. On the other hand, women stabilize at the same level of sexual activity as at the previous stage in the life cycle and often have a greater capacity for orgasm in middle adulthood than in young adulthood. This student statement indicates that learning has occurred.**

TEST-TAKING TIP: Review the changes related to sexuality that occur during the aging process, and note the differences between males and females.
Content Area: *Safe and Effective Care Environment; Management of Care;*
Integrated Process: *Nursing Process: Evaluation;*
Client Need: *Safe and Effective Care Environment; Management of Care:*
Cognitive Level: *Analysis;*
Concept: *Nursing Roles*

8. **ANSWERS: 1, 2, 4**
   Rationale:
   1. **Paraphilia identifies repetitive or preferred sexual fantasies or behaviors that involve nonhuman objects such as shoes.**
   2. **Paraphilia identifies repetitive or preferred sexual fantasies or behaviors that involve suffering or humiliation of oneself or one's partner.**
   3. Repetitive or preferred sexual fantasies or behaviors that involve a consenting 20- year-old would not be considered paraphilia. Because a 20-year-old has reached the age of consent, sexual behavior would not be considered pedophilia, the sexual arousal from prepubescent or early pubescent children.
   4. **Paraphilia identifies repetitive or preferred sexual fantasies or behaviors that involve suffering or humiliation of oneself or one's partner.**
   5. Sexual behavior with two concurrent consenting sexual contacts would not be considered a paraphilic disorder.
   TEST-TAKING TIP: Review the definition of paraphilia.
   Content Area: *Safe and Effective Care Environment; Management of Care;*
   Integrated Process: *Nursing Process: Assessment;*
   Client Need: *Safe and Effective Care Environment; Management of Care:*
   Cognitive Level: *Application;*
   Concept: *Assessment*

9. **ANSWER: 1**
   Rationale:
   1. **Currently sex with animals (zoophilic disorder) is classified as a paraphilic disorder.**
   2. Historically, oral-genital sexual behavior was viewed as unnatural. Currently this sexual behavior is not considered a disorder.
   3. Historically, anal sexual behavior (sodomy) was viewed as unnatural. Currently this sexual behavior is not considered a disorder.
   4. Historically, homosexual behavior was viewed as unnatural. Currently this sexual behavior is not considered a disorder.
   TEST-TAKING TIP: Review the sexual behaviors classified as paraphilic disorders.
   Content Area: *Safe and Effective Care Environment; Management of Care;*
   Integrated Process: *Nursing Process: Assessment;*
   Client Need: *Safe and Effective Care Environment; Management of Care:*
   Cognitive Level: *Application;*
   Concept: *Sexuality*

10. **ANSWER: 3**
Rationale:
1. Exhibitionistic disorder is characterized by recurrent and intense sexual arousal from the exposure of one's genitals to an unsuspecting individual. Pedophilic disorder is characterized by sexual arousal from prepubescent or early pubescent children that is equal to or greater than that derived from physically mature persons. This paraphilic disorder is incorrectly matched with its characteristic symptom.
2. Frotteuristic disorder is characterized by recurrent and intense sexual arousal involving touching and rubbing against a nonconsenting person. Sexual masochistic disorder is characterized by recurrent and intense sexual arousal from being humiliated, beaten, bound, or otherwise made to suffer. This paraphilic disorder is incorrectly matched with its characteristic symptom.
3. **Fetishistic disorder is characterized by recurrent and intense sexual arousal from the use of either nonliving objects or specific nongenital body parts. This paraphilic disorder is correctly matched with its characteristic symptom.**
4. Pedophilic disorder is characterized by sexual arousal from prepubescent or early pubescent children equal to or greater than that derived from physically mature persons. Frotteuristic disorder is characterized by recurrent and intense sexual arousal involving touching and rubbing against a nonconsenting person. This paraphilic disorder is incorrectly matched with its characteristic symptom.
TEST-TAKING TIP: Review the characteristic symptoms of the various paraphilic disorders.
Content Area: Safe and Effective Care Environment;
Management of Care;
Integrated Process: Nursing Process: Assessment;
Client Need: Safe and Effective Care Environment;
Management of Care:
Cognitive Level: Application;
Concept: Sexuality

11. **ANSWERS: 1, 2, 4**
Rationale:
1. **Speaking to a child in a sexual manner is a behavior that is classified as sexual abuse.**
2. **Indecent exposure and masturbation in the presence of a child are both behaviors that are classified as sexual abuse.**
3. Using profanity in the presence of a child is inappropriate but not classified as sexual child abuse.
4. **Inappropriate touching or acts of oral, vaginal, and/or anal penetration are classified as sexual child abuse.**
5. Exposing a child to parental alcohol and tobacco use can be detrimental, but the behavior is not classified as sexual child abuse.
TEST-TAKING TIP: Review the behaviors that are classified as sexual child abuse.
Content Area: Safe and Effective Care Environment;
Management of Care;
Integrated Process: Nursing Process: Evaluation;
Client Need: Safe and Effective Care Environment;
Management of Care:

Cognitive Level: Application;
Concept: Violence

12. **ANSWERS: 1, 2, 3**
1. **Most individuals with paraphilic disorders deny that they have a problem. This can be a challenge to the nursing care of these clients.**
2. **Most individuals with paraphilic disorders seek psychiatric care only after their inappropriate behavior comes to the attention of others. Illegal behaviors can cause intervention by law enforcement.**
3. **These clients should be referred to specialists who are accustomed to working with this special population. These referrals can complicate the nursing care.**
4. Clients diagnosed with paraphilic disorders are not typically suicidal or at risk for injury.
5. There are no specific medications prescribed for paraphilic disorders. There is no indication that these clients would be nonadherent with treatments.
TEST-TAKING TIP: Review the nursing care challenges that may occur when caring for clients diagnosed with paraphilic disorders.
Content Area: Safe and Effective Care Environment;
Management of Care;
Integrated Process: Nursing Process: Implementation;
Client Need: Safe and Effective Care Environment;
Management of Care:
Cognitive Level: Application;
Concept: Nursing

13. **ANSWERS: 1, 3, 4**
Rationale: Three major components of sexual development have been identified as: gender identity, sexual responsiveness, and the ability to establish relationships with others.
1. **The development of gender identity relates to one's sense of maleness or femaleness. Transvestic disorder is characterized by an intense sexual arousal from dressing in the clothes of the opposite gender. The development of gender identity may have been disturbed in transvestic disorder.**
2. Gynecomastia is abnormal enlargement of the breasts in men and may be a side effect of some antipsychotic medications. This is not a component of sexual development.
3. **The development of sexual responsiveness to appropriate stimuli may be disturbed in the case of the individual with fetishistic disorder, where the stimuli that causes sexual arousal is from the use of either nonliving objects or specific nongenital body parts.**
4. **In the case of individuals with exhibitionistic or the frotteuristic disorders, the development of the ability to form relationships may be disturbed.**
5. The development of appropriate moral behaviors is not a component of sexual development. In the case of individuals with frotteuristic disorders, the development of the ability to form relationships may be disturbed.
TEST-TAKING TIP: Review the components of sexual development and the paraphilic disorders that may result from deviations in this development.
Content Area: Safe and Effective Care Environment;
Management of Care;

Integrated Process: *Nursing Process: Assessment;*
Client Need: *Safe and Effective Care Environment;*
Management of Care:
Cognitive Level: *Application;*
Concept: *Development*

14. ANSWER: 4
Rationale:
1. *Primary erectile disorder* refers to cases in which the man has never been able to have intercourse. This sexual dysfunction is incorrectly matched with its characteristic symptom.
2. *Secondary erectile disorder* refers to cases in which the man has difficulty getting or maintaining an erection but has been able to have vaginal or anal intercourse at least once. This sexual dysfunction is incorrectly matched with its characteristic symptom.
3. Delayed ejaculation is characterized by marked delay in ejaculation or marked infrequency or absence of ejaculation during partnered sexual activity. Early (premature) ejaculation is persistent or recurrent ejaculation occurring within 1 minute of beginning partnered sexual activity and before the person wishes it. This sexual dysfunction is incorrectly matched with its characteristic symptom.
4. *Male hypoactive sexual desire disorder* **is a persistent or recurrent deficiency or absence of sexual fantasies and desire for sexual activity. This sexual dysfunction is correctly matched with its characteristic symptom.**
TEST-TAKING TIP: Review the types of sexual dysfunctions and their characteristic symptoms.
Content Area: *Safe and Effective Care Environment;*
Management of Care;
Integrated Process: *Nursing Process: Assessment;*
Client Need: *Safe and Effective Care Environment;*
Management of Care:
Cognitive Level: *Application;*
Concept: *Assessment*

15. ANSWER: 2
Rationale: Anorgasmia is a marked delay in, infrequency of, or absence of orgasm during sexual activity.
1. Impaired social interaction is defined as an insufficient or excessive quantity or ineffective quality of social exchange. Female orgasmic disorder (anorgasmia) is a specific sexual dysfunction, not a general problem with social interaction.
2. **Sexual dysfunction is defined as the state in which an individual experiences a change in sexual function during the sexual response phases of desire, excitation, and/or orgasm that is viewed as unsatisfying, unrewarding, or inadequate. This nursing diagnosis can be associated with the symptoms of female orgasmic disorder (anorgasmia) due to disturbances in the sexual response phase of orgasm.**
3. There is nothing presented in the question that would indicate that the client is at risk for self-mutilation.
4. Disturbed personal identity is defined as the inability to maintain an integrated and complete perception of self. This nursing diagnosis may apply when a client is diagnosed with gender dysphoria but does not address the symptoms of female orgasmic disorder (anorgasmia).

TEST-TAKING TIP: Review the key terms at the beginning of the chapter. Knowledge of terminology will help you choose the correct answer.
Content Area: *Safe and Effective Care Environment;*
Management of Care;
Integrated Process: *Nursing Process: Diagnosis (Analysis);*
Client Need: *Safe and Effective Care Environment;*
Management of Care:
Cognitive Level: *Analysis;*
Concept: *Critical Thinking*

16. ANSWER: 3
Rationale: Phimosis is a condition in which the foreskin of the penis cannot be pulled back causing pain during intercourse.
1. Impaired social interaction is defined as an insufficient or excessive quantity or ineffective quality of social exchange. Phimosis should not interfere with social interactions.
2. There is nothing presented in the question that would indicate that the client is at risk for self-mutilation. Self-mutilation does not address the pain caused by phimosis.
3. **Acute pain is defined as an unpleasant sensory and emotional experience arising from actual or potential tissue damage or described in terms of such damage. Because phimosis causes pain during intercourse, this nursing diagnosis is appropriate.**
4. Disturbed personal identity is defined as the inability to maintain an integrated and complete perception of self. This diagnosis does not address the pain caused by phimosis.
TEST-TAKING TIP: Understanding the meaning of phimosis is the key to correctly answering this question.
Content Area: *Safe and Effective Care Environment;*
Management of Care;
Integrated Process: *Nursing Process: Diagnosis (Analysis);*
Client Need: *Safe and Effective Care Environment;*
Management of Care:
Cognitive Level: *Analysis;*
Concept: *Critical Thinking*

17. ANSWER: 1
Rationale: Correctly written outcomes must be client centered, specific, realistic, and measurable and must also include a time frame.
1. **Sensate focus exercises are a treatment of choice for female sexual interest/arousal disorder. Understanding this therapy option is an appropriate outcome for this client. All the components of a correctly written outcome are included in this option.**
2. There are no specific medications approved for the treatment of female sexual interest/arousal disorder. Also, this outcome is incorrectly written because it does not include a time frame.
3. There may be relationship issues that could contribute to the diagnosis of female sexual interest/arousal disorder; however, there is no research to support that the male partner is primarily responsible for this disorder. Also, this outcome is incorrectly written because it does not include a time frame.
4. Increasing self-esteem in clients diagnosed with female sexual interest/arousal disorder is an appropriate outcome; however, "feeling better about self" is a vague statement.

The outcome must be stated in specific terms to be measured and evaluated.

TEST-TAKING TIP: Review the components of a correctly written outcome and understand the client problems that occur with the diagnosis of female sexual interest/arousal disorder.

Content Area: Safe and Effective Care Environment; Management of Care;
Integrated Process: Nursing Process: Planning;
Client Need: Safe and Effective Care Environment; Management of Care;
Cognitive Level: Application;
Concept: Critical Thinking

18. **ANSWER: 3**

Rationale: Correctly written outcomes must be client centered, specific, realistic, and measurable and must also include a time frame.

1. It is important to identify all sexual contacts to assess and treat potential infection, but compared with the other outcomes presented, this outcome does not take priority.
2. It is important to understand the consequences if the gonorrhea goes untreated to avoid future complications of the disease, but compared with the other outcomes presented, this outcome does not take priority. Also, this outcome is incorrectly written because it does not include a time frame.
3. Gonorrhea is a sexually transmitted disease (STD). Agreeing to refrain from unprotected sexual activity until laboratory work indicates that no gonorrhea is present must take priority to contain the transmission of this disease. All the components of a correctly written outcome are included in this option.
4. It is important to understand the need to complete a full course of medication treatment to successfully eradicate the disease, but compared with the other outcomes presented, this outcome does not take priority.

TEST-TAKING TIP: Review the components of a correctly written outcome and understand that prevention of the STD transmission must take priority.

Content Area: Safe and Effective Care Environment; Management of Care;
Integrated Process: Nursing Process: Planning;
Client Need: Safe and Effective Care Environment; Management of Care;
Cognitive Level: Application;
Concept: Critical Thinking

19. **ANSWERS: 3**

Rationale:
1. Clients diagnosed with gender dysphoria can experience impaired social interaction related to behaviors that are not socially accepted, but they should not have any problem maintaining eye contact. Therefore, this intervention is not correctly matched with the nursing diagnosis presented.

2. Clients diagnosed with gender dysphoria may experience low self-esteem due to nonacceptance by peers and family. This may put the client at risk for self-directed violence, but they are usually not prone to violence toward others. Also restraints should only be used when injury is imminent and all other avenues of intervention have been exhausted.
3. Clients diagnosed with gender dysphoria can experience disturbed personal identity due to discomfort and distress related to their assigned gender. Discussing with the client the types of behaviors that are more culturally acceptable and role-playing these behaviors allows the child to practice the behaviors he or she will attempt to generalize to life situations. This nursing diagnosis and nursing intervention are correctly matched.
4. Clients diagnosed with gender dysphoria can experience disturbed personal identity but are not so out of touch with reality as to experience altered body image. Also, a client's perception of reality should not be challenged. When caring for clients experiencing altered perceptions, the nurse should assess the client's perception of reality, present objective reality, and redirect the client to a neutral stimulus.

TEST-TAKING TIP: You must first determine the nursing diagnoses that would apply to a client diagnosed with gender dysphoria. Then you should evaluate the appropriateness of the nursing intervention presented.

Content Area: Safe and Effective Care Environment, Management of Care;
Integrated Process: Nursing Process: Diagnosis (Analysis);
Client Need: Safe and Effective Care Environment; Management of Care;
Cognitive Level: Analysis;
Concept: Critical Thinking

20. **ANSWER: Sadism**

Rationale: The essential feature of sexual sadism disorder, a paraphilic disorder, is a feeling of sexual excitement resulting from administering pain, suffering, or humiliation to another person. The pain, suffering, or humiliation inflicted on the other is real; it is not imagined and may be either physical or psychological in nature. A person with a diagnosis of sexual sadism disorder is sometimes called a sadist. The name of the disorder is derived from the name of the Marquis Donatien de Sade (1740–1814), a French aristocrat who became notorious for writing novels around the theme of inflicting pain as a source of sexual pleasure.

TEST-TAKING TIP: Review information about the paraphilic disorder of sexual sadism.

Content Area: Psychosocial Integrity;
Integrated Process: Nursing Process: Assessment;
Client Need: Psychosocial Integrity;
Cognitive Level: Knowledge;
Concept: Sexuality

CASE STUDY: Putting it All Together

Jamie, a 12-year-old, was wearing his twin sister's clothes and dancing in front of the mirror when he saw his mother standing in the doorway. Horrified, his mother yelled, "Jamie, how long has this been going on?" Jamie ripped off the dress, locked himself in his room, and refused to talk. When coaxing and pleading were met with continued silence, Jamie's mother made an appointment with the children's pediatrician.

Examination revealed a physically healthy 12-year-old boy. Laboratory reports ruled out adrenogenital disorders. The pediatrician called the East Meadow Psychiatric Solution Center, and a referral was made to Zac, a psychiatric nurse practitioner whose specialty was childhood deviations in sexual development. At the first meeting, Jamie's mother told Zac that her ex-husband deserted the family shortly after the twins' birth and that the twins never had a father figure or any significant male role models. She states that Jamie has shown no interest in masculine activities, such as playing with trucks, action figures, enjoying sport activities, or even roughhousing with peers. She reports that Jamie is a good student, respectful, quiet, and a basic loner. She tells Zac that Jamie spends most of his time reading, playing the piano, and cooking and baking with her. "Not that I mind; he's such good company," she declares. "No matter what, I love my son very much. I just want to know what I'm dealing with."

Jamie reluctantly, but with some sense of relief, agrees to talk to Zac. During the initial interview, Zac notes that Jamie is polite, reserved, and overwhelmingly sad. His shoulders are slumped, his eyes are downcast, and his affect is flat. After brief idle chitchat, Jamie, in anguish, opens up saying, "Well, now my mother knows!" Zac responds, "What exactly does she know?" Jamie begins to cry and shout, "She knows I'm weird! I just don't feel like a boy on the inside. I know I'm a big disappointment, and I don't know what to do about it. What's wrong with me?" After calming down, Jamie admits to having hated his body for as long as he can remember and tells Zac, "If I were a girl, my life would he happy and normal."

1. On the basis of Jamie's symptoms and actions, what medical diagnosis would Zac assign to Jamie?
2. What are Jamie's subjective symptoms that would lead to the determination of this diagnosis?
3. What are Jamie's objective symptoms that would lead to the determination of this diagnosis?
4. On the basis of Jamie's diagnosis, what treatments might Zac consider to relieve Jamie's symptoms?
5. What North American Nursing Diagnosis Association (NANDA) nursing diagnosis would be appropriate for Jamie?
6. On the basis of this nursing diagnosis, what short-term outcomes would be appropriate for Jamie?
7. On the basis of this nursing diagnosis, what long-term outcomes would be appropriate for Jamie?
8. List the nursing interventions (actions) that will assist Jamie in successfully meeting these outcomes.
9. List the questions that should be answered in determining the success of the nursing actions.

Chapter 19

Victims of Abuse or Neglect

KEY TERMS

Abuse—The maltreatment of one person by another

Battering—A pattern of coercive control founded on and supported by physical and/or sexual violence or threat of violence of an intimate partner; don't confuse with *battery,* the unconsented touching of another person

Emotional neglect—A chronic failure by the parent or caretaker to provide the child with the hope, love, and support necessary for the development of a sound, healthy personality

"Granny dumping"—The abandonment of elderly relatives by their caregivers; coined in the United States in the early 1990s when it was believed that elderly people were being deserted by their caregivers and left in hospitals or other public places where the authorities would find them and take responsibility for them

Incest—The occurrence of sexual contact or interaction between, or sexual exploitation of, close relatives, or between participants who are related to each other by a kinship bond that is regarded as a prohibition to sexual relations (e.g., caretakers, stepparents, stepsiblings)

Physical neglect—Refusal of or delay in seeking health care, abandonment, expulsion from the home, refusal to allow a runaway to return home, and inadequate supervision

Rape—The expression of power and dominance by means of sexual violence, most commonly by men over women, although men may also be rape victims

"Sandwich generation"—The generation of middle-aged individuals who are effectively "sandwiched" between the obligation to care for their aging parent who may be ill, unable to perform various tasks, or in need of financial support and children who require financial, physical, and emotional support

Survivor—A person who carries on despite hardships or trauma and remains functional

Victim—A person who suffers from a destructive or injurious action or agency; one who is harmed by or made to suffer under a circumstance or condition

Victimizer—Someone who treats another cruelly or unfairly by harming or committing a crime against others

Abuse is on the rise in this society. More injuries are attributed to intimate partner violence than to all stranger rapes, muggings, and automobile accidents combined. An increase in the incidence of child abuse and related fatalities has also been documented. Incidences of sexual assault are rising and, because of underreporting, these types of assault are often considered a silent-violent epidemic. Abuse affects all populations equally. It occurs among all races, religions, economic classes, ages, and educational backgrounds. The phenomenon is cyclical in that many abusers were themselves victims of abuse as children. Child abuse became a mandatory reportable occurrence in the United States in 1968. Responsibility for the protection of elders from abuse rests primarily with the states. Violence incurs physical, psychological, and social devastation that nurses can address in the care of this population.

I. Prevalence

A. Three in 10 women and 1 in 10 men in the United States report having been the victim of intimate partner violence

B. Rape is vastly underreported in the United States

C. In the United States, 1 in 5 women and 1 in 71 men report having been raped at some time in their lives

D. In 2010, an estimated 3.3 million cases of possible child abuse or neglect were reported to child protective services (about 25% of these cases were substantiated)

E. An estimated 1,560 children died from causes related to abuse or neglect in 2010

F. In 2012, the annual cost of intimate partner violence, measured in terms of medical care and lost productivity, was more than $406 billion

II. Predisposing Factors

A. Biological theories
   1. Neurophysiological influences: components of the neurological system have been implicated in the facilitation and inhibition of aggressive impulses.
      a. Temporal lobe.
      b. Limbic system.
      c. Amygdaloid nucleus.
   2. Biochemical influences.
      a. Various neurotransmitters (norepinephrine, dopamine, and serotonin) may play a role in the facilitation and inhibition of aggressive impulses.
      b. Findings consistent with "fight-or-flight" arousal as stress response.
      c. An explanation of these biochemical influences on violent behavior is presented in Figure 19.1.
   3. Genetic influences.
      a. Some studies linked increased aggressiveness with selective inbreeding in mice.
      b. Genetic karyotype XYY was thought to be linked to aggressive behavior, but this link has not been firmly established.
   4. Disorders of the brain implicated in violent behaviors.
      a. Brain tumors, particularly in the areas of the limbic system and the temporal lobes.
      b. Trauma to the brain, resulting in cerebral changes.
      c. Diseases (encephalitis, epilepsy—particularly temporal lobe epilepsy).

B. Psychological theories
   1. Psychodynamic theory.
      a. Unmet needs for satisfaction and security result in an underdeveloped ego and a weak superego.
      b. Immature ego cannot prevent dominant id behaviors from occurring.
      c. Weak superego is unable to produce feelings of guilt.
   2. Learning theory.
      a. Children learn to behave by imitating role models (usually parents).
      b. With maturity, imitate teachers, friends, and others.

MAKING THE CONNECTION

According to psychodynamic theory, when there is faulty ego development, the individual cannot effectively handle frustration and turns to aggression and violence. This violent behavior supplies the individual with power and prestige that boosts the self-image and validates a significance to his or her life that is lacking because of early unmet needs.

   c. May model behaviors after individuals observed on television/movies (using violence to triumph over villains).
   d. Imitation likely when models are perceived as prestigious or influential.
   e. Imitation likely when behavior is positively reinforced.
   f. With a biological predisposition toward aggressive behavior, may be more susceptible to negative role modeling.
   g. Individuals who were abused or who witnessed domestic violence as a child are more likely to behave in an abusive manner as adults.

C. Sociocultural theories
   1. Social scientists believe aggressive behavior is primarily a product of one's culture and social structure.
   2. Poverty and income are powerful predictors of homicide and violent crime.
   3. Violence may occur when individuals realize that their needs and desires are not being met relative to other people.

DID YOU KNOW?

Societal influences may contribute to violence. When poor and oppressed people find that they have limited access through legitimate channels, they are more likely to resort to delinquent behaviors in an effort to obtain desired ends.

III. Nursing Process: Assessment of Victims of Abuse or Neglect

A. Battering
   1. A pattern of behavior used to establish power and control through fear and intimidation.
   2. Threat of violence often used.
   3. The victim is in or has been in an intimate relationship with the victimizer.
   4. Battering happens when one person believes he or she is entitled to control another.

B. Intimate partner violence
   1. A pattern of abusive behavior that is used by an intimate partner to gain or maintain power and control over the other intimate partner.

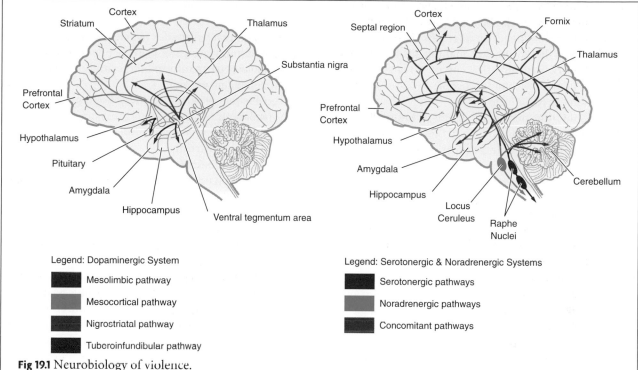

Fig 19.1 Neurobiology of violence.

Neurotransmitters

Neurotransmitters that have been implicated in the etiology of aggression and violence include serotonin (decreases) and norepinephrine and dopamine (increases) (Hollander et al., 2008; Tardiff, 2003).

Associated Areas of the Brain

- Limbic structures: emotional alterations
- Prefrontal and frontal cortices: modulation of social judgment
- Amygdala: anxiety, rage, fear
- Hypothalamus: stimulates sympathetic nervous system in "fight-or-flight" response
- Hippocampus: learning and memory

Medications Used to Modulate Aggression

1. Studies have suggested that selective serotonin reuptake inhibitors (SSRIs) may reduce irritability and aggression consistent with the hypothesis of reduced serotonergic activity in aggression.
2. Mood stabilizers that dampen limbic irritability may be important in reducing the susceptibility to react to provocation or threatening stimuli by overactivation of limbic system structures such as the amygdala (Siever, 2002). Carbamazepine (Tegretol), phenytoin (Dilantin), and divalproex sodium (Depakote) have yielded positive results. Lithium has also been used effectively in violent individuals (Schatzberg, Cole, & DeBattista, 2010).
3. Antiadrenergic agents such as beta blockers (e.g., propranolol) have been shown to reduce aggression in some individuals, presumably by dampening excessive noradrenergic activity (Schatzberg et al., 2010).
4. In their ability to modulate excessive dopaminergic activity, antipsychotics—both typical and atypical—have been helpful in the control of aggression and violence, particularly in individuals with comorbid psychosis.

2. Violence can be physical, sexual, emotional, economic, or psychological actions or threats of actions that influence another person. Includes behaviors that intimidate, manipulate, humiliate, isolate, frighten, terrorize, coerce, threaten, blame, hurt, injure, or wound someone.
3. Prevalence (data from 2012).
   a. Eighty-two percent of victims of intimate violence were women.
   b. Women aged 25 to 34 experienced the highest per capita rates of intimate partner violence.
   c. Intimate partners committed 2% of the nonfatal violence against men.
   d. Forty-nine percent of women and 72% of men reported the victimizations to the police.
   e. Most common reason for not reporting was because it was a "private or personal matter."
C. Profile of the typical victim
   1. The typical battered person is a woman from any age, racial, religious, cultural, educational, and socioeconomic group.
   2. May be married or single.
   3. Housewives or business executives.
   4. Typically have low self-esteem.
   5. Commonly adhere to feminine gender-role stereotypes.
   6. Often accept the blame for the batterer's actions.
   7. Feelings of guilt, anger, fear, and shame are common.
   8. May be isolated from family and support systems.
   9. May have grown up in an abusive home.
   10. May have left home, gotten married, at a very young age to escape abuse.
   11. Views her relationship as male dominant.
   12. With continued abuse, loses ability to see the options available to her and to make decisions concerning her life (and possibly those of her children).
   13. *Learned helplessness:* progressive inability to act on her own behalf; regardless of behavior, outcome is unpredictable and usually undesirable.
D. Profile of the typical **victimizer**
   1. Batterers are typically men who have low self-esteem and pathological jealousy.
   2. Presents with "dual personality" (one to the partner and one to the rest of the world).
   3. Often under a great deal of stress with limited coping skills.
   4. Very possessive and perceives spouse as a possession.
   5. Threatened when partner shows independence or attempts to share herself and her time with others.
   6. Often ignores small children.
   7. May target small children for abuse as the children grow older (particularly if they protect mother).

8. May emotionally abuse by threats of taking away children.
9. Continually degrades female partner by insulting and humiliating her at every opportunity.
10. Isolates partner from others until she is totally dependent on him.
11. Must know partner's whereabouts at every moment.
12. Achieves power and control through intimidation.
E. The cycle of battering
   1. Cycle of predictable behaviors that occur in three distinct phases, varying in time and intensity and repeated over time (see Fig. 19.2).
   2. Phase I: the tension-building phase.
      a. May last from a few weeks to many months or even years.
      b. Victim senses that the victimizer's tolerance for frustration is declining.
      c. Victimizer becomes angry with little provocation.
      d. After lashing out at victim, victimizer may be quick to apologize.
      e. Victim may become nurturing and compliant.
      f. Victim anticipates victimizer's every need to prevent escalating anger.
      g. Victim may just try to stay out of victimizer's way.
      h. Minor battering incidents may occur.
      i. Victim accepts abuse as legitimately directed toward self.
      j. Victim denies anger and rationalizes victimizer behavior.

DID YOU KNOW?
Examples of rationalizations used by the victim include the following: "I need to do better"; "He's under so much stress at work"; "It's the alcohol. If only he didn't drink." As part of rationalization, the victim assumes the guilt for the abuse, even reasoning that perhaps the victim *did* deserve the abuse, just as the aggressor suggests.

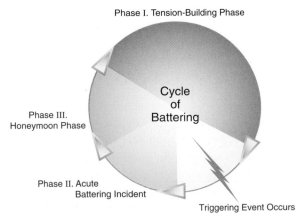

Fig 19.2 The cycle of battering.

    k. Victimizer fears that victim will leave.

    l. Victimizer's jealousy and possessiveness increase.

    m. Victimizer uses threats and brutality to keep victim in captivity.

    n. Battering incidents become more intense.

    o. Victim becomes less and less psychologically capable of restoring equilibrium.

    p. Victim withdraws from victimizer, which is misinterpreted as rejection, further escalating the victimizer's anger.

3. Phase II: the acute battering incident.

    a. Most violent phase and the shortest, usually lasting up to 24 hours.

    b. Begins with victimizer wanting to "just teach the victim a lesson" and justifying behavior to self.

    c. Victim may intentionally provoke the behavior.

    d. Victim's only option is to find a safe place to hide from the victimizer.

    e. Beating is severe.

    f. Victimizer generally minimizes the severity of the abuse.

    g. Victim seeks help only for severe injury or if the victim fears for life or lives of children.

    h. Victimizer cannot understand what has happened, only that in rage, control is lost over behavior.

4. Phase III: calm, loving, respite ("honeymoon") phase.

    a. Lasts somewhere between the lengths of time associated with Phases I and II; can be so short as to almost pass undetected.

    b. Victimizer becomes extremely loving, kind, and contrite.

    c. Victimizer promises that the abuse will never recur and begs victim's forgiveness.

    d. Victimizer is afraid victim will leave and uses every bit of charm to prevent victim from leaving.

    e. Victim believes victimizer can now control behavior.

    f. Victimizer believes victim will not "act up" again now that victimizer has "taught victim a lesson."

    g. Victimizer plays on victim's feelings of guilt.

    h. Victim desperately wants to believe victimizer.

    i. Victim relives original dream of ideal love and chooses to believe that victimizer is committed to a loving, healthy relationship.

    j. Victim hopes that previous phases will not be repeated; in most instances, the cycle soon begins again with renewed tensions and minor battering incidents.

    k. In an effort to return to the Phase III kind of loving, the battered victim becomes a collaborator in abusive lifestyle.

    l. Victim and victimizer become locked together in an intense, symbiotic relationship.

5. Why does victim stay?

    a. Fear of retaliation (threats of death or death of children).

    b. Low self-esteem and sense of powerlessness.

    c. No ability to see a way out.

    d. Fear of losing custody of the children.

    e. Lack of financial resources or job skills.

    f. Lack of support network.

    g. Pressure from family members to stay in the marriage and try to work things out.

    h. Religious convictions against divorce, believing that victim must save the marriage at all costs.

    i. Memory of good times and love in the relationship encourages hope that victimizer will change behavior and good times can develop again.

F. Child abuse

DID YOU KNOW?

Children are vulnerable and relatively powerless, and the effects of maltreatment are infinitely deep and long lasting. Child maltreatment typically includes physical or emotional injury, physical or emotional neglect, or sexual acts inflicted on a child by a caregiver.

1. Physical abuse.

    a. Any nonaccidental physical injury (minor bruises to severe fractures or death).

    b. Can be a result of:

        i. Punching

        ii. Beating

        iii. Kicking

        iv. Biting

        v. Shaking

        vi. Throwing

        vii. Stabbing

        viii. Choking

        ix. Hitting by:

            a) Hand

            b) Stick

            c) Strap

            d) Other object

        x. Burning

        xi. Otherwise harming

    c. Inflicted by parent, caregiver, or other person who has responsibility for the child.

    d. Maltreatment is considered whether or not the caretaker intended to cause harm.

    e. Even if the injury resulted from overdiscipline or physical punishment, the most obvious way to detect it is by outward physical signs; however, behavioral indicators also may be evident.

  f. Signs of physical abuse.
- i. The child:
  - a) Has unexplained burns, bites, bruises, broken bones, or black eyes
  - b) Has fading bruises or other marks noticeable after an absence from school
  - c) Seems frightened of the parents or caregivers and protests or cries when it is time to go home
  - d) Shrinks at the approach of adults
  - e) Reports injury by a parent or another adult caregiver
- ii. The parent or other adult caregiver:
  - a) Offers conflicting, unconvincing, or no explanation for child's injury
  - b) Describes the child as "evil," or in some other very negative way
  - c) Uses harsh physical discipline
  - d) Has a history of abuse as a child

2. Emotional abuse.
  a. A pattern of behavior on the part of the parent or caretaker that results in serious impairment of the child's social, emotional, or intellectual functioning.
  b. Examples include:
- i. Belittling or rejecting the child
- ii. Ignoring the child
- iii. Blaming the child for things over which he or she has no control
- iv. Isolating the child from normal social experiences
- v. Using harsh and inconsistent discipline

  c. Indicators may include:
- i. Showing extremes in behavior, such as overly compliant or demanding behavior, extreme passivity, or aggression
- ii. Acting either inappropriately adult (parenting other children) or inappropriately infantile (frequently rocking or head-banging)
- iii. Delays in physical or emotional development
- iv. Suicide attempts
- v. Reporting a lack of attachment to the parent

  d. Behaviors of the parent or other adult caregiver:
- i. Constantly blames, belittles, or berates the child
- ii. Is unconcerned about the child
- iii. Refuses to consider offers of help for the child's problems
- iv. Overtly rejects the child

3. Physical and emotional neglect.
  a. Indicators of neglect: the child.
- i. Is frequently absent from school
- ii. Begs or steals food or money
- iii. Lacks needed medical or dental care, immunizations, or glasses
- iv. Is consistently dirty and has severe body odor
- v. Lacks sufficient clothing for the weather
- vi. Abuses alcohol or other drugs
- vii. States that there is no one at home to provide care

  b. Indicators of neglect: the parent or other adult caregiver.
- i. Appears to be indifferent to the child
- ii. Seems apathetic or depressed
- iii. Behaves irrationally or in a bizarre manner
- iv. Is abusing alcohol or other drugs

4. Sexual abuse of a child
  a. Any sexual act with a child performed by an adult or an older child.
  b. Child sexual abuse could include a number of acts, including but not limited to:
- i. Sexual touching of any part of the body, clothed or unclothed
- ii. Penetrative sex, including penetration of the mouth
- iii. Encouraging a child to engage in sexual activity, including masturbation
- iv. Intentionally engaging in sexual activity in front of a child
- v. Showing children pornography, or using children to create pornography
- vi. Encouraging a child to engage in prostitution

  c. Sexual exploitation of a child.
- i. Child is induced or coerced into engaging in sexually explicit conduct for the purpose of promoting any performance
- ii. Child is being used for the sexual pleasure of an adult (parent or caretaker) or any other person

  d. Indicators of sexual abuse: the child.
- i. Has difficulty walking or sitting
- ii. Suddenly refuses to change for gym or to participate in physical activities
- iii. Reports nightmares or bedwetting
- iv. Experiences a sudden change in appetite
- v. Demonstrates bizarre, sophisticated, or unusual sexual knowledge or behavior
- vi. Becomes pregnant or contracts a venereal disease, particularly if younger than age 14 years
- vii. Runs away
- viii. Reports sexual abuse by a parent or another adult caregiver

  e. Indicators of sexual abuse: the parent or other adult caregiver:
- i. Is unduly protective of the child or severely limits the child's contact with other children, especially of the opposite sex

  ii. Is secretive and isolated
  iii. Is jealous or controlling with family members
  f. Characteristics of the abuser.
  i. Ninety percent of parents who abuse their children were severely physically abused by their own mothers or fathers
  ii. Experiencing a stressful life situation (unemployment, poverty)
  iii. Have few, if any, support systems, commonly isolated from others
  iv. Lack understanding of child development or care needs
  v. Lack adaptive coping strategies, anger easily, have difficulty trusting others
  vi. Expects the child to be perfect, may exaggerate any mild difference the child manifests from the "usual"
  g. Other risk factors for maltreatment include characteristics of the child, the parent, and the environment (These characteristics are presented in Box 19.1).
  h. When multiple factors coexist, the risk of child abuse increases.
5. The incestuous relationship.
  a. Incest may take many forms, with father daughter being the most common.
  b. Usually there is an impaired sexual relationship between the parents.
  c. Father is typically domineering, impulsive, and physically abusive.
  d. Mother is passive and submissive and denigrates her role as wife and mother.
  e. Mother often aware of, or strongly suspects, the incestuous behavior.
  f. May believe in or fear husband's absolute authority.
  g. May deny that daughter is being harmed.

  h. May be grateful that husband's sexual demands are reflected toward daughter.
  i. Onset of the incestuous relationship typically begins when daughter is 8 to 10 years old.
  j. Commonly begins with genital touching and fondling.
  k. Child may initially accept the sexual advances as signs of affection.
  l. With continued behavior, daughter usually becomes more bewildered, confused, and frightened, never knowing whether her father will be paternal or sexual in his interactions with her.
  m. Daughter's relationship with father may become love–hate.
  n. Strives for the ideal father–daughter relationship.
  o. Fearful and hateful of the sexual demands father places on her.
  p. Mother may be alternately caring and competitive.
  q. Father may interfere with daughter's normal peer relationships out of fear of exposure.
  r. Some fathers may have unconscious homosexual tendencies, and have difficulty achieving a stable heterosexual orientation.
  s. Some fathers have frequent sex with their wives and several of their own children.
  t. Oldest daughter most vulnerable.
  u. Some fathers form sequential relationships with several daughters.
  v. If incest has been reported with one daughter, it should be suspected with all of the other daughters.
6. The adult survivor of incest.
  a. Common characteristics.
  i. Lack of trust resulting from an unsatisfactory parent–child relationship
  ii. Low self-esteem and poor sense of identity
  iii. Often feels trapped

Box 19.1 Factors and Characteristics That Place a Child at Risk for Maltreatment

Child	Parent	Environment (Community and Society)
Emotional/behavioral difficulties	*Low self-esteem*	*Social isolation*
Chronic illness	*Poor impulse control*	*Poverty*
Physical disabilities	*Substance abuse/alcohol abuse*	*Unemployment*
Developmental disabilities	*Young maternal or paternal age*	*Low educational achievement*
Preterm birth	*Abused as a child*	*Single-parent home*
Unwanted	*Depression or other mental illness*	*Non–biologically related male living in the home*
Unplanned	*Poor knowledge of child development or unrealistic expectations of the child*	*Family or intimate partner violence*
	Negative perception of normal child behavior	

Source: Flaherty & Stirling (2010). Clinical report—The pediatrician's role in child maltreatment prevention. *Pediatrics*, *126*(4), 833-841. Reprinted with permission.

    iv. Experiences fear, even fear for their lives

    v. If victim reports the incest, particularly to the mother, he or she may not be believed

    vi. Results are self-doubt and the inability to trust his or her own feelings

    vii. Child develops feelings of guilt with realization that parents are using him or her to solve their own problems

    viii. Distortion of the development of a normal association of pleasure with sexual activity

    ix. Peer relationships delayed, altered, inhibited, or perverted

    x. May completely retreat from sexual activity and avoid all close interpersonal relationships throughout life

    xi. Women may experience diminished libido, pain/penetration disorder, nymphomania, or promiscuity

    xii. Males may experience impotence, premature ejaculation, or exhibitionism, or compulsive sexual conquests may occur

    xiii. Both male and female survivors may experience symptoms of:
      a) Posttraumatic stress disorder
      b) Sexual dysfunction
      c) Somatization disorders
      d) Compulsive sexual behaviors
      e) Depression
      f) Anxiety
      g) Eating disorders
      h) Substance disorders
      i) Intolerance of intimacy
      j) Constant search for intimacy

DID YOU KNOW?
The conflicts associated with pain (either physical or emotional) and sexual pleasure experienced by children who are sexually abused are commonly manifested symbolically in adult relationships. Women who were abused as children commonly enter into relationships with men who abuse them physically, sexually, or emotionally.

      k) Often estranged from nuclear family members
      l) May be blamed by family members for disclosing the "family secret" and often accused of overreacting to the incest

G. Sexual assault

  1. Any type of sexual act in which an individual is threatened, coerced, or forced to submit against his or her will.

  2. Rape, a type of sexual assault, occurs over a broad spectrum of experiences ranging from the surprise attack by a stranger to insistence on sexual intercourse by an acquaintance or spouse.

  3. Rape is an act of aggression, not one of passion.

  4. Rape can occur regardless of the victim's age.

DID YOU KNOW?
In a study of a prison sample of rapists, it was found that in *stranger rapes,* targets were not chosen for any reason having to do with appearance or behavior but simply because the individual happened to be in a certain place at a certain time.

  5. Types of rape
    a. **Acquaintance rape** applies to situations in which the rapist is acquainted with the victim.

DID YOU KNOW?
Date rape is a sexual assault that occurs during a social engagement agreed to by the victim. College campuses are the location for a staggering number of these types of rapes, a great many of which go unreported. An increasing number of colleges and universities are establishing programs for rape prevention and counseling for survivors of rape.

    b. **Marital rape** is the case in which a spouse may be held liable for sexual abuse directed at a marital partner against that person's will.

    c. **Statutory rape** is unlawful intercourse between a person who is older than the age of consent and a person who is younger than the age of consent.
      i. Legal age of consent varies from state to state, ranging from age 16 to 18
      ii. The older participant can be arrested for statutory rape even if sexual encounter was consensual

  5. Profile of the victimizer.
    a. Mother-dominated childhood continuing into adulthood.
    b. Mother possessive and seductive but rejecting.
    c. Overbearing mother who rescued child when delinquent acts created problems.
    d. Mother quick to withdraw love and attention when child goes against her wishes.
    e. Anger of child toward mother can be displaced onto other women.
    f. When seductive behavior is combined with parental encouragement of assaultive behavior, personality development in the child results in sadistic, homicidal sexual attacks on women in adolescence or adult life.
    g. Many rapists grow up in abusive homes.
    h. When parental brutality is discharged by the father, the anger may be directed toward the mother who did not protect child from physical assault.
    i. Feminist view suggests that rape is most common in societies that encourage aggressiveness

in males and have distinct gender roles and in which men regard women's roles as inferior.

j. Greatest number of rapists are between ages 25 and 44 years.

k. Fifty-four percent are white, 32% are African American, and the remainder are of other races, mixed race, or of unknown race.

l. Many are either married or cohabiting at the time of their offenses.

m. Most rapists do not have histories of mental illness.

n. Sixty-two percent of the rapists use a weapon (most frequently a knife).

o. The weapon is usually used to terrorize and subdue the victim, not to inflict serious injury.

6. Profile of the victim.
   a. Highest risk age-group is 16 to 34 years.
   b. Most sexual assault victims are single women.
   c. The attack frequently occurs in or close to the victim's own neighborhood.
   d. Choice of victim is based on chance availability.
   e. Rape survivors experience an overwhelming sense of violation and helplessness.
   f. Feelings begin with the powerlessness and intimidation experienced during the rape.
   g. Emotional patterns of response.
      i. *Expressed response pattern:* the survivor expresses feelings of fear, anger, and anxiety through such behaviors as crying, sobbing, smiling, restlessness, and tension
      ii. *Controlled response pattern:* feelings are masked or hidden, and a calm, composed, or subdued affect is seen
      iii. *Compounded rape reaction:* along with typical manifestations (described subsequently), additional symptoms such as depression and suicide, substance abuse, and even psychotic behaviors may be noted
      iv. *Silent rape reaction:* survivor tells no one about the assault; anxiety is suppressed and the emotional burden may become overwhelming

DID YOU KNOW?

Clients who experience a *silent rape reaction* may not reveal the unresolved sexual trauma until they are forced to face another sexual crisis in their life that reactivates the previously unresolved feelings. This may include the beginning of an intimate relationship or an anticipated pregnancy and childbirth.

h. The following manifestations may be evident in the days and weeks after the attack.
   i. Contusions and abrasions on various parts of the body
      ii. Headaches, fatigue, sleep pattern disturbances
      iii. Stomach pains, nausea and vomiting
      iv. Vaginal discharge and itching, burning upon urination, rectal bleeding and pain
      v. Rage, humiliation, embarrassment, desire for revenge, and self-blame
      vi. Fear of physical violence and death

H. Elder abuse (Detection of elder abuse is difficult)
   1. Prevalence.
      a. Between 1 and 2 million Americans aged 65 or older have been injured, exploited, or otherwise mistreated by someone on whom they depended for care or protection.
      b. Only 1 in 14 incidents (excluding self-neglect) are reported to authorities.
   2. Profile of abuser.
      a. Often a relative living with the elderly person (may be assigned caregiver).
      b. Characteristics:
         i. Under economic stress
         ii. Substance abusers
         iii. Themselves the victims of previous family violence
         iv. Exhausted and frustrated by the caregiver role
   3. Profile of victim.
      a. Being a white female aged 70 or older.
      b. Being mentally or physically impaired.
      c. Being unable to meet daily self-care needs.
      d. Often isolated and infirm.
      e. Having care needs that exceed the caretaker's ability.
      f. Often minimize or deny abuse.
      g. May fear retaliation.
      h. May be embarrassed about existence of abuse in family.
      i. May be protective toward family member.
      j. Often unwilling to pursue legal action.

MAKING THE CONNECTION

The long-term effects of sexual assault depend largely on the individual's ego strength and social support system and the way he or she was treated as a victim. Various long-term effects include increased restlessness, dreams and nightmares, and phobias (particularly those having to do with sexual interaction). Some women report that it takes years to get over the experience; they describe a sense of vulnerability and a loss of control over their own lives during this period. They feel defiled and unable to wash themselves clean, and some women are unable to remain living alone in their home or apartment.

DID YOU KNOW?

Abuse of elderly individuals may be psychological, physical, or financial. Neglect may be intentional or unintentional. Unintentional neglect is inadvertent, whereas intentional neglect is deliberate. In addition, elderly individuals may be the victims of sexual abuse, which is sexual intimacy between two persons that occurs without the consent of one of the persons involved.

4. Psychological abuse.
   a. Yelling.
   b. Insulting.
   c. Harsh commands.
   d. Threats.
   e. Silence.
   f. Social isolation.
5. Physical abuse.
   a. Striking.
   b. Shoving.
   c. Beating.
   d. Restraint.
6. Financial abuse.
   a. Misuse of finances, property, or material possessions.
   b. Theft of finances, property, or material possessions.
7. Neglect: failure to fulfill the physical needs of an individual who cannot achieve these independently.
8. "Granny-dumping."
   a. Abandoning elderly individuals at emergency departments, nursing homes, or other facilities.
   b. Leaving elderly in the hands of others when the strain of caregiving becomes intolerable.
9. Types of elder abuse are summarized in Box 19.2
10. Factors that contribute to elder abuse.
    a. Longer life.
       i. Population older than age 75 increasing rapidly
       ii. Older population more likely to be physically/mentally impaired
       iii. Most likely to need assistance
    b. Dependency.

DID YOU KNOW?

Changes associated with normal aging or induced by chronic illness often result in loss of self-sufficiency in elderly persons, requiring that they become dependent on another for assistance with daily functioning. Long life may also consume finances to the point that the elderly individual becomes financially dependent.

    c. Stress.
       i. Stress inherent in the caregiver role is a factor in most abuse cases

---

Box 19.2 Examples of Elder Abuse

Physical Abuse

Striking, hitting, beating
Shoving
Bruising
Cutting
Restraining

Psychological Abuse

Yelling
Insulting, name-calling
Harsh commands
Threats
Ignoring, silence, social isolation
Withholding of affection

Neglect (intentional or unintentional)

Withholding food and water
Inadequate heating
Unclean clothes and bedding
Lack of needed medication
Lack of eyeglasses, hearing aids, false teeth

Financial Abuse or Exploitation

Misuse of the elderly person's income by the caregiver
Forcing the elderly person to sign over financial affairs to another person against his or her will or without sufficient knowledge about the transaction

Sexual Abuse

Sexual molestation; rape
Any type of sexual intimacy against the elderly person's will

---

Sources: Murray, Zentner, & Yakimo (2009); Sadock & Sadock (2007); and Stanley, Blair, & Beare (2005).

       ii. May be due to family psychopathology
      iii. Healthy family members can become abusive as the result of the exhaustion and acute stress caused by overwhelming caregiving responsibilities
    d. Learned violence.
       i. Children who have been abused or witnessed abusive and violent parents are more likely to evolve into abusive adults
      ii. In some families, abusive behavior is the normal response to tension or conflict
      iii. This type of behavior can be transmitted from one generation to another

---

MAKING THE CONNECTION

The stress of caring for aging family members is compounded in an age group that has been dubbed the "**sandwich generation**"—those individuals who elected to delay childbearing so that they are now at a point in their lives when they are "sandwiched" between providing care for their children and providing care for their aging parents.

iv. Abuse may stem from unresolved family conflicts or retaliation for previous maltreatment

11. Identifying elder abuse.

    a. Indicators of psychological abuse.

        i. Depression

        ii. Withdrawal

        iii. Anxiety

        iv. Sleep disorders

        v. Increased confusion

        vi. Agitation

    b. Indicators of physical abuse.

        i. Bruises

        ii. Welts

        iii. Lacerations

        iv. Burns

        v. Punctures

        vi. Evidence of hair pulling

        vii. Skeletal dislocations

        viii. Fractures

    c. Manifestations of neglect.

        i. Consistent hunger

        ii. Poor hygiene

        iii. Inappropriate dress

        iv. Consistent lack of supervision

        v. Consistent fatigue (listlessness)

        vi. Unattended physical problems

        vii. Unattended medical needs

        viii. Abandonment

    d. Manifestations of sexual abuse.

        i. Pain or itching in genital area

        ii. Bruising or bleeding in external genitalia, vaginal, or anal areas

        iii. Unexplained sexually transmitted disease

    e. Indications of financial abuse.

        i. Obvious disparity between assets and satisfactory living conditions

        ii. Complaints of lack of funds for daily living expenses

    f. Nurse's responsibilities.

        i. Responsible for reporting any suspicions of elder abuse

        ii. Every effort must be made to ensure the client's safety

---

MAKING THE CONNECTION

A competent elderly person has the right to choose his or her health-care options. As inappropriate as it may seem, some elderly individuals choose to return to the abusive situation. In this instance, he or she should be provided with names and phone numbers to call for assistance if needed. The nurse should refer for a follow-up visit by an adult protective service representative.

IV. Nursing Process: Diagnosis (Analysis)

Based on data collected during the nursing assessment, possible nursing diagnoses for the client who has survived abuse include:

A. Rape-trauma syndrome related to (R/T) sexual assault as evidence by (AEB) verbalizations of the attack; bruises and lacerations over areas of body; severe anxiety

B. Powerlessness R/T cycle of battering evidenced by verbalizations of abuse; bruises and lacerations over areas of body; fear for safety and that of children; verbalizations of no way to get out of the relationship.

C. Risk for delayed development R/T abusive family situation.

V. Nursing Process: Planning

A. The following outcomes may be developed to guide the care of a client who has been sexually assaulted: **The client will:**

  1. No longer experience panic anxiety.

  2. Demonstrate a degree of trust in the primary nurse.

  3. Receive immediate attention to physical injuries.

  4. Initiate behaviors consistent with the grief response.

B. The following outcomes may be developed to guide the care of a client who has been physically battered: **The client will:**

  1. Receive immediate attention to physical injuries.

  2. Verbalize assurance of his or her immediate safety.

  3. Discuss life situations with primary nurse.

  4. Verbalize choices from which he or she may receive assistance.

C. The following outcomes may be developed to guide the care of a child who has been abused: **The child will:**

  1. Receive immediate attention to physical injuries.

  2. Demonstrate trust in primary nurse by discussing abuse through the use of play therapy.

  3. Demonstrate a decrease in regressive behaviors.

VI. Nursing Process: Implementation for Clients Who Have Survived Abuse

A. Interventions for clients who are experiencing rape-trauma syndrome

  1. It is important to communicate the following to the individual who has been sexually assaulted:

    a. You are safe here.

    b. I'm sorry that it happened.

    c. I'm glad you survived.

    d. It's not your fault. No one deserves to be treated this way.

    e. You did the best that you could.

Someone who has been sexually assaulted fears for his or her life and must be reassured of his or her safety. He or she may also be overwhelmed with self-doubt and self-blame, and it is important to instill trust and validate self-worth.

2. Explain every assessment procedure that will be conducted and why it is being conducted.
3. Ensure that data collection is conducted in a caring, nonjudgmental manner.
4. Ensure that the client has adequate privacy for all immediate postcrisis interventions.
5. Try to have as few people as possible providing the immediate care or collecting immediate evidence.
6. Encourage the client to give an account of the assault; listen but do not probe.
7. Discuss with the client whom to call for support or assistance.
8. Provide information about referrals for aftercare.

DID YOU KNOW?

It is critical to provide referral information in writing for later reference (psychotherapist, mental health clinic, community advocacy group). A client experiencing high levels of anxiety may have trouble focusing, concentrating, and remembering this important information.

B. Interventions for clients who are victims of battering and are experiencing powerlessness
   1. In collaboration with physician, ensure that all physical wounds, fractures, and burns receive immediate attention; take photographs if the individual permits.

Nonjudgmental listening provides an avenue for catharsis that the client needs to begin healing. A detailed account may be required for legal follow-up, and a caring nurse, as client advocate, may help to lessen the trauma of evidence collection.

If the victim is accompanied by the person who did the battering, the victim is not likely to be truthful about the injuries.

2. Take the client to a private area to do the interview.
3. If the victim has come alone or with children, assure the victim of safety.
4. Encourage the victim to discuss the battering incident.
5. Ask questions about whether this has happened before, whether the victimizer takes drugs, whether the victim has a safe place to go, and whether victim wants to consider pressing charges.
6. Ensure that "rescue" efforts are not attempted by the nurse; offer support, but remember that the final decision must be made by the client.

DID YOU KNOW?

When victims make their own decisions, they will gain a sense of control over their life situations. Imposing judgments and giving advice are nontherapeutic.

7. Stress to the individual the importance of safety.

🛑 The battered victim must be made aware of the variety of resources that are available. These may include crisis hot lines, community groups for women who have been abused, shelters, counseling services, and information regarding the victim's rights in the civil and criminal justice system. After a discussion of these available resources, the victim may choose for himself or herself. If her decision is to return to the marriage and home, this choice must be respected.

C. Interventions for children who are experiencing risk for delayed development
   1. Perform complete physical assessment.
   2. Take particular note of bruises (in various stages of healing), lacerations, and client complaints of pain in specific areas.
   3. Do not overlook or discount the possibility of sexual abuse.
   4. Assess for nonverbal signs of abuse: aggressive conduct, excessive fears, extreme hyperactivity, apathy, withdrawal, age-inappropriate behaviors.
   5. Conduct an in-depth interview with the parent or adult who accompanies the child.
      a. If the injury is being reported as an accident, is the explanation reasonable?
      b. Is the injury consistent with the explanation?
      c. Is the injury consistent with the child's developmental capabilities?
   6. Use games or play therapy to gain child's trust.
   7. Use games or play therapy to assist the child in describing his or her side of the story.
   8. Determine whether the nature of the injuries warrants reporting to authorities.

MAKING THE CONNECTION

A report is commonly made if there is reason to suspect that a child has been injured as a result of physical, mental, emotional, or sexual abuse. "Reason to suspect" exists when there is evidence of a discrepancy or inconsistency in explaining a child's injury. Most states require that the following individuals report cases of suspected child abuse: all health-care workers, all mental health therapists, teachers, child-care providers, firefighters, emergency medical personnel, and law enforcement personnel. Reports are made to the Department of Health and Human Services or a law enforcement agency.

MAKING THE CONNECTION

Specific state statutes must enter into the decision of whether to report suspected child abuse. Individual state statutes regarding what constitutes child abuse and neglect may be found at http://www.childwelfare.gov/systemwide/laws_policies/state

---

VII. Nursing Process: Evaluation

A. *Short-term* evaluation of the nursing actions for the client who has survived abuse may be facilitated by gathering information using the following types of questions:
1. Has the individual been reassured of his or her safety?
2. Is this evidenced by a decrease in panic anxiety?
3. Have wounds been properly cared for and provision made for follow-up care?
4. Have emotional needs been attended to?
5. Has trust been established with at least one person to whom the client feels comfortable relating the abusive incident?
6. Have available support systems been identified and notified?
7. Have options for immediate circumstances been presented?

B. *Long-term* evaluation of the nursing actions for the client who has survived abuse may be facilitated by gathering information using the following types of questions:
1. Is the individual able to conduct activities of daily living satisfactorily?
2. Have physical wounds healed properly?
3. Is the client appropriately progressing through the behaviors of grieving?
4. Is the client free of sleep disturbances (nightmares, insomnia), psychosomatic symptoms (headaches, stomach pains, nausea/vomiting), regressive behaviors (enuresis, thumb sucking, phobias), and psychosexual disturbances?
5. Is the individual free from problems with interpersonal relationships?
6. Has the individual considered the alternatives for change in his or her personal life?
7. Has a decision been made relative to the choices available?
8. Is he or she satisfied with the decision that has been made?

VIII. Treatment Modalities

A. Crisis intervention
1. Crisis intervention is time limited (6–8 weeks).
2. Resurfaced problems, beyond this time frame, need to be addressed by other agencies (long-term psychotherapy from a psychiatrist or mental health clinic).
3. Crisis counselor will attempt to help the individual draw on previous successful coping strategies to regain control over his or her life.
4. Crisis intervention if client has been sexually assaulted:
   a. The focus of initial interview and follow-up is on the rape incident alone.
   b. Problems identified but unassociated with the rape are not dealt with at this time.
   c. Goal of crisis intervention is to help survivors return to their previous lifestyle as quickly as possible.
   d. Client should be involved in the intervention.
      i. Promotes a sense of competency, control, and decision making
      ii. Decreases powerlessness and validates personal worth
      iii. Helps to begin the recovery process
   e. Crisis counselor will address symptoms common to the post-trauma client.
      i. Difficulty making decisions
      ii. Extreme or irrational fears
      iii. General mistrust

DID YOU KNOW?
Observable manifestations of posttrauma clients may include stark hysteria, expressions of anger and rage, or silence and withdrawal.

      iv. Guilt and feelings of responsibility for the rape
      v. Numerous physical manifestations
   f. Crisis intervention if client is victim of domestic violence:
      i. Counselor ensures that client is given various resources and options to make informed

           personal decisions regarding what she
           wishes to do with her life

    ii. Support groups help reduce isolation and
       teach new strategies for coping with the
       aftermath of physical or sexual abuse

B. Safe house or shelter

  1. Available in most major cities in the United
     States.

  2. Where victims can go to be assured of protection
     for them and their children (haven for physical
     safety).

  3. Provides a variety of services.

  4. Victims receive emotional support from staff and
     each other.

  5. Avenue for expression of intense emotions.

  6. Victims allowed to grieve for what has been lost
     and for what was expected but not achieved.

  7. Provides help to overcome tremendous guilt
     associated with self-blame; difficult to overcome
     guilt when responsibility has been taken for
     another's behavior over a long period.

  8. Shelter may provide individual and group
     counseling.

  9. Help with bureaucratic institutions such as the
     police, legal representation, and social services.

  10. May provide child care and children's
      programming.

  11. May provide employment counseling and link-
      ages with housing authorities.

  12. Usually run by a combination of professional
      and volunteer staff (nurses, psychologists,
      lawyers, and others).

DID YOU KNOW?

Individuals who themselves were previously abused
are often among the volunteer staff members at safe
houses or battered victim shelters.

MAKING THE CONNECTION

Group work is an important part of the service of shelters. Victims in residence range from those in the immediate crisis phase to those who have progressed through
a variety of phases of the grief process. Those newer
members can learn a great deal from the victims who
have successfully resolved similar problems.

  13. Length of stay varies depending on outside sup-
      port network, financial situation, and personal
      resources.

  14. New arrivals given time to experience relief of a
      safe and secure environment.

  15. Making decisions is discouraged during the
      period of immediate crisis and disorganization.

  16. Once the victim's emotions are stabilized, planning
      for the future begins.

  17. Victim makes own decision about "where he or
      she wants to go from here."

  18. He or she is accepted and supported in whatever
      he or she chooses to do.

C. Family therapy

  1. Focuses on helping families develop democratic
     ways of solving problems; with more frequent use
     of democratic means of conflict resolution, physi-
     cal violence decreases.

  2. Encourages conflict resolution that produces
     mutual benefits for all concerned, rather than
     engaging in power struggles.

  3. Teaches more effective methods of disciplining
     children.

    a. Time-out techniques.

    b. Methods that emphasize positive reinforcement
      for acceptable behavior; to succeed, family
      members must be committed to consistent use
      of these behavior modification techniques.

  4. Teaches parents what to expect from children at
     various stages of development.

  5. Provides anticipatory guidance to deal with the
     crises commonly associated with these stages.

  6. Includes therapy sessions with all family members
     related to communication.

    a. Encourages expression of honest feelings in a
      manner that is nonthreatening to other family
      members.

    b. Teaches active listening, assertiveness tech-
      niques, and respecting the rights of others.

    c. Identifies and seeks to resolve barriers to
      effective communication.

  8. May refer to agencies that promote effective
     parenting skills (parent effectiveness training).

  9. May refer to agencies that may relieve the stress
     of parenting ("Mom's Day Out" programs, sitter-
     sharing organizations, and day-care institutions).

  10. May refer to support groups for abusive parents.

REVIEW QUESTIONS

1. The occurrence of sexual contacts or interaction between, or sexual exploitation of, close relatives, or between participants who are related to each other by a kinship bond that is regarded as a prohibition to sexual relations is termed _____.

2. Abuse is on the rise in this society. From a biological perspective, which of the following factors may predispose individuals to aggressive and violent behavior? **Select all that apply:**
   1. A decrease in serotonin and an increase in norepinephrine and dopamine are implicated in the etiology of aggression.
   2. Some scientists believe that aggressive behavior is primarily a product of one's culture and social structure.
   3. The chromosomal aberration karyotype XYY syndrome may be linked to aggressive and deviant behavior.
   4. Organic brain syndromes associated with various cerebral disorders have been implicated in the predisposition to aggressive behavior.
   5. Parents who display aggressive and violent behavior may produce children who display the same behaviors as adults.

3. A nursing instructor is teaching students about the characteristics of a child abuser. Which of the following student statements indicates that learning has occurred? **Select all that apply.**
   1. It is reported that 60% of parents who abuse their children were severely physically abused by their own parents.
   2. Often abusers lack support systems and are commonly isolated from others.
   3. Abusers often experience stressful life situations such as unemployment and poverty.
   4. Abusers lack coping strategies, have anger issues, and have difficulty trusting others.
   5. Abusers have low expectations of their children and seldom compare their child's behavior to other children's.

4. In writing a plan of care for a child who has been physically abused, the nurse would consider which intervention a priority?
   1. Conduct an in-depth interview with the parent or adult who accompanies the child
   2. Perform complete physical assessment of the child
   3. Determine whether the nature of the injuries warrant reporting to the authorities
   4. Use games or play therapy to gain the child's trust

5. A young woman is brought to the emergency department (ED) after being attacked and violently raped. She screams, "I'll kill him with my bare hands." At this time, which priority nursing diagnosis would the nurse assign to this client?
   1. Rape-trauma syndrome
   2. Risk for suicide
   3. Sexual dysfunction
   4. Risk for other-directed violence

6. A nurse documents the following nursing diagnosis: *risk for delayed development.* Which client symptom led to this evaluation?
   1. A female with repressed anxiety and unmet dependency needs
   2. Dysfunctional grieving process and lifestyle of helplessness
   3. A child with unexplained burns, bites, bruises, and broken bones
   4. A foul-smelling, disheveled male

7. A timid 4-year-old child has recently been hospitalized with unexplained bruises, burns, and welts on back, buttocks, and legs. Which priority nursing diagnosis would the nurse assign to this child?
   1. Risk for self-mutilation
   2. Risk for other-directed violence
   3. Risk for delayed development
   4. Risk for suicide

8. When establishing a plan of care for a client with a nursing diagnosis of rape-trauma syndrome, which is an appropriate outcome?
   1. The client will demonstrate behaviors consistent with age-appropriate growth and development.
   2. The client will exhibit physical wound healing without complications.
   3. The client will verbally acknowledge misconception of body image.
   4. The client will verbalize aspects about sexuality that he or she would like to change.

9. A 25-year-old woman has been admitted to the hospital after being physically battered by her husband. When writing a plan of care, which client outcome should the nurse prioritize?
   1. The client will discuss life situations with the nurse.
   2. The client will make appropriate choices to access assistance.
   3. The client will verbalize assurance of her immediate safety.
   4. The client will receive immediate attention to physical injuries.

10. After a female victim of battering has been medically treated and advised of available resources, the victim decides to return to the marriage and home. Which appropriate plan of action should the nurse pursue?
    1. Notify the Family Violence Law Center of this client's decision.
    2. Enroll the client in a victim/victimizer support group.
    3. Respect the victim's decision to return to her marriage and husband.
    4. Make an immediate referral to a domestic violence therapist.

11. A sexually assaulted female has been treated in the ED for multiple cuts and abrasions. Now, in an attempt to calm and comfort this frightened client, which nursing intervention would take priority?
    1. Communicate to the client that it was not her fault.
    2. Communicate to the client that you are sorry it happened.
    3. Communicate to the client that you are glad she survived.
    4. Communicate to the client that she is safe at this time.

12. An ED nurse suspects that a child has been physically abused. Which of the following signs and symptoms should the nurse recognize as reflective of the nursing diagnosis: *Risk for injury R/T abusive family situation*? **Select all that apply.**
    1. A child clutching and clinging to parent
    2. A child exhibiting unexplained burns, bites, bruises, broken bones, or black eyes
    3. A child with fading bruises or other marks noticeable after an absence from school
    4. A child protesting or crying when it is time to go home
    5. A child shrinking away at the approach of adults

13. A pattern of coercive control founded on and supported by physical and/or violence or threat of violence on an intimate partner is termed _____.

14. After a month's observation, the school nurse suspects that a 7-year-old child is being emotionally abused at home. Which of the following signs and symptoms would have led the school nurse to this conclusion? **Select all that apply.**
    1. The child seems frightened and resists going home from school.
    2. The child shows extremes in passive or aggressive behavior.
    3. The child has attempted suicide.
    4. The child has delays in physical and emotional development.
    5. The child reports hearing voices and seeing angry ghosts.

15. An instructor is teaching students about what signs to look for when child physical and emotional neglect is suspected. Which of the following student statements indicates that learning has occurred? **Select all that apply.**
    1. "A child is frequently absent from school."
    2. "A child begs or steals food or money."
    3. "A child contracts a venereal disease."
    4. "A child lacks sufficient clothing for the weather."
    5. "A child uses alcohol or other drugs."

16. The expression of power and dominance by means of sexual violence, most commonly by men over women, although men may also be victims is termed _____.

17. A seventh-grade teacher asks the school nurse, "What should I look for if I suspect that a child is being sexually abused?" The nurse's response should include which of the following signs and symptoms? **Select all that apply.**
    1. A child has difficulty walking or sitting
    2. A child suddenly refuses to change for gym or participate in activities
    3. A child is constantly dirty and has severe body odor
    4. A child suddenly experiences a change in appetite
    5. A child reports nightmares or bedwetting

18. A pediatric postgraduate nursing student is writing a research thesis on the signs and symptoms that are characteristic of emotionally abused children. Which of the following should be included in the research thesis? **Select all that apply.**
    1. Extremes in behavior, for example, compliant or demanding behavior, extreme passivity or aggression
    2. Acting either inappropriately adult (parenting other children) or inappropriately infantile
    3. Participating in frequent rocking or head banging
    4. Frequently begging or stealing food
    5. Reporting a lack of attachment to the parent

19. A female client is an adult survivor of incest and has just been hospitalized with severe depression. Which of the following signs and symptoms would the nurse expect to assess? **Select all that apply.**
    1. Self-care deficit
    2. Agoraphobia
    3. Low self-esteem and poor sense of identity
    4. Feelings of guilt
    5. Distorted association of pleasure with sexual activity

20. Which of the following characteristics would a nurse understand as common to the profile of a victim of rape? **Select all that apply.**
    1. Likely to have been acquainted with the victimizer
    2. Likely to be over age 40
    3. Likely to have been attacked close to home
    4. Likely to have been threaten and subdued by a knife
    5. Likely to be a single woman

REVIEW ANSWERS

1. ANSWER: incest

Rationale: Incest is sexual activity between family members or close relatives. This typically includes sexual activity between people in a consanguineous relationship (blood relations) and sometimes those related by affinity, such as individuals of the same household, step relatives, those related by adoption or marriage, or members of the same clan or lineage.

TEST-TAKING TIP: Review key terms at beginning of chapter.
Content Area: Psychosocial Integrity;
Integrated Process: Nursing Process: Assessment;
Client Need: Psychosocial Integrity;
Cognitive Level: Knowledge;
Concept: Sexuality

2. ANSWERS: 1, 3, 4

Rationale:

1. **From a biological perspective, studies show that various neurotransmitters—in particular serotonin, norepinephrine, and dopamine—may play a role in the facilitation and inhibition of aggressive behaviors.**

2. From a sociocultural, not biological, perspective, scientists believe that aggressive behavior is primarily a product of one's culture and social structure.

3. **From a biological perspective, chromosomal aberration karyotype XYY syndrome has been found to contribute to aggressive behavior in a small percentage of cases.**

4. **From a biological perspective, organic brain syndromes associated with various cerebral disorders have been implicated in the predisposition to aggressive and violent behavior.**

5. From a learning, not biological, perspective, parents who display aggressive and violent behavior may produce children who display the same behaviors as adults.

TEST-TAKING TIP: Review the etiological implications that predispose individuals to be abusive. Note that all answers are correct; however, only Options 1, 3, and 4 are based from a biological perspective.
Content Area: Psychosocial Integrity;
Integrated Process: Nursing Process: Assessment;
Client Need: Psychosocial Integrity;
Cognitive Level: Application;
Concept: Violence

3. ANSWERS: 2, 3, 4

Rationale:

1. It has been reported that 90%, not 60%, of parents who abuse their children were severely physically abused by their own parents. This student's statement indicates that further instruction is needed.

2. **It has been noted that child abusers lack support systems and are commonly isolated from others. This student's statement indicates that learning has occurred.**

3. **Unemployment and poverty are common stressors that child abusers often experience. This student's statement indicates that learning has occurred.**

4. **Child abusers often lack coping strategies, have anger issues, and have difficulty trusting others. This student's statement indicates that learning has occurred.**

5. Child abusers have high, not low, expectations of their child. In fact, they expect their child to be perfect and may exaggerate any mild behavioral difference their child manifests. This student's statement indicates that further instruction is needed.

TEST-TAKING TIP: Review the profile of a child abuser.
Content Area: Safe and Effective Care Environment: Management of Care;
Integrated Process: Nursing Process: Implementation;
Client Need: Safe and Effective Care Environment: Management of Care;
Cognitive Level: Application;
Concept: Nursing Roles

4. ANSWER: 2

Rationale:

1. Conducting an in-depth interview with the parent or the adult who accompanies the child is an important intervention; however, the priority safety intervention is to determine the extent of the child's injuries.

2. **An accurate and thorough physical assessment is necessary to detect any life-threatening injuries and provide needed care. This intervention prioritizes client safety.**

3. Determining whether the nature of the injuries warrants reporting to the authorities is an important intervention; however, the priority safety intervention is to determine the extent of the child's injuries.

4. Using games or play therapy to establish a trusting relationship with an abused child is an important intervention; however, the priority safety intervention is to determine the extent of the child's injuries.

TEST-TAKING TIP: Interventions that provide client safety are always prioritized when planning client care.
Content Area: Safe and Effective Care Environment: Management of Care;
Integrated Process: Nursing Process: Planning;
Client Need: Safe and Effective Care Environment: Management of Care;
Cognitive Level: Analysis;
Concept: Nursing

5. ANSWER: 1

Rationale:

1. **Rape-trauma syndrome is defined as a sustained maladaptive response to a forced, violent sexual penetration against the victim's will and consent. The client in the question has been attacked and violently raped and therefore meets the criteria for this priority nursing diagnosis.**

2. There is nothing presented in the question to indicate that this client is suicidal. Therefore, a *Risk for Suicide* nursing diagnosis would not apply.

3. Sexual dysfunction is defined as the state in which an individual experiences a change in sexual function during a sexual response phase of desire, excitation, and/or orgasm, which is viewed as unsatisfying, unrewarding, or inadequate. There is nothing in the question indicating that the client is experiencing sexual dysfunction.

4. Threats of violence directed at others must be reported, but, *at this time,* while being treated in the ED, these threats cannot be accomplished. If the client continues to voice homicidal ideations, it then becomes a priority concern.

TEST-TAKING TIP: Note the wording in the question, *priority* and *at this time*, which will lead to determining the nursing diagnosis of rape-trauma syndrome.
Content Area: *Safe and Effective Care Environment: Management of Care;*
Integrated Process: *Nursing Process: Diagnosis (Analysis);*
Client Need: *Safe and Effective Care Environment: Management of Care;*
Cognitive Level: *Analysis;*
Concept: *Critical Thinking*

6. **ANSWER: 3**
Rationale:
1. The nursing diagnosis of *ineffective coping*, not *risk for delayed development*, would document and address a client's repressed anxiety and unmet dependency needs.
2. The nursing diagnosis of *powerlessness*, not *risk for delayed development*, would document and address a client's dysfunctional grieving process and lifestyle of helplessness.
3. The nursing diagnosis of *risk for delayed development* would document and address a situation in which family members have been abusive to a child, causing burns, bites, bruises, and broken bones. This abuse would possibly lead to the delayed development of this child.
4. The nursing diagnosis of *self-care deficit*, not *risk for delayed development*, would document and address a client's inability to meet the requirements for personal hygiene.
TEST-TAKING TIP: Familiarize yourself with symptoms associated with the nursing diagnosis of *risk for delayed development* and recognize that child abuse can delay normal development.
Content Area: *Safe and Effective Care Environment: Management of Care;*
Integrated Process: *Nursing Process: Diagnosis (Analysis);*
Client Need: *Safe and Effective Care Environment: Management of Care;*
Cognitive Level: *Analysis;*
Concept: *Critical Thinking*

7. **ANSWER: 3**
Rationale:
1. There is nothing in the question indicating that this child is self-mutilating. The welts on back and buttocks would make self-infliction improbable.
2. There is nothing in the question indicating that this child is at risk for inflicting bodily harm to others. Being timid and 4 years old, child would not be likely to strike out at others.
3. If there has been a pattern of abuse associated with this child's injuries, the child is at risk for delayed development. Compared with the other nursing diagnoses presented, *risk for delayed development* would be the first concern and the priority nursing diagnosis.
4. There is nothing in the question indicating that this child is at risk for suicide. At age 4, suicide would not be associated with behaviors or thoughts consistent with age-appropriate actions.
TEST-TAKING TIP: Review the victims of abuse section in the chapter and familiarize yourself with nursing diagnoses associated with the abused child. The key word "timid" helps to eliminate Option 2.

Content Area: *Safe and Effective Care Environment: Management of Care;*
Integrated Process: *Nursing Process: Diagnosis (Analysis);*
Client Need: *Safe and Effective Care Environment: Management of Care;*
Cognitive Level: *Analysis;*
Concept: *Critical Thinking*

8. **ANSWER: 2**
Rationale:
1. The outcome of demonstrating behaviors consistent with age-appropriate growth and development would be created for the nursing diagnosis of *risk for delayed development*, not *rape-trauma syndrome*.
2. The outcome of having physical wounds heal without complications is an appropriate outcome for an individual with the nursing diagnosis of *rape-trauma syndrome*.
3. The outcome of verbally acknowledging the misconception of body image would be created for the nursing diagnosis of *disturbed body image* associated with an eating disorder, not a nursing diagnosis of *rape-trauma syndrome*.
4. The outcome of verbalizing aspects about sexuality that he or she would like to change would be created for the nursing diagnosis of *ineffective sexuality pattern*, not a nursing diagnosis of *rape-trauma syndrome*.
TEST-TAKING TIP: Review the victims of rape section presented in the chapter and familiarize yourself with the outcome criteria for various problems facing these individuals.
Content Area: *Safe and Effective Care Environment: Management of Care;*
Integrated Process: *Nursing Process: Planning;*
Client Need: *Safe and Effective Care Environment: Management of Care;*
Cognitive Level: *Application;*
Concept: *Critical Thinking*

9. **ANSWER: 4**
Rationale: Psychologist Abraham Maslow defined basic human needs as a hierarchy, a progression from simple physical needs to more complex emotional needs. These basic physiological needs have a greater priority over those higher on the pyramid.
1. Although it is important that the client be able to discuss life situations with the nurse, physical safety is a basic human need and must take priority.
2. Although it is important that the client make appropriate choices to receive assistance, receiving immediate attention to physical injuries is always the priority.
3. Although it is important that the client be able to verbalize understanding of her immediate safety, receiving immediate attention to physical injuries is always the priority.
4. Receiving immediate attention to physical injuries is the priority outcome to maintain client safety.
TEST-TAKING TIP: Review the victims of battering section presented in the chapter and familiarize yourself with the outcome criteria for these individuals. Also review Maslow's Hierarchy of Needs.
Content Area: *Safe and Effective Care Environment: Management of Care;*
Integrated Process: *Nursing Process: Planning;*

Client Need: Safe and Effective Care Environment: Management of Care;
Cognitive Level: Application;
Concept: Critical Thinking

10. **ANSWER: 3**
Rationale:
1. After all available resources have been explored, the client's choice to return to the marriage and home must be respected. The nurse should not usurp the client's decision by notifying the Family Violence Law Center.
2. After all available resources have been explored, the client's choice to return to the marriage and home must be respected. The nurse should not usurp the client's decision by enrolling the client in a victim/victimizer support group.
3. The battered victim must be made aware of the variety of resources that are available. These may include crisis hot lines, community groups for victims who have been abused, shelters, counseling services, and information regarding the victim's rights in the civil and criminal justice system. After a discussion of these available resources, the victim may choose for herself. If her decision is to return to the marriage and home, this choice must be respected.
4. After all available resources have been explored, the client's choice to return to the marriage and home must be respected. The nurse should not usurp the client's decision by making an immediate referral to a domestic violence therapist.
TEST-TAKING TIP: Review the victims of battering section presented in the chapter and become familiar with the guidelines that would assist the nurse in appropriately caring for a victim of abuse. Remember, regardless of a client's poor decisions, the nurse must respect client choices.
Content Area: Safe and Effective Care Environment: Management of Care;
Integrated Process: Nursing Process: Planning;
Client Need: Safe and Effective Care Environment: Management of Care;
Cognitive Level: Application;
Concept: Nursing

11. **ANSWER: 4**
Rationale:
1. It is important to communicate to the individual who has been sexually assaulted that the attack was not her fault; however, the priority intervention in this situation is to reassure the victim that she is safe. Unless this frightened victim is assured of her safety, high anxiety levels will prevent the effectiveness of other interventions.
2. It is important to show empathy by communicating to the client that you are sorry the sexual assault happened; however, the priority intervention in this situation is to reassure the victim that she is safe. Unless this frightened victim is assured of her safely, high anxiety levels with prevent the effectiveness of other interventions.
3. It is important to show empathy by communicating to the client that you are glad that she survived; however, the priority intervention in this situation is to reassure the victim that she is safe. Unless this frightened victim is

assured of her safely, high anxiety levels with prevent the effectiveness of other interventions.
4. Once the victim's physical wounds are treated, communicating to the client that she is safe is the priority nursing intervention. Unless this frightened victim is assured of her safely, all other interventions will have little or no value.
TEST-TAKING TIP: Remember that high levels of anxiety affect a client's ability to concentrated, communicate, and understand directions, skills needed to benefit from important nursing care.
Content Area: Safe and Effective Care Environment: Management of Care;
Integrated Process: Nursing Process: Implementation;
Client Need: Safe and Effective Care Environment: Management of Care;
Cognitive Level: Application;
Concept: Nursing

12. **ANSWERS: 2, 3, 4, 5**
Rationale:
1. A nurse who suspects child abuse would expect fearful, not clutching and clinging, behaviors toward parental figures.
2. A nurse who suspects child abuse would expect a child to exhibit evidence of unexplained burns, bites, bruises, broken bones, or black eyes.
3. A nurse who suspects child abuse would expect a child to show evidence of fading bruises or other marks noticeable after an absence from school.
4. A nurse who suspects child abuse would expect a child to be frightened of the parents and protest or cry when it is time to go home.
5. A nurse who suspects child abuse would expect a child to shrink away at the approach of adults.
TEST-TAKING TIP: Familiarize yourself with the symptoms associated with physical abuse of a child.
Content Area: Safe and Effective Care Environment: Management of Care;
Integrated Process: Nursing Process: Evaluation;
Client Need: Safe and Effective Care Environment: Management of Care;
Cognitive Level: Application;
Concept: Assessment

13. **ANSWER: battering**
Rationale: Battering is a pattern of repeated physical assault usually of a woman by her spouse or intimate partner. Men are also battered, although this occurs much less frequently.
TEST-TAKING TIP: Review key terms at beginning of chapter.
Content Area: Psychosocial Integrity;
Integrated Process: Nursing Process: Assessment;
Client Need: Psychosocial Integrity;
Cognitive Level: Knowledge;
Concept: Violence

14. **ANSWERS: 2, 3, 4**
Rationale:
1. The school nurse might observe this behavior when a child frightened of going home is being physically, not emotionally, abused.

2. The school nurse would suspect emotional abuse if a child shows extremes in behavior, such as overly compliant or demanding behavior, extreme passivity, or aggression.

3. The school nurse would suspect emotional abuse if a child has attempted suicide.

4. The school nurse would suspect emotional abuse if a child has delays in physical or emotional development.

5. If a child reports hearing voices and seeing angry ghosts, the school nurse might suspect a sensory perception disorder, not emotional abuse.

TEST-TAKING TIP: Familiarize yourself with the signs and symptoms associated with emotional abuse. Remember that child maltreatment typically includes physical or emotional injury, physical or emotional neglect, or sexual acts inflicted on a child by a caregiver.

Content Area: Safe and Effective Care Environment: Management of Care;
Integrated Process: Nursing Process: Assessment;
Client Need: Safe and Effective Care Environment: Management of Care;
Cognitive Level: Application;
Concept: Assessment

15. **ANSWERS: 1, 2, 4, 5**
Rationale:

1. Frequent absences from school may indicate that a child is experiencing physical or emotional neglect. This student's statement indicates that learning has occurred.

2. A child begging or stealing food or money may indicate that a child is experiencing physical or emotional neglect. This student's statement indicates that learning has occurred.

3. A child contracting a venereal disease may be a sign that the child is experiencing sexual abuse, not physical or emotional neglect. This student's statement indicates that further instruction is needed.

4. When a child lacks sufficient clothing for the weather, the child may be experiencing physical or emotional neglect. This student's statement indicates that learning has occurred.

5. When a child uses alcohol or other drugs, the child may be experiencing physical or emotional neglect. This student's statement indicates that learning has occurred.

TEST-TAKING TIP: Review the physical and emotional neglect section of the chapter. Remember that child maltreatment typically includes physical or emotional injury, physical or emotional neglect, or sexual acts inflicted on a child by a caregiver.

Content Area: Safe and Effective Care Environment: Management of Care;
Integrated Process: Nursing Process: Implementation;
Client Need: Safe and Effective Care Environment: Management of Care;
Cognitive Level: Application;
Concept: Nursing Roles

16. **ANSWER: rape**
Rationale: Rape is a type of sexual assault usually involving sexual intercourse or other forms of sexual penetration perpetrated against a person without that person's consent. The act may be carried out by physical force, coercion, abuse of authority or against a person who is incapable of valid consent, such as one who is unconscious, incapacitated, or below the legal age of consent. The term *rape* is sometimes used interchangeably with the term *sexual assault.*

TEST-TAKING TIP: Review key terms at beginning of chapter.
Content Area: Psychosocial Integrity;
Integrated Process: Nursing Process: Assessment;
Client Need: Psychosocial Integrity;
Cognitive Level: Knowledge;
Concept: Violence

17. **ANSWERS: 1, 2, 4, 5**
Rationale:

1. The teacher might suspect sexual abuse if she notices that the child has difficulty walking or sitting.

2. The teacher might suspect sexual abuse if she notices that the child suddenly refuses to change for gym or participate in activities.

3. A child who is constantly dirty and has severe body odor would be suspected of being physically or emotionally neglected, not sexually abused.

4. The teacher might suspect sexual abuse if she notices that the child suddenly experiences a change in appetite.

5. The teacher might suspect sexual abuse if the child suddenly reports nightmares or bedwetting.

TEST-TAKING TIP: Review the sexual abuse of a child section in the chapter. Remember that child maltreatment typically includes physical or emotional injury, physical or emotional neglect, or sexual acts inflicted upon a child by a caregiver.
Content Area: Safe and Effective Care Environment: Management of Care;
Integrated Process: Nursing Process: Implementation;
Client Need: Safe and Effective Care Environment: Management of Care;
Cognitive Level: Application;
Concept: Assessment

18. **ANSWERS: 1, 2, 3, 5**
Rationale:

1. Extremes in behavior might be indicative of a child that is being emotionally abused. This symptom should be included in the student's thesis.

2. Acting either inappropriately adult or infantile might be indicative of a child that is being emotionally abused. This symptom should be included in the student's thesis.

3. Participating in frequent rocking or head banging might be indicative of a child that is being emotionally abused. This symptom should be included in the student's thesis.

4. Frequently begging or stealing food might be indicative of a child that is being physically neglected, not emotionally abused. This symptom should not be included in the student's thesis.

5. A lack of attachment to the parent might be indicative of a child that is being emotionally abused. This symptom should be included in the student's thesis.

TEST-TAKING TIP: Review the emotional abuse of a child section in the chapter. Remember that child maltreatment

typically includes physical or emotional injury, physical or emotional neglect, or sexual acts inflicted on a child by a caregiver.
Content Area: Safe and Effective Care Environment: Management of Care;
Integrated Process: Nursing Process: Implementation;
Client Need: Safe and Effective Care Environment: Management of Care;
Cognitive Level: Application;
Concept: Violence

19. **ANSWERS: 3, 4, 5**
Rationale:
1. Survivors of incest can experience severe depression leading to an impaired ability to perform or complete activities of daily living independently; however, *self-care deficit* is a nursing diagnosis, not a sign or symptom that reflects this client's problem. The symptoms of self-care deficit might include disheveled appearance, body odor, and/or halitosis.
2. A survivor of incest may exhibit many symptoms of anxiety, but agoraphobia is not typically experienced. *Agoraphobia* is defined as the fear of being in places or situations in which escape might be difficult or in which help might not be available in the event of a panic attack.
3. Survivors of incest have a history of unsatisfactory parent-child relationships leading to a low self-esteem and a poor sense of identity.
4. Survivors of incest develop feelings of guilt with the realization over the years that the parents are using them in an attempt to solve their own problems.
5. Survivors of incest commonly have distorted development of a normal association of pleasure and sexual activity. Peer relationships are often delayed, altered, inhibited, or perverted. They may completely retreat from sexual activity and avoid all close interpersonal relationships throughout life.

Review the adult survivor of incest section in this chapter. When asked for a sign or symptom, assessment data is required.
Content Area: Safe and Effective Care Environment: Management of Care;
Integrated Process: Nursing Process: Assessment;
Client Need: Safe and Effective Care Environment: Management of Care;
Cognitive Level: Application;
Concept: Assessment

20. **ANSWERS: 3, 4, 5**
Rationale:
1. Choice of victim is based on chance availability, not previous acquaintance. In a study of a prison sample of rapists, it was found that victims were not chosen for any reason having to do with appearance or behavior but simply because the individual happened to be in a certain place at a certain time.
2. Although rape can occur at any age, the highest risk age-group is between ages 16 and 34 years, not over age 40.
3. Most rape victims are single women, and the attack frequently occurs in or close to the victim's own neighborhood.
4. It has been found that 62% of rapists use a weapon, most frequently a knife. They use the weapon to terrorize and subdue the victim but not to inflict serious injury.
5. Statistics show that most sexual assault victims are single women.
TEST-TAKING TIP: Review the characteristics of victims of rape.
Content Area: Safe and Effective Care Environment: Management of Care;
Integrated Process: Nursing Process: Assessment;
Client Need: Safe and Effective Care Environment: Management of Care;
Cognitive Level: Application;
Concept: Violence

CASE STUDY: Putting it All Together

Allie is a petite, shy 6-year-old. At this time, she is sitting in a puddle of urine in the emergency department (ED), sucking her thumb while holding and rubbing her arm. As she cries out in pain, her mother, Carol, sits close and attempts to comfort her. As the ED nurse approaches, Allie grimaces, cries, "No," and shrinks away.

This is not Allie's first ED visit. History reveals that at 9 months, Allie was treated for burns on her chest and abdomen when she reportedly pulled a cup of hot coffee off an end table. At 3 years of age, she reportedly fell down a flight of stairs and fractured her femur. X-rays now reveal a fractured left ulna midway between the wrist and elbow. It is noted that handprint bruising encircles the fracture. Also noted are new and old pencil eraser–sized scars and burns on Allie's legs, arms, and buttocks.

When asked how her arm got hurt, Allie says, "Go away," hides behind her mother, and refuses to talk. Carol quickly says, "I was in the house when she fell off the swing in the back yard. You know how kids are." When asked about the handprint bruising, her mother states, "That's probably where I grabbed her arm to break the fall." When the nurse reminds Carol that she reported being in the house when the fall occurred, she begins to cry, "I didn't mean to hurt her. I really didn't."

A call is placed to the hospital's psychiatric nurse practitioner (PNP), Macie. While Allie's mother fills out paperwork for a complete physical and x-rays, Macie takes Allie aside, cleans her up, and begins gently talking to her. Macie tells Allie what a brave girl she is and how some day she'd like a little girl just like her. Allie warms up immediately and says, "Maybe I could go home with you and be your little girl."

As Allie's arm is being casted, Macie interviews Carol. Still tearful, Carol talks about living in poverty and being physically and sexually abused as a child. She admits that her pregnancy with Allie resulted in a split from her boyfriend and her resentful feelings toward the unborn child. "I do love her, though," Carol wails. "Allie was potty trained by 2; but, all of a sudden, she's now wetting her pants. When she doesn't act like other normal kids, I just lose it!" On the basis of physical evidence and inconsistencies in the reporting of the event by the mother, Macie notifies the Department of Health and Human Services.

1. On the basis of Allie's symptoms, past history of injuries, and reporting inconsistencies, what medical diagnosis would Macie assign to Allie?
2. What are Allie's subjective symptoms that would lead to the determination of this diagnosis?
3. What are Allie's objective symptoms that would lead to the determination of this diagnosis?
4. What inconsistency, revelation, and characteristic profile did Carol present that might have led the PNP to notify the Department of Health and Human Services?
5. On the basis of Allie's diagnosis, what treatment might Macie consider to address Allie's situation?
6. On the basis of Carol's behavior, what treatments might Macie consider to assist with Carol's problems?
7. What North American Nursing Diagnosis Association (NANDA) nursing diagnosis would be appropriate for Allie?
8. On the basis of this nursing diagnosis, what short-term outcomes would be appropriate for Allie?
9. On the basis of this nursing diagnosis, what long-term outcomes would be appropriate for Allie?
10. List the nursing interventions (actions) that will assist Allie in successfully meeting these outcomes.
11. List the questions that should be answered in determining the success of the nursing actions.

Chapter 20

Comprehensive Final Examination

1. A mental disorder is defined as a health condition characterized by significant dysfunction in which of the following? **Select all that apply.**
   1. Emotions
   2. Values
   3. Cognitions
   4. Behaviors
   5. Ethics

2. Which of the following are characteristics of mild anxiety? **Select all that apply.**
   1. Mild anxiety enhances learning.
   2. Mild anxiety leads to confusion and loss of concentration.
   3. Mild anxiety increases motivation.
   4. Mild anxiety requires problem-solving assistance.
   5. Mild anxiety prepares people for action.

3. Which immediate biological responses are associated with fight-or-flight syndrome?
   1. Bronchioles in the lungs dilate, and respiration rate increases.
   2. Vasopressin increases fluid retention and vasoconstriction, increasing blood pressure.
   3. Hormones stimulate the thyroid gland to increase metabolic rate.
   4. Gonadotropins cause a decrease in secretion of sex hormone and produce impotence.

4. Which individual would be at the highest risk for a diagnosis of mental illness?
   1. An individual who sees situations as either all good or all bad.
   2. An individual who drinks alcohol but is never late for work.
   3. An individual who is estranged from alcoholic relatives.
   4. An individual who steadfastly defends a pro-life stance.

5. A client expresses frustration and hostility toward the nursing staff regarding the lack of care a recently deceased parent received. According to Kübler-Ross, which stage of grief is this client experiencing?
   1. Anger
   2. Disequilibrium
   3. Developing awareness
   4. Bargaining

6. A 9-year-old child tells the nurse that she has been chosen as captain of her soccer team. According to Peplau, which psychological stage of development should the nurse determine that this child has completed?
   1. "Learning to count on others."
   2. "Learning to delay satisfaction."
   3. "Identifying oneself."
   4. "Developing skills in participation."

7. After studying the concepts of personality development, the nursing student understands that Peplau is to nursing theory as Freud is to:
   1. Psychosocial theory
   2. Psychoanalytic theory
   3. Interpersonal theory
   4. Object relations theory

8. Order the stages of cognitive development according to Jean Piaget.
   1. _____ Formal operations
   2. _____ Preoperational
   3. _____ Sensorimotor
   4. _____ Concrete operations

9. Mahler would assign the term _____ _____ to a 4-year-old child who is completely emotionally attached to mother and reacts stressfully if the possibility of separation occurs.

10. A 16-year-old mother brings her malnourished, irritable, and dirty 10-week-old infant to the clinic. A diagnosis of "failure to thrive" is assigned. According to Erikson, this child is at risk for developing which negative outcome?
    1. Guilt
    2. Inferiority
    3. Shame and doubt
    4. Mistrust

11. A nurse is teaching a parent whose child has been diagnosed with schizophrenia. Which of the following information should the nurse include about the National Alliance on Mental Illness (NAMI)? **Select all that apply.**
    1. NAMI advocates for access to services for the mentally ill.
    2. NAMI provides free education about mental illness.
    3. NAMI supplies prescribed antipsychotic drugs.
    4. NAMI provides affordable housing for the mentally ill.
    5. NAMI supports research related to mental illness.

12. According to the public health model, an intervention that is aimed at minimizing early symptoms of psychiatric illness and directed toward reducing the prevalence and duration of the illness is referred to as _____ prevention.

13. A psychiatrist who embraces the psychological recovery model tells the nurse that a client is in the *Rebuilding* stage. What should the nurse expect to find when assessing this client?
    1. A client feeling a sense of personal empowerment
    2. A client setting realistic goals
    3. A client resolving to begin the work of recovery
    4. A client who is confident in managing symptoms

14. As a basic concept of the recovery model, the _____ maintains primary control over clinical decision making.

15. As part of discharge planning, a nurse is teaching a client's family about possible reasons for medication nonadherence. Which of the following should the nurse include? **Select all that apply.**
    1. Adverse side effects can cause medication nonadherence.
    2. Medication cost can be a factor in medication nonadherence.
    3. As symptoms decrease, clients may feel no need for continued medication.
    4. It may be difficult for the client to accept a diagnosis of mental illness.
    5. Misunderstanding of instructions can contribute to nonadherence.

16. Order the following behaviors that typically occur in the three phases of the group development process.
    1. _____ The members may experience stages of the grief process.
    2. _____ The members are overly polite due to fear of rejection by the group.
    3. _____ The members turn to each other rather than the leader for guidance.

17. Which nursing diagnosis should a nurse identify as being correctly formulated?
    1. Bipolar disorder R/T biochemical alterations AEB manic behavior
    2. Disturbed sleep pattern R/T hyperactivity AEB midnight awakenings
    3. Anxiety R/T racing thoughts
    4. Risk for injury R/T sleep deprivation AEB unsteady gait

18. In teaching a nursing student about the African American cultural group, which information should the nursing instructor include?
    1. The majority of African Americans place little value on strong religious beliefs.
    2. Sickle cell anemia occurs predominantly in African Americans.
    3. Many African American households are headed by men.
    4. In the Deep South, the African American folk practitioner is known as a shaman.

19. Which of the following describe nonverbal communication? **Select all that apply.**
    1. Written documentation
    2. Gestures
    3. Body posture
    4. General appearance
    5. Colloquialisms

20. Which of the following contributes to nonverbal communication? **Select all that apply.**
    1. Vocal cues
    2. Topic of discussion
    3. Open posture
    4. Eye contact

21. When communicating with each other in public, Arab Americans may stand close together, maintain steady eye contact, and _____ only members of the same sex.

22. A client states, "Since I don't know why I have to attend group therapy, I won't be there today." Which is an example of the nontherapeutic communication block of "requesting an explanation"?
    1. "You must attend group to get the benefit of this therapy."
    2. "Your psychiatrist wouldn't include group in your plan of care if it was not beneficial."
    3. "Why do you feel this way about attending group therapy?"
    4. "Your psychiatrist has prescribed group therapy to provide an opportunity for you to interact with others experiencing similar problems."

23. A nursing instructor is teaching about nonverbal communication. Which student statement indicates a need for further instruction?
    1. "Nonverbal communication makes up the majority of all effective communication."
    2. "Touch is a form of nonverbal communication, and its use is culturally determined."
    3. "Nonverbal communication should be congruent with verbal communication."
    4. "Physical appearance is not considered a component of nonverbal communication."

24. In response to the client's statement, "I'm disappointed that my antidepressant medication isn't working yet," the nurse states, "A lot of clients expect a quick fix." The nurse has used the nontherapeutic block of _____ feelings.

25. Which is an example of the communication technique of "focusing"?
    1. Client: "I'm just not as sharp as I used to be."
       Nurse: "I'm not sure what you mean when you use the word 'sharp.'"
    2. Client: "When I am faced with failure, I can't seem to be able to experience any emotions."
       Nurse: "Feeling nothing must make you feel empty."
    3. Client: "My anger makes me want to quit my job. I need the money. I'm powerless over this situation."
       Nurse: "Let's talk about what precipitates your anger."
    4. Client: "I can't feel anything."
       Nurse: "You can't feel anything?"

26. A nursing instructor provides the following nurse-client interactions and asks a student to choose examples of *reflection*. Which student choice indicates that further instruction is needed?
    1. Client: "I hate that this arthritis is crippling me."
       Nurse: "You're angry that your disease is limiting your functioning?"
    2. Client: "The doctor said that schizophrenia will be with me for my whole life."
       Nurse: "Sounds like you are disappointed that this disease is not curable."
    3. Client: "I can't believe I yelled at my roommate last night."
       Nurse: "Sounds like you are embarrassed by your behavior."
    4. Client: "I attended every group therapy session this week."
       Nurse: "I am very pleased that you took my advice and attended those activities."

27. Which situation exemplifies an ethical egoism perspective?
    1. A teenager abides by the curfew set by his or her parents because disappointing them would make the teenager feel guilty.
    2. A teenager abides by the curfew set by his or her parents because not doing so is against the house rules.
    3. A teenager abides by the curfew set by his or her parents because he or she would not want to hurt the parents' feelings.
    4. A teenager abides by the curfew set by parents because he or she wants to maintain his or her set allowance and other privileges.

28. A nursing instructor is teaching about ethical dilemmas that may arise in a clinical setting. Which of the following student statements indicate that learning has occurred? **Select all that apply.**
    1. "Within an ethical dilemma, there is evidence of both moral 'rightness' and 'wrongness' of an action."
    2. "In an ethical dilemma, there is conscious conflict regarding an individual's decision making."
    3. "In an ethical dilemma, a choice must be made between two equally favorable alternatives."
    4. "In an ethical dilemma, often the reasons supporting each side of the argument for action are illogical and inappropriate."
    5. "In most situations that involve an ethical dilemma, taking no action is considered an action taken."

29. Which situation exemplifies the ethical principle of veracity?
    1. A nurse uses verbal strategies instead of forced seclusion to calm an agitated client.
    2. A nurse talks with a client's physician to gain permission for the client to attend an upcoming fieldtrip.
    3. A nurse encourages a client diagnosed with dementia to choose what to wear for the day.
    4. A nurse teaches a client about the chronic nature of his or her diagnosis of schizophrenia.

30. A despondent client diagnosed with schizophrenia has an interaction with a nurse. Although the client shies away, the nurse gives the client a reassuring hug at the end of their conversation. With which legal action may the nurse be charged?
    1. Breach of confidentiality
    2. Battery
    3. Assault
    4. Defamation of character

31. An instructor is teaching students about The Joint Commission's standards regarding the use of restraints and/or seclusion. Which student statement indicates that learning has occurred?
    1. "For adults 18 years and older, orders for restraint or seclusion must be renewed every 24 hours."
    2. "For children and adolescents aged 9 to 17, orders for restraint or seclusion must be renewed every 12 hours."
    3. "For children younger than 9 years, orders for restraint or seclusion must be renewed every 2 hours."
    4. "Seclusion or restraints must be discontinued at the earliest possible time regardless of when the order is scheduled to expire."

32. A client has been involuntarily committed to a psychiatric unit. Which right does the nurse expect the client to retain?
    1. The right to an immediate court hearing
    2. The right to choose staff for treatment
    3. The right to refuse psychotropic medications
    4. The right to be released within 24 hours of a written request

33. A nurse is caring for a client who is suspected of having the diagnosis of hair-pulling disorder, or trichotillomania. What condition must be ruled out before a definitive diagnosis of this disorder?
    1. Bipolar disorder
    2. Alopecia areata
    3. Post-traumatic stress disorder (PTSD)
    4. Body dysmorphic disorder (BDD)

34. Which of the following situations is a common reason for the elderly to experience sleep disturbances? **Select all that apply.**
    1. Discomfort or pain
    2. Dementia
    3. Inactivity
    4. Anxiety
    5. Medications

35. A client diagnosed with generalized anxiety disorder complains of feeling out of control and states, "I just can't do this anymore." Which nursing action takes priority at this time?
    1. Ask the client, "Are you thinking about harming yourself?"
    2. Remove all potentially harmful objects from the milieu.
    3. Place the client on a one-to-one observation status.
    4. Encourage the client to verbalize feelings during the next group.

36. Structural brain imaging indicates that clients diagnosed with generalized anxiety and panic disorders have pathological involvement of the _____ lobes of the brain.

37. From a psychoanalytic theory prospective, which of the following predisposing factors offer insight into the etiology of phobias? **Select all that apply.**
    1. Phobias come from faulty processing of the Oedipal/Electra complex.
    2. Unconscious fears expressed in a symbolic manner prevent confrontation of real fear.
    3. A stressful stimulus produces an "unconditioned" response of fear, resulting in a phobia.
    4. Avoidance behaviors used to prevent anxiety reactions lead to phobias.
    5. Innate fears are characteristics or tendencies with which one is born.

38. A despondent college student being treated for a panic disorder tells the nurse, "I've had it! For no reason, my heart pounds, and I can't seem to breathe. Life's just not worth living!" On the basis of this information, which nursing diagnosis takes priority?
    1. Ineffective airway clearance
    2. Ineffective coping
    3. Risk for suicide
    4. Knowledge deficit

39. A type of behavioral therapy used for clients diagnosed with trauma-related disorders that is somewhat similar to implosion therapy, or flooding, is called _____ _____ therapy.

40. A nursing instructor is teaching students about the major goals of the treatment for adjustment disorders. Which of the following statements indicate that learning has occurred? **Select all that apply.**
    1. "A major goal is to relieve symptoms associated with a stressor."
    2. "A major goal is to reduce flashbacks and psychotic thoughts."
    3. "A major goal is to improve coping with stressors that can't be reduced or removed."
    4. "A major goal is to establish support systems that can help maximize adaptation."
    5. "A major goal is to reduce avoidance behaviors and psychic numbing."

41. In which phase of eye movement desensitization and reprocessing (EMDR) is it critical for the client to develop a sense of trust in the therapist?
    1. The assessment phase
    2. The preparation phase
    3. The desensitization phase
    4. The installation

42. A child witnesses a parent being taken away by ambulance after a fatal accident. Now each time the child hears a siren, he or she reacts with uncontrollable anxiety. What type of crisis is this child experiencing?
    1. Maturational/developmental crisis
    2. Dispositional crisis
    3. Crisis resulting from traumatic stress
    4. Crisis reflecting psychopathology

43. In an effort to maintain safety, a nurse should evaluate a client's potential for violence. Which factors should the nurse consider during this assessment? **Select all that apply.**
    1. Past history of violent behavior
    2. Feelings of power and control
    3. A diagnosis of bipolar disorder
    4. A diagnosis of Munchausen's syndrome
    5. Symptoms of dementia

44. A child has been diagnosed with an adjustment disorder. The parent asks the nurse why no medications have been prescribed. Which of the following are appropriate nursing responses? **Select all that apply.**
    1. "Psychoactive drugs carry the potential for physiological dependence."
    2. "Psychoactive drugs carry the potential for psychological dependence."
    3. "Specific medications will soon be prescribed for your child's disorder."
    4. "Medication effects may be temporary and mask the real problem."
    5. "Only adults receive medications specifically for adjustment disorders."

45. A nursing instructor is about to meet with a student diagnosed with a gambling disorder. When discussing the student's history, which of the following is the nurse likely to assess? **Select all that apply.**
    1. Absences from school due to gambling
    2. Willingness to seek help
    3. Lack of parental discipline
    4. A family with materialistic values
    5. Close family members who have similar gambling problems

46. Addiction is a potential problem for some nurses. What percentages of nurses suffer from a substance use disorder, and which is the chemical most widely abused?
    1. 5%–10% using anxiolytics
    2. 5%–10% using opioids
    3. 10%–15% using cannabis
    4. 10%–15% using alcohol

47. The physiological and mental readjustment that accompanies the discontinuation of an addictive substance is defined as _____.

48. A mother asks the nurse how best to help her teenager deal with the consequences of her husband's heavy and prolonged drinking problem. Which nursing statement would be most appropriate?
    1. "Your son may find an Alateen support group helpful."
    2. "You should get your son involved in monitoring your husband's drinking."
    3. "Encourage your son to confront his father and not tolerate increased drinking."
    4. "Tell your son that he should tolerate the drinking because addiction is a disease."

49. A nursing instructor is teaching about inhalant use disorder. Which of the following student statements indicate that more instruction is needed? **Select all that apply.**
    1. "'Huffing' is a procedure in which the substance is placed in a paper or plastic bag and inhaled from the bag by the user."
    2. "Inhalants generally act as central nervous system depressants."
    3. "Neurological damage can occur with inhalant use."
    4. "Inhalant substances are not readily available and are illegal and expensive."
    5. "'Bagging' is a procedure in which a rag soaked with the substance is applied to the mouth and nose and the vapors are breathed."

50. A mute client experiencing catatonia has been admitted to the inpatient psychiatric unit with a diagnosis of schizophrenia. What would the nurse expect to observe?
    1. Frenzied and purposeless movements
    2. Exaggerated suspiciousness
    3. Stuporous withdrawal
    4. Sexual preoccupation

51. _____ symptoms of schizophrenia spectrum disorder tend to reflect a diminution or loss of normal functions.

52. A client has been involuntarily committed to a forensic unit for stalking the president. The client states, "He is in love with me. What's the problem?" Which subtype of delusional disorder is associated with the client's presenting symptom?
    1. Erotomanic type
    2. Grandiose type
    3. Jealous type
    4. Persecutory type

53. Which of the following are anatomical abnormalities seen in clients diagnosed with schizophrenia? **Select all that apply.**
    1. Ventricular enlargement
    2. Sulci enlargement
    3. Cerebellar atrophy
    4. Decreased cerebral size
    5. Increased intracranial size

54. A nursing instructor is teaching about antipsychotic drugs and their side effects. Which of the following student statements indicate that learning has occurred? **Select all that apply.**
    1. "Blockage of the dopamine receptors controls positive symptoms."
    2. "Dry mouth and constipation can be caused by cholinergic blockade."
    3. "Histamine blockade can cause orthostatic hypotension and tremors."
    4. "Dopamine blockage can result in extrapyramidal symptoms."
    5. "Weight gain can result from alpha-adrenergic receptor blockage."

55. The physician informs the client that succinylcholine chloride (Anectine) will be administered before electroconvulsive therapy (ECT). The client asks, "Why must I take this medication?" Which is the appropriate nursing response?
    1. "To help settle your stomach before the procedure."
    2. "To facilitate prolonged muscular activity during the procedure."
    3. "To relax skeletal muscles during the ECT procedure."
    4. "To control your respirations during ECT."

56. A client is scheduled for electroconvulsive therapy (ECT). Before the client's ECT treatment, what should the nurse teach the client?
    1. General anesthesia and muscle relaxants will be used during treatment.
    2. It will take 4 to 5 hours to recover from the procedure.
    3. ECT has been used since the 1930s. There is absolutely no risk involved.
    4. Permanent memory loss is a major side effect.

57. A student nurse hears a physician instruct a client not to consume foods containing the amino acid tyramine. Which antidepressant medication would the student expect to see ordered on the client's medication administration record?
    1. Phenelzine (Nardil)
    2. Clomipramine (Anafranil)
    3. Citalopram (Celexa)
    4. Venlafaxine (Effexor)

58. _____ is described as a behavioral expression of emotions.

59. Substance intoxication or withdrawal may evoke mood symptoms. Which of the following substances can be associated with the diagnosis of substance-induced depression? **Select all that apply.**
    1. Alcohol
    2. Amphetamines
    3. Nonopioid analgesics
    4. Phencyclidine-like substances
    5. Hallucinogens

60. A 48-year-old depressed man is admitted with a superficial gunshot wound to the head. He insists that it was an accident. Which priority nursing diagnosis would be entered in this client's record?
    1. Risk for post-trauma syndrome R/T misinterpretation of reality AEB superficial self-inflicted gunshot wound to head
    2. Ineffective coping R/T an impulse control disorder AEB self-inflicted gunshot wound to head
    3. Risk for suicide R/T failed suicide attempt
    4. Ineffective denial R/T denial of problems

61. What differentiates occasional spontaneous behaviors of childhood and behaviors associated with bipolar disorder? **Select all that apply.**
    1. In bipolar disorder, symptoms occur most days in a week.
    2. In bipolar disorder, symptoms are severe enough to cause a moderate disturbance in two or more domains.
    3. In bipolar disorder, symptoms occur three or four times a week.
    4. In bipolar disorder, symptoms occur four or more hours a day.
    5. In bipolar disorder, symptoms are severe enough to cause an extreme disturbance in one domain.

62. A nurse documents a client's problem with the following nursing diagnosis: *disturbed sensory-perception.* Which client symptom led to this conclusion?
    1. Manipulation of others
    2. Delusions of grandeur
    3. Auditory and visual hallucinations
    4. Extreme hyperactivity

63. Bipolar II disorder is characterized by recurrent bouts of severe depression with episodic occurrences of _____.

64. Which action should the nurse prioritize when caring for a newly diagnosed client experiencing bipolar mania?
    1. Advise client that liquids will be restricted and monitored.
    2. Provide client with finger foods that are nutritious and easy to handle.
    3. Inform client that sodium intake will be continuously restricted.
    4. Place client on suicide precautions until mood has been stabilized.

65. A nurse is documenting care for a client diagnosed with bipolar I disorder who is experiencing extreme mania. *Risk for injury* is documented on the client's plan of care. What is the rationale for this nursing diagnosis? **Select all that apply.**
    1. During mania, the client experiences extreme hyperactivity that can lead to injury.
    2. During mania, rationality is impaired, and the client may injure self inadvertently.
    3. During mania, due to racing, disorganized thoughts, the client may become suicidal.
    4. During mania, the client is extremely distractible and responses are exaggerated, which can lead to injury.
    5. During mania, hyperactivity and distractibility impair a client's focus and may lead to accidents such as falls.

66. Which medication is classified as an anticonvulsant but used as a mood-stabilizing agent in the treatment of bipolar disorder?
    1. Lamotrigine (Lamictal)
    2. Donepezil (Aricept)
    3. Risperidone (Risperdal)
    4. Imipramine (Tofranil)

67. Which therapeutic communication technique is being used in this interaction with a client diagnosed with borderline personality disorder?
    Client: "Every time I get angry with someone, I always have this need to take a razor blade to my arms and legs."
    Nurse: "Can you describe the triggers that initiate your anger?"
    1. Encouraging comparison
    2. Exploring
    3. Formulating a plan of action
    4. Making observations

68. A client diagnosed with a personality disorder is self-centered and has an exaggerated sense of self-worth. The nurse recognizes that this behavior is symptomatic of which personality disorder?
    1. Schizoid personality disorder
    2. Narcissistic personality disorder
    3. Borderline personality disorder
    4. Antisocial personality disorder

69. A nursing instructor is teaching students about clients diagnosed with narcissistic personality disorder and the quality of their relationships. Which student statement indicates that learning has occurred?
    1. "Their close relationships are viewed in extremes of idealization and devaluation and alternate between overinvolvement and withdrawal."
    2. "Their interpersonal relationships are constrained by having little genuine interest in others."
    3. "Exploitation is their primary means of relating to others, including deceit and coercion."
    4. "They have marked impairments in close relationships, associated with mistrust and anxiety."

70. The predisposing factors of parental antagonism, harassment, and aggression are to the development of paranoid personality disorder as the predisposing factor of parental judgment in pointing out transgressions is to the development of:
    1. Obsessive-compulsive personality disorder
    2. Narcissistic personality disorder
    3. Avoidant personality disorder
    4. Schizotypal personality disorder

71. _____ _____
    describes parents who are overprotecting, overcontrolling, and too involved in their child's life.

72. The mother of a female client diagnosed with a borderline personality disorder asks what the term "splitting" means. Which is the nurse's best response?
    1. "The term 'splitting' means that the individual feels that she cannot split from or exist without her significant other."
    2. "The term 'splitting' means the individual perceives that her mind is splitting in two separate parts."
    3. "The term 'splitting' means that the individual feels abandoned and must split her loyalties equally between her mother and father."
    4. "The term 'splitting' means that the individual idealizes another and tends to see them as all good or all bad."

73. From an epidemiological perspective, which of the following factors accurately describe the prevalence of bulimia nervosa? **Select all that apply.**
    1. Onset of this disorder occurs from age 10 years through adolescence.
    2. This disorder is more prevalent than anorexia nervosa.
    3. This disorder affects up to 4% of young women.
    4. This disorder occurs where a scant amount of food is available.
    5. This disorder occurs primarily in societies that place emphasis on thinness.

74. After a client diagnosed with anorexia nervosa has been physically stabilized, which nursing intervention should take priority?
    1. Teaching the client about food and new recipes
    2. Encouraging verbalization of feelings related to family dynamics
    3. Administering medications specifically targeted for eating disorders
    4. Enforcing a rigid daily schedule

75. A client diagnosed with bulimia nervosa has frequent episodes of binging and purging. Which charting entry documents another symptom that this client is likely to experience?
    1. "Thoughts are tangential, with flight of ideas."
    2. "Rates mood 2 out of 10."
    3. "Midnight awakenings due to recurrent nightmares."
    4. "Aggressive and hostile toward other clients in milieu."

76. From a psychoanalytical perspective, which is a predisposing factor to obesity?
    1. Twin studies support the implication of heredity as a predisposing factor.
    2. Hypothyroidism interferes with basal metabolism leading to obesity.
    3. Obese individuals have unresolved dependency needs.
    4. Obesity occurs when caloric intake exceeds caloric output.

77. From an epidemiological perspective, which of the following factors accurately describe the prevalence of obesity? **Select all that apply.**
    1. Greater rates of obesity are associated with higher levels of education.
    2. 68.5% of 20-year-olds are overweight, and 35% are in the obese range.
    3. 6.3% of the U.S. adult population may be categorized as extremely obese.
    4. Higher rates of obesity occur in African Americans and Latino Americans than in whites.
    5. Greater rates of obesity exist among higher socioeconomic groups.

78. A client diagnosed with anorexia nervosa is assigned the nursing diagnosis *imbalanced nutrition: less than body requirements.* Which of the following are appropriate nursing interventions to deal with this problem? **Select all that apply.**
    1. Monitor ordered nasogastric tube feeding per hospital protocol.
    2. Talk about foods the client enjoys to encourage consumption.
    3. Consult with dietitian to determine appropriate number of calories required to provide adequate nutrition and realistic weight gain.
    4. Using the same scale, weigh client daily on arising and after first voiding.
    5. Assess moistness and color of oral mucous membranes.

79. _____ is a condition that can follow extreme weight loss in women diagnosed with anorexia nervosa.

80. Which symptoms should a nurse recognize as differentiating a client diagnosed with pseudodementia from a client diagnosed with neurocognitive disorder (NCD)?
    1. There is no change in appetite in NCD, whereas appetite is diminished in pseudodementia.
    2. Remote memory loss is greater than recent memory loss in NCD, whereas recent and remote memory loss are equal in pseudodementia.
    3. Confabulation occurs with pseudodementia, whereas confabulation does not occur with NCD.
    4. Attention and concentration are impaired in pseudodementia, whereas attention and concentration are intact in NCD.

81. A nurse is scoring a mental status examination to assess for a neurocognitive disorder. The client tested is 55 years of age. Which mean score is normal for this age range?
    1. 82.3
    2. 75.5
    3. 66.9
    4. 67.9

82. A client diagnosed with NCD due to Alzheimer's disease is currently in the second stage of the disease process. On the basis of symptoms typical of this stage, which of the following nursing diagnoses would be assigned? **Select all that apply.**
    1. Anxiety R/T loss of short-term memory
    2. Ineffective role performance R/T cognitive symptoms
    3. Low self-esteem R/T feelings of shame
    4. Risk for injury R/T impairments in cognitive and psychomotor functioning
    5. Nutrition: less than body requirements R/T diminished mental capacity

83. Symptoms of depression that mimic those of neurocognitive disorder are termed _____.

84. A mother suddenly has no memory of her identity or her home location after learning that her son has been captured during combat. The psychiatric nurse practitioner would assign which medical diagnosis to this client?
    1. Dissociative amnesia disorder
    2. Depersonalization-derealization disorder
    3. Conversion disorder (functional neurological symptom disorder)
    4. Dissociative identity disorder

85. A condition in which an individual has nearly all the signs and symptoms of pregnancy but is not pregnant is called _____.

86. Which of the following diagnoses would be classified as a somatic symptom disorder? **Select all that apply.**
    1. Illness anxiety disorder
    2. Dissociative amnesia
    3. Depersonalization-derealization disorder
    4. Conversion disorder (functional neurological symptom disorder)
    5. Munchausen disorder

87. Which of the following client behaviors associated with a dissociative disorder are correctly matched with the nursing diagnosis that addresses the behavior? **Select all that apply.**
    1. Verbalization of physical complaints without pathology: chronic pain
    2. Alteration in experiencing the environment: disturbed sensory perception
    3. Feigning of psychological symptoms: ineffective coping
    4. Loss of physical functioning without pathology: fear
    5. Presence of more than one personality: disturbed personal identity

88. On the basis of epidemiological statistics, which client would a nurse recognize as most likely to be diagnosed with conversion disorder (functional neurological symptom disorder)?
    1. A young woman from an rural area
    2. An older woman from a urban area
    3. A young man from an urban area
    4. An older man from a rural area

89. Excessive psychomotor activity that may be purposeful or aimless, accompanied by physical movements and verbal utterances that are usually more rapid than normal, is called _____.

90. A child has been prescribed methylphenidate transdermal system (Daytrana). Which medication information should the nurse provide the family?
    1. The patch should be placed on the same spot daily to avoid skin irritation.
    2. To avoid irritation when changing the patch, remove the old patch quickly.
    3. Mild skin redness or itching can be expected at the patch site.
    4. To avoid irritation, powder the area before applying the patch.

91. A client is diagnosed with attention deficit-hyperactivity disorder (ADHD) and is prescribed atomoxetine HCL (Strattera). What is the advantage of taking this medication?
    1. Strattera is safe to take when a client has cardiovascular disease.
    2. Clients diagnosed with bipolar disorder can also be prescribed atomoxetine.
    3. It is not necessary to monitor for suicidal ideations.
    4. Risk for abuse or misuse is low.

92. Which of the following factors should a nurse recognize as characteristic of oppositional defiant disorder (ODD)? **Select all that apply.**
    1. It is characterized by a pattern of behavior in which the basic rights of others or major age-appropriate societal norms or rules are violated.
    2. Specific phobias are not uncommon (fear of the dark, ghosts, animals).
    3. Maladaptive behaviors may interfere with social, educational, occupational, or other important areas of functioning.
    4. Common comorbid disorders include attention-deficit disorder and anxiety and mood disorders.
    5. In some cases of ODD, there may be a progression to conduct disorder.

93. A nursing instructor is teaching about trends related to extramarital sex. Which student statement indicates that learning has occurred?
    1. "The incidence of extramarital sex for males is on the rise."
    2. "The incidence of extramarital sex for females is holding constant."
    3. "Most individuals believe the goal in marriage should be sexual exclusivity."
    4. "Fifty percent of all divorces are caused by infidelity and/or adultery."

94. Which of the following paraphilic disorders is correctly matched with its characteristic symptom? **Select all that apply.**
    1. Sexual sadistic disorder: sexual arousal of being humiliated, beaten, bound, or otherwise made to suffer
    2. Transvestic disorder: sexual arousal from the physical or psychological suffering of another individual
    3. Voyeuristic disorder: sexual arousal involving the act of observing an unsuspecting individual who is naked
    4. Fetishistic disorder: sexual arousal from the use of either nonliving objects or specific, nongenital body parts
    5. Exhibitionistic disorder: sexual arousal from the exposure of one's genitals to an unsuspecting individual

95. A woman is diagnosed with female sexual interest/arousal disorder. On the basis of an understanding of the characteristic symptoms of this disorder, which nursing diagnosis should the nurse assign to this client?
    1. Risk for self-directed or other-directive violence
    2. Impaired social interaction
    3. Disturbed personal identity
    4. Sexual dysfunction

96. Which of the following interventions should a nurse anticipate when planning care for a male client diagnosed with erectile disorder? **Select all that apply.**
    1. Behavior therapy
    2. Cognitive therapy
    3. Systematic desensitization
    4. Group therapy
    5. Sensate focus therapy

97. The condition of experiencing recurring and intense sexual arousal in response to enduring extreme pain, suffering, or humiliation is termed, sexual _____ disorder.

98. Which of the following characteristics would a nurse understand as common to the profile of a sexual victimizer? **Select all that apply.**
    1. Most victimizers have a history of mental illness.
    2. Mothers of victimizers are possessive and seductive, but rejecting.
    3. Many victimizers grow up in abusive homes.
    4. The greatest number of victimizers are between the ages of 25 and 44.
    5. Sixty-two percent of victimizers use a weapon (most frequently a gun).

99. A form of child maltreatment in which there is a deficit in meeting a child's basic needs, including the failure to provide basic health care, supervision, nutrition, education, and/or safe housing needs is termed _____ _____.

100. From a sociocultural perspective, which of the following factors may predispose individuals to aggressive and violent behavior? **Select all that apply.**
    1. Studies show that various neurotransmitters may play a role in the facilitation and inhibition of aggressive impulses.
    2. Theorists have suggested that children imitate the abusive behavior of their parents.
    3. Studies show that poverty and income are strong predictors of abuse and violent behavior.
    4. American society was founded on a general acceptance of violence as a means of solving problems.
    5. Societal influences may contribute to violence when individuals perceive that their needs and desires are not being met relative to other people.

REVIEW ANSWERS

1. ANSWERS: 1, 3, 4

Rationale: A mental disorder can be defined as a health condition characterized by significant dysfunction in an individual's cognitions, emotions, or behaviors that reflects a disturbance in the psychological, biological, or developmental process underlying mental functioning.

1. Significant dysfunction in emotions is a characteristic of a mental disorder.

2. Significant dysfunction in values is not necessarily a characteristic of a mental disorder.

3. Significant dysfunction in cognitions is a characteristic of a mental disorder.

4. Significant dysfunction in behaviors is a characteristic of a mental disorder.

5. Significant dysfunction in ethics is not necessarily a characteristic of a mental disorder.

TEST-TAKING TIP: Review the definition of a mental disorder.
Content Area: Safe and Effective Care Environment;
Integrated Process: Nursing Process: Assessment;
Client Need: Safe and Effective Care Environment: Management of Care;
Cognitive Level: Application;
Concept: Assessment

2. ANSWERS: 1, 3, 5

Rationale:

1. Mild anxiety sharpens the senses and therefore enhances learning.

2. Mild anxiety sharpens the senses and does not lead to confusion and loss of concentration.

3. Mild anxiety does increase motivation and prepares people for action.

4. Moderate, not mild, anxiety requires problem-solving assistance.

5. Mild anxiety does increase motivation and prepares people for action.

TEST-TAKING TIP: Understand that mild anxiety sharpens the senses, increases motivation for productivity, increases perceptual field, and heightens awareness in the environment.
Content Area: Physiological Integrity;
Integrated Process: Nursing Process: Assessment;
Client Need: Physiological Integrity: Physiological Adaptation;
Cognitive Level: Application;
Concept: Stress

3. ANSWER: 1

Rationale: During the immediate "fight-or-flight" response, the hypothalamus stimulates the sympathetic nervous system resulting in various physical effects. During the sustained fight-or-flight response, the hypothalamus stimulates the pituitary gland to release hormones that result in other various physical effects.

1. During the immediate response of fight or flight, the bronchioles in the lungs dilate, and respiration rate increases. This reaction immediately allows the individual to have the oxygen levels in the blood to decide whether he or she needs to fight or flee the area. Other immediate responses by the body include the following: the adrenal medulla releases norepinephrine and epinephrine into the bloodstream; the pupils of the eyes dilate; secretion from the lacrimal glands increases; the force of cardiac contraction and output increases; and heart rate, blood pressure, and sweat gland secretions increase.

2. This response is associated with the sustained, not immediate, response to stress.

3. This response is associated with the sustained, not immediate, response to stress.

4. This response is associated with the sustained, not immediate, response to stress.

TEST-TAKING TIP: Understand that the fight-or-flight response includes immediate and sustained stress responses. The sustained response maintains the body in an aroused condition for extended periods. Note the keywords in this question, "immediate response," which determine the correct answer.
Content Area: Physiological Integrity;
Integrated Process: Nursing Process: Assessment;
Client Need: Physiological Integrity: Physiological Adaptation;
Cognitive Level: Application;
Concept: Stress

4. ANSWER: 1

Rationale:

1. Black and Andreasen define mental health as a state of being that is relative rather than absolute. An individual who sees situations as either all good or all bad is at risk for a diagnosis of mental illness.

2. Maslow defined mental health in the context of individual functioning. An individual who drinks alcohol but is never late for work is demonstrating that alcohol consumption has not negatively affected his or her functioning. This individual is not currently at risk for mental illness.

3. Black and Andreasen define mental health as the successful performance of mental functions shown by the establishment of fulfilling relationships. An individual who is estranged from alcoholic relatives has distanced himself or herself from a dysfunctional family, and this does not necessarily put him or her at risk for mental illness.

4. Townsend defines mental health as the successful adaptation to stressors evidenced by thoughts, feelings, and behaviors that are age-appropriate and congruent with local and cultural norms. An individual who steadfastly defends a pro-life stance is adhering to his or her moral convictions, and this does not necessarily put him or her at risk for mental illness.

TEST-TAKING TIP: Be able to differentiate between the concepts of mental health and mental illness.
Content Area: Psychosocial Integrity;
Integrated Process: Nursing Process: Evaluation;
Client Need: Psychosocial Integrity;
Cognitive Level: Application;
Concept: Assessment

5. ANSWER: 1

Rationale: Kübler-Ross's five stages of grief consist of denial, anger, bargaining, depression, and acceptance.

1. The client in the question is exhibiting anger surrounding the death of a parent. Kübler-Ross describes anger as the second stage in the normal grief response. This stage occurs when clients experience the reality of

the situation. Feelings associated with this stage include sadness, guilt, shame, helplessness, and hopelessness.

2. Disequilibrium is a stage in Bowlby's, not Kübler-Ross's, model of the normal grief response. Bowlby's model consists of four stages of grief, including numbness or protest, disequilibrium, disorganization and despair, and reorganization.

3. Developing awareness is a stage in Engel's, not Kübler-Ross's, model of the normal grief response. Engel's model consists of five stages of grief, including shock/disbelief, developing awareness, restitution, resolution of loss, and recovery.

4. The client in the question is exhibiting signs of anger, not bargaining. Bargaining is the third stage of Kübler-Ross's model of the normal grief response.

TEST-TAKING TIP: Review all of the models related to the normal grief response and be able to distinguish between them.

Content Area: Psychosocial Integrity;
Integrated Process: Nursing Process: Assessment;
Client Need: Psychosocial Integrity;
Cognitive Level: Application;
Concept: Grief and Loss

6. **ANSWER: 4**
Rationale:
1. According to Peplau, the "Learning to count on others" stage occurs during infancy. The major developmental task of this stage is learning to communicate in various ways with the primary caregiver to have comfort needs fulfilled. The age of the child presented in the question rules out the "Learning to count on others" stage.
2. According to Peplau, the "Learning to delay satisfaction" stage occurs during toddlerhood. The major developmental task of this stage is learning the satisfaction of pleasing others by delaying self-gratification in small ways. The age of the child presented in the question rules out the "Learning to delay satisfaction" stage.
3. According to Peplau, the "Identifying oneself " stage occurs during early childhood. The major developmental task of this stage is learning appropriate roles and behaviors by acquiring the ability to perceive the expectations of others. The age of the child presented in the question rules out the "Identifying oneself" stage.
4. **According to Peplau, the "Developing skills in participation" stage occurs during late childhood. The major developmental task of this stage is learning the skills of compromise, competition, and cooperation with others; establishing a more realistic view of the world and a feeling of one's place in it. The age of the child presented in the question indicates that she is in the "Developing skills in participation" stage.**

TEST-TAKING TIP: Be familiar with the developmental tasks in the four stages of Peplau's interpersonal theory of personality development.

Content Area: Psychosocial Integrity;
Integrated Process: Nursing Process: Evaluation;
Client Need: Psychosocial Integrity;
Cognitive Level: Analysis;
Concept: Evidenced-based Practice

7. **ANSWER: 2**
Rationale: Peplau developed the nursing theory that promotes the nurse-client relationship by applying interpersonal theory to nursing practice. Key concepts include the nurse as a resource person, a counselor, a teacher, a leader, a technical expert, and a surrogate.

1. Erikson developed psychosocial theory as a further expansion of Freud's psychoanalytic theory. Erikson's theory is based on developmental task completion during eight stages of personality development throughout the life cycle: trust versus mistrust, autonomy versus shame and doubt, initiative versus guilt, industry versus inferiority, identity versus role confusion, intimacy versus isolation, generativity versus stagnation, and ego integrity versus despair.

2. **Freud developed psychoanalytic theory. He is known as the father of psychiatry, and he developed and organized the structure of the personality into three components: the id, ego, and superego. He also described the formation of personality through five stages of psychosexual development: oral, anal, phallic, latency, and genital.**

3. Sullivan developed interpersonal theory based on the belief that individual behavior and personality development are the direct results of interpersonal relationships. According to Sullivan, there are six stages of development: infancy, childhood, juvenile, preadolescence, early adolescence, and late adolescence.

4. Mahler developed object relations theory (birth to 36 months), which describes the separation–individuation process of the infant from the maternal figure. Using three phases, Mahler described the autistic phase, the symbiotic phase, and the separation–individuation phase. Mahler's theory of object relations aids the nurse in assessing the client's level of individuation from primary caregivers.

TEST-TAKING TIP: The focus of this question is the basic concepts of the theoretical models presented. Freud developed psychoanalytic theory on the basis of psychosexual development, whereas the concept of the nurse-client relationship is the basis of Peplau's nursing theory model.

Content Area: Psychosocial Integrity;
Integrated Process: Nursing Process: Evaluation;
Client Need: Psychosocial Integrity;
Cognitive Level: Analysis;
Concept: Evidenced-based Practice

8. **ANSWER: The correct order is 4, 2, 1, 3**
Rationale: Jean Piaget believed that human intelligence progresses through a series of stages that are related to age, demonstrating at each successive stage a higher level of logical organization than at the previous stages. The stages of cognitive development occur in the following order:
1. Sensorimotor (0–2 years)
2. Preoperational (2–7 years)
3. Concrete operations (7–11 years)
4. Formal operations (11 years–adulthood)

TEST-TAKING TIP: Review Piaget's stages of cognitive development and recognize the age ranges designated for each stage.

Content Area: Psychosocial Integrity;
Integrated Process: Nursing Process: Assessment;
Client Need: Psychosocial Integrity;
Cognitive Level: Analysis;
Concept: Evidenced-based Practice

9. ANSWER: symbiotic psychosis
Rationale: Mahler suggests that absence of, or rejection by, the maternal figure at the symbiotic phase can lead to **symbiotic psychosis.** Symbiotic psychosis occurs between the ages of 2 to 5 years. The child is completely emotionally attached to mother and reacts stressfully if the possibility of separation occurs.
TEST-TAKING TIP: Review Mahler's object relations theory of personality development.
Content Area: Psychosocial Integrity;
Integrated Process: Nursing Process: Assessment;
Client Need: Psychosocial Integrity;
Cognitive Level: Knowledge;
Concept: Evidenced-based Practice

10. ANSWER: 4
Rationale:
1. Guilt is the negative outcome of Erikson's "late-childhood" stage of development, initiative versus guilt. This stage ranges from 3 to 6 years of age. The major developmental task for late childhood is to develop a sense of purpose and the ability to initiate and direct one's own activities. The child described does not fall within the age range of the late-childhood stage.
2. Inferiority is the negative outcome of Erikson's "school-age" stage of development, industry versus inferiority. This stage ranges from 6 to 12 years of age. The major developmental task for school age is to achieve a sense of self-confidence by learning, competing, performing successfully, and receiving recognition from significant others, peers, and acquaintances. The child described does not fall within the age range of the school-age stage.
3. Shame and doubt are the negative outcomes of Erikson's "early-childhood" stage of development, autonomy versus shame and doubt. This stage ranges from 18 months through 3 years of age. The major developmental task for early childhood is to gain some self-control and independence within the environment. The child described does not fall within the age range of the early-childhood stage.
4. Mistrust is the negative outcome of Erikson's "infancy" stage of development, trust versus mistrust. This stage ranges from birth to 18 months of age. The major developmental task for infancy is to develop a basic trust in the parenting figure and be able to generalize it to others. The infant in the question is at risk for the negative outcome of mistrust due to the primary caregiver's failure to respond to the infant's basic needs.
TEST-TAKING TIP: When assessing for signs of mistrust, look for an infant with unmet needs due to lack of response from the mothering figure. The age of the infant presented in the question should alert you to the developmental task conflict experienced.
Content Area: Psychosocial Integrity;
Integrated Process: Nursing Process: Assessment;
Client Need: Psychosocial Integrity;
Cognitive Level: Application;
Concept: Critical Thinking

11. ANSWERS: 1, 2, 5
Rationale: National Alliance on Mental Illness (NAMI) is the nation's largest grassroots mental health organization dedicated to building better lives for the millions of Americans affected by mental illness.
1. NAMI advocates for access to services and treatment for the mentally ill.
2. NAMI provides free education, advocacy, and support group programs for the mentally ill.
3. NAMI does not supply prescribed antipsychotic drugs. NAMI may assist with discovering resources for medication access but does not directly provide antipsychotic medications.
4. NAMI does not provide affordable housing for the mentally ill. NAMI may assist with discovering resources for housing access but does not directly provide housing for the mentally ill.
5. NAMI supports research related to mental illness and is committed to raising awareness and building a community of hope for the mentally ill.
TEST-TAKING TIP: Familiarize yourself with NAMI and how this organization contributes to the welfare of the mentally ill.
Content Area: Safe and Effective Care Environment: Management of Care;
Integrated Process: Nursing Process: Assessment;
Client Need: Safe and Effective Care Environment: Management of Care;
Cognitive Level: Application;
Concept: Nursing Roles

12. ANSWER: secondary
Rationale: Secondary prevention is health care that is directed at reduction of the prevalence of psychiatric illness by shortening the course (duration) of the illness. This is accomplished through early identification of problems and prompt initiation of treatment.
TEST-TAKING TIP: Understand that the secondary level of prevention deals with minimizing symptoms after the problem has been identified.
Content Area: Safe and Effective Care Environment: Management of Care;
Integrated Process: Nursing Process: Assessment;
Client Need: Safe and Effective Care Environment: Management of Care;
Cognitive Level: Knowledge;
Concept: Promoting Health

13. ANSWER: 2
Rationale: Andresen and associates have conceptualized a five-stage model of recovery called the psychological recovery model. The stages are as follows: Stage 1—Moratorium; Stage 2—Awareness; Stage 3—Preparation; Stage 4—Rebuilding; and Stage 5: Growth.
1. In the Awareness stage, a consumer feels a sense of personal empowerment.
2. In the Rebuilding stage, the consumer controls life and sets realistic goals.
3. In the Preparation stage, a consumer resolves to begin the work of recovery.
4. In the Growth stage, a consumer is confident in managing symptoms.
TEST-TAKING TIP: Review the five stages of the psychological recovery model as described by

Andresen and the consumer behaviors that occur within each stage.
Content Area: Safe and Effective Care Environment: Management of Care;
Integrated Process: Nursing Process: Assessment;
Client Need: Safe and Effective Care Environment: Management of Care;
Cognitive Level: Analysis;
Concept: Assessment

14. **ANSWER: Client or Consumer**
    Rationale: The basic concept of a recovery model is empowerment of the consumer (client). The recovery model is designed to allow consumers primary control over decisions about their own care.
    TEST-TAKING TIP: Understand that recovery must be person-driven, self-determined, and self-directed. These are the foundations for recovery.
    Content Area: Safe and Effective Care Environment: Management of Care;
    Integrated Process: Nursing Process: Assessment;
    Client Need: Safe and Effective Care Environment: Management of Care;
    Cognitive Level: Knowledge;
    Concept: Evidenced-based Practice

15. **ANSWERS: 1, 2, 3, 4, 5**
    Rationale:
    1. **Adverse side effects, such as weight gain and sexual dysfunction, can cause medication nonadherence.**
    2. **Psychotropic medications can be extremely expensive. This cost can be a factor in medication nonadherence.**
    3. **As psychotropic medications begin to improve symptoms, clients may feel no need for continued medication use. This can be exacerbated by any thought disorders the client may be experiencing.**
    4. **Taking psychotropic medications is a daily reminder of the presence of a chronic mental illness. Medication nonadherence can be a way for the client to deny his or her diagnosis.**
    5. **Forgetfulness or misunderstanding of medication instructions can contribute to nonadherence. This can be exacerbated by any thought disorders the client may be experiencing.**
    TEST-TAKING TIP: Review the definition of the term *nonadherence. Nonadherence* has replaced the older term *noncompliance.*
    Content Area: Safe and Effective Care Environment: Management of Care;
    Integrated Process: Nursing Process: Implementation;
    Client Need: Safe and Effective Care Environment: Management of Care;
    Cognitive Level: Application;
    Concept: Medication

16. **ANSWER: The correct order is 3, 1, 2**
    Rationale: The three phases of group development proceed from initial or orientation phase, through middle or working phase, to final or termination phase.
    1. In the initial or orientation phase, members have not yet established trust and will respond to this lack of trust

by being overly polite. These behaviors are generated by a fear of rejection by the group.
2. In the middle or working phase, the members turn to each other rather than the leader for guidance. These behaviors are due to the establishment of trust within the group.
3. In the Final or Termination phase, the group members may express surprise over the actual materialization of the end. These behaviors represent the grief process of denial, which may then progress to anger.
TEST-TAKING TIP: Be able to identify the three phases of group development and the members' behaviors that may occur in each phase.
Content Area: Psychosocial Integrity;
Integrated Process: Nursing Process: Assessment;
Client Need: Psychosocial Integrity;
Cognitive Level: Analysis;
Concept: Collaboration

17. **ANSWER: 2**
    Rationale:
    1. A nursing diagnostic statement should never contain a medical diagnosis (bipolar disorder). A nursing diagnosis is a statement of the client's problem for which a nurse can intervene.
    2. **The nurse should determine that the correct diagnosis would be *disturbed sleep pattern R/T hyperactivity AEB midnight awakening*. A nursing diagnosis should describe the client's problem using NANDA nomenclature. The diagnosis should facilitate the development of appropriate nursing interventions.**
    3. This actual nursing diagnosis does not contain an "as evidenced by" statement and therefore is incorrectly written.
    4. This potential nursing diagnosis contains an "as evidenced by" statement. If evidence of the client's problem is present, the diagnosis would be considered actual and not a "risk for" or potential diagnosis.
    TEST-TAKING TIP: Understand that a correctly written actual nursing diagnosis must include an accepted NANDA-I stem, a "related-to" statement, and an "as-evidenced-by" statement. A potential or "risk for" diagnosis does not contain an "as evidenced by" statement because the problem has not yet occurred.
    Content Area: Safe and Effective Care Environment: Management of Care;
    Integrated Process: Nursing Process: Analysis;
    Client Need: Safe and Effective Care Environment: Management of Care;
    Cognitive Level: Analysis;
    Concept: Critical Thinking

18. **ANSWER: 2**
    Rationale:
    1. The majority of African Americans are devoted to their churches and religious organizations, with the vast majority practicing some form of Protestantism.
    2. **Sickle cell anemia, which is genetically derived, occurs predominantly in African Americans.**
    3. Many African American households are headed by women, not men.

4. A shaman is the medicine man or woman in the Native American, not African American, culture.
TEST-TAKING TIP: Familiarize yourself with the diversity of cultural groups. A review of Table 5-4 ("Summary of Six Cultural Phenomena in Comparison of Various Cultural Groups") in Chapter 5 of this text will help you to correctly answer this question.
Content Area: Psychosocial Integrity;
Integrated Process: Nursing Process: Assessment;
Client Need: Psychosocial Integrity;
Cognitive Level: Application;
Concept: Diversity

19. **ANSWERS: 2, 3, 4**
Rationale:
1. The product of the communication process is the message. Words, either verbal or written, are the primary channels for verbal, not nonverbal, communication.
2. Gestures are the mannerisms that modify a verbal communication and are considered nonverbal in nature.
3. The way in which an individual positions his or her body nonverbally communicates messages regarding self-esteem, gender identity, status, and interpersonal warmth or coldness.
4. General appearance and dress are part of the total nonverbal stimuli that influence interpersonal responses.
5. Colloquialisms are verbal, not nonverbal, expressions of regional words and phrases.
TEST-TAKING TIP: Review the various aspects of nonverbal communication and distinguish them from verbal communication.
Content Area: Psychosocial Integrity;
Integrated Process: Nursing Process: Assessment;
Client Need: Psychosocial Integrity;
Cognitive Level: Application;
Concept: Communication

20. **ANSWERS: 1, 3, 4**
Rationale:
1. Vocal cues consist of pitch, tone, and loudness of spoken messages. These vocal cues greatly influence the way individuals interpret verbal messages.
2. The topic of discussion relates to what is being verbalized and does not contribute to nonverbal communication.
3. Open posture contributes to nonverbal communication. The way in which an individual positions his or her body communicates messages regarding self-esteem, gender identity, status, and interpersonal warmth or coldness.
4. Eye contact contributes to nonverbal communication. Eyes have been called "the windows of the soul." It is through eye contact that individuals view and are viewed by others in a revealing way.
5. Vocabulary is defined as all the words of a language and relates to what is being verbalized; it does not contribute to nonverbal communication.
TEST-TAKING TIP: Review the various components of nonverbal communication.
Content Area: Safe and Effective Care Environment;
Integrated Process: Nursing Process: Assessment;
Client Need: Safe and Effective Care Environment: Management of Care;

Cognitive Level: Application;
Concept: Communication

21. **ANSWER: touch**
Rationale:
When communicating with each other, Arab Americans may stand close together, maintain steady eye contact, and **touch** only members of the same sex.
TEST-TAKING TIP: Review the various communication behaviors that are influenced by culture.
Content Area: Safe and Effective Care Environment;
Integrated Process: Nursing Process: Assessment;
Client Need: Safe and Effective Care Environment: Management of Care;
Cognitive Level: Knowledge;
Concept: Diversity

22. **ANSWER: 3**
Rationale:
1. This is an example of "giving advice," which blocks communication by concluding prematurely the client's personal decisions.
2. This is an example of "defending," which blocks communication by placing the client and nurse in adversarial positions.
3. This is an example of the nontherapeutic communication block of "requesting an explanation," in which the nurse unrealistically expects the client to provide information of which the client may not be cognitively aware. This block often puts the client on the defensive.
4. This is an example of the therapeutic communication technique of "giving information." Giving information provides the client with accurate data on which realistic decisions can be made.
TEST-TAKING TIP: Any communication response that contains the word "why" in any place in the sentence can be classified as a nontherapeutic block to communication.
Content Area: Safe and Effective Care Environment;
Integrated Process: Nursing Process: Implementation;
Client Need: Safe and Effective Care Environment: Management of Care;
Cognitive Level: Application;
Concept: Communication

23. **ANSWER: 4**
Rationale:
1. Nonverbal communication makes up between 70% to 90% of all effective communication. This student statement indicates that learning has occurred.
2. Touch is a powerful communication tool. It is a basic form of nonverbal communication, and the appropriateness of its use is culturally determined. This student statement indicates that learning has occurred.
3. Verbal and nonverbal communication must match. Behaviors can change a verbal message. For example, a client is unlikely to believe a nurse who says, "Please call me if you need something" while frowning and using a harsh tone of voice. This student statement indicates that learning has occurred.
4. Physical appearance and dress are part of the total nonverbal stimuli that influence interpersonal responses,

and, under some conditions, they are the primary determinants of such responses. This student statement indicates a need for further instruction.
TEST-TAKING TIP: Review the components of nonverbal communication.
Content Area: Safe and Effective Care Environment;
Integrated Process: Nursing Process: Evaluation;
Client Need: Safe and Effective Care Environment:
Management of Care;
Cognitive Level: Application;
Concept: Communication

24. **ANSWER: belittling**
Rationale:
In response to the client's statement, "I'm disappointed that my antidepressant medication isn't working yet," the nurse states, "A lot of clients expect a quick fix." The nurse has used the nontherapeutic block of *belittling* feelings. The use of this nontherapeutic block to communication lumps the client with "a lot of clients" and does not consider the client's individuality.
TEST-TAKING TIP: The question itself eliminates the choice of any therapeutic communication technique.
Content Area: Safe and Effective Care Environment;
Integrated Process: Nursing Process: Assessment;
Client Need: Safe and Effective Care Environment:
Management of Care;
Cognitive Level: Knowledge;
Concept: Communication

25. **ANSWER: 3**
Rationale:
1. "Clarification" is used by a nurse to check the understanding of what has been said by the client and helps the client make his or her thoughts or feelings more explicit. The communication exchange presented is an example of the therapeutic technique of "clarification," not "focusing."
2. "Reflection" is used when directing back what the nurse understands in regard to ideas, feelings, questions, and content. The communication exchange presented is an example of the therapeutic technique of "reflection," not "focusing.
3. The communication exchange presented is an example of the therapeutic communication technique of "focusing," which poses a statement that helps an individual expand on a specific topic of importance.
4. "Restatement" is used by a nurse to repeat to the client the main thought that the client has expressed. This lets the client know that the nurse is focused and engaged in the communication process. The communication exchange presented is an example of the therapeutic technique of "restatement," not "focusing."
TEST-TAKING TIP: Familiarize yourself with the therapeutic communication technique of "focusing."
Content Area: Safe and Effective Care Environment;
Integrated Process: Nursing Process: Evaluation;
Client Need: Safe and Effective Care Environment:
Management of Care;
Cognitive Level: Application;
Concept: Communication

26. **ANSWER: 4**
Rationale:
The therapeutic communication technique of "reflection" refers questions and feelings back to the client so that they may be recognized and accepted. Also, the client may recognize that his or her point of view has value.
1. This nurse-client exchange is an example of "reflection." The choice of this example would indicate that learning had occurred.
2. This nurse-client exchange is an example of "reflection." The choice of this example would indicate that learning had occurred.
3. This nurse-client exchange is an example of "reflection." The choice of this example would indicate that learning had occurred.
4. This nurse-client exchange is an example of the nontherapeutic communication technique of "giving approval," not the therapeutic technique of "reflection." "Giving approval" is when the nurse sanctions the client's ideas or behavior. This implies that the nurse has the right to pass judgment. The choice of this example would indicate that further instruction is needed.
TEST-TAKING TIP: Review the communication technique of "reflection" and the communication block of "giving approval" and distinguish between the two.
Content Area: Safe and Effective Care Environment;
Integrated Process: Nursing Process: Evaluation;
Client Need: Safe and Effective Care Environment:
Management of Care;
Cognitive Level: Application;
Concept: Communication

27. **ANSWER 4**
Rationale:
1. The basis of utilitarianism is "the greatest-happiness principle." Actions are right if they promote happiness and wrong if they produce the reverse of happiness. The guilt the teenager expects to feel has prompted the action of abiding by his or her curfew. This action is based on the principles of utilitarianism, not ethical egoism.
2. The basis of Kantianism is that ethical decisions are made out of respect for moral law. It is a moral duty to follow the law. The teenager in this situation is following the house rules by abiding by his or her curfew and is prompted to do this from a Kantianism, not ethical egoism, perspective.
3. Christian ethics approaches ethical decision making on the basis of love, forgiveness, and honesty. The basic principle is the golden rule: "Do unto others as you would have them do unto you." The decision of the teenager to abide by his or her curfew to avoid hurting the parent's feelings is based on the principles of Christian ethics, not ethical egoism.
4. Ethical egoism approaches ethical decision making on the basis of what is best for the individual making the decision. The teenager maintains curfew only for his or her individual benefit, which is maintenance of allowance and privileges. This decision is prompted from an ethical egoism perspective.
TEST-TAKING TIP: Review principles incorporated in various ethical theories and match the situation presented in the question with the theory it exemplifies.

Content Area: Safe and Effective Care Environment: Management of Care;
Integrated Process: Nursing Process: Implementation;
Client Need: Safe and Effective Care Environment: Management of Care;
Cognitive Level: Application;
Concept: Ethics

28. **ANSWERS: 1, 2, 5**
Rationale:
1. Within an ethical dilemma, evidence exists to support both moral "rightness" and moral "wrongness" related to a certain action. This student statement indicates that learning has occurred.
2. In an ethical dilemma, the individual that must make the choice experiences conscious conflict regarding the decision. Ethical dilemmas generally create a great deal of emotion. This student statement indicates that learning has occurred.
3. In an ethical dilemma, a choice must be made between two equally unfavorable, not favorable, alternatives. This student statement indicates a need for further instruction.
4. An ethical dilemma arises when there is no clear reason to choose one action over another. Often the reasons supporting each side of the argument for action are logical and appropriate, not illogical and inappropriate. This student statement indicates a need for further instruction.
5. It is true that in most situations involving ethical dilemmas, taking no action is considered an action taken. This student statement indicates that learning has occurred.
TEST-TAKING TIP: Review the concepts of an ethical dilemma. If reasons for decision making are illogical and inappropriate, the decision maker would have an easier time making an appropriate choice. This logic would eliminate Option 4.
Content Area: Safe and Effective Care Environment: Management of Care;
Integrated Process: Nursing Process: Implementation;
Client Need: Safe and Effective Care Environment: Management of Care;
Cognitive Level: Application;
Concept: Ethics

29. **ANSWER 4**
Rationale:
1. Nonmaleficence is the ethical principle that requires health care providers to do no harm to their clients. When a nurse uses verbal strategies, instead of forced seclusion, to calm an agitated client, the nurse is implementing the ethical principle of nonmaleficence, not veracity.
2. Beneficence is the ethical principle that refers to one's duty to benefit or promote the good of others. When a nurse advocates for a client, the nurse is implementing the ethical principle of beneficence, not veracity.
3. Autonomy is the ethical principle that respects an individual's right to determine his or her destiny. This principle presumes that the individual is capable of making independent choices for himself or herself. When a nurse supports a competent client's right to refuse offered

medications, the nurse is implementing the ethical principle of autonomy, not veracity.
4. Veracity is the ethical principle that refers to one's duty to always be truthful and not deceive or mislead. When a nurse teaches a client about the chronic nature of his or her diagnosis of schizophrenia, the nurse is implementing the ethical principle of veracity. Being honest is not always easy, but clients have the right to know about their diagnosis, treatment, and prognosis.
TEST-TAKING TIP: Review the ethical principles of autonomy, beneficence, nonmaleficence, justice, and veracity.
Content Area: Safe and Effective Care Environment: Management of Care;
Integrated Process: Nursing Process: Assessment;
Client Need: Safe and Effective Care Environment: Management of Care;
Cognitive Level: Application;
Concept: Ethics

30. **ANSWER: 2**
Rationale:
1. Breach of confidentiality is a common law tort that refers to disobedience of the set laws that govern the privacy of personal information. The nurse in the question has not breached client confidentiality.
2. Battery is the unconsented touching of another person. Charges can result when treatment that includes touching is administered to a client against his or her wishes and outside of an emergency situation. When the nurse in the question hugs the client without consent, the nurse has committed battery.
3. Assault is an act that results in a person's genuine fear and apprehension that he or she will be touched without consent. The nurse in the question did not commit assault.
4. Defamation of character occurs when a person shares detrimental information about another. When the information is shared verbally, it is called slander. When the information is in writing, it is called libel. The nurse in the question has not defamed the character of the client.
TEST-TAKING TIP: Review the types of lawsuits that may occur in the psychiatric setting and be aware of the types of behaviors that may result in charges of malpractice.
Content Area: Safe and Effective Care Environment: Management of Care;
Integrated Process: Nursing Process: Evaluation;
Client Need: Safe and Effective Care Environment: Management of Care;
Cognitive Level: Application;
Concept: Ethics

31. **ANSWER: 4**
Rationale:
1. According to The Joint Commission standards, orders for restraint or seclusion must be renewed every 4, not 24, hours for adults 18 years and older. This student statement indicates that further instruction is needed.
2. According to the Joint Commission standards, orders for restraint or seclusion must be renewed every 2, not 12, hours for children and adolescents aged 9 to 17. This student statement indicates that further instruction is needed.

3. According to The Joint Commission standards, orders for restraint or seclusion must be renewed every 1 hour, not every 2 hours, for children younger than 9 years. This student statement indicates that further instruction is needed.

4. The Joint Commission has established specific standards regarding the use of seclusion and restraints. A current example of these standards is that the secluding or restraining of an individual must be discontinued at the earliest possible time, regardless of when the order is scheduled to expire. This student statement indicates that learning has occurred.

TEST-TAKING TIP: Review the current and specific standards established by The Joint Commission regarding the use of seclusion and restraints of an individual.

Content Area: Safe and Effective Care Environment: Management of Care;
Integrated Process: Nursing Process: Implementation;
Client Need: Safe and Effective Care Environment: Management of Care;
Cognitive Level: Application;
Concept: Regulations

32. **ANSWER: 3**
Rationale:
1. Emergency commitments are time limited and state law determined. A court hearing for an involuntarily committed individual is scheduled, usually within 72 hours, not immediately.
2. Neither voluntarily admitted nor involuntarily committed clients have the right to determine who on the staff will be assigned to their care. Client assignments are generally made by the charge nurse with consideration for client need, staff expertise, and continuity of care.
3. An involuntarily committed client has the right to refuse psychotropic medications. There are exceptions to this, which include an immediate danger of violence toward self or others, legally determined incompetence, an inability to care for self, and a specifically defined status of "gravely disabled."
4. An involuntarily commitment status results in substantial restrictions of the rights of an individual. An involuntarily committed client has lost the right to leave the psychiatric facility by his or her own volition. A court proceeding, with input from the entire treatment team, will determine when this client can safely be discharged.
TEST-TAKING TIP: Review the rights that a mentally ill client retains when admitted either voluntarily or involuntarily for psychiatric care.

Content Area: Safe and Effective Care Environment: Management of Care;
Integrated Process: Nursing Process: Assessment;
Client Need: Safe and Effective Care Environment: Management of Care;
Cognitive Level: Application;
Concept: Ethics

33. **ANSWER: 2**
Rationale:
1. Bipolar disorder is characterized by mood swings from profound depression to extreme euphoria (mania) with

intervening periods of normalcy. Psychotic symptoms may or may not be present. This disorder is not associated with trichotillomania and would not need to be ruled out before the diagnosis.
2. Alopecia areata is a dermatological condition that results in hair loss in sharply defined patches, involving hairy areas of the body, usually the scalp or beard. This condition must be ruled out to establish the diagnosis of hair-pulling disorder or trichotillomania.
3. PTSD is a syndrome of symptoms that develops after a psychologically distressing event that is outside the range of usual human experience (e.g., rape, war). This disorder is not associated with trichotillomania and would not need to be ruled out before the diagnosis.
4. BDD is characterized by the exaggerated belief that the body is deformed in some specific way. This disorder is not associated with trichotillomania and would not need to be ruled out before the diagnosis.
TEST-TAKING TIP: Review the definition of alopecia areata.

Content Area: Psychosocial Integrity;
Integrated Process: Nursing Process: Assessment;
Client Need: Psychosocial Integrity;
Cognitive Level: Application;
Concept: Stress

34. **ANSWERS: 1, 2, 3, 4, 5**
Rationale: Sleep disturbances include hypersomnia (excessive sleepiness or seeking excessive amounts of sleep) and insomnia (difficulty initiating or maintaining sleep).
1. Chronic conditions, such as arthritis and joint and muscle discomfort and pain, represent some of the many reasons why elderly clients are at an increased risk for sleep disturbances.
2. Confusion and wandering as a result of dementia can be a reason why elderly clients are at an increased risk for sleep disturbances.
3. Inactivity and other psychosocial concerns, such as loneliness or boredom, can be a reason why elderly clients are at an increased risk for sleep disturbances.
4. Increased anxiety is a reason why elderly clients can be at an increased risk for sleep disturbances.
5. Medications have many side effects, including insomnia, and medications are metabolized differently in elderly clients. Many elderly clients experience polypharmacy in the treatment of chronic conditions, and so they are at higher risk for sleep disturbances.
TEST-TAKING TIP: Understand the different biological and psychosocial factors that may influence the sleep patterns of elderly clients.

Content Area: Psychosocial Integrity;
Integrated Process: Nursing Process: Assessment;
Client Need: Psychosocial Integrity;
Cognitive Level: Application;
Concept: Sleep, Rest, and Activity

35. **ANSWER: 1**
Rationale:
1. The nurse should recognize the statement, "I can't do this anymore," as evidence of hopelessness and further assess the suicidal ideations potential.

2. Removing all potentially harmful objects from the milieu can be an appropriate intervention, but only after the severity of client risk is determined. This assessment is critical for the nurse to intervene appropriately and in a timely manner.

3. Placing the client on a one-to-one observation status can be an appropriate intervention, but only after the severity of client risk is determined. This assessment is critical for the nurse to intervene appropriately and in a timely manner.

4. Although it is important for the client to verbalize feelings, this does not take priority at this time. Suicidal risk needs to be determined to ensure client safety by implementation of appropriate and timely nursing interventions.

TEST-TAKING TIP: Review the steps of the nursing process. Assessment is the first step. A nurse must initially assess a situation before determining appropriate nursing interventions.

Content Area: *Safe and Effective Care Environment: Management of Care;*
Integrated Process: *Nursing Process: Implementation;*
Client Need: *Safe and Effective Care Environment: Management of Care;*
Cognitive Level: *Application;*
Concept: *Critical Thinking*

36. **ANSWER: temporal**
Rationale: Structural brain imaging indicates that clients diagnosed with generalized anxiety and panic disorders have pathological involvement of the temporal lobes of the brain. Emotional states are affected by lower brain centers including the limbic system, thalamus, hypothalamus, and reticular formation.

TEST-TAKING TIP: Review the biological theory related to the etiology of generalized anxiety and panic disorder.

Content Area: *Safe and Effective Care Environment: Management of Care;*
Integrated Process: *Nursing Process: Assessment;*
Client Need: *Safe and Effective Care Environment: Management of Care;*
Cognitive Level: *Knowledge;*
Concept: *Stress*

37. **ANSWERS: 1, 2**
Rationale:
1. **From a psychoanalytic theory perspective, Freud thought that phobias come from faulty processing of the Oedipal/Electra complex. He also believed that incestuous feelings and fear of retribution from the same-gender parent results in repression and displacement on to something safe and neutral, the phobic stimulus.**
2. **From a psychoanalytic theory perspective, although modern-day psychoanalysts believe in Freud's concept of phobic development, psychoanalysts also believe that unconscious fears prevent confrontation of real fear and may be expressed in a symbolic manner, such as phobias.**
3. From a learning theory, not psychoanalytic, perspective, classical conditioning in the case of phobias may be explained as follows: by a stressful stimulus producing an "unconditioned" response of fear.

4. From a cognitive theory, not psychoanalytic theory, perspective, avoidance behaviors used to prevent anxiety reactions lead to phobias.
5. From a biological theory, not psychoanalytic theory, perspective, innate fears represent a part of the overall characteristics or tendencies with which one is born.

TEST-TAKING TIP: Review the various theories of origin associated with phobias and be able to match the theories with the answer choices presented.

Content Area: *Psychosocial Integrity;*
Integrated Process: *Nursing Process: Assessment;*
Client Need: *Psychosocial Integrity;*
Cognitive Level: *Application;*
Concept: *Evidenced-based Practice*

38. **ANSWER: 3**
Rationale:
1. Ineffective airway clearance is defined as the inability to clear secretions or obstructions from the respiratory tract. There is nothing in the question to indicate that the client has an obstructed airway. Hyperventilating during a panic attack will cause shortness of breath and is most probably the reason the client is experiencing feelings of air deprivation.
2. Ineffective coping is the inability to form a valid appraisal of the stressors, inadequate choices of practiced responses, and/or inability to use available resources. How an individual copes with stress is a conscious choice. The physiological response of a panic attack is precipitated by anxiety but is not consciously chosen; therefore, this nursing diagnosis does not apply.
3. **Because the client is despondent and makes statements such as "Life's just not worth living!" and "I've had it!" an indication of self-harm must be considered. Although other nursing diagnoses may be valid and appropriate, the safety of the client is always the nurse's first priority.**
4. The client statement "For no reason, my heart pounds, and I can't seem to breathe" indicates that the client does not understand the physiological response to severe levels of anxiety. Helping the client to understand cause and effect will be beneficial; however, when the client is experiencing high levels of anxiety, it is not an appropriate time to teach. The nursing diagnosis of knowledge deficit, although applicable at a future time, is not a priority.

TEST-TAKING TIP: Understand that any time a client would indicate either overtly or covertly the potential for self-harm, the nursing diagnosis of *Risk for Suicide* must take priority.

Content Area: *Safe and Effective Care Environment: Management of Care;*
Integrated Process: *Nursing Process: Analysis;*
Client Need: *Safe and Effective Care Environment: Management of Care;*
Cognitive Level: *Application;*
Concept: *Critical Thinking*

39. **ANSWER: prolonged exposure**
Rationale: Prolonged exposure therapy is a type of behavioral therapy used for clients diagnosed with trauma-related disorders. It is somewhat similar to implosion

therapy, or flooding. During this type of therapy, the individual is exposed to repeated and prolonged mental recounting of the traumatic experience. This intense emotional processing of the traumatic event serves to neutralize the memories so that they no longer result in anxious arousal or escape or avoidance behaviors.
TEST-TAKING TIP: Review the types of behavioral therapy used in the treatment of trauma related disorders.
Content Area: Safe and Effective Care Environment: Management of Care;
Integrated Process: Nursing Process: Assessment;
Client Need: Safe and Effective Care Environment: Management of Care;
Cognitive Level: Knowledge;
Concept: Evidenced-based Practice

40. ANSWERS: 1, 3, 4
Rationale:
1. To relieve symptoms associated with a stressor is a major goal of adjustment disorder treatment. This student statement indicates that learning has occurred.
2. To reduce flashbacks and psychotic thoughts is a major goal of post-traumatic stress disorder (PTSD) treatment. This student statement indicates that further instruction is needed.
3. To improve coping with stressors that can't be reduced or removed is a major goal of adjustment disorder treatment. This student statement indicates that learning has occurred.
4. To establish support systems that maximize adaptation is a major goal of adjustment disorder treatment. This student statement indicates that learning has occurred.
5. To reduce avoidance behaviors and psychic numbing is a major goal of PTSD treatment. This student statement indicates that further instruction is needed.
TEST-TAKING TIP: Differentiate between the major goals of the treatment for adjustment disorders and PTSD.
Content Area: Safe and Effective Care Environment: Management of Care;
Integrated Process: Nursing Process: Planning;
Client Need: Safe and Effective Care Environment: Management of Care;
Cognitive Level: Application;
Concept: Stress

41. ANSWER: 2
Rationale:
1. In the assessment phase of EMDR, the client identifies a specific scene from the target event that best represents the memory. Although the establishment of trust is important in any client–therapist relationship, it is critical in the *preparation phase* of EMDR.
2. In the preparation phase of EMDR, the therapist teaches the client certain self-care techniques (e.g., relaxation techniques) for dealing with emotional disturbances that may arise during or between sessions. It is critical for the client to develop a sense of trust in the therapist during this phase of EMDR.
3. In the desensitization phase of EMDR, the client gives attention to the negative beliefs and disturbing emotions associated with the traumatic event while focusing his or her vision on the back-and-forth motion of the therapist's finger. Although the establishment of trust is important in any client–therapist relationship, it is critical in the *preparation phase* of EMDR.
4. In the installation phase of EMDR, the client gives attention to the positive belief that he or she has identified to replace the negative belief associated with the trauma. Although the establishment of trust is important in any client–therapist relationship, it is critical in the *preparation phase* of EMDR.
TEST-TAKING TIP: Understand that teaching self-care techniques in the preparation phase of EMDR requires that the client trust the therapist.
Content Area: Safe and Effective Care Environment: Management of Care;
Integrated Process: Nursing Process: Implementation;
Client Need: Safe and Effective Care Environment: Management of Care;
Cognitive Level: Application;
Concept: Nursing

42. ANSWER: 3
Rationale:
1. Maturational/developmental crises occur in response to situations that trigger emotions related to unresolved conflicts in one's life. The situation presented in the question is not reflective of this type of crisis.
2. Dispositional crises occur when there is an acute response to an external stressor such as when an individual experiences a traumatic stressor and violently displaces it onto another person. The situation presented in the question is not reflective of this type of crisis.
3. Crises resulting from traumatic stress occur when the crisis is precipitated by unexpected external stresses over which the individual has little or no control and from which he or she feels emotionally overwhelmed and defeated. The situation presented in the question is reflective of this type of crisis.
4. Crises reflecting psychopathology occur when preexisting psychopathology has been instrumental in precipitating the crisis or when psychopathology significantly impairs or complicates adaptive resolution. The situation presented in the question is not reflective of this type of crisis.
TEST-TAKING TIP: Review the six classes of emotional crises and be able to match a situation to the appropriate crisis type.
Content Area: Psychosocial Integrity;
Integrated Process: Nursing Process: Evaluation;
Client Need: Psychosocial Integrity;
Cognitive Level: Application;
Concept: Trauma

43. ANSWERS: 1, 3, 5
Rationale:
1. A past history of violence is one of the factors that have been identified as an important consideration in assessing for potential violence.
2. The individual who becomes violent usually feels an underlying helplessness, not feelings of power and control.

3. Diagnoses that have a strong association with violent behavior are schizophrenia, major depression, bipolar disorder, and substance use disorders. Substance abuse, in addition to mental illness, compounds the increased risk of violence.

4. Munchausen's disorder is a factitious disorder that involves the conscious, intentional feigning of physical or psychological symptoms. A diagnosis of Munchausen's syndrome is not typically associated with violent behavior.

5. Dementia and antisocial, borderline, and intermittent explosive personality disorders have also been associated with a risk for violent behavior.

TEST-TAKING TIP: Review the factors that have been identified as important considerations in assessing for potential violence.
Content Area: Safe and Effective Care Environment: Management of Care;
Integrated Process: Nursing Process: Assessment;
Client Need: Safe and Effective Care Environment: Management of Care;
Cognitive Level: Application;
Concept: Assessment

44. **ANSWERS: 1, 2, 4**
Rationale:
1. Adjustment disorder is not commonly treated with medications because psychoactive drugs carry the potential for physiological dependence.
2. Adjustment disorder is not commonly treated with medications because psychoactive drugs carry the potential for psychological dependence.
3. Adjustment disorder is not commonly treated with medications. Antianxiety or antidepressant medication may be used for symptoms of anxiety or depression.
4. Adjustment disorder is not commonly treated with medications because medication effects may be temporary and mask the real problem.
5. Adjustment disorder is not commonly treated with medications for both adults and children.

TEST-TAKING TIP: Understand that no specific medications are prescribed for clients diagnosed with adjustment disorder.
Content Area: Safe and Effective Care Environment: Management of Care;
Integrated Process: Nursing Process: Implementation;
Client Need: Safe and Effective Care Environment: Management of Care;
Cognitive Level: Application;
Concept: Stress

45. **ANSWERS: 1, 3, 4, 5**
Rationale:
1. Clients who are diagnosed with a gambling disorder present with impairment in occupational functioning because of absences from work or school to gamble.
2. Most pathological gamblers deny that they have a problem, making treatment difficult because of their unwillingness to seek help.

3. Inappropriate parental discipline such as absence, inconsistency, or harshness has been linked to an increased prevalence of gambling disorder.
4. A family emphasis on material and financial symbols has been linked to an increased prevalence of gambling disorder.
5. Familial and twin studies show an increased prevalence of pathological gambling in family members of individuals diagnosed with the disorder.

TEST-TAKING TIP: Review factors that may indicate a predisposition to a gambling disorder.
Content Area: Safe and Effective Care Environment: Management of Care;
Integrated Process: Nursing Process: Assessment;
Client Need: Safe and Effective Care Environment: Management of Care;
Cognitive Level: Application;
Concept: Assessment

46. **ANSWER: 4**
Rationale:
1. It is estimated that 10% to 15%, not 5% to 10%, of nurses suffer from substance use disorder and that alcohol, not anxiolytics, is most widely abused.
2. It is estimated that 10% to 15%, not 5% to 10%, of nurses suffer from substance use disorder and that alcohol, not opioids, is most widely abused.
3. It is estimated that 10% to 15% of nurses suffer from substance use disorder but, alcohol, not cannabis, is most widely abused.
4. It is estimated that 10% to 15% of nurses suffer from substance use disorder and alcohol is the most widely abused drug, followed closely by narcotics.

TEST-TAKING TIP: Review the prevalence of substance use disorder in nurses and recognize that alcohol is the most widely abused substance.
Content Area: Safe and Effective Care Environment: Management of Care;
Integrated Process: Nursing Process: Assessment;
Client Need: Safe and Effective Care Environment: Management of Care;
Cognitive Level: Application;
Concept: Addiction

47. **ANSWER: withdrawal**
Rationale: The physiological and mental readjustment that accompanies the discontinuation of an addictive substance is defined as withdrawal. Substance withdrawal occurs upon abrupt reduction or discontinuation of a substance that has been used regularly over a prolonged period of time. The substance-specific syndrome includes clinically significant physical signs and symptoms as well as psychological changes such as disturbances in thinking, feeling, and behavior.

TEST-TAKING TIP: Review the definition of *withdrawal* in the context of substance abuse.
Content Area: Psychosocial Integrity;
Integrated Process: Nursing Process: Assessment;
Client Need: Psychosocial Integrity;
Cognitive Level: Knowledge;
Concept: Addiction

48. ANSWER: 1

Rationale:

1. This therapeutic response addresses the wife's concerns by giving information about Alateen. Alateen is a community-based organization of teenaged children of alcoholics, which shares the philosophical and organizational structure of Alcoholics Anonymous. Alateen is the youth version of Al-Anon.

2. This is an inappropriate, nontherapeutic nursing response that gives incorrect advice. A client diagnosed with alcohol use disorder must be responsible for his or her continued sobriety, and a teenager should not be burdened with this responsibility.

3. This inappropriate, nontherapeutic nursing response gives advice and gives inappropriate responsibility to the teenager.

4. Even though addiction is a disease, this inappropriate, nontherapeutic nursing response indirectly reinforces the father's behavior.

TEST-TAKING TIP: Look for an appropriate therapeutic communication technique that does not place responsibility on the teenage son.

Content Area: Safe and Effective Care Environment: Management of Care;

Integrated Process: Nursing Process: Implementation;

Client Need: Safe and Effective Care Environment: Management of Care;

Cognitive Level: Application;

Concept: Addiction

49. ANSWERS: 1, 4, 5

Rationale:

1. "Huffing" is a procedure in which a rag soaked with the substance is applied to the mouth and nose and the vapors are breathed. This student statement indicates a need for further instruction.

2. It is true that inhalants generally act as central nervous system depressants. This student statement indicates that learning has occurred.

3. Neurological damage, such as ataxia, peripheral and sensorimotor neuropathy, speech problems, and tremor, can occur with inhalant use. This student statement indicates that learning has occurred.

4. Inhalant substances are readily available, legal, and inexpensive, making inhalants a drug of choice for poor people, children, and young adults. This student statement indicates a need for further instruction.

5. "Bagging" is a procedure in which the substance is placed in a paper or plastic bag and inhaled from the bag by the user. This student statement indicates a need for further instruction.

TEST-TAKING TIP: Review information about inhalant use disorder.

Content Area: Safe and Effective Care Environment: Management of Care;

Integrated Process: Nursing Process: Evaluation;

Client Need: Safe and Effective Care Environment: Management of Care;

Cognitive Level: Application;

Concept: Addiction

50. ANSWER: 3

Rationale:

1. A nurse would observe frenzied and purposeless movements in a client experiencing catatonic excitement. The client's mutism indicates catatonic stupor, not catatonic excitement.

2. Exaggerated suspiciousness is a characteristic of the symptom of paranoia, not catatonia.

3. The client's mutism indicates catatonic stupor. This client would be noted to have extreme psychomotor retardation, and efforts to move the individual may be met with bodily resistance.

4. Sexual preoccupation is generally associated with sexual disorders and the manic phase of bipolar disorder. The nurse would not expect to observe sexual preoccupation in a client experiencing catatonia.

TEST-TAKING TIP: The symptom of mutism indicates that the client's problem is catatonic stupor, which immediately eliminates Option 2.

Content Area: Safe and Effective Care Environment: Management of Care;

Integrated Process: Nursing Process: Assessment;

Client Need: Safe and Effective Care Environment: Management of Care;

Cognitive Level: Application;

Concept: Cognition

51. ANSWER: Negative

Rationale: Negative symptoms of schizophrenias tend to reflect a diminution or loss of normal functions. Negative symptoms are difficult to treat and respond less well to antipsychotics than positive symptoms. They are also the most destructive because they render the patient inert and unmotivated. Examples of negative symptoms include apathy, anergia, and anhedonia.

TEST-TAKING TIP: Review the classification of schizophrenia symptoms and be able to differentiate between negative and positive symptoms.

Content Area: Psychosocial Integrity;

Integrated Process: Nursing Process: Assessment;

Client Need: Psychosocial Integrity;

Cognitive Level: Knowledge;

Concept: Assessment

52. ANSWER: 1

Rationale:

1. While experiencing an erotomanic type of delusion, the individual believes that someone, usually of a higher status, is in love with him or her. Famous persons are often the subjects of erotomanic delusions. The situation presented in the question is an example of an erotomanic delusion.

2. While experiencing a grandiose type of delusion, an individual has irrational ideas regarding his or her own worth, talent, knowledge, or power. The situation presented in the question is not an example of a grandiose delusion.

3. An individual experiencing a jealous type of delusion irrationally and without cause believes that his or her sexual partner is unfaithful. The situation presented in the question is not an example of a jealous delusion.

4. An individual experiencing a persecutory type of delusion irrationally and without cause believes that he or she is being persecuted or malevolently treated in some way. The situation presented in the question is not an example of a persecutory delusion.
TEST-TAKING TIP: Review the positive symptoms of schizophrenia and be able to distinguish the various types of delusions.
Content Area: Safe and Effective Care Environment: Management of Care;
Integrated Process: Nursing Process: Assessment;
Client Need: Safe and Effective Care Environment: Management of Care;
Cognitive Level: Application;
Concept: Cognition

53. **ANSWERS: 1, 2, 3, 4**
Rationale:
1. Ventricular enlargement is the most consistent finding in clients diagnosed with schizophrenia.
2. Sulci enlargement is seen in clients diagnosed with schizophrenia.
3. Cerebellar atrophy is seen in clients diagnosed with schizophrenia.
4. Decreased cerebral size is seen in clients diagnosed with schizophrenia.
5. Decreased, not increased, intracranial size is seen in clients diagnosed with schizophrenia.
TEST-TAKING TIP: Review the anatomical abnormalities associated with a diagnosis of schizophrenia.
Content Area: Psychosocial Integrity;
Integrated Process: Nursing Process: Assessment;
Client Need: Psychosocial Integrity;
Cognitive Level: Application;
Concept: Cognition

54. **ANSWERS: 1, 2, 4**
Rationale:
1. Blockage of dopamine receptors does control positive symptoms of schizophrenia. This student statement indicates that learning has occurred.
2. Cholinergic blockade causes anticholinergic side effects (dry mouth, blurred vision, constipation, urinary retention, tachycardia). This student statement indicates that learning has occurred.
3. Blockage of the alpha-adrenergic receptors, not histamine blockade, produces dizziness, orthostatic hypotension, tremors, and reflex tachycardia. This student statement indicates the need for further instruction.
4. Dopamine blockage can result in extrapyramidal symptoms (EPS) and prolactin elevation (galactorrhea, gynecomastia). This student statement indicates that learning has occurred.
5. Weight gain and sedation can result from histamine blockade, not alpha-adrenergic receptor blockage. This student statement indicates the need for further instruction.
TEST-TAKING TIP: Review the action mechanisms of antipsychotic medications and the potential resulting side effects.
Content Area: Psychosocial Integrity;
Integrated Process: Nursing Process: Assessment;

Client Need: Psychosocial Integrity;
Cognitive Level: Application;
Concept: Medication

55. **ANSWER: 3**
Rationale:
1. Succinylcholine chloride is not given as an antiemetic but rather to relax the skeletal muscles during the ECT procedure.
2. Succinylcholine chloride is rapidly destroyed in the body, thus making the onset rapid and the action brief. Rather than stimulating muscular activity, it acts to relax skeletal muscles.
3. Succinylcholine chloride is the medication of choice used to relax the skeletal muscles and prevent severe muscle contractions and potential skeletal fractures during the seizure induced by ECT.
4. Succinylcholine chloride is not administered to control respirations. Because succinylcholine chloride relaxes all skeletal muscles, including respiratory muscles, the client must be oxygenated with pure oxygen during and after ECT until spontaneous respirations return.
TEST-TAKING TIP: Review intravenous medications that are associated with ECT. Understand the implication of administering succinylcholine chloride.
Content Area: Safe and Effective Care Environment: Management of Care;
Integrated Process: Nursing Process: Implementation;
Client Need: Safe and Effective Care Environment: Management of Care;
Cognitive Level: Application;
Concept: Medication

56. **ANSWER: 1**
Rationale:
1. According to the American Psychiatric Association standards, ECT should be given under general anesthesia with the use of a muscle relaxant drug.
2. Recovery from ECT does not take 4 to 5 hours. Clients resume normal activity soon after the treatment is completed.
3. ECT has been in use since the 1930s. However, there is some degree of risk with any procedure requiring general anesthesia.
4. There are no reliable research data showing that ECT therapy causes permanent memory loss.
TEST-TAKING TIP: Review the mechanisms and actions, side effects, and risks associated with ECT treatment.
Content Area: Safe and Effective Care Environment: Management of Care;
Integrated Process: Nursing Process: Implementation;
Client Need: Safe and Effective Care Environment: Management of Care;
Cognitive Level: Application;
Concept: Nursing Roles

57. **ANSWER: 1**
Rationale:
1. Phenelzine (Nardil) is an antidepressant classified as a monoamine oxidase inhibitor (MAOI). Hypertensive crisis may occur with the ingestion of foods or other

products containing high concentrations of the amino acid tyramine.

2. Clomipramine (Anafranil) is an antidepressant classified as a tricyclic (TCA). There are no dietary restrictions associated with this medication.

3. Citalopram (Celexa) is an antidepressant classified as a selective serotonin reuptake inhibitor (SSRI). There are no dietary restrictions associated with this medication.

4. Venlafaxine (Effexor) is an antidepressant classified as a serotonin-norepinephrine reuptake inhibitor (SNRI). There are no dietary restrictions associated with this medication.

TEST-TAKING TIP: Review Table 11-3 ("Diet and Drug Restrictions for Clients on MAOI Therapy") in Chapter 11 of this text. Note the various classifications of antidepressant drugs.

Content Area: Safe and Effective Care Environment: Management of Care;
Integrated Process: Nursing Process: Evaluation;
Client Need: Safe and Effective Care Environment: Management of Care;
Cognitive Level: Analysis;
Concept: Medication

58. **ANSWER: Affect**
Rationale: Affect is the behavioral expression of emotion; it may be appropriate (congruent to the situation), constricted or blunted (diminished range of intensity), or flat (absence of emotional expression).

TEST-TAKING TIP: Review the definition of the term *affect.*
Content Area: Psychosocial Integrity;
Integrated Process: Nursing Process: Assessment;
Client Need: Psychosocial Integrity:
Cognitive Level: Knowledge;
Concept: Mood

59. **ANSWERS: 1, 2, 4, 5**
Rationale:
1. Alcohol can induce intoxication and withdrawal symptoms; therefore, alcohol can be associated with the diagnosis of substance-induced depression.
2. Amphetamines can induce intoxication and withdrawal symptoms; therefore, amphetamines can be associated with the diagnosis of substance-induced depression.
3. Nonopioid analgesics are pain medications for mild to moderate pain. Nonopioid analgesics include ibuprofen, acetaminophen, and aspirin and are not associated with intoxication or withdrawal symptoms.
4. Phencyclidine-like substances can induce intoxication and withdrawal symptoms; therefore, phencyclidine-like substances can be associated with the diagnosis of substance-induced depression.
5. Hallucinogens can induce intoxication and withdrawal symptoms; therefore, hallucinogens can be associated with the diagnosis of substance-induced depression.

TEST-TAKING TIP: Review the etiology of substance-induced depressive disorder. Memorize the list of substances that may evoke intoxication or withdrawal symptoms.
Content Area: Safe and Effective Care Environment: Management of Care;

Integrated Process: Nursing Process: Evaluation;
Client Need: Safe and Effective Care Environment: Management of Care;
Cognitive Level: Analysis;
Concept: Mood

60. **ANSWER: 3**
Rationale:
1. *Risk for post-trauma syndrome* is a NANDA nursing diagnosis that may eventually correspond to this client's behavior; however, *risk for suicide* takes priority because client safety is always the first consideration. Note that "risk for" any nursing diagnosis would not have an AEB statement because the problem has not yet occurred.
2. *Ineffective coping R/T an impulse control disorder* is a NANDA nursing diagnosis that may correspond to this client's behavior; however, *risk for suicide* takes priority, as client safety is always the first consideration.
3. **Risk for suicide R/T failed suicide attempt is the priority NANDA nursing diagnosis that corresponds to this client's behavior. An attempt at suicide validates that the client is actively suicidal, and maintaining client safety takes priority.**
4. *Ineffective denial R/T denial of problems* is a NANDA nursing diagnosis that may correspond to this client's behavior; however, *risk for suicide* takes priority because client safety is always the first consideration. Note that this is an incorrectly written NANDA nursing diagnosis because the required AEB statement has not been included.

TEST-TAKING TIP: A suicidal attempt will justifiably lead to a nursing diagnosis of *risk for suicide.* It is appropriate and crucial to prioritize this "risk for" diagnosis. All other diagnoses become a moot point if suicide becomes a reality.
Content Area: Safe and Effective Care Environment; Management of Care;
Integrated Process: Nursing Process: Diagnosis (Analysis);
Client Need: Safe and Effective Care Environment: Management of Care;
Cognitive Level: Analysis;
Concept: Critical Thinking

61. **ANSWERS: 1, 2, 4, 5**
Rationale:
1. Symptoms of bipolar disorder occur most days in a week.
2. Symptoms of bipolar disorder are severe enough to cause extreme disturbance in one domain or moderate disturbance in two or more domains.
3. Symptoms of bipolar disorder occur three or four times a day, not three or four times a week.
4. Symptoms of bipolar disorder occur 4 or more hours a day.
5. Symptoms of bipolar disorder are severe enough to cause extreme disturbance in one domain or moderate disturbance in two or more domains.

TEST-TAKING TIP: Review the FIND (frequency, intensity, number, and duration) strategy used to evaluate symptoms to diagnose bipolar disorder in children and adolescents.
Content Area: Psychosocial Integrity;
Integrated Process: Nursing Process: Evaluation;
Client Need: Psychosocial Integrity;

Cognitive Level: Application;
Concept: Development

62. ANSWER: 3
Rationale:
1. The nursing diagnosis of *impaired social interaction,* not *disturbed sensory-perception,* would document the client's manipulation of others.
2. The nursing diagnosis of *disturbed thought processes,* not *disturbed sensory-perception,* would document the client's delusions of grandeur.
3. The nursing diagnosis of *disturbed sensory-perception* would document the client's auditory and visual hallucinations.
4. The nursing diagnosis of *risk for injury,* not *disturbed sensory-perception,* would document the client's behavior of extreme hyperactivity.
TEST-TAKING TIP: Review Table 12-1 ("Assigning Nursing Diagnoses to Behaviors Commonly Associated with Bipolar Mania") in Chapter 12 of this text to familiarize yourself with behaviors that are associated with nursing diagnoses for bipolar mania.
Content Area: Safe and Effective Care Environment: Management of Care;
Integrated Process: Nursing Process: Diagnosis (Analysis);
Client Need: Safe and Effective Care Environment: Management of Care;
Cognitive Level: Analysis;
Concept: Critical Thinking

63. ANSWER: hypomania
Rationale: Bipolar II disorder is characterized by recurrent bouts of severe depression with episodic occurrences of **hypomania.** The individual who is assigned this diagnosis may present with symptoms (or history) of depression or hypomania.
TEST-TAKING TIP: Review the symptoms of bipolar II disorder and remember that experiencing a full manic episode would lead to a diagnosis of bipolar I, not bipolar II, disorder.
Content Area: Psychosocial Integrity;
Integrated Process: Nursing Process: Assessment;
Client Need: Psychosocial Integrity;
Cognitive Level: Knowledge;
Concept: Mood

64. ANSWER: 2
Rationale:
1. Fluid and sodium intake is addressed when the mood stabilizer lithium carbonate is prescribed for bipolar mania. A client is then instructed to consume a diet adequate, not restricted, in sodium as well as 2,500 to 3,000 mL of fluid per day.
2. Clients experiencing mania may be at increased risk for nutrition deficits because of increased metabolic rates that accompany mania. Providing finger foods that are nutritious and easy to consume during manic hyperactivity will assist the client to maintain adequate caloric intake.
3. Fluid and sodium intake is addressed when the mood stabilizer lithium carbonate is prescribed for bipolar mania. A client is then instructed to consume a diet

adequate, not restricted, in sodium as well as 2,500 to 3,000 mL of fluid per day.
4. Clients diagnosed with bipolar mania may be at an increased risk for suicide during the depressive phase of the disorder. The client in the question is in the manic, not depressive, phase of bipolar disorder.
TEST-TAKING TIP: Review the nursing actions for treating a client diagnosed with bipolar mania. Review the nursing implications when administering lithium carbonate to recognize incorrect information concerning fluids and sodium.
Content Area: Safe and Effective Care Environment: Management of Care;
Integrated Process: Nursing Process: Implementation;
Client Need: Safe and Effective Care Environment: Management of Care;
Cognitive Level: Analysis;
Concept: Nursing

65. ANSWERS: 1, 2, 4, 5
Rationale:
1. During mania the client experiences extreme hyperactivity, which can lead to injury.
2. During mania rationality is impaired, and the client may injury self inadvertently.
3. During mania the client's mood is characterized by euphoria and elation. It is during the depressive phase of bipolar disorder that the client may be at risk for suicide.
4. During mania the client is extremely distractible, and responses to even the slightest stimuli are exaggerated. This can lead to injury.
5. During mania hyperactivity and distractibility impair a client's focus and concentration and can lead to accidents such as falls.
TEST-TAKING TIP: Review the NANDA definition for the nursing diagnosis of *risk for injury.*
Content Area: Safe and Effective Care Environment: Management of Care;
Integrated Process: Nursing Process: Diagnosis (Analysis);
Client Need: Safe and Effective Care Environment: Management of Care;
Cognitive Level: Application;
Concept: Critical Thinking

66. ANSWER: 1
Rationale:
1. Lamotrigine (Lamictal) is classified as an anticonvulsant and used as a mood-stabilizing agent in the treatment of bipolar disorder.
2. Donepezil (Aricept) is classified as a cholinesterase inhibitor and is not used in the treatment of bipolar disorder.
3. Risperidone (Risperdal) is classified as an antipsychotic but can be used as a mood-stabilizing agent.
4. Imipramine (Tofranil) is classified as a tricyclic antidepressant and is not used in the treatment of bipolar disorder.
TEST-TAKING TIP: Review Table 12-2 ("Mood-Stabilizing Agents") in Chapter 12 of this text for the classification and use of mood-stabilizing agents.
Content Area: Safe and Effective Care Environment: Management of Care;
Integrated Process: Nursing Process: Evaluation;

Client Need: Safe and Effective Care Environment:
Management of Care;
Cognitive Level: Application;
Concept: Medication

67. **ANSWER: 2**
Rationale:
1. Encouraging comparison is the therapeutic communication technique of asking the client to compare similarities and differences in ideas, experiences, or interpersonal relationships. The nurse's question to the client does not reflect this therapeutic technique.
2. When the nurse asks, "Can you describe the triggers that initiate your anger?" The nurse is using the therapeutic technique of "exploring." Exploring is the technique of delving further into a subject, idea, or even a relationship. In this case, the nurse is possibly exploring with the client the connection between feelings of rejection and abandonment and the maladaptive coping pattern of self-injurious behavior.
3. Formulating a plan of action occurs when a client is encouraged to formulate a plan for dealing with a stressful situation. The nurse's question to the client does not reflect this therapeutic technique.
4. Making observations occurs when the nurse verbalizes what is observed or perceived. The nurse's question to the client does not reflect this therapeutic technique.
TEST-TAKING TIP: Review the characteristics of borderline personality to understand the need to explore the client's anger as it relates to feelings of rejection and abandonment.
Content Area: Safe and Effective Care Environment: Management of Care;
Integrated Process: Nursing Process: Implementation;
Client Need: Safe and Effective Care Environment: Management of Care;
Cognitive Level: Application;
Concept: Communication

68. **ANSWER: 2**
Rationale:
1. The clinical picture of a client diagnosed with schizoid personality disorder includes a marked withdrawal from social contact, avoidance of others, and a cold, aloof persona. The client behaviors presented in the question are indicative of narcissistic, not schizoid, personality.
2. Being self-centered and having an exaggerated sense of self-worth is a characteristic of a narcissistic personality disorder. These individuals also lack empathy and are hypersensitive to the evaluation of others.
3. The clinical picture of a client diagnosed with borderline personality disorder includes a pattern of intense and chaotic relationships with affective instability and fluctuating attitudes toward others. The client behaviors presented in the question are indicative of narcissistic, not borderline, personality.
4. The clinical picture of a client diagnosed with antisocial personality disorder includes a lack of empathy and remorse. They are callously unconcerned for the feelings of others. These individuals use manipulation to control others. The client behaviors presented in the question are indicative of narcissistic, not antisocial, personality.

TEST-TAKING TIP: Review the clinical pictures and recognize the many characteristics that contribute to each of the 10 personality disorders.
Content Area: Safe and Effective Care Environment: Management of Care;
Integrated Process: Nursing Process: Assessment;
Client Need: Safe and Effective Care Environment: Management of Care;
Cognitive Level: Application;
Concept: Self

69. **ANSWER: 2**
Rationale:
1. Close relationships that are viewed in extremes of idealization and devaluation and that alternate between overinvolvement and withdrawal is associated with borderline, not narcissistic, personality disorder. This student's statement indicates that further instruction is needed.
2. Interpersonal relationships that are constrained by having little genuine interest in others describes relationships associated with narcissistic personality disorder. This student's statement indicates that learning has occurred.
3. Using exploitation, deceit, and coercion as primary means of relating to others describes an antisocial, not narcissistic, personality disorder. This student's statement indicates that further instruction is needed.
4. Having marked impairments in close relationships associated with mistrust and anxiety describes paranoid, not narcissistic, personality disorder. This student's statement indicates that further instruction is needed.
TEST-TAKING TIP: Review the definition and clinical picture for narcissistic personality disorder to recognize characteristic behaviors of this disorder.
Content Area: Safe and Effective Care Environment: Management of Care;
Integrated Process: Nursing Process: Evaluation;
Client Need: Safe and Effective Care Environment: Management of Care;
Cognitive Level: Analysis;
Concept: Self

70. **ANSWER: 1**
Rationale:
1. Predisposing factors in the development of obsessive-compulsive personality disorder include parental judgments in pointing out transgressions and rule infractions. Children are reared by over controlling parents, and praise for positive behaviors is bestowed on the child less frequently than punishment for undesirable behaviors.
2. Predisposing factors in the development of narcissistic, not obsessive-compulsive, personality disorder include overly critical parents who demand perfection and have unrealistic expectations.
3. Predisposing factors in the development of avoidant, not obsessive-compulsive, personality disorder include parental and/or peer rejection and censure.
4. Predisposing factors in the development of schizotypal, not obsessive-compulsive, personality disorder include parental indifference, impassivity, or formality, leading

to a pattern of discomfort with personal affection and closeness.
TEST-TAKING TIP: Review the various predisposing factors that contribute to the development of personality disorders.
Content Area: Safe and Effective Care Environment: Management of Care;
Integrated Process: Nursing Process: Evaluation;
Client Need: Safe and Effective Care Environment: Management of Care;
Cognitive Level: Analysis;
Concept: Self

71. **ANSWER: Helicopter parenting**
Rationale: *Helicopter parenting* describes parents who pay overly close attention to their child's experiences and problems. These parents hover over their children and become too involved in their lives, including interfering in college or career decisions later in life.
TEST-TAKING TIP: Review the definition of *helicopter parenting* and understand how parental overprotection and overcontrol might affect the direction of a child's personality.
Content Area: Psychosocial Integrity;
Integrated Process: Nursing Process: Assessment;
Client Need: Psychosocial Integrity;
Cognitive Level: Knowledge;
Concept: Development

72. **ANSWER: 4**
Rationale:
1. The term "splitting" refers to when an individual idealizes another and tends to see them as all good or all bad; it does not mean split from, or existing without, a significant other.
2. The term "splitting" refers to when an individual idealizes another and tends to see them as all good or all bad; it is not a perception that the client's mind is splitting in two separate parts.
3. The term "splitting" refers to when an individual idealizes another and tends to see them as all good or all bad; it is not a feeling that the client must split her loyalties equally between her mother and father.
4. **The term "splitting" means that the individual idealizes another and tends to see them as all good or all bad. An individual diagnosed with borderline personality disorder tends to regress during stressful times and will often resort to splitting, denial, projection, and injurious behavior such as self-mutilation.**
TEST-TAKING TIP: Review the definition of "splitting" in the context of the diagnosis of borderline personality disorder.
Content Area: Safe and Effective Care Environment: Management of Care;
Integrated Process: Nursing Process: Implementation;
Client Need: Safe and Effective Care Environment: Management of Care;
Cognitive Level: Application;
Concept: Assessment

73. **ANSWERS: 2, 3, 5**
Rationale:
1. The onset of bulimia nervosa occurs not from age 10 years through adolescence, but in late adolescence or early adulthood.

2. **Bulimia nervosa is more prevalent than anorexia nervosa.**
3. **Bulimia nervosa affects up to 4% of young women.**
4. Bulimia nervosa occurs where abundant, not scant, food is available.
5. **Bulimia nervosa occurs primarily in societies that place emphasis on thinness as the model of attractiveness for women.**
TEST-TAKING TIP: Review the epidemiological factors related to bulimia nervosa.
Content Area: Psychosocial Integrity;
Integrated Process: Nursing Process: Assessment;
Client Need: Psychosocial Integrity;
Cognitive Level: Application;
Concept: Nutrition

74. **ANSWER: 2**
Rationale:
1. A client diagnosed with anorexia nervosa has an obsession with food. Teaching the client about food and new recipes would reinforce this obsession rather than help the client explore more adaptive coping strategies.
2. **Family relationships of clients diagnosed with anorexia nervosa often show unhealthy involvement between the members (enmeshment). The members strive to maintain "appearances," and the parents endeavor to retain the child in a dependent position. Conflict avoidance may be a strong factor in the interpersonal dynamics. Because these problems may be the ultimate cause of the eating disorder, after physiological stabilization, assisting the client to verbalize feelings related to family dynamics should be the priority nursing intervention.**
3. There are no medications specifically indicated for eating disorders. Various medications have been prescribed for associated symptoms such as anxiety and depression.
4. A flexible routine, rather than a rigid schedule, would encourage a sense of client responsibility and control. Control issues are central to the etiology of eating disorders. For treatment programs to be successful, the client must perceive that he or she is in control of the treatment.
TEST-TAKING TIP: Review nursing interventions for clients diagnosed with anorexia nervosa.
Content Area: Safe and Effective Care Environment: Management of Care;
Integrated Process: Nursing Process: Implementation;
Client Need: Safe and Effective Care Environment: Management of Care;
Cognitive Level: Analysis;
Concept: Nursing

75. **ANSWER: 2**
Rationale:
1. Clients diagnosed with eating disorders do not typically experience thought disorders such as tangential thinking or flight of ideas.
2. **Clients diagnosed with eating disorders are at high risk for experiencing feelings of depression and anxiety. A mood rating of 2/10 is an objective symptom of depression. This documentation reflects another symptom of bulimia nervosa that this client is likely to experience.**

3. Clients diagnosed with eating disorders do not typically experience midnight awakenings due to recurrent nightmares. This is a symptom typically experienced by clients diagnosed with post-traumatic stress disorder (PTSD).

4. Clients diagnosed with eating disorders do not typically experience aggression and hostility toward others. Because of an altered body image, these clients may tend to avoid others because they typically binge and purge in secret.

TEST-TAKING TIP: Review the background assessment data for bulimia nervosa, and note the symptoms that a client would likely experience.

Content Area: Safe and Effective Care Environment: Management of Care;
Integrated Process: Nursing Process: Assessment;
Client Need: Safe and Effective Care Environment: Management of Care:
Cognitive Level: Application;
Concept: Assessment

76. ANSWER: 3

Rationale:

1. Studies of twins and adoptees reared by normal and overweight parents have supported the implication of heredity as a predisposing factor to obesity. This etiological implication is from a biological, not a psychoanalytical, perspective.

2. It is true that hypothyroidism is a problem that interferes with basal metabolism, leading to obesity. This etiological implication is from a biological, not a psychoanalytical, perspective.

3. **The psychoanalytical view of obesity proposes that obese individuals have unresolved dependency needs and are fixed in the oral stage of psychosexual development.**

4. Obesity results from an ingestion of a greater number of calories than are expended. Many overweight individuals lead sedentary lifestyles, making it difficult to burn off calories. This etiological implication is from a biological, not a psychoanalytical, perspective.

TEST-TAKING TIP: Review the background assessment data for obesity and note the key words *psychoanalytical perspective* in the question.

Content Area: Psychosocial Integrity;
Integrated Process: Nursing Process: Assessment;
Client Need: Psychosocial Integrity;
Cognitive Level: Application;
Concept: Evidenced-based Practice

77. ANSWERS 2, 3, 4

Rationale:

1. Greater rates of obesity are associated with lower, not higher, levels of education

2. **68.5% of 20-year-olds are overweight, and 35% are in the obese range. This accurately describes the prevalence of obesity.**

3. **6.3% of the U.S. adult population may be categorized as *extremely* obese (a body mass index greater than 40). This accurately describes the prevalence of obesity.**

4. **There are higher rates of obesity in African Americans and Latino Americans than in whites. This accurately describes the prevalence of obesity.**

5. There are greater rates of obesity among lower, not higher, socioeconomic groups. This accurately describes the prevalence of obesity.

TEST-TAKING TIP: Review the epidemiological factors related to obesity.

Content Area: Psychosocial Integrity;
Integrated Process: Nursing Process: Assessment;
Client Need: Psychosocial Integrity;
Cognitive Level: Application;
Concept: Evidenced-based Practice

78. ANSWERS: 1, 3, 4, 5

Rationale:

1. **For the client who is emaciated and is unable or unwilling to maintain an adequate oral intake, the physician may order a liquid diet to be administered via nasogastric tube. Nursing care of the individual receiving tube feedings should be administered according to established hospital protocol.**

2. Do not focus on food and eating. The real issues related to refusal of food have little to do with its consumption. The nursing focus should be on control issues that precipitate these behaviors.

3. **For the client who is able and willing to consume an oral diet, the dietitian will determine the appropriate number of calories required to provide adequate nutrition and realistic weight gain.**

4. **Weigh client daily, immediately on arising and after first voiding. Always use same scale, if possible. These assessments are important measurements of nutritional status and provide guidelines for treatment.**

5. **Assess moistness and color of oral mucous membranes. Assess skin turgor and integrity regularly. These assessments are important measurements of nutritional status and provide guidelines for treatment.**

TEST-TAKING TIP: Review the appropriate interventions for clients diagnosed with anorexia nervosa that have been assigned the nursing diagnosis: *imbalanced nutrition: less than body requirements.*

Content Area: Safe and Effective Care Environment: Management of Care;
Integrated Process: Nursing Process: Implementation;
Client Need: Safe and Effective Care Environment: Management of Care;
Cognitive Level: Application;
Concept: Nursing

79. ANSWER: Amenorrhea

Rationale: Extreme weight loss that results from anorexia nervosa can cause amenorrhea. When amenorrhea occurs, body mass index (BMI) is rarely greater than 19, and at least 10% of normal body weight has been lost. When amenorrhea occurs, anorexia nervosa should be considered.

TEST-TAKING TIP: Review the symptoms of anorexia nervosa including amenorrhea.

Content Area: Psychosocial Integrity;
Integrated Process: Nursing Process: Assessment;
Client Need: Psychosocial Integrity;
Cognitive Level: Knowledge;
Concept: Nutrition

80. ANSWER: 1
Rationale:
1. With neurocognitive disorder, appetite is unchanged. With pseudodementia, appetite is diminished.
2. Recent, not remote, memory loss is greater in pseudodementia, whereas recent and remote memory loss is equal in NCD.
3. Confabulation to deal with memory gaps occurs with NCD, whereas confabulation does not occur with pseudodementia.
4. Attention and concentration are impaired in NCD, whereas attention and concentration are intact in pseudodementia.
TEST-TAKING TIP: Review Table 15-1 ("A Comparison of Neurocognitive Disorder and Pseudodementia") in Chapter 15 of this text.
Content Area: Safe and Effective Care Environment: Management of Care;
Integrated Process: Nursing Process: Evaluation;
Client Need: Safe and Effective Care Environment: Management of Care;
Cognitive Level: Analysis;
Concept: Cognition

81. ANSWER: 1
Rationale:
1. 82.3 is the mean score for normal individuals in the age group 50 to 59.
2. 75.5 is the mean score for normal individuals in the age group 60 to 69.
3. 66.9 is the mean score for normal individuals in the age group 70 to 79.
4. 67.9 is the mean score for normal individuals in the age group 80 to 89.
TEST-TAKING TIP: Review Box 16-2 in Chapter 16 of this text (Mental Status Examination for Neurocognitive Disorder (NCD)).
Content Area: Safe and Effective Care Environment: Management of Care;
Integrated Process: Nursing Process: Assessment;
Client Need: Safe and Effective Care Environment: Management of Care;
Cognitive Level: Application;
Concept: Assessment

82. ANSWERS: 1, 3
Rationale:
1. In the second stage of the disease process, a client diagnosed with NCD due to Alzheimer's disease (AD) may experience *anxiety R/T short-term memory loss*. In this stage, the individual begins to lose things and forget names of people, which in turn may cause apprehension and fear.
2. The nursing diagnosis of *ineffective role performance R/T symptoms interfering with work performance* would address problems beginning in the third, not the second, stage of the AD process.
3. In the second stage of the disease process, a client diagnosed with AD may develop low self-esteem because of impaired cognition fostering a negative view of self, leading to feelings of shame. In this stage, the individual

becomes aware of the intellectual decline and may feel **humiliated, anxious, and depressed.**
4. The nursing diagnosis of *risk for injury R/T impairments in cognitive and psychomotor functioning* would address problems beginning in the sixth, not the second, stage of the AD process.
5. The nursing diagnosis of *nutrition: less than body requirements R/T diminished mental capacity* would address problems beginning in the seventh stage, not the second stage, of the AD process.
TEST-TAKING TIP: Review the progression of AD and then match the AD stage with the appropriate nursing diagnoses that address the problems of that stage.
Content Area: Safe and Effective Care Environment: Management of Care;
Integrated Process: Nursing Process: Diagnosis (Analysis);
Client Need: Safe and Effective Care Environment: Management of Care;
Cognitive Level: Analysis;
Concept: Critical Thinking

83. ANSWER: pseudodementia
Rationale: Pseudodementia is a condition of extreme apathy, which outwardly resembles dementia but is not the result of actual mental deterioration. Pseudodementia is not permanent; once a person's depression is successfully treated, his or her cognitive symptoms will go away as well.
TEST-TAKING TIP: Review the definition of *pseudodementia*.
Content Area: Psychosocial Integrity;
Integrated Process: Nursing Process: Assessment;
Client Need: Psychosocial Integrity;
Cognitive Level: Knowledge;
Concept: Cognition

84. ANSWER: 1
Rationale:
1. The client in the question is exhibiting symptoms of dissociative amnesia. Dissociative amnesia is characterized by the inability to recall important personal information, usually of a traumatic or stressful nature, that is too extensive to be explained by ordinary forgetfulness and is not due to the direct effects of substance use or a neurological or other medical conditions.
2. Depersonalization-derealization disorder is characterized by a temporary change in the quality of self-awareness, which often takes the form of feelings of unreality, changes in body image, feelings of detachment from the environment, or a sense of observing oneself from outside the body. The client in the question is exhibiting problems with memory due to a traumatic event, which is not associated with depersonalization-derealization disorder.
3. Conversion disorder (functional neurological symptom disorder) is characterized by a loss of or change in body function that cannot be explained by any known medical disorder or pathophysiological mechanism. The client in the question is exhibiting problems with memory due to a traumatic event, which is not associated with conversion disorder.
4. Dissociative identity disorder is characterized by the existence of two or more personalities in a single individual. Sufferers of this rare condition are usually victims of

severe abuse. The client in the question is exhibiting problems with memory due to a traumatic event, which is not associated with dissociative identity disorder.
TEST-TAKING TIP: Review the symptoms associated with dissociative amnesia.
Content Area: Safe and Effective Care Environment: Management of Care;
Integrated Process: Nursing Process: Assessment;
Client Need: Safe and Effective Care Environment: Management of Care;
Cognitive Level: Application;
Concept: Assessment

85. **ANSWER: pseudocyesis**
Rationale: Pseudocyesis is a condition in which an individual has nearly all the signs and symptoms of pregnancy but is not pregnant. This is classified as a conversion disorder. A conversion disorder is a loss of or change in body function that cannot be explained by any known medical disorder or pathophysiological mechanism. This symptom may represent a strong desire to be pregnant.
TEST-TAKING TIP: Review the definition of *pseudocyesis.*
Content Area: Psychosocial Integrity;
Integrated Process: Nursing Process: Assessment;
Client Need: Psychosocial Integrity;
Cognitive Level: Knowledge;
Concept: Cognition

86. **ANSWERS: 1, 4**
Rationale: Somatic symptom disorder is a mental disorder characterized by physical symptoms that suggest physical illness or injury. Symptoms cannot be explained fully by a general medical condition or by the direct effect of a substance and are not attributable to another mental disorder.
1. Illness anxiety disorder may be defined as an unrealistic or inaccurate interpretation of physical symptoms or sensations, leading to preoccupation with and fear of having a serious disease. This disorder is classified as a somatic symptom disorder.
2. Dissociative amnesia may be defined as an inability to recall important personal information, usually of a traumatic or stressful nature, that is too extensive to be explained by ordinary forgetfulness and is not due to the direct effects of substance use or a neurological or other medical condition. This disorder is classified as a dissociative disorder, not a somatic symptom disorder.
3. Depersonalization-derealization disorder is characterized by a temporary change in the quality of self-awareness, which often takes the form of feelings of unreality, changes in body image, feelings of detachment from the environment, or a sense of observing oneself from outside the body. This disorder is classified as a dissociative disorder, not a somatic symptom disorder.
4. Conversion disorder (functional neurological symptom disorder) is characterized by a loss of or change in body function that cannot be explained by any known medical disorder or pathophysiological mechanism. This disorder is classified as a somatic symptom disorder.
5. Munchhausen's disorder involves conscious, intentional feigning of physical or psychological symptoms. Individuals diagnosed with Munchhausen's disorder pretend to be ill

to receive emotional care and support commonly associated with the role of "patient." This disorder is classified as a factitious disorder, not a somatic symptom disorder.
TEST-TAKING TIP: Review the characteristics associated with somatic symptom disorder and differentiate between the various disorder classifications.
Content Area: Psychosocial Integrity;
Integrated Process: Nursing Process: Evaluation;
Client Need: Psychosocial Integrity;
Cognitive Level: Comprehension;
Concept: Assessment

87. **ANSWERS: 2, 5**
Rationale:
1. Clients diagnosed with the somatic symptom disorder of illness anxiety, which is not a dissociative disorder, often verbalize numerous physical complaints in the absence of any pathophysiological evidence. These clients experience pain, but there is no underlying pathology to support the complaints.
2. Clients diagnosed with depersonalization-derealization disorder, a dissociative disorder, can experience a temporary disturbance in the perception of the external environment (derealization). Disturbed sensory perception is correctly matched with this symptom.
3. Ineffective coping is a nursing diagnosis that reflects the behavior of consciously feigning psychological symptoms to gain attention. But this behavior is a characteristic of a factitious disorder, not a dissociative disorder.
4. Loss of physical functioning is a characteristic of conversion disorder (functional neurological symptom disorder), a somatic symptom disorder, not a dissociative disorder. Also the diagnosis of conversion disorder is incorrectly matched with the loss of physical functioning because clients with conversion disorder show little concern related to their loss of function ("la belle indifférence").
5. The presence of more than one personality within an individual is a symptom of dissociative identity disorder, a dissociative disorder. The nursing diagnosis of disturbed personal identity is correctly matched with this symptom.
TEST-TAKING TIP: Match the diagnosis with the client behavior that indicates a dissociative disorder. Other types of disorders should not be considered.
Content Area: Safe and Effective Care Environment: Management of Care;
Integrated Process: Nursing Process: Diagnosis (Analysis);
Client Need: Safe and Effective Care Environment: Management of Care;
Cognitive Level: Analysis;
Concept: Critical Thinking

88. **ANSWER: 1**
Rationale:
1. Conversion disorder (functional neurological symptom disorder) occurs more frequently in adolescents and young adults than in other age groups and more frequently in women than in men. Higher prevalence exists in lower socioeconomic groups, rural populations, and among those with less education. Compared with the others presented, this client would have the

highest chance of being diagnosed with conversion disorder.
2. Younger, not older, clients from rural, not urban, areas have a higher incidence of a conversion disorder diagnosis. Compared with the others presented, this client would not have the highest chance of being diagnosed with conversion disorder.
3. Women, not men, from rural, not urban, areas have a higher incidence of a conversion disorder diagnosis. Compared with the others presented, this client would not have the highest chance of being diagnosed with conversion disorder.
4. Younger, not older, women, not men, have a higher incidence of a conversion disorder diagnosis. Compared with the others presented, this client would not have the highest chance of being diagnosed with conversion disorder.
TEST-TAKING TIP: Review the epidemiological statistics for the diagnosis of conversion disorder.
Content Area: Safe and Effective Care Environment: Management of Care;
Integrated Process: Nursing Process: Evaluation;
Client Need: Safe and Effective Care Environment: Management of Care;
Cognitive Level: Application;
Concept: Cognition

89. **ANSWER: hyperactivity**
Rationale: The term "hyperactivity" is used to define excessive psychomotor activity that may be purposeful or aimless, accompanied by physical movements and verbal utterances that are usually more rapid than normal. Inattention and distractibility are common with hyperactive behavior.
TEST-TAKING TIP: Review the definition of *hyperactivity.*
Content Area: Psychosocial Integrity;
Integrated Process: Nursing Process: Assessment;
Client Need: Psychosocial Integrity;
Cognitive Level: Knowledge;
Concept: Assessment

90. **ANSWER: 3**
Rationale: Methylphenidate transdermal system (Daytrana) is a patch given to children to address symptoms associated with attention deficit-hyperactivity disorder (ADHD).
1. It is suggested that the patch should be placed 1 day on the left hip and the next day on the right hip. The patch placement should be rotated to avoid skin irritation.
2. The old patch should be removed gently, not quickly, and if needed an oil-based product such as petroleum jelly or mild soaps can be used.
3. There may be mild skin redness (light pink to red) or itching at the patch site. Typically, skin irritation disappears within 24 hours. However, if there is more intense redness that does not improve within 48 hours or spreads beyond the patch, then the patch should be discontinued and the physician notified.
4. A new patch should be applied to nonirritated and intact, clean, dry skin without powder, oil, or lotion.
TEST-TAKING TIP: Review Table 17-3 ("Medications for Attention Deficit-Hyperactivity Disorder") in Chapter 17 of this text.

Content Area: Safe and Effective Care Environment: Management of Care;
Integrated Process: Nursing Process: Implementation;
Client Need: Safe and Effective Care Environment: Management of Care;
Cognitive Level: Application;
Concept: Medication

91. **ANSWER: 4**
Rationale: Atomoxetine HCL (Strattera) is a medication used to treat clients diagnosed with attention deficit-hyperactivity disorder (ADHD). Atomoxetine, unlike stimulants, is not a scheduled substance.
1. The U.S. Food and Drug Administration (FDA) has issued warnings associated with central nervous system stimulants and atomoxetine for the risk of sudden death in clients who have cardiovascular disease. Clients with known serious structural cardiac abnormalities, cardiomyopathy, serious heart rhythm abnormalities, or serious cardiac abnormalities should not be prescribed atomoxetine.
2. Atomoxetine can induce a mixed/manic episode in clients diagnosed with bipolar disorder. Therefore, clients diagnosed with bipolar disorder should not be prescribed atomoxetine.
3. The FDA has issued a black box warning associated with atomoxetine for an increased risk of suicidal ideation in children or adolescents. Therefore, it is necessary to monitor for these symptoms and behaviors in client prescribed this medication.
4. Unlike other treatments approved for ADHD, atomoxetine does not have abuse potential and is not a scheduled substance.
TEST-TAKING TIP: Review Table 17-3 ("Medications for Attention Deficit-Hyperactivity Disorder" in Chapter 17 of this text).
Content Area: Safe and Effective Care Environment: Management of Care;
Integrated Process: Nursing Process: Evaluation;
Client Need: Safe and Effective Care Environment: Management of Care;
Cognitive Level: Analysis;
Concept: Medication

92. **ANSWERS: 3, 4, 5**
Rationale:
1. Oppositional defiant disorder (ODD) is characterized by a persistent pattern of angry mood and defiant behavior that occurs more frequently than is usually observed in individuals of comparable age and developmental level. Individuals diagnosed with conduct disorder, not ODD, have a persistent pattern of behavior in which the basic rights of others or major age-appropriate societal norms or rules are violated.
2. Specific phobias such as fear of the dark, ghosts, and animals are common in children diagnosed with separation anxiety disorder, not ODD.
3. Oppositional and defiant behaviors often interfere with social, educational, occupational, or other important areas of functioning in children and adolescents diagnosed with ODD.

4. Common comorbid disorders with the diagnosis of ODD include attention deficit-hyperactivity disorder and anxiety and mood disorders.

5. In some cases of ODD, there may be a progression to conduct disorder. Conduct disorder and ODD show high levels of overlap, and both diagnoses show substantial comorbidity with other non–antisocial disorders.

TEST-TAKING TIP: Review the factors and characteristics associated with ODD.

Content Area: Safe and Effective Care Environment: Management of Care;
Integrated Process: Nursing Process: Assessment;
Client Need: Safe and Effective Care Environment: Management of Care;
Cognitive Level: Application;
Concept: Assessment

93. **ANSWER: 3**
Rationale: About a third of married men and a fourth of married women have engaged in extramarital sex at some time during their marriages.

1. The incidence of extramarital sex for men is holding constant, not increasing. This student statement indicates that further instruction is needed.

2. Evidence suggests that extramarital sex is increasing for women, not holding constant. This student statement indicates that further instruction is needed.

3. Attitudes toward extramarital sex remain relatively stable, and most individuals believe the goal in marriage should be sexual exclusivity. This student statement indicates that learning has occurred.

4. Twenty percent, not 50%, of all divorces are caused by infidelity or adultery. This student statement indicates that further instruction is needed.

TEST-TAKING TIP: Review the trends related to extramarital sex.

Content Area: Safe and Effective Care Environment: Management of Care;
Integrated Process: Nursing Process: Evaluation;
Client Need: Safe and Effective Care Environment: Management of Care;
Cognitive Level: Application;
Concept: Sexuality

94. **ANSWERS: 3, 4, 5**
Rationale:
1. Sexual sadistic disorder is the recurrent and intense sexual arousal from the physical or psychological suffering of another individual. Sexual masochistic disorder is sexual arousal from being humiliated, beaten, bound, or otherwise made to suffer. This paraphilic disorder is incorrectly matched with its characteristic symptom.

2. Transvestic disorder is characterized by the recurrent and intense sexual arousal from dressing in the clothes of the opposite gender. Sexual sadistic disorder is the recurrent and intense sexual arousal from the physical or psychological suffering of another individual. This paraphilic disorder is incorrectly matched with its characteristic symptom.

3. Voyeuristic disorder is characterized by recurrent and intense sexual arousal involving the act of observing an unsuspecting individual who is naked, in the process of

disrobing, or engaging in sexual activity. This paraphilic disorder is correctly matched with its characteristic symptom.

4. Fetishistic disorder is characterized by recurrent and intense sexual arousal from the use of either nonliving objects or specific nongenital body parts. This paraphilic disorder is correctly matched with its characteristic symptom.

5. Exhibitionistic disorder is characterized by sexual arousal from the exposure of one's genitals to an unsuspecting individual. This paraphilic disorder is correctly matched with its characteristic symptom.

TEST-TAKING TIP: Review the characteristic symptoms of the various paraphilic disorders.

Content Area: Safe and Effective Care Environment: Management of Care;
Integrated Process: Nursing Process: Assessment;
Client Need: Safe and Effective Care Environment: Management of Care;
Cognitive Level: Application;
Concept: Sexuality

95. **ANSWER: 4**
Rationale:
1. There is nothing in the question that indicates that this woman has any intention of harming self or others; therefore, this nursing diagnosis is inappropriate and would not be assigned.

2. Impaired social interaction is defined as an insufficient or excessive quantity or ineffective quality of social exchange. Female sexual interest/arousal disorder is characterized by reduced or absent frequency or intensity of interest or pleasure in sexual activity. Just because a woman has reduced or absent sexual drive does not mean she has a social interaction problem.

3. Disturbed personal identity is defined as the inability to maintain an integrated and complete perception of self. This diagnosis may apply when a client is diagnosed with gender dysphoria, not female sexual interest/arousal disorder.

4. Sexual dysfunction is defined as the state in which an individual experiences a change in sexual function during the sexual response phases of desire, excitation, and/or orgasm, which is viewed as unsatisfying, unrewarding, or inadequate. This nursing diagnosis can be associated with the symptoms of female sexual interest/arousal disorder.

TEST-TAKING TIP: Review the symptoms of female sexual interest/arousal disorder and consider the possible nursing diagnoses that would reflect these symptoms.

Content Area: Safe and Effective Care Environment: Management of Care;
Integrated Process: Nursing Process: Diagnosis (Analysis);
Client Need: Safe and Effective Care Environment: Management of Care;
Cognitive Level: Analysis;
Concept: Critical Thinking

96. **ANSWERS: 3, 4, 5**
Rationale:
1. Behavior therapy is a form of psychotherapy, the goal of which is to modify maladaptive behavior patterns by

reinforcing more adaptive behaviors. This type of therapy does not apply to the diagnosis of erectile disorder.

2. Cognitive therapy is a type of therapy in which the client is taught to control thought distortions. Thought distortion is not a symptom of erectile dysfunction; therefore, this therapy would not be appropriate for a client diagnosed with this disorder.

3. Systematic desensitization has been used successfully in decreasing the anxiety that may contribute to erectile difficulties. Clinicians widely agree that even when significant organic factors have been identified, psychological factors may also be present and must be considered in treatment.

4. Group therapy has been used successfully in decreasing the anxiety that may contribute to erectile difficulties. Clinicians widely agree that even when significant organic factors have been identified, psychological factors may also be present and must be considered in treatment.

5. Sensate focus therapy is a therapeutic technique used to treat individuals and couples with sexual dysfunction. It has been used successfully in decreasing the anxiety that may contribute to erectile difficulties. Clinicians widely agree that even when significant organic factors have been identified, psychological factors may also be present and must be considered in treatment.

TEST-TAKING TIP: Review general therapeutic approaches that treat various sexual dysfunctions.
Content Area: Safe and Effective Care Environment: Management of Care;
Integrated Process: Nursing Process: Planning;
Client Need: Safe and Effective Care Environment: Management of Care;
Cognitive Level: Application;
Concept: Male Reproduction

97. **ANSWER: masochism**
Rationale: The identifying feature of sexual masochism disorder, a paraphilic disorder, is gaining gratification from pain, deprivation, degradation, or other experiences generally considered aversive or unpleasant inflicted or imposed on oneself, either as a result of one's own actions or the actions of others.
TEST-TAKING TIP: Review information about the paraphilic disorder of sexual masochism disorder.
Content Area: Psychosocial Integrity;
Integrated Process: Nursing Process: Assessment;
Client Need: Psychosocial Integrity;
Cognitive Level: Knowledge;
Concept: Sexuality

98. **ANSWERS: 2, 3, 4**
Rationale:
1. Most victimizers do not have a history of mental illness.
2. The mother figure of a sexual victimizer is noted to be domineering and seductive, but rejecting.
3. Many victimizers report growing up in abusive homes.
4. Statistics show that the greatest number of victimizers are between the ages of 25 and 44.
5. Sixty-two percent of victimizers do use a weapon, but the weapon most frequently used is a knife, not a gun.

TEST-TAKING TIP: Review the characteristics of a sexual victimizer.
Content Area: Safe and Effective Care Environment: Management of Care;
Integrated Process: Nursing Process: Assessment;
Client Need: Safe and Effective Care Environment: Management of Care;
Cognitive Level: Application;
Concept: Violence

99. **ANSWER: physical neglect**
Rationale: Physical neglect is the persistent failure to meet a child's basic physical and/or psychological needs. Physical neglect is likely to result in the serious impairment of the child's health or development. Neglect may occur during pregnancy as a result of maternal substance abuse. Once a child is born, neglect may involve a parent or caregiver failing to provide adequate food, clothing and shelter (including exclusion from home or abandonment); failing to protect a child from physical and emotional harm or danger; failing to ensure adequate supervision (including the use of inadequate caregivers); or failing to ensure access to appropriate medical care or treatment. It may also include neglect of, or unresponsiveness to, a child's basic emotional needs.
TEST-TAKING TIP: Review the definition of *physical neglect*.
Content Area: Psychosocial Integrity;
Integrated Process: Nursing Process: Assessment;
Client Need: Psychosocial Integrity;
Cognitive Level: Knowledge;
Concept: Violence

100. **ANSWERS: 3, 4, 5**
Rationale:
1. From a biological, not sociocultural, perspective, various neurotransmitters—in particular norepinephrine, dopamine, and serotonin—may play a role in the facilitation and inhibition of aggressive impulses.
2. From a learning, not sociocultural, perspective, children learn to behave by imitating their role models, who are usually their parents. Individuals who were abused as children or who witnessed domestic violence as a child are more likely to behave in an abusive manner as adults.
3. From a sociocultural perspective, studies have shown that poverty and income are strong predictors of abuse and violent behavior.
4. From a sociocultural perspective, American society was founded essentially on a general acceptance of violence as a means of solving problems.
5. From a sociocultural perspective, societal influences may contribute to violence when individuals realize that their needs and desires are not being met relative to other people.
TEST-TAKING TIP: Review the etiological implications that predispose individuals to be abusive. Note that all answers are correct; however, only Options 3, 4, and 5 are based on a sociocultural prospective.
Content Area: Psychosocial Integrity;
Integrated Process: Nursing Process: Assessment;
Client Need: Psychosocial Integrity;
Cognitive Level: Application;
Concept: Violence

Putting It All Together
Case Study Answers

Chapter 7

1. Based on Addy's symptoms and actions, Gavin would assign the medical diagnosis of phobic disorder.
2. The term mysophobia describes the fear of dirt, germs, and contamination.
3. Addy's subjective symptoms include her statement "The filthy world is a dangerous place" as well as her disclosures that she rarely has contact with people other than her immediate family and that she cannot maintain employment due to her fears.
4. Addy's objective symptoms include fidgeting behavior, continuous washing of hands and disinfecting surfaces, and an apprehensive affect with minimal eye contact.
5. Certain early experiences may set the stage for phobic reactions later in life. Some researchers believe that phobias, particularly specific phobias, are symbolic of original anxiety-producing objects or situations that have been repressed. Addy's early experience with her younger brother's death and the family's quarantine could have been repressed leading to Addy's projected, irrational fear of all germs.
6. Habit-reversal therapy
   Systematic desensitization
   Implosion therapy (flooding)
7. Gavin might prescribe a variety of anxiolytics that are used for specific phobic disorders. Gavin might consider the benzodiazepine alprazolam to treat Addy's severe anxiety.
8. Specific phobias are generally not treated with medication unless panic attacks accompany the phobia. Gavin might consider the use of antidepressants, such as tricyclics, monoamine oxidase inhibiters (MAOIs), or selective serotonin reuptake inhibitors (SSRIs) for long-term therapy to diminish Addy's anxiety symptoms.
   Antihypertensive agents, such as beta-blockers, can be used in long-term therapy to diminish anxiety symptoms.
9. Fear R/T dirt, germs, and possible contamination AEB apprehensive affect, fidgeting behavior, and client statements.
10. Addy will discuss fear of dirt, germs, and contamination with her PCP within two days of treatment.
11. Addy will be able to function in the presence of dirt, germs, and contamination without experiencing panic anxiety by the time of discharge from treatment.
12. Appropriate nursing interventions may include:
    a. Reassuring Addy that she is safe.
    b. Exploring Addy's perception of the threat to physical integrity or threat to self concept.
    c. Discussing reality of the situation with Addy to recognize aspects that can be changed and those that cannot.
    d. Including Addy in making decisions related to selection of alternative coping strategies. (e.g., Addy may choose either to avoid the phobic stimulus or to attempt to eliminate the fear associated with it.)
    e. If Addy elects to work on elimination of the fear, techniques of desensitization or implosion therapy may be employed.
    f. Encouraging Addy to explore underlying feelings that may be contributing to irrational fears and to face them rather than suppress them.
    g. Exploring Addy's perception of the threat to physical integrity or threat to self-concept.
13. Evaluation of the nursing actions for Addy may be facilitated by gathering information using the following types of questions.
    a. Can Addy recognize signs and symptoms of escalating anxiety?
    b. Can Addy use skills learned to interrupt the escalating anxiety before it reaches the panic level?
    c. Can Addy demonstrate the activities most appropriate for her that can be used to maintain anxiety at a manageable level (relaxation techniques, physical exercise)?
    d. Can Addy maintain anxiety at a manageable level without medication?
    e. Can Addy verbalize a long-term plan for preventing panic anxiety in the face of a stressful situation?

f. Can Addy discuss the phobic object or situation without becoming anxious?

g. Can Addy function in the presence of the phobic object or situation without experiencing panic anxiety?

Chapter 8

1. Based on Bobby's symptoms and actions, Willie would assign a medical diagnosis of post-traumatic stress disorder (PTSD).

2. Bobby's subjective symptoms include his description of frequent nightmares from which he awakens in a cold sweat with heart palpitations, always being terrified, feelings of emotional detachment from family, and the belief that he is unable to prevent his family from burning up in a fire.

3. Bobby's objective symptoms include hyper-vigilant behavior, flat affect, and pacing and wringing his hands.

4. Willie would consider individual therapy, which may include cognitive therapy and/or prolonged exposure therapy. Also used in the treatment of PTSD is group/family therapy and Eye Movement Desensitization and Reprocessing (EMDR) therapy.

5. Willie recognizes selective serotonin reuptake inhibitors (SSRI) as a first-line treatment for PTSD. Other antidepressants, such as tricyclics, and monoamine oxidase inhibitors (MAOI) have also been effective. Anxiolytics, antihypertensives, and mood stabilizers have been effective in controlling symptoms.

6. Post trauma syndrome R/T fighting a 3-alarm fire that resulted in two deaths AEB nightmares, hyper-vigilance, emotional detachment, and pacing.

7. Bobby will be able to talk about the traumatic event and demonstrate the ability to cope with emotional reactions in an individually appropriate manner by discharge.

8. Bobby will be able to reestablish and restore family relationships, integrate the traumatic experience into his persona, and renew and establish meaningful goals after discharge.

9. Appropriate nursing interventions may include:

a. Assigning the same staff to Bobby as often as possible.

b. Using a nonthreatening, matter of fact, but friendly approach.

c. Being consistent; keeping all promises; conveying acceptance; spending time with Bobby.

d. Staying with Bobby during periods of nightmares. Offering reassurance of safety and security and assuring Bobby that his symptoms are not uncommon following a trauma of this magnitude.

e. Encouraging Bobby to talk about the trauma at his own pace.

f. Obtaining accurate history from Bobby's wife about the trauma and Bobby's specific response.

g. Discussing coping strategies used in response to trauma.

h. Assisting Bobby to comprehend the trauma if possible. Discussing feelings of vulnerability and Bobby's "place" in the world following the trauma.

10. Evaluation of the nursing actions for Bobby may be facilitated by gathering information using the following types of questions.

a. Can Bobby discuss the traumatic event without experiencing panic anxiety?

b. Can Bobby discuss changes that have occurred in his life because of the traumatic event?

c. Does Bobby continue to have nightmares?

d. Has Bobby learned and can he demonstrate new adaptive coping strategies?

e. Has Bobby regained a satisfactory relationship with his wife and children?

Chapter 9

1. Steve's symptoms meet the requirements for the diagnosis of substance use disorder.

2. The following predisposing factors may have led to Steve's diagnosis:

a. Alcoholic father.

b. Dysfunctional parenting.

c. Antisocial personality traits.

3. Steve's subjective symptoms are as follows:

a. States his father was an alcoholic and beat his mother.

b. Blames overcritical boss for drinking binge.

c. Requests money and discharge from PNP.

d. States he is depressed and down on his luck.

e. Denies previous intoxication and legal problems.

4. Steve's objective symptoms are as follows:

a. Blood alcohol level of 0.08%.

b. Detoxed without complication.

c. Documented history of long-term alcohol abuse.

d. A documented long rap sheet including extortion, domestic violence, delinquent child support, and two previous DUIs.

5. Therapies may include Alcoholics Anonymous (AA), individual and family counseling, disulfiram (Antabuse), acamprosate (Campral), and group therapy.

6. Ineffective denial R/T inadequate coping skills AEB statements that he has no problem with alcohol.

7. Within 5 days, Steve will begin to recognize the effect alcohol has had on his life.

8. By time of discharge, Steve will be willing to attend AA meetings as part of the recovery process.

9. The nurse should employ the following interventions:
   a. Accept client unconditionally.
   b. Identify ways in which use of alcohol has contributed to maladaptive behaviors.
   c. Do not allow client to blame others for behaviors associated with alcohol abuse.
   d. Set limits on manipulative behavior.
   e. Practice alternative, more adaptive, coping strategies.
   f. Give positive feedback for delaying gratification and using adaptive coping strategies.
   g. Assess client's level of knowledge and readiness to learn.
   h. Include significant others in teaching.
   i. Provide information about physical effects of alcohol on body.
   j. Teach about possibility of using disulfiram.
   k. Encourage continued participation in long-term treatment.
   l. Promote participation in outpatient support system (e.g., AA).
   m. Assist client to identify alternative sources of satisfaction.
   n. Provide support for health promotion and maintenance.
10. The following questions can help determine the success of the nursing actions:
    a. Is the client still in denial?
    b. Does the client accept responsibility for his own behavior? Has he acknowledged a personal problem with substances?
    c. Has a correlation been made between personal problems and the use of substances?
    d. Does the client still make excuses or blame others for use of substances?
    e. Has the client remained substance-free during hospitalization?
    f. Does the client cooperate with treatment?
    g. Does the client refrain from manipulative behavior and violation of limits?
    h. Is the client able to verbalize alternative adaptive coping strategies to substitute for substance use? Has the use of these strategies been demonstrated? Does positive reinforcement encourage repetition of these adaptive behaviors?
    i. Is the client able to verbalize the effects of substance abuse on the body?
    j. Does the client verbalize that he wants to recover and lead a life free of alcohol?
11. Complications may include: peripheral neuropathy, alcoholic myopathy, Wernicke's encephalopathy, Korsakoff's psychosis, alcoholic cardiomyopathy, esophagitis, gastritis, pancreatitis, alcoholic hepatitis, cirrhosis of the liver, leukopenia, thrombocytopenia, sexual dysfunction.
12. Steve is using the defense mechanisms of denial and projection.
13. Steve is exhibiting the personality traits of manipulation and exploitation.
14. During the detoxification phase, anxiolytics are titrated to prevent central nervous system overstimulation during alcohol withdrawal. During the recovery phase, medications such as naltrexone and acamprosate are used to decrease craving. Disulfiram may be used as a deterrent to alcohol consumption. Antidepressants can be prescribed to deal with depressive symptoms, and anxiolytics may be used for anxiety but must be used with caution because of their addictive properties.

Chapter 10

1. On the basis of Monique's symptoms and actions, Ms. Williams would assign a medical diagnosis of schizophrenia.
2. A family history of schizophrenia is a predisposing factor that may have led to acquiring the disorder. Monique's father's institutionalization for "bizarre" behavior would validate this family history. Statistically, offspring with one parent who has schizophrenia have a 5% to 6% chance of developing the disorder.
3. The following are Monique's subjective symptoms: Monique has been threatening suicide ever since losing custody of her three young children to her ex-husband. Monique's statement: "Are you the one having an affair with my husband, or are you the one who kidnapped my kids?" She also stated that she hates taking her medications because they increase appetite and decrease libido. She states, "The voices are telling me that my ex has paid off someone to kill me. First I lost my husband and then my kids. I just don't care anymore."
4. The following are Monique's objective symptoms: Monique attempted suicide by overdose. She has stopped taking her prescribed medications. Monique has a history of paranoia and command hallucinations. Her affect is hostile, her eyes dart around the room, and her lips silently move as if interacting with someone.
5. Altered sensory perception R/T brain chemical imbalance and current stressors of divorce and child custody loss and med nonadherence AEB hearing voices telling her that her ex has paid off someone to kill her.
6. Client will discuss content of hallucinations with nurse, express feelings generated by hallucinations, and be adherent to medication regime within 1 week.
7. Client will be able to define and test reality and recognize that the hallucinations are a result of her illness, by 6-month follow-up visit.

8. After stabilization of acute symptoms, the PNP might employ individual psychotherapy, group therapy (with emphasis on social interaction and reality testing), behavior therapy (with emphasis on positive reinforcement of adaptive behaviors), and social skills training (with emphasis on functional skills relevant to activities of daily living).

9. The PNP is likely to prescribe a second generation atypical antipsychotic to treat Monique's positive symptoms. These medications (olanzapine [Zyprexa], quetiapine [Seroquel], or risperidone [Risperdal]) have fewer side effects than older typical antipsychotics and are effective in treating the positive symptoms of schizophrenia.

10. The following nursing interventions can be helpful for a client who is actively hallucinating:
    a. Observe client for signs of hallucinations (listening pose, laughing or talking to self, stopping in midsentence).
    b. Avoid touching the client without warning.
    c. Accept the client and encourage her to share the content of hallucinations.
    d. Do not reinforce the hallucination. Use "the voices" instead of words like "they" that imply validation.
    e. Let client know that you do not share the perception. Say, "Even though I realize the voices are real to you, I do not hear any voices speaking."
    f. Help the client understand the connection between increased anxiety and the presence of hallucinations.
    g. Distract the client from the hallucination.
    h. For persistent hallucinations, encourage client to listen to the radio, watch television, or hum a tune to distract the client from the voices.

11. Evaluation of the nursing actions for the client with schizophrenia may be facilitated by gathering information using the following types of questions:
    a. Has the client established trust with at least one staff member?
    b. Is the anxiety level maintained at a manageable level?
    c. Is delusional thinking still prevalent?
    d. Is hallucinogenic activity evident? Does the client share content of hallucinations, particularly if commands are heard?
    e. Is the client able to interrupt escalating anxiety with adaptive coping mechanisms?
    f. Is the client easily agitated?
    g. Is the client able to interact with others appropriately?
    h. Does the client voluntarily attend therapy activities?
    i. Is the client compliant with medication? Does the client verbalize the importance of taking medication regularly and on a long-term basis? Does he or she verbalize understanding of possible side effects and when to seek assistance from the physician?
    j. Does the client spend time with others rather than isolating self?
    k. Does the family have information regarding support groups in which they may participate and from which they may seek assistance in dealing with their family member who is ill?
    l. If the client lives alone, does she have a source for assistance with home maintenance and health management?

Chapter 11

1. On the basis of Melanie's symptoms and actions, Jim would assign a medical diagnosis of major depressive disorder (MDD).

2. Melanie's subjective symptoms include her description of insomnia, tearfulness, and suicidal thoughts of wishing to die and be with her deceased son.

3. Melanie's objective symptoms include weight loss, a doleful expression, shaky voice, crying inconsolably, blaming self for son's suicide because she failed to read the "black box" antidepressant warning.

4. The PNP would consider individual psychotherapy, which would focus on helping Melanie to resolve complicated grief reactions. Cognitive therapy, which focuses on changing "automatic thoughts," would help Melanie control negative thought distortions. Group therapy should be considered once the acute phase of the illness has passed. An antidepressant such as a selective serotonin reuptake inhibitor (SSRI) or a tricyclic could be prescribed.

5. Risk for suicide R/T blaming self for son's death.

6. Melanie will seek out staff when feeling the urge to harm self during hospitalization.

7. Melanie will not blame self for son's death by outpatient follow-up appointment in 6 weeks.

8. Appropriate nursing interventions may include:
    a. Create safe environment for Melanie by removing all potentially harmful objects.
    b. Formulate a short-term written safety plan that Melanie will not harm self during a specific time period.
    c. Convey an accepting attitude and enable Melanie to express feelings openly.
    d. Help Melanie to explore angry feelings so that they may be directed externally.
    e. Once she is stabilized, teach Melanie the normal stages of grief and behaviors associated with each stage.

f. Identify sources that Melanie may use after discharge when feelings of suicide prevail.

g. Help Melanie identify areas of life situation that are under her control.

9. Evaluation questions may include the following:

a. Have suicidal ideations subsided?

b. Does Melanie know where to seek assistance outside the hospital when suicidal thoughts occur?

c. Has Melanie discussed the recent loss with staff and family members?

d. Can Melanie verbalize feelings and behaviors associated with each stage of the grieving process and recognize her position in the process?

e. Is anger expressed appropriately?

f. Can Melanie identify areas of life situation over which she has control?

Chapter 12

1. On the basis of Rick's symptoms and actions, Melanie would assign a medical diagnosis of bipolar I (acute mania).

2. Rick's subjective symptoms include:

a. "I always 'crash' into despair."

b. "I took out a second mortgage on our house and opened three law offices."

c. "Then the bills were coming in faster than I could pay them."

d. "I tell her I don't need to eat, and sleeping is such a waste of time."

e. "Her parents never liked me, and I'll bet they're telling her things about me that aren't true."

f. "I don't seem to be able to complete plans that I set in motion before my world turns upside down".

g. "I stay awake at night just basking in my own brilliance."

3. Rick's objective symptoms include:

a. Emaciation (wife states that client has not eaten or slept in days).

b. Inappropriate dress.

c. Suggestive sexual remarks (calling the nurse "honey" and "darlin'").

d. Loud voice and rapid pressured speech.

e. Flight of ideas.

f. Pacing, banging fist on table.

g. Remarks suggest persecutory delusions.

h. Remarks suggest grandiose thinking.

4. The NP would consider individual therapy, which focuses on interpersonal deficiencies and treatment adherence. After the acute phase of the illness has passed, group therapy should be considered to provide Rick an opportunity to discuss troubling issues in his life. Family therapy would aid in restoring adaptive family functioning, and cognitive therapy would assist Rick in identifying dysfunctional patterns of thinking and behaving. Tranquilizing medications may be ordered to address acute manic symptoms for the first week of hospitalization, and mood stabilizing agents such as lithium carbonate could be prescribed for controlling symptoms. Client teaching should emphasize client medication adherence and include information on medication side effects, lithium toxicity, and the need for periodic blood tests.

5. Imbalanced nutrition: less than body requirements R/T increased metabolic need secondary to hyperactivity, refusal to eat, and inability to sit still long enough to eat AEB weight loss and emaciation.

6. Short-term goal: Client will consume sufficient foods and between-meal snacks to meet increased caloric needs by discharge.

7. Long-term goal: Client will exhibit no symptoms of malnutrition by 6-week follow-up appointment.

8. The nursing interventions (actions) that will assist Rick to successfully meet these outcomes include:

a. Offering high protein, high calorie fingers foods.

b. Make available juice and snacks on unit.

c. Input and output, calorie count, daily weights.

d. Assess and provide favorite foods.

e. Supplement with vitamins and minerals.

f. Sit with client during meals.

9. To evaluate the success of nursing interventions, the following questions should be asked:

a. Has client gained (maintained) weight during hospitalization?

b. Is client able to verbalize importance of adequate nutrition and fluid intake?

c. Have nutritional status and weight been stabilized to the point that client can be safely discharged?

d. Is the client willing and able to select foods to maintain adequate nutrition?

Chapter 13

1. Emily's symptoms meet the requirements for the diagnosis of borderline personality disorder.

2. The following predisposing factors may have led to Emily's diagnosis:

a. Poor relationships with parents.

b. Parental abandonment as a toddler.

c. Self-absorbed mother.

3. Emily's subjective symptoms are as follows:

a. States she now hates the nurses that she once adored.

b. Attempts to seduce her nurse, Scott, when he caught her with alcohol.

c. Poor family relationships. States, "My mother only cares about herself."

d. Admits to feelings of depression and anxiety.

e. States that cutting and alcohol consumption make her feel less hollow.

4. Emily's objective symptoms are as follows:

a. Razor cuts to arms and legs.

b. Attempts to bring alcohol onto unit.

c. Cannot make friends on unit.

d. Becomes angry when not the center of attention.

e. Angry affect and piercing eye contact.

5. Dialectic behavioral therapy has been used as a treatment for the self-injurious and parasuicidal behavior of client's with borderline personality disorder. Although medication has no effect in the direct treatment of personality disorders, symptomatic treatment may include antipsychotics and selective serotonin reuptake inhibitors.

6. Impaired social interaction R/T extreme fears of abandonment AEB alternating clinging and distancing behaviors, staff splitting, and inability to establish relationships.

7. Within 5 days, Emily will discuss with her nurse behaviors that impede the development of satisfactory interpersonal relationships.

8. By discharge, Emily will interact appropriately with others in the therapy setting in both social and therapeutic activities.

9. The nurse should employ the following interventions:

a. Convey an accepting attitude.

b. Identify ways for Emily to discharge pent-up anger appropriately such as brisk exercise.

c. Help Emily explore true source of anger, such as toddler abandonment issues.

d. Set limits on acting-out behavior.

e. Recognize splitting behaviors and discourage Emily's staff criticism or praise.

f. Help Emily understand how splitting behaviors interfere with satisfactory relationships.

g. Role-play appropriate interpersonal interactions.

10. The following questions can help determine the success of the nursing actions:

a. Does the client recognize when anger is getting out of control?

b. Can the client seek out staff instead of expressing anger in an inappropriate manner?

c. Can the client use other sources for rechanneling anger (e.g., physical activities)?

d. Can the client follow rules and regulations of the therapeutic milieu with little or no reminding?

e. Can the client verbalize which behaviors are appropriate and which are not?

f. Does the client express a desire to change?

g. Can the client delay gratifying own desires in deference to those of others when appropriate?

h. Does the client refrain from manipulating others to fulfill own desires?

Chapter 14

1. On the basis of Shannon's symptoms and actions, Sean would assign a medical diagnosis of anorexia nervosa.

2. The following are the predisposing psychodynamic influences which may have led to Shannon's disorder:

a. Her mother responded to Shannon's physical and emotional needs with food.

b. Shannon may have had a delayed ego development and an unfulfilled sense of separation-individuation.

c. Shannon's threatened ego may have led to a lack of control over her body.

d. Shannon is unable to control behaviors associated with food and eating.

e. Shannon exhibits unhealthy enmeshment with her mother.

f. Shannon's mother kept her in a dependent position.

g. Shannon places a high value on perfectionism.

3. The following are Shannon's subjective symptoms: Shannon states that she no longer feels hungry. She has thoughts of being a fat failure when she was actually underweight. She asked the nurse about the calories in the intravenous fluid. She states that she never had time for friends, play dates, or outside activities. She related being devastated when her mother's Olympic dream was dashed. She stated that she was not satisfied with her and Jack's relationship.

4. The following are Shannon's objective symptoms: she presented with less than 85% of expected weight for her height and a BMI of 17. Assessment revealed hypotension and bradycardia, poor skin turgor, dry, pale oral mucosa, dehydration, electrolyte imbalance, and lanugo.

5. Imbalanced nutrition: less than body requirements R/T refusal to eat and drink AEB less than 85% of expected weight for her height, a BMI of 17, and lanugo. Deficient fluid volume R/T refusal to eat and drink AEB hypotension, bradycardia, poor skin turgor, and dry, pale oral mucosa.

6. Shannon will gain 2 pounds a week during hospitalization. Shannon will drink 125 mL each hour during waking hours while hospitalized.

7. Shannon will exhibit no signs or symptoms of malnutrition or dehydration by discharge.

8. The PNP might employ behavior modification to change maladaptive eating behaviors. Cognitive and/or cognitive-behavioral therapy would help Shannon confront irrational thinking. Family therapy would educate family members about the disorder's manifestations, possible etiology, and prescribed treatment.

9. There is no specific classification of medications used exclusively for the treatment of eating disorders. There are medication trials and off-label use of various drugs to treat these disorders. Medications can be prescribed for associated symptoms such as anxiety and depression.

10. The following nursing interventions can be helpful for a client who has been diagnosed with anorexia nervosa:
    a. Consult with dietitian to determine appropriate number of calories required to provide adequate nutrition and realistic weight gain.
    b. Mutually develop a contract related to privileges and restrictions based on compliance with treatment and direct weight gain.
    c. Do not focus on food and eating.
    d. Weigh client daily in morning after first voiding, using the same scale.
    e. Keep a strict record of intake and output.
    f. Regularly assess skin turgor and integrity.
    g. Assess moistness and color of oral mucous membranes.
    h. Stay with client during established mealtimes (usually 30 minutes) and for at least 1 hour after meals.
    i. If weight loss occurs, enforce contract restrictions.
    j. Implement interventions and communicate with family in a matter-of-fact, nonpunitive way.
    k. Encourage client to explore and identify true feelings and fears.
11. Evaluation of the nursing actions for the client diagnosed with anorexia nervosa may be facilitated by gathering information using the following types of questions:
    a. Has the client steadily gained 2 to 3 pounds per week to at least 80% of body weight for age and size?
    b. Is the client free of signs and symptoms of malnutrition and dehydration?
    c. Does the client consume adequate calories as determined by the dietitian?
    d. Have there been any attempts to hide food from the tray to discard later?
    e. Has the client admitted that a problem exists and that eating behaviors are maladaptive?
    f. Have behaviors aimed at manipulating the environment been discontinued?
    g. Is the client willing to discuss the real issues concerning family roles, sexuality, dependence/independence, and the need for achievement?
    h. Does the client understand how he or she has used maladaptive eating behaviors in an effort to achieve a feeling of some control over life events?
    i. Has the client acknowledged that perception of body image as "fat" is incorrect?

Chapter 15

1. On the basis of Jack's history and symptoms, Eve would assign a medical diagnosis of neurocognitive disorder.

2. The MRI might indicate degenerative pathology of the brain that includes atrophy, widening cortical sulci, and enlarged cerebral ventricles, which would change the diagnosis to NCD due to Alzheimer's disease.
3. The results of the mental status examinations indicate that Jack has progressed from stage I to stage II of NCD due to Alzheimer's disease.
4. Eve understands that Jack is using confabulation to deny a memory problem by filling in gaps with imaginary events.
5. Eve would understand that the focus of treatment is general supportive care, with provisions for security, stimulation, patience, and nutrition.
6. Eve might prescribe a cholinesterase inhibitor such as donepezil (Aricept) to treat Jack's cognitive impairment, an antipsychotic such as risperidone (Risperdal) to treat Jack's agitation, an antidepressant such as sertraline (Zoloft) to treat Jack's possible depression, an anxiolytic such as lorazepam (Ativan) to treat Jack's anxiety, and a sedative hypnotic such as temazepam (Restoril) to treat Jack's possible insomnia.
7. Jack's subjective symptoms include the following: claiming that confusion and forgetfulness is nothing more than normal aging, that being admitted to an assisted living facility is a big mistake and insisting that he doesn't belong, denying problems regarding driving and becoming lost, and filling in memory gaps with imaginary events.
8. Jack's objective symptoms include the following: family and close friends noting progressively more and more forgetfulness and confusion; his son finding his father's door open, the stove burner on, and Jack not home; reports of Jack getting lost while driving; results from the two mental status examinations and the MRI.
9. Disturbed thought processes; impaired memory R/T cerebral degeneration AEB disorientation, confusion, memory deficits, and inaccurate interpretation of the environment.
10. Short-term outcome: Jack will utilize provided clocks, calendars, and room identification to maintain reality orientation.
11. Long-term outcome: Jack will maintain reality orientation to the best of his ability.
12. The following are interventions used to assist Jack in successfully meeting these outcomes:
    a. Frequently orient Jack to reality. Use clocks and calendars with large numbers that are easy to read. Use notes and large signs as reminders. Allow Jack to have personal belongings.
    b. Keep explanations simple. Use face-to-face interactions. Speak slowly and do not shout.

    c. Discourage rumination of delusional thinking. Talk about real events and real people. Remember that the Jack's level of reality is different from the nurse's. Do not lie to him. May need to use validation therapy and redirection.

    d. Monitor Jack for medication side effects.

    e. Encourage Jack to view old photographs.

13. The following questions may be used for measurement of outcomes in Jack's care:

    a. Has Jack experienced physical injury?

    b. Has Jack harmed self or others?

    c. Has Jack maintained reality orientation to the best of his capability?

    d. Is Jack able to communicate with consistent caregiver?

    e. Is Jack able to fulfill activities of daily living with assistance?

    f. Can Jack discuss positive aspects about self and life?

Chapter 16

1. On the basis of Megan's symptoms and actions, Jessie would assign a medical diagnosis of conversion disorder (functional neurological symptom disorder).

2. Megan has learned that through paralysis, she can avoid stressful obligations and postpone unwelcomed challenges. This will be a *primary gain* for Megan.

3. Jessie understands that aiding Megan by pushing her wheelchair may encourage manipulation, dependence, and unnecessary attention. This would foster a secondary gain which would encourage continuation of symptoms.

4. Megan is experiencing "la belle indifference." This is a term that defines a disproportionate degree of unconcern, or complacency about, symptoms such as paralysis or loss or sensation in part of the body, associated with conversion disorder (functional neurological symptom disorder). Physical symptoms are unconsciously used to relieve anxiety and therefore are viewed by Megan as nonthreatening.

5. Megan's subjective symptoms include her admission that her legs became paralyzed two times before stressful ballet performances; being unconcerned about her condition and the effect on her dancing career; and her stating that she is under a great deal of stress, and that she doesn't want to disappoint her parents by not meeting their high expectations.

6. Megan's objective symptoms include loss of purposeful movement involving both legs; presenting as a well-nourished, attractive young woman; neurological tests results being within normal limits; and having a flat, sad affect of 2/10 and an apathetic indifference to her surroundings.

7. Disturbed sensory perception R/T repressed severe anxiety AEB loss of leg function without evidence of organic pathology.

8. Megan will verbalize understanding of emotional problems as a contributing factor to the alteration in physical functioning by day 5.

9. Megan will demonstrate recovery of lost or altered function by discharge.

10. The PNP might employ the following treatment modalities:

    a. Individual psychotherapy to help Megan develop healthy and adaptive behaviors, to encourage her to move beyond her somatic symptoms, and manage her life more effectively.

    b. Group psychotherapy to help Megan share her experiences of illness, learn to verbalize thoughts and feelings, and to experience confrontation by group members and leaders when she rejects responsibility for maladaptive behaviors.

    c. Behavior therapy to focus on rewarding Megan's autonomy, self sufficiency, and independence, thereby decreasing Meagan's need for secondary gains.

11. The following nursing interventions can be helpful for a client diagnosed with conversion disorder (functional neurological symptom disorder) and experiencing disturbed sensory perception:

    a. Monitor physician's ongoing assessments, laboratory reports, and other data to ensure that possibility of organic pathology is clearly ruled out.

    b. Identify primary or secondary gains that the physical symptoms may be providing Megan (increased dependency, attention, protection from experiencing a stressful event).

    c. Do not focus on the disability, and encourage client to be as independent as possible. Intervene only when Megan requires assistance.

    d. Maintain nonjudgmental attitude when providing assistance to Megan. The physical symptom is not within Megan's conscious control and is very real to her.

    e. Do not allow Megan to use the disability as a manipulative tool to avoid participation in therapeutic activities. Withdraw attention if Megan continues to focus on physical limitations.

    f. Encourage Megan to verbalize fears and anxieties. Help identify physical symptoms as a coping mechanism that is used in times of extreme stress.

    g. Help Megan identify coping mechanisms that she could use when faced with stressful situations, rather than retreating from reality with a physical disability.

    h. Give positive reinforcement for identification or demonstration of alternative, more adaptive coping strategies.

12. Evaluation of the nursing actions for the client diagnosed with disturbed sensory perception may be facilitated by gathering information using the following types of questions:
    a. Can Megan recognize signs and symptoms of escalating anxiety?
    b. Can Megan intervene with adaptive coping strategies to interrupt the escalating anxiety before physical symptoms are exacerbated?
    c. Can Megan verbalize an understanding of the correlation between physical symptoms and times of escalating anxiety?
    d. Does Megan have a plan for dealing with increased stress to prevent exacerbation of physical symptoms?
    e. Does Megan demonstrate full recovery from previous loss or alteration of physical functioning?

Chapter 17

1. On the basis of symptoms and actions, Tessa would assign a medical diagnosis of oppositional defiant disorder (ODD).
2. Enforced authority, conflict over control, and Elise's demand for autonomy are predisposing factors that may have led to her oppositional, defiant, and negative behavior.
3. Stating that she doesn't have a problem; feeling that skipping school isn't a big deal; thinking all questions being asked are stupid; calling her mother "holier than thou" and a bitch; thinking her family feels she's an embarrassment, and stating, "I plan to live my life my way" are Elise's subjective symptoms.
4. Elise's objective symptoms are reported by her mother as starting in the second grade with Elise becoming disruptive and refusing to do class work. These behaviors progressed through the years with more absenteeism than attendance. She reports that Elise is sullen, belligerent, strong willed, and defiant at home. Elise has had several run-ins with the authorities and lately is sneaking out at night and not returning until the next day.
5. Defensive coping R/T low self-esteem; unsatisfactory parent-child relationship AEB oppositional and defiant behavior.
6. Elise will verbalize personal responsibility for difficulties experienced in interpersonal relationships within 5 days of hospitalization.
7. Elise will accept responsibility for her own behaviors and interact with others without becoming defensive by discharge.
8. The following nursing interventions can be helpful for a client who has been diagnosed with ODD:
    a. Help Elise recognize that feelings of inadequacy provoke defensive behavior, such as blaming others for problems and the need to "get even."
    b. Provide immediate, nonthreatening feedback for passive-aggressive behavior.
    c. Help identify situations that provoke defensiveness and practice through role-play more appropriate responses.
    d. Provide immediate positive feedback for acceptable behavior.
9. Tessa might employ the following treatment modalities:
    a. Behavior therapy is based on the concepts of classical and operant conditioning. Behavior therapy rewards appropriate behavior and withholds rewards when behaviors are disruptive or otherwise inappropriate.
    b. Family therapy can be employed to identify and resolve problem areas between family members by improving family interactions, social functioning and, parental self-control.
    c. Group therapy provides children the opportunity to learn to tolerate and accept differences in others, to offer and receive support from others.
10. The following questions should be asked to evaluate the success of the nursing actions in achieving the goals of therapy:
    a. Is Elise cooperating with a schedule of therapeutic activities? Is her level of participation adequate?
    b. Is Elise's attitude toward therapy less negative?
    c. Is Elise accepting responsibility for problem behavior?
    d. Is Elise verbalizing the unacceptability of her passive-aggressive behavior?
    e. Is Elise able to identify which behaviors are unacceptable and substitute more adaptive behaviors?
    f. Is Elise able to interact with staff and peers without defending behavior in an angry manner?
    g. Is Elise able to verbalize positive statements about self?
    h. Is increased self-worth evident with fewer manifestations of manipulation?
    i. Is Elise able to make compromises with others when issues of control emerge?
    j. Are anger and hostility expressed in an appropriate manner?
    k. Can Elise verbalize ways of releasing anger adaptively?
    l. Is Elise able to verbalize true feelings instead of allowing them to emerge through use of passive-aggressive behaviors?

Chapter 18

1. On the basis of Jamie's symptoms and actions, Zac would assign a medical diagnosis of gender dysphoria in children.

2. Jamie's subjective symptoms include crying and shouting, "Well, now my mother knows I'm weird! I just don't feel like a boy on the inside. I know I'm a big disappointment, and I don't know what to do about it. What's wrong with me?" Jamie admits to having hated his body for as long as he can remember and tells Zac, "If I was a girl, my life would be happy and normal."

3. Jamie's objective symptoms as reported by his mother include shutting himself away after being caught dressing in his sister's clothes and showing little interest in gender-appropriate activities and toys. She also reports that Jamie has never had a father figure or any male role models. Medical examination and laboratory findings reveal a physically health 12-year-old boy with no adrenogenital disorders. Zac notes that Jamie is polite, reserved, and overwhelmingly sad. His shoulders are slumped, his eyes are downcast, and his affect is flat.

4. On the basis of Jamie's diagnosis, Zac might consider behavior modification therapy. This treatment would serve to help Jamie embrace the games and activities of his assigned gender and promote development of friendships with same-gender peers. The goal is acceptance of a culturally appropriate self-image without mental health concerns from discomfort associated with the assigned gender.

   An additional treatment model Zac might recommend is pubertal delay for Jamie, who has suffered with extreme lifelong gender dysphoria and who has a supportive mother who will encourage Jamie to pursue a desired change in gender. A gonadotropin-releasing hormone agonist would be administered, which suppresses pubertal changes. The treatment is reversible if Jamie decides later not to pursue the gender change. When the medication is withdrawn, external sexual development would proceed, and Jamie would have avoided permanent surgical intervention. If Jamie decides as an adult to advance to the surgical intervention, the proponents of the hormonal treatment suggest that initiating pubertal delay at an early age will result in high percentages of individuals who will more easily pass into the opposite gender role than when treatment commenced well after the development of secondary sexual characteristics.

5. Disturbed personal identity R/T biological factors and family dynamics AEB discomfort and distress related to assigned gender.

6. If Jamie is treated with behavior modification therapy in order to embrace his own gender, Jamie's short-term outcome may be that he will be able to verbalize knowledge of behaviors that are appropriate and culturally acceptable for his assigned gender. If Jamie is treated with pubertal delay hormonal therapy, Jamie's short-term outcome may be that he will express acceptance and comfort with potential gender change.

7. If Jamie is treated with behavior modification therapy to embrace his assigned gender, Jamie's long-term outcome may be that he will demonstrate behaviors that are appropriate and culturally acceptable for that gender. If Jamie is treated with pubertal delay hormonal therapy, Jamie's long-term outcome may be that he will express personal satisfaction and acceptance of gender change choice.

8. Appropriate nursing interventions may include:
   a. Spending time with Jamie and showing positive regard.
   b. Being aware of personal feelings and attitudes toward Jamie's behavior.
   c. Allowing Jamie to describe his perception of the problem.
   d. Discussing with Jamie the types of behaviors that are more culturally acceptable.
   e. Practicing these behaviors through role-playing or with play therapy strategies (male and female dolls).
   f. Positive reinforcement or social attention for using appropriate behaviors. No response is given for stereotypical opposite-gender behaviors.
   g. The objective in working for behavioral change in a child who has gender dysphoria is to enhance culturally appropriate same-gender behaviors, but not necessarily to extinguish all coexisting opposite-gender behaviors.
   h. Supporting Jamie and his family in any decision related to gender change.
   i. Providing resources to support Jamie's choice of therapy.
   j. Referring Jamie and his family to an appropriate outpatient facility based on Jamie's choice of treatment.

9. Evaluation of the nursing actions for Jamie may be facilitated by gathering information using the following type of questions:
   a. Does Jamie perceive that a problem existed that requires a change in behavior for resolution?
   b. Does Jamie demonstrate use of behaviors that are culturally accepted for his assigned gender?
   c. Can Jamie use these culturally accepted behaviors in interactions with others?
   d. Is Jamie accepted by peers when same-gender behaviors are used?
   e. If Jamie is refusing to change behaviors, what is the peer reaction?
   f. What is Jamie's response to negative peer reaction?
   g. Can Jamie verbalize positive statements about self?
   h. Can Jamie discuss past accomplishments without dwelling on the perceived failures?
   i. Has Jamie shown progress toward accepting self as a worthwhile person regardless of others' responses to his behavior?

j. Has Jamie considered the reactions of others to a gender change?

k. Does Jamie understand the consequences and ramifications related to a change in gender?

Chapter 19

1. On the basis of Allie's symptoms, past history of injuries, and reporting inconsistencies, Macie would assign a medical diagnosis of "fractured ulna of the left arm with possible child abuse as a contributing factor."

2. Allie's subjective symptoms include crying out in pain and saying, "No, go away," and hiding behind her mother when the nurse asked questions about her injuries. She displays regressive symptoms of wetting her pants and thumb-sucking. Allie suggests to the PNP, "Maybe I could go home with you and be your little girl."

3. Allie's objective symptoms include numerous emergency department (ED) visits to treat burns along with femur and ulna fractures. Examination also reveals handprint bruising at ulna facture site and old and new pencil-eraser-sized burns and scars on her body.

4. Carol first states that she was in the kitchen when Allie fell off the swing and then states the handprint bruising happened when she tried to break Allie's fall from the swing. When caught in the discrepancy, Carol reveals that she did hurt Allie but tries to justify her violent actions by complaining about Allie's behavior. Carol's victimizer profile includes being sexually and physically abused as a child, living in poverty, having resentment toward her child, and having unrealistic child expectation issues.

5. Crisis intervention would be most beneficial for Allie. After her physical needs have been met and because Allie is vulnerable and powerless, the PNP would focus on maintaining Allie's safety by coordinating interventions and referrals to prevent future abuse. The principles of crisis intervention could be used to stabilize Allie emotionally and physically, and future individual and family therapy may be indicated. The Department of Health and Human Services may provide a safe environment by the use of foster care until allegations of child abuse are investigated.

6. Family therapy would be most beneficial for Carol. This therapy may include:

a. Assisting Carol in developing democratic ways of solving problems as a means of conflict resolution.

b. Assisting Carol in learning more effective methods of disciplining Allie, aside from physical punishment.

c. Teaching Carol methods that emphasize the importance of positive reinforcement for acceptable behavior and making sure that Carol is committed to consistent use of this behavior modification technique so it can be successful.

d. Referring Carol to agencies that promote effective parenting skills and ways to relieve the stress of parenting.

e. Encouraging Carol to join support groups for abusive parents.

7. Risk for injury R/T abusive family situation.

8. Allie's short-term outcome will be to remain safe and free from physical and emotional harm.

9. Allie's long-term outcome will be to experience a safe and nurturing family environment.

10. Appropriate nursing interventions may include:

a. Performing complete physical assessment on Allie. Take particular note of bruises (in various stages of healing) and Allie's complaints of pain in specific areas. Do not overlook or discount the possibility of sexual abuse. Assess for nonverbal signs of abuse: aggressive conduct, excessive fears, extreme hyperactivity, apathy, withdrawal, regression, and age-inappropriate behaviors.

b. Conduct an in-depth interview with Allie's mother, Carol. If the injury is being reported as an accident, consider whether the explanation is reasonable. Is the injury consistent with the explanation? Is the injury consistent with Allie's developmental capabilities?

c. Use games or play therapy to gain Allie's trust. Use these techniques to assist in describing her side of the story.

d. Determine whether the nature of the injuries warrants reporting to authorities. Specific state statutes must enter into the decision of whether to report suspected child abuse.

11. Evaluation of the nursing actions for Allie may be facilitated by gathering information using the following type of questions:

a. Has Allie received immediate attention to physical injuries?

b. Does Allie demonstrate trust in the primary nurse by discussing abuse through the use of play therapy?

c. Is Allie demonstrating a decrease in regressive behaviors?

d. Has Allie been reassured of her safety?

e. Have wounds been properly cared for and provision made for follow-up care?

f. Have emotional needs been met?

g. Have available support systems been identified and notified?

Index

Page numbers followed by "f" denote figures, "t" denote tables, and "b" denote boxes